MW00767866

Breast Cancer Management

Application of Evidence to Patient Care

Breast Cancer Management

Application of Evidence to Patient Care

Edited by

Jean-Marc Nabholtz MD
Cross Cancer Institute
Edmonton, Canada

Katia Tonkin MD
Cross Cancer Institute
Edmonton, Canada

Matti S Aapro MD
Multidisciplinary Institute of Oncology
Clinique de Genolier
Genolier, Switzerland

Aman U Buzdar MD
Department of Breast Medical Onology
University of Texas
MD Anderson Cancer Center
Houston, USA

MARTIN DUNITZ

© Martin Dunitz Ltd 2000

First published in the United Kingdom in 2000 by

Martin Dunitz Ltd
The Livery House
7–9 Pratt Street
London NW1 0AE

Tel: +44-(0)20-7482-2202
Fax: +44-(0)20-7267-0159
E-mail: info.dunitz@tandf.co.uk
Website: http://www.dunitz.co.uk

Reprinted 2001

A CIP catalogue record for this book is available from the British Library

ISBN 1-85317-915-9

Distributed in the United States by:
Blackwell Science Inc.
Commerce Place, 350 Main Street
Malden, MA 02148, USA
Tel: 1-800-215-1000

Distributed in Canada by:
Login Brothers Book Company
324 Salteaux Cresent
Winnipeg, Manitoba R3J 3T2
Canada
Tel: 1-204-224-4068

Distributed in Brazil by:
Ernesto Reichmann Distribuidora de Livros, Ltda
Rua Coronel Marques 335, Tatuape 03440-000
Sao Paulo,
Brazil

Composition by Wearset, Boldon, Tyne and Wear.
Printed and bound in Great Britain by
Biddles Ltd, Guildford and King's Lynn

CONTENTS

Preface

Breast cancer is a major health problem throughout the Western world. It accounts for 32% of all female cancers in the USA and 18% of all cancer deaths, a figure surpassed only by lung cancer mortality. In the USA in 1996, there were 185 000 new cases and 44 000 deaths from breast cancer. Although the lifetime risk for breast cancer is 1 in 9, or 11%, almost half of this risk occurs after the age of 65. Breast cancer is, however, the most common cause of death in women aged 40–55.

Thus, there is an urgent need to take data derived from clinical trials in a timely fashion and apply them to our treatment algorithms for breast cancer patients. We need to speed up the process required to design clinical trials, execute them swiftly and publicize widely those results that impact directly on patient care. The fundamental process driving this publication is the desire to take clinical trial evidence, as it is, integrate the knowledge and apply it to the clinical situation. This is particularly important for phase III data, which provide the most powerful evidence that we have. Well-designed randomized clinical trials with clear hypotheses and appropriately defined outcome criteria give results that drive the future clinical use of any new drug/biologic therapy in oncology.

The initiative for this book has come directly from the Breast Cancer International Research Group (BCIRG). This Academic Global Virtual Group (AGVG) exists to undertake breast cancer trials of innovative treatments in a more timely way than possible through existing cooperative groups. It is an innovative and exciting new paradigm for clinical trial design and execution, and led to the First International BCIRG Conference on Breast Cancer, 'Towards Evidence-Based Paradigms', held in Edmonton, Canada, in June 1998. At this forum researchers delivered papers on the current and future prospects for breast cancer therapy. This led to the Second International BCIRG Conference, 'Application of New Evidence to Patient Treatment', which was held in Edmonton, in June 2000.

The future for oncology research lies in global strategies. BCIRG is the first Academic Global Virtual Group – a new paradigm in clinical trial organization in oncology. BCIRG arose from an academic initiative, and it fills the gap between the pharmaceutical industry (which has the means to develop and market new drugs) and government-funded cooperative groups, which are known for the quality of their work but also for their slowness in developing and executing clinical trials. New drug development is an arena where time and patient numbers are crucial. The best way to obtain appropriate data in order to register a new therapy is to undertake appropriate clinical trials in a timely fashion. This is achievable only with worldwide cooperation of investigators and sophisticated state-of-the-art data monitoring and management.

At the present time, we appear fortunate in having the opportunity to test many new and innovative approaches to treat breast cancer. However, this plethora of treatments reinforces the important challenge of investigator collaboration. New methods are being developed to test therapies that need evaluation in ways unlike those traditionally used for new drug development. In this complex arena, the ability to rapidly apply the evidence from clinical trials to our patients in the clinic is paramount.

The following are fundamental concepts that underpin the BCIRG:

1. *Academic and independent:* a group of academic investigators in various countries known for commitment, quality of data produced (FDA level) with high potential for patient accrual. The focus is on phase III studies, although the group has the potential for phase I–II seeding programs.
2. *Global:* a group operating on several continents simultaneously (as distinct from most cooperative groups, which are usually organized in one country or continent), using available communication technology to link a network of academic investigators to support such an organization. The advantages of this type of group are:
   - Access to investigators from countries well known for research (North America and western Europe) but also from countries that are not traditionally involved in co-operative research programs (eastern Europe, Middle East, South Africa and South America). This allows good investi-

gators around the world the best opportunity to demonstrate their outstanding ability and commitment.
   - Speed of action is the essence of the Academic Global Virtual Group: initiating a phase III trial in the adjuvant setting is usually a long process (12–18 months) and accrual time can be as long as 3–5 years. The BCIRG has already successfully completed its first trial with a start-up time of 6 months and accrued 1500 patients in 12 months. This is a major factor in the rapid availability of pivotal data, crucial for our patients, and meets the goals of research industry.
3. *Virtual:* a group based on a flexible selection of academic investigators according to the strategy and type of trials being performed (phase I–II, preparatory phase III, and pivotal phase III).

The BCIRG has developed pragmatic clinical strategies for promising new therapies on a global scale. This has accelerated the availability of pivotal data in breast cancer treatments. Having already been a major player in the development of the taxanes and, more recently, in pure antiestrogens and a new polyfunctional cytocykine, BCIRG has turned its attention to gene therapy.

Herceptin is the latest and most promising targeted therapy for women whose tumors express the antigen c-ErbB-2 on the surface of their tumors. The overexpression of this antigen, which occurs in about 25% of tumors, has led to registration trials in metastatic breast cancer. These data have demonstrated survival advantage for a combination of Herceptin and chemotherapy over chemotherapy alone. This warrants swift action to move this compound into the adjuvant setting. BCIRG is in the process of completing two phase II studies to determine the best platinum salt to add to Herceptin, before embarking on a major phase III adjuvant program. This is a demonstration of the BCIRG philosophy of swift academic global action.

We are all aware of the statistics that drive us to improve the current treatment of breast cancer. The worldwide incidence of this disease has been increasing since the 1960s. Despite perceptions to the contrary, the 5-year survival rate of all breast cancer patients in 1995 was 94%, compared with 78% in 1940. Breast cancer mortality has therefore decreased in the face of an increasing incidence. This is certainly the result of advances in patient awareness, leading to early reporting of symptoms, improved methods of detection and a genuine treatment effect.

This book is intended to be an invaluable reference for all surgical, radiation and medical oncologists treating breast cancer. The introductory chapters in the book introduce the available tools and necessary concepts currently used to analyze the medical literature. They also introduce the reader to the benefits and potential limitations of each approach. The middle sections (2–8) of the book consist of chapters that focus on the available published data as it is, particularly on level I evidence from phase III trials. Using the levels of evidence outlined in Chapter 2, each author has reviewed the literature for their particular topic and produced a clear and concise review of the available data for each therapy. This allows readers to decide for themselves which therapy has the most evidence

to support it. The final sections (9–11) review the available evidence for treatment strategies in breast cancer therapy. In balancing these two main parts of the book – the state-of-the-art knowledge based on available evidence, and the expert opinions assessing this evidence – practicing oncologists can decide how best they should treat their patients.

This new millennium will be witness to the rapid evolution of new approaches in breast cancer therapy. In a short space of time clinical trials will have tested numerous new approaches. We are progressing toward individualized treatments that will involve the rational use of prognostic and predictive factors. We are witnessing the beginning of potentially long-term suppressive rather than curative therapies, in both the adjuvant and the metastatic setting. These new challenges will require even more cooperation among all specialties involved in the diagnosis and treatment of breast cancer. The team of medical oncologist, pathologist, surgeon and radiation oncologist, with research nurses, clinical nurse specialists and others must work closely together with our pharmaceutical and biotechnology industry partners to ensure rapid and appropriate utility of new therapies.

J-M Nabholtz
K Tonkin
MS Aapro
AU Buzdar

Contributors

Matti S Aapro, MD
Multidisciplinary Institute of Oncology
Clinique de Genolier
1 Rte de Muids
CH-1272 Genolier
Switzerland

Susan G Arbuck MD
Investingational Drug Branch
National Cancer Institute
6130 Executive Blvd N. Rm 715
Rockville, MD 20852-4910
USA

Colin Baigent BM BCh
Clinical Trial Service Unit &
Epidemiological Studies Unit (CTSU)
University of Oxford
Radcliffe Infirmary
Oxford OX2 6HE
UK

Harry D Bear MD PhD
Division of Surgical Oncology &
The Massey Cancer Center
Medical College of Virginia
Virginia Commonwealth University
PO Box 980011
Richmond, VA 23298-0011
USA

Hervé Bonnefoi MD
Hôpitaux Universitaires de Genève
Rue Micheli de Crest 24
CH-1211 Geneva 14
Switzerland

Andrew Bottomley MD
EORTC Quality of Life Unit
EORTC Data Center
Avenue E Mounier, 83
B-1200 Brussels
Belgium

George P Browman MD
Professor, Department of Clinical
Epidemiology & Biostatistics
McMaster University
Hamilton Regional Cancer Centre
699 Concession Street
Hamilton, ON L8V 5C2
Canada

Heather Bryant, MD
Alberta Cancer Board
382 Heritage Medical
Research Bldg
Calgary, AB T2N 4N1
Canada

Aman U Buzdar MD
Department of Breast Medical Oncology
University of Texas
MD Anderson Cancer Center
1515 Holcombe Blvd
Houston, TX 77030-4009
USA

Fatima Cardoso MD
Chemotherapy Unit
Jules Bordet Institute
125 Bd de Waterloo
1000 Brussels
Belgium

John Crown MD
Consultant Medical Oncologist
St Vincent's University Hospital
Elm Park
Dublin 4
Ireland

Janet Dancey MD
Senior Investigator
Investigational Drug Branch
National Cancer Institute
6130 Executive Blvd, EPN 7115
Rockville, MD 20852-7426
USA

Andrea Decensi MD
European Institute of Oncology
Via Ripamonti 435
20141 Milan
Italy

Angelo Di Leo MD
Chemotherapy Unit
Jules Bordet Institute
125 Bd de Waterloo
1000 Brussels
Belgium

Elizabeth A Eisenhauer MD FRCP(C)
Director, Investigational New Drug Program
National Cancer Institute of Canada
Clinical Trials Group
Queen's University
82–84 Barrie Street
Kingston, ON K7L 3N6
Canada

Ian O Ellis FRCPath
Reader in Pathology
Department of Histopathology
Nottingham City Hospital
Hucknall Road
Nottingham NG5 1PB
UK

Christopher W Elston FRCPath
Consultant Histopathologist
Department of Histopathology
Nottingham City Hospital
Hucknall Road
Nottingham NG5 1PB
UK

Antonio Fabiano Ferreira Filho MD
Chemotherapy Unit
Jules Bordet Institute
125 Bd de Waterloo
1000 Brussels
Belgium

Bernard Fisher MD
NSAPB Scientific Director's Office
Four Allegheny Center, Suite 602
Pittsburgh, PA 15212-5234
USA

David Gancberg MD
Chemotherapy Unit
Jules Bordet Institute
125 Bd de Waterloo
1000 Brussels
Belgium

Bruce G Haffty MD
Associate Professor
Department of Therapeutic Radiology
Yale University School of Medicine
333 Cedar Street
New Haven, CT 06520-3206
USA

Gabriel N Hortobagyi MD
Professor of Medicine & Chairman
Department of Breast Medical Oncology
University of Texas
MD Anderson Cancer Center
1515 Holcombe Blvd
Houston, TX 77030-4009
USA

Anthony Howell MD
Professor of Medical Oncology
Christie Hospital NHS Trust
Wilmslow Road
Manchester M20 4BX
UK

Clifford A Hudis MD
Chief, Breast Cancer Medicine Service
Memorial Sloan-Kettering Cancer Center
1275 York Avenue
New York, NY 10021-6007
USA

Judith Hugh MD
Department of Medicine
Cross Cancer Institute
11560 University Avenue
Edmonton, AB T6G
Canada

Mien-Chie Hung MD
Department of Molecular & Cellular Oncology
University of Texas
MD Anderson Cancer Center
1515 Holcombe Blvd
Houston, TX 77030-4009
USA

Richard Iggo PhD
Swiss Institute for Experimental Cancer Research
(ISREC)
Oncogene Group
Chemin des Boveresses 155
CH-1066 Epalinges
Switzerland

Stewart M Jackson MD
British Columbia Cancer Agency
600 W 10th Ave
Vancouver, BC V5Z 4E6
Canada

Philip Jacobs
Department of Public Health Sciences
University of Alberta
13-130C Clinical Sciences Bldg
Edmonton, AB T6G 2G3
Canada

Gottfried E Konecny MD
Department of Medicine
Division of Hematology/Oncology
UCLA School of Medicine
Los Angeles, CA 90095
USA

Sheryl Koski MD
Department of Medicine
Cross Cancer Institute
11560 University Avenue
Edmonton, AB T6G 1Z2
Canada

David N Krag MD
SD Ireland Professor of Surgical Oncology
University of Vermont
Given Bldg Room E309
Burlington, VT 05405-0068
USA

Michael D Lagios MD
Medical Director
Breast Cancer Consultation Service
St Mary's Medical Center
450 Stanyan Street
San Francisco, CA 94117
USA

Denis Larsimont MD
Anatomy Pathology
Jules Bordet Institute
125 Bd de Waterloo
1000 Brussels
Belgium

Andrew HS Lee MRCPath
Consultant Histopathologist
Department of Histopathology
Nottingham City Hospital
Hucknall Road
Nottingham NG5 1PB
UK

Mary-Ann Lindsay BSc(Pharm) Pharm D
BCIRG
Cross Cancer Institute
11560 University Ave
Edmonton, AB T6G 1Z2
Canada

Gershon Y Locker MD
Chief, Division of Hematology-Oncology
Evanston Northwestern Healthcare
2650 Ridge Ave, Room 2220
Evanston, IL 60091
USA

Caroline Lohrisch MD
Investigational Drug Branch for Breast Cancer
Institut Jules Bordet
Bd de Waterloo 125
1000 Brussels
Belgium

Nadine MacLean BA
Institute of Health Economics
Cross Cancer Institute
#1200, 10405 Jasper Avenue
Edmonton, AB T5J 3N4
Canada

Eleftherios P Mamounas MD MPH FACS
Medical Director
Mt Saini Center for Breast Health
Mt Sinai Cancer Centre
26900 Cedar Road
Beachwood, OH 44122-1148
USA

Miguel Martín MD
Hospítal Universitario San Carlos
Cuidad Universitaria S/N
28040 Madrid
Spain

Anthony B Miller MB FRCP
Head, Division of Clinical Epidemiology
Deutsches Krebsforschungszentrum
Im Neuenheimer Feld 28
D-69120 Heidelberg
Germany

Kathy D Miller MD
Division of Hematology & Oncology
Indiana University School of Medicine
535 Barnhill Drive, RT-473
Indianapolis, IN 46202
USA

Frederick L Moffat Jr MD
Associate Professor of Surgery
Division of Surgical Oncology
University of Miami School of Medicine
Sylvester Comprehensive Cancer Center
1475 NW 12th Ave, Room 3550
Miami, FL 33136
USA

Pamela N Munster MD
Memorial Sloan-Kettering Cancer Center
1275 York Avenue
New York, NY 10021
USA

Jean-Marc Nabholtz MD
Senior Medical Oncologist
Chairman, Breast Cancer International
Research Group (BCIRG)
Cross Cancer Institute
11560 University Avenue
Edmonton, AB T6G 1Z2
Canada

Joyce A O'Shaughnessy MD
US Oncology Research
3535 Worth Street, Collins 5
Dallas, TX 75246
USA

Alexander HG Paterson MD
Tom Baker Cancer Centre
Department of Medicine
1331 29 St. NW
Calgary, AB T2N 4N2
Canada

Mark D Pegram MD
Division of Hematology/Oncology
UCLA School of Medicine
10833 Le Conte Ave, Room 11-934
Los Angeles, CA 90095
USA

Sir Richard Peto FRS
Clinical Trial Service Unit &
Epidemiological Studies Unit (CTSU)
University of Oxford
Radcliffe Infirmary
Oxford OX2 6HE
UK

Martine J Piccart MD PhD
Chemotherapy Unit
Institut Jules Bordet
125 Bd de Waterloo
1000 Brussels
Belgium

Sarah E Pinder MRCPath
Senior Lecturer
Department of Histopathology
Nottingham City Hospital
Hucknall Road
Nottingham NG5 1PB
UK

Joseph Ragaz MD
British Columbia Cancer Agency
600 W 10th Ave
Vancouver, BC V5Z 4E6
Canada

Lewis Rowett MD
Education & Information Coordinator
European Society for Medical Oncology
Via Soldino 22
6900 Lugano
Switzerland

Dennis J Slamon MD
Division of Hematology/Oncology
UCLA School of Medicine
10833 Le Conte Ave, Room 11-934
Los Angeles, CA 90095
USA

George W Sledge MD
Division of Hematology & Oncology
Indiana University School of Medicine
535 Barnhill Drive, RT-473
Indianapolis, IN 46202
USA

Ian E Smith MD FRCP FRCPE
Department of Medical Oncology
The Breast Unit
The Royal Marsden Hospital
Fulham Road
London SW3 6JJ
UK

Michael Smylie MD
Department of Medicine
Cross Cancer Institute
11560 University Ave
Edmonton, AB T6G 1Z2
Canada

Barbara Conner-Spady PhD
University of Alberta
Centre for Research in Applied Measurement
and Evaluation
Department of Educational Psychology
Edmonton, AB T6G 1Z2
Canada

Marc Spielmann MD
Head, Breast Cancer Department
Institut Gustave Roussy
39 Rue Camille Desmoulins
F-94805 Villejuif
France

Edward A Stadtmauer MD
Associate Professor of Medicine
Director, Bone Marrow & Stem Cell Transplant
Program
University of Pennsylvania Cancer Center
16 Penn Tower
3400 Spruce Street
Philadelphia, PA 19104
USA

Justin Stebbing MA MRCP
Department of Medical Oncology
The Breast Unit
The Royal Marsden Hospital
Fulham Road
London SW3 6JJ
UK

Patrick Therasse, MD
EORTC Data Centre
Ave E Mounier 83/Bte 11
Brussels 1200
Belgium

Ann D Thor MD
Department of Pathology and Surgery
Evanston Northwestern Healthcare
Northwestern University Medical School
2650 Ridge Avenue
Evanston, IL 60201
USA

Katia Tonkin MD
Senior Medical Oncologist
Department of Medicine
Cross Cancer Institute
11560 University Avenue
Edmonton, AB T6G 1Z2
Canada

Naoto T Ueno MD
Department of Blood and Marrow
Transplantation
University of Texas
MD Anderson Cancer Center
1515 Holcombe Blvd, #65
Houston, TX 77030
USA

Peter Venner MD
Department of Medicine
Cross Cancer Institute
11560 University Avenue
Edmonton, AB T6G 1Z2
Canada

Umberto Veronesi MD
European Institute of Oncology
Via Ripamonti 435
20141 Milan
Italy

Laurent Zelek MD
Medical Oncologist
Breast Cancer Department
Institut Gustave Roussy
39 Rue Camille Desmoulins
F-94805 Villejuif
France

Acknowledgements

This publication was brought together in record time. This was only possible with enormous amounts of cooperation from a lot of people, not all of whom can be mentioned here. Special thanks go to all our authors and section editors who suffered a barrage of e-mails and phone calls. Also special thanks to Alison Campbell of Martin Dunitz Publishers, who was knowledgeable and calm even when things got really tight for time.

Above all we need to acknowledge our patients, because it is for them that we continue to strive to learn more about breast cancer. It is for the patients' sake that we need to understand and apply our knowledge as fast as we can so that we can limit their suffering. It is the patients who take part in the clinical trials, and without them little progress would be made. Heartfelt thanks to each and every one of you, your families and friends.

PART I
Available Tools and Their Application

1
History of the use of evidence in medicine

Jean-Marc Nabholtz, Katia Tonkin

HISTORICAL PERSPECTIVE

Clinical medicine has for most of its history been practiced at the bedside. Although several journals can claim publishing dates before 1900, rigorous clinical trials, as we now understand them, are a relatively new phenomenon. It is likely that one of the earliest trials took place around AD 1200.[1] Frederick II, Emperor of Rome, decided to study the effects of exercise on the digestion of food. He fed two knights the same food and while one slept the other went out hunting. He had both killed after several hours and found that the sleeping knight had digested more food – surely not a study approved by an ethics committee and certainly one without informed consent.

In the seventeenth century, Jan Baptista van Helmont[1] planned a large study of 200–500 people. He was a philosopher and physician who did not believe in the practice of blood letting. He intended to divide the patients into two groups by casting lots, with only one group allowed treatment with blood letting. He planned to assess the number of funerals as an end-point. Unfortunately, for unknown reasons this experiment, incorporating large numbers, randomization and statistical analysis, never took place.

In 1753, Lind planned a comparative trial of the most promising treatments for scurvy. He studied 12 individuals with the disease and divided them into six groups of two, devising a different diet for each group.[2] The two sailors given oranges and lemons had improved within 6 days – one was fit enough to report for duty and the other was appointed nurse to the rest. Unfortunately, Lind himself did not fully believe his own results and promoted fresh air as the primary recommendation, with fruits and vegetables secondarily. The British Navy did not implement his findings for 50 years when they eventually began to supply lemon juice to their ships. Although there are still delays in putting findings from modern trials into everyday practice, 50 years does seem extreme.

Perhaps the true beginning of modern scientific medicine with statistical analysis began in Paris in the nineteenth century with Pierre Charles Alexandre Louis.[3] He discussed the foundation of counting the number of individuals who benefited from a treatment and compared these with a second group given a different therapy. Thus, he established a numerical method and the concept of two groups of patients with a disease being compared in a trial of therapies. He discussed the need for exact patient observation, knowledge of the natural history of the disease when untreated and careful observation of deviations from the intended treatment. Louis showed that blood letting was a useless practice by studying patients with a wide variety of diseases, including pneumonia, erysipelas and throat inflammation, which led eventually to a decline in the practice. His experiments were very influential in France, Britain and the USA, and he can be considered a founding figure in the establishment of clinical trials and epidemiology as scientific practices.

Another important figure in France in the nineteenth century was Claude Bernard. In addition to his work on physiology, he was a firm believer in objectivity and set down standards for future experimentalists in the book *An Introduction to the Study of Experimental Medicine* in 1865.[4]

However, few clinicians embraced the idea of trials testing clinical outcome until after the work of the mathematician and geneticist Ronald Fisher in the 1920s. Fisher is of course responsible for Fisher's exact test, which is a non-parametric test for comparing two proportions from independent samples. It is called Fisher's exact test because the probability of observing a value as extreme, or more extreme than the one observed for the test statistic, is calculated from a 2×2 contingency table with fixed row and column totals. Fisher was born in London in 1890. He was educated at Harrow and Cambridge and did his most important statistical work while he was statistician of the Rothamsted Research Station from 1919. He refined the student t-test and, while Galton Professor at University College, published *The Design of Experiments* (1935),[5] which has profoundly influenced experimental method. He is best known, perhaps, for his clarification of the rhesus (Rh) blood groups. This happened because Fisher had moved to take the Chair of Genetics at Cambridge in 1943, where he stayed until his retire-

ment in 1957. The confusing results of the Rh story were largely elucidated over discussions with colleagues in a local pub. The data were presented in the USA in 1946 and the definitive article was eventually published in 1947 in *Scientific American*.[6] Interestingly, he challenged the conclusion that smoking causes lung cancer from the observations that Doll and Hill made in 1956 from studies of British family physicians. Fisher said that there were three ways to interpret the meaning of an association between A and B: A can cause B; B can cause A; or some other factor can cause A and B. Fisher was outraged that scientists would select such an interpretation of the smoking issue and force it on the public without better evidence. He thought Doll and Hill were pseudoscientists who assumed something that was not known. He never tried to review later evidence and the suggestion that his arguments lost value because he was employed as a consultant to the tobacco firms was felt by medical historians to be unjust. He disliked and mistrusted puritanical tendencies of all kinds.

The discovery of penicillin at the beginning of the 1940s was such an important therapeutic advance that clinical trials were unnecessary. The trial of the effect of penicillin on war wounds in north Africa showed its superiority, even though penicillin was given to the most serious cases because the surgeons did not want to deny them therapy. In this way penicillin was given a very biased test, but it still proved to be superior.

The first clinical trial with a properly randomized control group was for streptomycin in the treatment of pulmonary tuberculosis. The Medical Research Council undertook the study under the direction of individuals such as Sir Austin Bradford Hill and published it in 1948. Several centers were involved and at each center patients were randomized to streptomycin and bed-rest or bed-rest alone. Evaluation of radiographs was done independently by two radiologists and a clinician unaware of the treatment allocation or the assessment of the other physician involved. Outcome evaluation included survival and radiological improvement. In particular, the blinded assessment of results is especially innovative for its time and even now considered important in obtaining unbiased results. The *British Medical Journal* report[7] cites statistically significant differences in mortality at the level of $p = 0.001$ and significant differences in the primary outcome measure of radiological improvements. The two groups were well balanced on admission for characteristics that were likely to influence outcome, such as fever, and the results were evaluated according to the gravity of the illness.

The Medical Research Council (MRC) followed this trial with a double-blind randomized evaluation of antihistamines for the common cold, using a placebo control. Patients were asked to evaluate their own improvement and over 20% failed to comply with treatment or evaluation. The clear rejection of antihistamines was achieved only through the use of such rigorous methodology.

Sir Austin Bradford Hill had a major impact on oncology as a result of his publications with Richard Doll on 'Mortality in relation to smoking: ten years' observation of British doctors' published in 1964[8] in the *British Medical Journal*. Their original work was published in 1954 and 1956,[9] and was a mammoth survey of 59 600 men and women on the British Medical Register. By limiting their questions, they were able to get responses from 40 637 individuals, which in itself is a major achievement. Amazingly, all but 2% of the original sample alive and on the Register replied to the second questionnaire. They also went to great lengths to discover the accurate causes of deaths for all those individuals who had died between the two intervals. They showed that the total mortality rate was 28% higher among cigarette smokers – this was not only higher among

those who were continuing to smoke but even higher in those who smoked larger numbers of cigarettes. Not surprisingly, the difference in mortality between smokers and non-smokers is significant at the $p \leq 0.001$ level. To their credit, they also examined confounding factors such as alcohol or the possibility that smoking habits might have been determined by other environmental or constitutional factors. They showed an increase in cancers of the lung and upper aerodigestive tract, other respiratory illness and cardiovascular disease.

Hill continued to have a major influence on clinical trials performed by the MRC into the 1960s, publishing articles on the conduct of clinical trials that argued for the use of concurrent controls, randomization, definition of eligible patients, definition of treatment schedule, objective evaluation and statistical analysis.

The largest field trial ever of 1.8 million children was undertaken in 1954 to assess the efficacy of the Salk vaccine. As the annual incidence of polio was only 1 in 2000 and clear evidence of treatment effect was needed as soon as possible, a large trial was needed. Although the positive results led to the widespread use of the killed-virus vaccine, it was later replaced by the safer live Sabin vaccine.

Hill's efforts led to other trials by others, most notably the British epidemiologists Archibald Cochrane and Sir Richard Doll. Cochrane was interested in epidemiology, particularly of pneumoconiosis, and later in health services research. He became honorary director of the MRC's epidemiology unit and promoted the randomized clinical trial to determine treatment and optimum length of stay. In 1972, he wrote *Effectiveness and Efficiency: Random Reflections on Health Services*,[10] which had a widespread effect. His name is now synonymous with examination of evidence since the inception of the Cochrane Collaboration, which undertakes meta-analysis of clinical questions in order to provide practicing physicians with guidance in their everyday practice.

In oncology, the first level V reports of effectiveness of chemotherapy came from responses to aminopterin in children with acute leukemia in 1948. After this, there were a number of studies without controls, which were thought to be unnecessary because of the universally fatal outcome of the disease. In 1954, Emil Frei and the National Cancer Institute (NCI) organized the first randomized clinical oncology trial in acute lymphocytic leukemia (ALL) with two schedules of 6-mercaptopurine and methotrexate. A total of 56 patients were accrued from five centers. This was a randomized phase III trial, which provided level 1 evidence. The success of the organization of this trial quickly led to two cooperative groups being formed. The first the Children's Cancer Study Group and the second the Cancer and Leukemia Group B (CALGB).

The nitrogen mustards were being used early in the 1950s against solid tumors. This led five institutions on the east coast of the USA to form the Eastern Solid Tumor Group in 1955 and, supported by the NCI, they investigated nitrogen mustard and thiotepa in solid malignancies. This group later became the Eastern Cooperative Oncology Group (ECOG). The early promising results led to an expansion of cooperative groups, to a total of 21 by 1960, most of them investigating chemotherapy although some were evaluating radiation or surgery. Until the 1970s, however, most of the research would not be considered adequate by modern standards because patients with advanced disease and a poor outlook were being evaluated, with only temporary shrinkage of tumors occurring. Patient survival was rarely an outcome and patients were usually followed for only a few months.

In breast cancer, Dr Gianni Bonadonna's Milan group and the National Surgical Adjuvant Breast and Bowel Project (NSABP), under the guidance of Dr Bernard Fisher, performed the most notable early trials. They showed that chemotherapy after mastectomy improved not only disease-free, but ultimately overall, survival, an effect that persists for more than 15 years of follow-up. These early promising results were followed by many trials, which examined the role of chemotherapy in the adjuvant treatment of breast cancer. Such a large body of data was produced that the Oxford Clinical Trial Group set up the Early Breast Cancer Cooperative Trialists Group (EBCCTG) and undertook a meta-analysis of all the available data. This has recently been updated and now includes second-generation trials using anthracycline-based regimens. A further update will be available in September 2000.

In the last 30 years, American cancer trials have undertaken the largest number of randomized clinical studies ever in a single disease area. The quality of the data has been steadily improving, with attention to detail in data collection and analysis. This has allowed long-term survival and toxicity information to be obtained on many thousands of patients. In addition to clinical information, more recently pathological data have been collected, so that molecular and other tumor-specific information can be evaluated within the trial framework. This information is part of the scientific rationale leading to strategies that will enable us to give targeted treatments in the future.

EVIDENCE-BASED MEDICINE: PAST AND PRESENT USES

Evidence-based medicine (EBM) was developed to answer problems that physicians have had in deciding on a clinical treatment when there have been two or more opposing views about the appropriate therapy. Physicians need regularly updated, relevant, clinical information and an ability to extrapolate from experimental reports to actual clinical practice. Evidence-based medicine involves the integration of clinical expertise and patient values with available research evidence.

In practical terms EBM requires the following:

- The conversion of the need for information into answerable questions.
- The ability to search for the best available evidence with which to answer the questions.
- A critical appraisal of the evidence with respect to its validity, importance and applicability.
- The ability to integrate the evidence with clinical knowledge and individual patient needs.
- Evaluation of our ability to execute the first four steps, and improving on them for the future.

Evidence-based medicine has been made easier as international groups have undertaken systematic reviews of the literature. Evidence-based journals have sprung up, and search strategies and electronic searching services have allowed us more efficient use of available literature. It recognizes that we need to integrate our clinical expertise, which takes account of our skill to identify the patient's health state, individual risks and benefits of an intervention, as well as the values and expectations of the intervention. Without clinical judgment, EBM can become useless because even the best evidence may not apply to an individual patient. The best evidence incorporates clinical trial data, hopefully on a group of patients with similar characteristics to the individual whom the physician wishes to treat. The rapid rise of EBM is linked to the use of randomized controlled trials in the last two decades. These trials have linked pathophysiologic questions to clinical interventions and in many cases have demonstrated that what had seemed to be clinically obvious could not be proved in well-controlled studies. Professor Gordon Guyatt and his groups at McMaster University in Hamilton, Ontario coined the term 'EBM' in 1992. There has been an exponential increase in the interest in the subject, which has led to the establishment of six evidence-based journals.

Despite the rise of EBM, recent surveys of general practitioners in the UK and internists in Canada and the USA have demonstrated that physicians still rely on their colleagues, review articles and textbooks. As the volume of clinical literature expands almost exponentially, we have less and less time to read all the information and, the further we are from graduation, the more likely we are to have diminishing clinical performance and diminishing clinically important knowledge. In addition, research advances are inconsistently applied both geographically and according to the age of the patient.

Evidence-based medicine has been shown to be feasible, but as yet there are no data on the effect of EBM on outcomes. Evidence-based medicine has limitations, such as difficulty in describing information to the patient in intelligible concise ways, including the risks and benefits, the patient's values of potential outcomes and the side effects. Clinicians need to be able to use these methods at the bedside, which is not yet possible despite the development of a series of decision aids. Evidence-based medicine still has a long way to go with respect to its practicability, intelligibility and the speed with which the information can be found, as well as its use at the bedside.

USE OF OPINION LEADERS AND EXPERTS

Those whom we regard as world experts have always influenced our thinking. They have driven the clinical trial agenda and therefore the questions asked within those trials. They have sometimes been extraordinarily innovative and at other times have followed one line of thinking over many years and trials. The cooperative group trials currently progress at what appears to be a slow pace. This may result partly from numerous competing trials with many interesting questions occurring over a short period of time in breast cancer. It may also reflect an increasing bureaucracy within the large cooperative group structure and difficulty in getting all the factions to agree on one particular trial design.

The answers from their own trials have the greatest influence on the opinions of experts. It is a rare individual who can give a true overview of the work of others, especially in the light of competing results.

Individual oncologists are frequently participants in large multicenter, and more recently multinational, clinical trials. Not surprisingly, therefore, they are likely to change their practice based on results of the trials in which they participate. This also influences the ability of the oncologist to accept an expert opinion, especially if it is contrary to the studies in which they have participated.

NEW APPROACH: APPLICATION OF NEW EVIDENCE TO PATIENT TREATMENT

Although we continue with more complex clinical practices, there is an ever-increasing and daunting volume of clinical literature to assimilate. We are in desperate need of methods to understand and integrate all the new information presented to us on a daily basis. We have not only to review all the standard medical journals, but also to integrate new methods that information technology presents to us. We recognize that patients have become more educated, and that the pharmaceutical industry and others bypass the physician, reaching to patients directly with appealing new advertisements in magazines and on the television. We need at least to keep ahead of the Internet and the other sources of information that our patients access.

We have to answer several questions before we should think of applying new information to our clinical practice:

- What is relevant to our particular patient group?
- What other evidence needs consideration before we accept the results of the latest trial?
- Is this information in line with other data or is it a contrary opinion?
- Do we need to wait for confirmatory data from other trials?

We need to determine first that the data are relevant to our own patients. Then we examine the evidence according to guidelines outlined in the rest of Part I of this book (Chapters 2–7). We can then review the data in both Parts II (Chapters 8–29) and III (Chapters 30–41) to evaluate available evidence and expert opinion. Once the data pass scrutiny under these stringent conditions, we are obliged to incorporate it into our therapeutic algorithm.

Even those who have been instrumental in the acceptance of the traditional evidence-based approach have recently begun to question a slavish adherence to its use.[11] Browman, who can be considered one of the pioneers of evidence-based approaches, endorses the use of clinical judgment when considering the validity and applicability of research evidence. For an individual patient, the factors that influence an evidence-based decision differ from the broader policy context, with legitimate differences in recommendations based on the same information. Used properly, therefore, the case report can be a powerful tool to illustrate complex clinical decision phenomena.

In reality, EBM involves the integration of our

clinical knowledge of our patients' values and available research data. We need to use our clinical experience to determine a patient's overall health, individual risks, and benefits and expectations. Even excellent evidence cannot always be applied to an individual patient.[12]

We need to search for the best evidence with which to answer the appropriate clinical question for an individual patient. We then need to appraise the results in a critical manner, especially with knowledge of other relevant data in the field, and apply the information to the patient whom we are treating.

The model of the Academic Global Virtual Group (AGVG) is a powerful new tool to assist us not only in the dissemination and understanding of new ideas, but also in their rapid testing in the framework of clinical trials. Thus, new data from the laboratory can be brought into the clinical trial arena in the quickest time possible and, once information from several phase II studies is available, rational design of phase III studies can be undertaken. The following are keys to the AGVG:

- Globalization, allowing worldwide access to patients and to subgroups for specific subgroup studies within main studies.
- A new close direct relationship between the pharmaceutical industry and clinical researchers.
- Partnerships, with an academically controlled global development strategy for promising new agents.
- Independent process.
- Quality of data.
- Modern means of communication, allowing for a virtual process in the group structure.

The AGVG is crucial to the development of oncology because there are vast numbers of new drugs and gene-based therapies that will become available within the next 5–10 years. The research groups that have the fastest track to patients will control trials of the future. The Breast Cancer International Research Group (BCIRG) is the first such AGVG in breast cancer and is making contributions to trials of taxanes, antiestrogens, cytokines and herceptin. All of this clinical trial activity, amazingly, has occurred within 3 years. The potential for this group using the AGVG style is almost limitless.

The aim is to develop biologically based and therefore individualized therapies. We will use new treatment paradigms to move far beyond our traditional systemic approach of chemotherapy versus hormone therapy or their combination. There is a strong potential within the BCIRG to have multiple concurrent phase II trials. As results of several different strategies mature at the same time, new generations of phase III trials can therefore be developed at a much faster pace than has occurred using the traditional cooperative group model.

We hope that you will find this new approach to the treatment of breast cancer useful. We intend it, above all else, to be a practical guide for you to use in your everyday clinical practice. We hope that some of the new gene-based approaches stimulate your interest. They are indeed, we believe, the light at the end of the tunnel. We await their speedy application in the clinic, after appropriate clinical trials.

In the end, we hope that it will be our patients who benefit from our work, because it is for them that all of this effort is intended. We remember each of their stories and their strength, and we fervently wish to do all that we can to be part of the processes that speed up bringing better treatments to them.

REFERENCES

1. Greenhalgh T, *How to Read a Paper: The Basics of Evidence Based Medicine.* London: BMJ Publishing Company, 1997.
2. Lind J, *A Treatise of the Scurvy.* Reprinted in *Lind's Treatise on Scurvy* (eds CP Stewart, D Guthrie). Edinburgh: Edinburgh University Press, 1953.
3. Lyons AS, Petricelli RJ, New York: Harry N Abrams, 1978: 513.
4. Bernard C, *An Introduction to the Study of Experimental Medicine.* Paris: Henry Schuman Inc, 1949. (Latest edition of original 1865 publication.)
5. Fisher RA, *The Design of Experiments.* Edinburgh: Oliver and Boyd, 1935.
6. Fisher RA, The Rhesus factor – A study in scientific method. *Sci Am* 1947; **35**:95–103.
7. Medical Research Council Investigations, Streptomycin Treatments of Pulmonary Tuberculosis. *BMJ* 1948; **4582**:769–82.
8. Doll R, Bradford-Hill A, Mortality in relation to smoking: Ten years' observation of British doctors. *BMJ* 1964; **1**:1399–410.
9. Doll R, Bradford-Hill A, Lung cancer and other causes of death in relation to smoking. *BMJ* 1956; **1**:1071–81.
10. Cochrane A, *Effectiveness and Efficiency: Random Reflections on Health Services.* Oxford: Oxford Nuffield Provincial Hospitals Trust, 1972.
11. Browman GP, Essence of evidence-based medicine: A case report. *J Clin Oncol* 1999; **17**:1969–73.
12. Straus SE, McAlister FA, Evidence based medicine: past, present and future. *Ann R Coll Physicians* 1999; **32**:260–4.

2
Clinical practice guidelines

George P Browman

DEFINITIONS

Clinical practice guidelines have been defined as systematically developed statements to assist practitioner and patient decisions about appropriate health care for specific clinical circumstances.[1] This definition implies many important principles. It prescribes a systematic and, therefore, a transparent process for developing guidelines. It acknowledges guidelines as tools, not rules, for practice, which are intended to assist clinical judgments, not replace them. The definition respects the input of patients in clinical decision-making. Finally, in addressing 'specific' clinical circumstances, the definition suggests that guidelines be designed to avoid vague generalizations that focus on the generic patient at the expense of the specific circumstances in question.

Evidence-based medicine has been defined as the explicit, systematic and judicious application of the best available evidence from health research in the management of individual patients.[2] This definition likewise implies principles that are often forgotten in the formulaic approach used by many guideline developers and decision-makers. As with guidelines, the definition demands a systematic process that implies transparency in how recommendations are built

from evidence. The definition calls for the 'judicious' use of the evidence, thus respecting the role of clinical judgment; it is implied that clinicians will value other inputs into their decisions that place a context around the evidence. The term 'best available' evidence should be distinguished from 'truth'. In making our decisions, we can do only the best with the evidence that is before us. We cannot predict how the evidence might change; thus, decisions based on high-quality evidence cannot be fairly judged in retrospect. However, the phrase 'best available' evidence also holds decision-makers accountable for considering all the evidence, rather than selecting the evidence based on personal beliefs, or based solely on their informal awareness of some of the evidence. Finally, the definition of 'evidence-based medicine' clearly places emphasis on evidence from the research domain, which is not intended to exclude information of other types.

Thus, decision-makers ought to be accountable only for considering the evidence, because it cannot always be applied in the clinical context of concern. Thus, a better definition of evidence-based medicine might be: the explicit *consideration* of the best available research evidence and its judicious application in the management of individual patients.

EVIDENCE-BASED CLINICAL PRACTICE GUIDELINES

Several methods have been used to develop clinical practice guidelines (CPGs). These can be generally classified as 'opinion based', 'consensus based' and 'evidence based'.[3] The main problem with 'opinion-based' CPGs, even from experts, is that they are not generally transparent in how the evidence was considered along the path to making recommendations. Even if the evidence is considered, the lack of transparency makes it difficult to know whether all the evidence was considered, whether the right evidence was considered, and whether there was bias in how the evidence was considered and used. Although expert opinion alone is legitimate as a clinical decision process for one's own patients, with whom there are implicit contractual arrangements, it is insufficient for making broader recommendations, which may affect the treatment of others outside of one's own practice. Here, the level of accountability ought to be greater. The role of the expert is to provide input into the interpretation of evidence that has been synthesized using explicit and rigorous methods.

'Consensus-based' CPGs rely mainly on group consensus methods which may, or may not, include the explicit consideration of best available evidence for making clinical recommendations. One of the criticisms of purely consensus methods is that, when consensus is the main goal of the process, it may often be achieved at the expense of what the evidence suggests.[4] The strength of consensus methods is that they harness the views of a variety of legitimate stakeholders. Consensus processes should be considered useful for improving evidence-based CPGs because evidence does not necessarily speak for itself. Consensus approaches can assist with the interpretation of the evidence from different perspectives, and for defining the clinical circumstances to which the evidence can be generalized. Thus, the combination of consensus and evidence-based methods is ideal for CPG development.

The process of 'evidence based' CPG development simply means that there was an explicit, and systematic, consideration of the 'best available' evidence, using rigorous methods such as the systematic review of the literature, which is designed to minimize bias in the location, selection and synthesis of the evidence.[5]

A simplistic evaluation of the evidence-based approach would question whether all the effort is worth it if, in the end, the recommendations produced are the same as those of other, less costly approaches. It is fair to assume that evidence-based and expert-based (or opinion-based) CPG development strategies are likely to produce the same or similar recommendations for a very high proportion of topics. After all, experts do not practice willful neglect of the evidence. However, accountability demands that we be more explicit in how we consider evidence when making recommendations.

In the longer term, evidence-based approaches may be more efficient than those that are opinion based, if we recognize that CPGs are living documents that require continuous refreshing (i.e. updating) as the evidence evolves. Explicit and transparent documents, which were developed systematically, are more amenable to modification over time using the same methods that were originally applied. In the absence of documented systematic methods for arriving at recommendations, new evidence that is based on expert opinion alone would not be able to benefit from a baseline inventory of processes and knowledge. This would require 'starting from scratch', especially if different experts are consulted when updating is needed.

THE HALLMARK OF THE EVIDENCE-BASED GUIDELINE AND LEVELS OF EVIDENCE

How would one judge whether a CPG is evidence based? The hallmark of an evidence-based CPG is the use of the systematic review, with an explicit method for synthesizing the entire body of evidence (using either qualitative or quantitative methods) in informing the clinical recommendations. A systematic review is not a CPG. It is only that part of the CPG that brings the clinical research evidence into the mix of other inputs. Furthermore, systematic reviews, as randomized trials themselves, can be of variable quality.[6]

Any CPG that does not provide a list of citations to support its clinical recommendations, based on evidence, cannot be considered to be evidence based because it asks the reader to 'trust' the author(s). Evidence-based CPGs ought to allow readers to delve into the evidence as deeply as they can, in the same way that the guideline developers did.

The use of 'levels of evidence'[7] is *not* the hallmark of an evidence-based approach, and the absence of 'levels of evidence' is not sufficient to reject a guideline because it is not evidence based. (Actually, the term 'evidence informed' is probably better than 'evidence based' in conveying the role of research evidence in clinical decisions or recommendations.) The term 'levels of evidence' was conceived as descriptive shorthand. It was intended to convey or categorize the quality of evidence, based on the rigor of the design used to generate it. This speaks to the validity of the conclusions based on the research. 'Levels of evidence' can be thought of as an ordinal classification of the quality of the research information available.

The use of 'levels of evidence' is, furthermore, intended to convey the nature of the best available evidence that addresses a particular problem. For example, if there are results from large randomized controlled trials of drug x versus a control for a given condition, then the level of evidence is level I based on most classifications. This evidence trumps lower quality evidence so that it is unnecessaary, in fact redundant, to classify such a recommendation as having, for example, level I plus levels II, III and IV evidence. Yet, many existing guidelines use this approach.

The use of 'levels of evidence' as a shorthand descriptive tool was never intended to provide only positive support for interventions. For example, level V evidence (case reports or case series depending on the classification used) is usually a flag that the evidence ought to be seriously challenged as a support for a positive recommendation. Yet, many guideline developers, in their enthusiasm, use level V evidence as justification to recommend an intervention, as opposed to justifying its rejection. Some guideline development groups actually categorize 'expert opinion' as level V evidence. This may provide a veneer of rigor that does not actually exist, and reduces the usefulness of the 'levels of evidence' approach. Level V evidence has also been used to attach to a recommendation a level of evidence for the apparent sake of completeness. Often, such a recommendation (such as a chest radiograph for staging breast cancer) will never be tested in a trial, and does not require slavish adherence to a formula. On the other hand, a recommendation such as an annual chest radiograph in otherwise healthy low-risk people ought to be supported by rigorous evidence before it is implemented.

As a result of these concerns, Cancer Care Ontario's guideline development initiative[8] has stopped using levels of evidence as a tool, choosing instead to use the richness and subtlety of language to express the full meaning of the intended message. Shorthand monikers are useful communications tools when properly used, but can deteriorate to a level of absurdity when abused.

THE BENEFITS AND LIMITATIONS OF THE CLINICAL PRACTICE GUIDELINE AS A DECISION AID

Benefits

Clinical practice guidelines serve as useful reference tools for helping clinicians and patients make clinical decisions. Evidence-based CPGs provide a valid and reliable summary of the available evidence. Given that the peer review literature is poorly organized for clinical decision-making, the CPG can be the vehicle for consolidating evidence related to a particular clinical problem, and highlighting the gaps in knowledge and where further research is needed.

Clinical practice guidelines may be useful to those responsible for organizing and paying for health-care services. An inventory of properly developed, credible, clinical guidelines serves to highlight where investments in health services are needed and justified.

Clinical practice guidelines also serve as a baseline inventory of knowledge that can foster dialogue among clinicians, patients, the public, health-care managers and payers, so that appropriate health care can be debated on the substantive issues. In Ontario, the cancer guideline initiative has elevated the level of discussion among several stakeholder groups.[8–10] This has resulted in increases rather than reductions in funding for cancer care services, especially in the approval for new and emerging chemotherapy and supportive care agents.

The use of a consensus mechanism around a rigorous evidence-based process has had the effect of 'changing the culture' of the cancer care system, improving communication among oncol-

ogists, and increasing the expertise of clinicians in searching for, evaluating and interpreting the evidence from health-care research. This has led to the awarding of CME (Continuing Medical Education) credits to clinicians who engage in the process of CPG development. Disease Site Groups have also invited oncology trainees to join them, which has provided a rich educational environment and opportunities for productive research. Some oncology residency and fellowship training programs have used Ontario cancer guidelines as part of their educational materials. In sum, it could be argued that the *process* of a rigorous and inclusive guideline development program adds at least, if not more, value to the system than the final product, the guideline itself.

Limitations

The main limitations of evidence-based guidelines relate to: the effort and cost of their development; duplication of effort; inadequate investments in implementation strategies; difficulties in evaluation; slow adoption of innovations as a side effect; and guideline abuse.

Effort and cost of development

Properly constructed evidence-based CPGs take a lot of time to develop. This means relatively high costs. Those who commission CPGs and expect high-quality products need to be patient. There are few available short cuts that will not in some way erode either the validity or the credibility of a guideline and therefore its effectiveness. Thus, 'cheap' CPGs will not add value to the health system.

Duplication of effort

Given the cost of their development, one of the most frustrating aspects of the guideline development 'industry' is the hubris of different organizations in wanting to be the main sponsor of a

CPG. This has led to unnecessary duplication of efforts in aspects of CPG development where cooperation is possible and preferable. Lack of cooperation has led to a wastage of funding for a very expensive resource. Given that CPGs need to be continuously updated, continued independent programs will waste even more resources on their updating processes. Strategies can be developed to pool resources and cooperate in the development and updating of CPGs, and in their implementation and evaluation.

Inadequate investment in implementation strategies

Although tremendous efforts and resources have been expended by a variety of groups to develop CPGs, these commitments have not been matched by support for implementation or evaluation. As for any other health-care innovation, CPGs will not be adopted if they are not made available to clinicians at the point of care to assist them with their decision-making. Passive dissemination and peer review publications are insufficient strategies to ensure that CPGs get used. The importance of implementation has been highlighted in a recent review about why physicians do not follow guidelines.[11]

Difficulties in evaluation

Efforts to evaluate the influence of CPGs on practice patterns, patient outcomes or both are currently in their early stages, and such evaluations are difficult to design and expensive to carry out. Strategies such as clinician surveys are very prone to bias, because it has been shown that how clinicians think they practice is quite different from how they do practice.[12,13] Audits of clinical records[14] and population data examining patterns of practice in relation to the timing of the release of a CPG may provide valuable information on the consistency of practice with a CPG, but will not provide direct evidence of whether a CPG is being consulted in the clinic. Only rigorous trials and, eventually, clinical information systems in the form of electronic medical records will yield direct information on whether clinicians consult CPGs, and whether they abide by their recommendations. Such information could, in the longer term, be related to patient outcomes. It is reasonable to ask at this time whether large investments in complex trials to evaluate CPGs can be justified when we are facing imminent dramatic changes in health records systems that will do the same job at less expense.

Slow adoption of innovations

The evidence-based approach can legitimately be criticized for its conservatism in recommending the adoption of new and promising, but not proven, interventions. The evidence-based proponents would argue that, for these interventions, research is what is required. This is a reaction to legitimate concerns in health care of the premature adoption of many innovative ideas, which were subsequently found to be less beneficial than advertised and often even harmful to patients. Notwithstanding the validity of this last claim, the evidence-based approach may be casting a pall over the spirit of innovation in oncology. Cancer is as much an investigative discipline as it is an evidence-based one. Although evidence-based principles embrace the investigative spirit in theory, there is concern that its application in practice may be having a dampening effect on innovation and its adoption, especially in publicly funded systems. This issue should not be minimized, and may contribute to the unwillingness of payers to support research-based practice in oncology, which is the life blood of the discipline.

Guideline abuse

The definitions of CPGs and evidence-based medicine are consistent in relating these concepts to the management of individual patient care. However, CPGs are being promoted more by managers and payers as vehicles to control practice and reduce costs. Nevertheless, in Ontario, CPGs have actually resulted in increased funding to the cancer care system. Although CPGs are intended as clinical tools, they are being used as policy tools. It is still not clear whether the decision context of the clinical encounter can be scaled up to the boardroom in terms of the utility of the evidence-based approach. In a recent article, it was pointed out how identical interpretation of the same research evidence by a clinician in a clinical context and a manager in a policy context could produce opposite courses of action, both of which are defensible.[15] We are still in the early learning phase in knowing how best to apply CPGs in clinical practice and policy.

Simplistic notions of evaluation of clinical practice also threaten CPGs. It seems perfectly clear, at this time, that the same research evidence can produce conflicting clinical recommendations, and that conflicts between clinical and policy recommendations can be defensible and legitimate (discussed below). Nevertheless, some managers and payers are intent on developing intrusive strategies that can interfere with good judgment about how to manage an individual patient. Data about variations between practice and guidelines ought to be interpreted as flags to the practitioner, not judgments of the practitioner. A well-implemented CPG that does not influence practice is as likely to signal a badly designed CPG as it is inappropriate practice.

In an instructive example, recommendations for the surgical management of stage I breast cancer, according to the Canadian Steering Committee, identify lumpectomy (breast-conserving surgery) followed by local radiation as the preferred option.[16] At the same time, Ontario's CPG recommends that either mastectomy or lumpec-

tomy followed by radiation is acceptable, but that the patient should be offered a choice.[17] These CPGs are consistent with one another, but clearly have different implications in terms of how they would be evaluated. Of interest, when a decision tool was developed in Ontario to help patients decide with their surgeons about which approach to take, the rate of breast-conserving surgery (BCS) actually fell for those surgeons who were more frequently offering BCS before the development of the decision aid (personal communication).

CONTRASTING CANADIAN AND AUSTRALIAN GUIDELINES ON BREAST CANCER

To highlight some of the principles discussed above, it is instructive to examine differences between guidelines on the same topic produced by two different organizations, both of which used a rigorous evidence-based approach. Here, the author has selected national guidelines from Canada and Australia for the management of early stage breast cancer. For additional insights, some guideline statements from the Cancer Care Ontario guideline initiative have also been included (Tables 2.1–2.4).

Table 2.1 highlights some of the fundamental differences between the Australian and Canadian national guidelines, both of which are evidence based. The most obvious feature distinguishing the sets of guidelines is that the Australian guidelines do not make any prescriptive statements at all, simply describing the nature of the evidence. Thus, they are devoid of any recommendations. Both the Canadian and the Ontario guidelines make recommendations for practice. The guideline statements in Tables 2.2 and 2.3 illustrate these differences. Note also, in Table 2.2, how the difference in the recommendations for the surgical management of early stage breast cancer

Table 2.1   Contrasting Canadian and Australian Breast Cancer Guidelines
Canadian breast cancer guidelines tend to be more prescriptive. Australian guidelines present the evidence.
Canadian breast CPGs follow a more traditional medical orientation. Australian guidelines stress communication, psychosocial issues, etc.
Canadian breast CPGs are formatted for quick reference to be used at point of care. Australian CPGs serve more as background reference material, although selected issues are highlighted.
Australian guidelines are more comprehensive in the material they cover.
Recommendations from both countries are generally consistent with the evidence. Differences seem to reflect local organizational and cultural (medical and societal) issues and perspectives.

Table 2.2   Contrasting guideline statements: mastectomy or lumpectomy
Canada: For patients with stage I or II breast cancer, BCS followed by radiotherapy **is generally recommended** . . .
Ontario: Women with stage I or II breast cancer who are candidates for BCS **should be offered the choice** of either BCS or modified . . .
Australia: There is **no difference in the rate of survival or** distant metastasis between women having mastectomy and those having BCS where appropriate.

reveals different values for patient choice between Canada and Ontario.

Table 2.4 demonstrates interesting differences in perspective between the Australian and Canadian guidelines in terms of the topics included for the management of early stage breast cancer. The medical orientation of the Canadian guidelines contrasts with the broader perspective of those produced in Australia. However, despite these noticeable differences in approach and style, there is overall consistency in the substance of the guidelines from the two countries.

TOOLS FOR GUIDELINES

Well-conceived, cancer-related, evidence-based CPGs are produced by a variety of sources, many of which have developed their own websites for reference. Useful websites for consulting guidelines on breast cancer include the Cancer Care Ontario Guideline Initiative <http://www.hiru.mcmaster.ca/ccopgi/>, the American Society of Clinical Oncology <http://www.asco.org/> and the Australian NHMRC National Breast Cancer Centre <http://www.nbcc.org.au/>. The National Comprehensive Cancer Network (NCCN) in the USA produces useful guidelines in the form of clinical algorithms. These guidelines are developed through expert consensus, and their publication does not include a comprehensive list of citations, so that to date they cannot be classified as evidence based.

Table 2.3   Contrasting guideline statements: radiotherapy after lumpectomy (BCS)

Canada:
Women who undergo BCS **should be advised to have** postoperative breast radiotherapy (RT). Omission of RT increases risk of local recurrence. Local breast RT should begin . . . not later than 12 weeks, but the optimal interval is not defined.

Ontario:
Women . . . who have undergone BCS **should be offered** postoperative breast irradiation. Optimal schedule not established. RT should begin . . . within 12 weeks, but window of safety is unknown.

Australia:
Radiotherapy after lumpectomy **significantly reduces the risk of local recurrence**. Omission of RT, leads to increased risk of local recurrence. 'While it is not uncommon clinical practice to omit RT in . . . selected cases . . . the decision requires the woman to weigh . . .'

A relatively new website sponsored by the US Agency for Health Research and Quality (AHRQ) uses specific eligibility criteria for evidence-based guidelines, before it will include them in its website. The website promises to help clinicians and policy-makers be aware of guidelines and determine the strengths and weaknesses among several different CPGs on the same topic, so that the most appropriate can be used in the circumstances. The website address for the US Guideline Clearinghouse is: <http://www.guideline.gov/index.asp>. The Canadian Medical Association also provides an inventory of guidelines in Canada, with links to original websites. The CMA website address is <http://www.cma.ca/cpgs/index.htm>. Some guideline programs produce CD-ROM versions of their products. One such program is the *Standards, Options and Recommendations* of the excellent evidence-based French oncology guideline initiative, which also provides a website: <http://www.fnclcc.fr/>. A commercial CD-ROM product with an extensive inventory of guide-

Table 2.4 Contrasting guideline topics: early stage disease	
Canadian Consensus Document	**Australian NHMRC Guidelines**
1. The palpable breast lump	1. Counseling issues
2. Investigation of mammography detected lesions	2. Volume/outcome considerations
3. Mastectomy or lumpectomy?	3. Navigating the health system
4. Axillary dissection	4. Role of surgery in mammography detected lesions
5. Management of DCIS	5. Simple vs radical mastectomy
6. Breast radiotherapy after BCS	6. Mastectomy vs BCS
7. Adjuvant systemic therapy for node-negative disease	7. Local radiotherapy after BCS
8. Adjuvant systemic . . . node-positive	8. Adjuvant therapy for node-positive and node-negative disease
9. Follow-up after treatment for . . .	9. Management of DCIS and LCIS
10. Management of chronic pain . . .	10. Follow-up after treatment

DCIS, ductal carcinoma in situ; LCIS, lobar carcinoma in situ; BCS, breast-conserving surgery.

lines is available from Faulkner & Gray, and guidelines are regularly updated at <http://www.guidelines.faulknergray.com>.

CONCLUSION

Clinical practice guidelines share the characteristics of other health-care innovations. Their introduction will be associated with some benefits, and their limitations will be recognized. But, as for other innovations, they need to be allowed to evolve as we learn more about how to use them in the most appropriate way. Progress in the application of clinical practice guidelines will require research if they are to evolve and improve in the same way as other health-care technologies.[18]

REFERENCES

1. Field MJ, Lohr KM. eds. *Institute of Medicine. Guidelines for Medical Practice: From development to use.* Washington DC: National Academy Press, 1992.
2. Sackett DL, Rosenberg WMC, Gray MJA et al, Evidence-based medicine: what it is and what is isn't. *BMJ* 1996; **312**:71–2.
3. Browman GP, Evidence-based paradigms and opinions in clinical management and cancer research. *Semin Oncol* 1999; **26**(suppl 8):9–13.
4. Wortman PM. Vinokur A, Sechrest L, Do consensus conferences work? A process evaluation of the NIH consensus development program. *J Health Politics, Policy Law* 1988; **13**:469–98.
5. Mulrow CD, Rationale for systematic reviews. *BMJ* 1994; **309**:597–9.
6. Jadad AR, Cook DJ, Jones A et al, Methodology and reports of systematic reviews and meta-analyses: a comparison of Cochrane reviews with articles published in paper-based journals. *JAMA* 1998; **280**:278–80.
7. Cook DJ, Guyatt GH, Laupacis A et al, Clinical recommendations using levels of evidence for antithrombotic agents. *Chest* 1995; **108**(4 suppl):227S–30S.
8. Browman GP, Levine MN, Mohide EA et al, The practice guidelines development cycle: A conceptual tool for practice guidelines development and implementation. *J Clin Oncol* 1995; **13**:502–12.
9. Evans WK, Newman TE, Graham I et al, Lung cancer practice guidelines: Lessons learned and issues addressed by the Ontario Lung Cancer Disease Site Group. *J Clin Oncol* 1997; **15**:3049–59.
10. Browman GP, Newman TE, Mohide EA et al, Progress of clinical oncology guidelines development using the practice guidelines development cycle: The role of practitioner feedback. *J Clin Oncol* 1998; **16**:1226–31.
11. Cabana MD, Rand CS, Powe NR et al, Why don't physicians follow clinical practice guidelines? *JAMA* 1999; **282**:1458–65.
12. Lomas J, Anderson GM, Domnick-Pierre K et al, Do practice guidelines guide practice? The effect of a consensus statement on the practice of physicians. *N Engl J Med* 1989; **321**:1306–11.
13. Rosser WW, Dissemination of guidelines on cholesterol. Effects on patterns of practice of general practitioners and family physicians in Ontario. *Can Fam Physician* 1993; **39**:280–4.
14. Ray-Coquard I, Philip T, Lehmann M et al, Impact of a clinical guidelines program for breast and colon cancer in a French cancer center. *JAMA* 1997; **278**:1591–5.
15. Browman GP. Essence of evidence-based medicine: A case report. *J Clin Oncol* 1999; **17**:1969–73.
16. Steering Committee on Clinical Practice Guidelines for the Care and Treatment of Breast Cancer, Mastectomy or lumpectomy? The choice of operation for clinical stage I and II breast cancer. *Can Med Assoc Journal* 1998; **158**(3 suppl):S15–21.

17. Mirsky D, O'Brien SE, McCready DR et al, Surgical management of early stage invasive breast cancer (stage I and II). *Cancer Prevention Control* 1997; 1:10–16.

18. Browman GP, Levine MN, Graham I et al, The clinical practice guideline: an evolving health care technology. *Cancer Prevention Control* 1997; 1:7–8.

3

Economic evaluation analysis in breast cancer therapy: From evidence to practice

Philip Jacobs, Nadine MacLean, Barbara Conner-Spady, Katia Tonkin

Economic evaluation analysis deals with the study of interventions, the focus of which is on the quantity of resources used in the management of patients in relation to outcomes. As a result of the rapidly changing technologies that are used in breast, as well as in other, cancer therapies, costs of treatment have risen substantially in recent years. In response to these cost increases, governments and insurers around the world have been seeking various means of containing costs. Drug formularies and clinical practice guideline programs are examples of initiatives that have been undertaken to control the use of new technologies. Economic analysis is an information tool that can be used by those who undertake these initiatives.

When we deal with resource issues, there are several different types of questions that we can address. First, we can compare alternative interventions that are focused on *the same* indications (e.g. metastatic breast cancer), addressing the question: 'What are the cost and outcome implications of using different interventions?' Alternatively, we can compare different interventions that focus on *different* indications of disease (e.g. breast cancer and colorectal cancer). The research question would be the same as above, but the context differs. Finally, we can address

the issue of whether we should treat breast cancer at all. The research question in this instance might be phrased as: 'Are the benefits that are gained from treating the patient (with a given technology) greater than the costs?'

In this chapter we focus on the first of these questions, which deals with the comparison of alternative interventions in breast cancer therapy. We discuss the comparison of costs and outcomes for these interventions. However, when addressing this question, we face some daunting problems. We first provide an overall framework for dealing with the general research question that we have just identified. Next, we summarize the results from the literature on cost-effectiveness in breast cancer therapy. In particular, we demonstrate how these results can be interpreted by users of data.

ELEMENTS OF COST-EFFECTIVENESS ANALYSIS IN BREAST CANCER THERAPY

Overview

The general elements for a cost-effectiveness analysis are set out in several textbooks[1-3] and in guidelines that have been issued to standardize methodologies.[4,5] The authors of the guidelines recommend that the following analytical elements should be specified in a cost-effectiveness analysis:

- Treatment indications should be identified.
- Alternative interventions should be clearly specified, including a 'do-nothing' alternative, if appropriate.
- A perspective or viewpoint should be chosen; this can be the patient's own perspective, the viewpoint of the payer (whether the third party insurers or the government health program); that of a single provider such as a hospital; or the broadest viewpoint, being the societal perspective, which includes all payers, including the patient and caregivers.
- A time horizon that incorporates beginning and ending time lines of the study should be selected. It is recommended that the time frame of the study be long enough to capture all downstream events (i.e. events subsequent to the intervention) that are associated with the study interventions.
- Appropriate outcome measures should be selected (see below).
- Sources of clinical data, which have been used to derive efficacy or effectiveness measures, should be specified.
- Resources and their related costs should be specified.

Following the application of these guidelines, a cost-effectiveness ratio, which summarizes the differences in costs and outcomes, can be derived. This ratio is made up of the net difference in costs between interventions divided by the net difference in outcomes between interventions.

Quality of information

Cost-effectiveness analyses can be conducted with data from both randomized clinical trials and administrative databases, or they can be constructed in the form of a 'decision analysis',

which is a modeling exercise using data from diverse sources (including clinical trials). However conducted, these analyses are subject to validity criteria which are similar to the standards used to gauge other clinical and economic data. These criteria are referred to as the level of evidence criteria. The level of evidence in cost-effectiveness analysis is made up of three criteria: the criterion used to assess the method of establishing effectiveness, the measure of outcome used and the method of measuring cost.[6]

Methods of establishing effectiveness

Most investigators accept the view that large, well-designed, randomized clinical trials are the gold standard in terms of establishing effectiveness.[7] Recently, however, investigators in the area of critical care medicine have put forward the view that studies that use observational databases can, if appropriately conducted, approach the level of evidence of randomized clinical trials.[8] Indeed, in recent years, observational databases have improved dramatically in terms of their quality, and statistical techniques used to control for self-selection bias have been adopted in ground breaking studies.[9] Data based on clinical opinion, rather than observation, are on the bottom rung in terms of quality of evidence.

Outcome measures

Although the definitions of health-related quality of life (HRQL) vary, most HRQL measures assess three broad areas of health: physical, psychological and social functioning.[10–13] Authors of health economics guidelines recommend that three different types of outcome measures be used in economic evaluations: generic health quality-of-life measures, disease-specific measures and preference-based measures.

Generic measures or non-condition-specific measures are designed to apply to a wide variety of populations and contain a broad spectrum of items. They are generally not as responsive as disease-specific instruments, but can be used to compare relative impacts of health programs across various populations. Preference-based measures are types of generic measure that produces a single index score for use in economic evaluation. Preference-based measures (sometimes called utility measures) require a weighting system to be applied to a health state. This process involves a number of steps, which are used to derive the single index score: the measurement of HRQL of the target population, the measurement of preferences, and the assignment of preferences to the health states of individuals.[10]

A special kind of index is the quality adjusted life year (QALY) index, which assigns the number 0 to a health 'state' of death and the number 1 to the state of 'perfect' health. A QALY can be derived from generic or preference measures, using processes that require the investigator to make additional assumptions. Although these assumptions are often artificial, QALY indexes have an advantage of allowing the investigator to incorporate the health status of the patient while he or she is alive (usually valued at >0) with that after death (valued at 0) up to the final point of observation. This, the QALY is a very useful tool to use when comparing outcomes of individuals with varying survival times.

Instruments of HRQL should be chosen so that the inferences drawn from the scores are valid and not open to misinterpretation. Thus, sufficient data should have been published to provide suitable reliability estimates and evidence of validity. Ideally, this data should have been collected for a similar purpose and within a similar group to that for which the tool will be used. In choosing a HRQL instrument, there are several criteria to consider, including applicability to purpose, reliability, validity and feasibility. The HRQL instrument should meet the purpose

of the study, e.g. to assess different aspects of HRQL over time, a cancer-specific HRQL instrument would be the most appropriate. Reliability reflects the consistency and stability of a measurement. Estimates of reliability are dependent on the method of estimation, the number of items in the instrument and the variability of the sample. Validity is a continuing process of evaluation of the degree to which empirical evidence and theoretical rationales coincide and support the adequacy and appropriateness of interpretations and actions based on a score.[14]

The kinds of evidence of validity that are important depend on the intended use of the HRQL scores: the content of the questionnaire should be based on a theoretical rationale; the dimensions should be representative of HRQL as it is conceptualized; the scoring model should be congruent with the underlying conceptual model; the items should be clear, unambiguous and relevant to the patient population; and the time frame should be clearly defined and relevant to the study. An important aspect of the validity of tools used in outcome research is responsiveness – the ability of an HRQL to respond to an underlying clinically relevant change. Other kinds of evidence of validity include comparisons of different groups that are expected to differ on aspects of HRQL, convergent and discriminant evidence, and evidence of the relevance and usefulness of the scores for their applied purposes. Finally, feasibility reflects the need for the questionnaire to be short enough to reduce respondent and staff burden, for the questionnaire to be standardized, easy to code and score, and for the resources to be available to ensure rigorous data collection.

There has been considerable discussion about the source of the HRQL data. There is a general consensus that HRQL indices should represent the views of the patients, not those of the providers. However, the argument has been put forward that the general public, who pay for health care, should have *their* preferences for different health states expressed. One problem with this viewpoint is that the general public may not be able to imagine what certain illness experiences are really like; thus, their preferences for imaginary health states might differ considerably from those that were actually experienced.

Examples of outcome measures in breast cancer

The Functional Living Index – Cancer (FLIC)[15] and the QLQ-C30[16] are two examples of cancer-specific HRQL tools. The FLIC is a widely used, 22-item, cancer-specific tool which was designed to produce an overall global measure of the effect of cancer on patient function. It has acceptable reliability, and the evidence supports responsiveness, and convergent and discriminant validity in the breast cancer population. The QLQ-C30, a 30-item instrument, was designed for evaluating the quality of life of patients participating in international clinical trials. It includes six functional subscales, three symptom scales and six single items. Although the initial psychometric studies for the QLQ-C30 were conducted in lung cancer patients, several studies have supported aspects of validity in the breast cancer population. The QLQ-B23,[17] a supplementary module to the QLQ-C30 for use in breast cancer patients, measures body image, sexuality and symptoms specific to breast cancer.

The EQ-5D, a generic, preference-based HRQL tool, was designed to be used alongside condition-specific measures as an outcome measure in evaluative studies.[18] It has five questions and an accompanying visual analog scale. Although reliability estimates of the EQ-5D are acceptable, validity evidence is inconsistent and its usefulness as a HRQL measure in clinical trials of breast cancer patients has not been established. Several measurement issues affect the validity of EQ-5D index scores, including: broadness of levels,[19] ceiling effects in patient and population groups,[20,21] less responsiveness than other measures[22–24] and unresolved issues in the measurement of preferences.

In spite of the weak validity evidence, an increasing number of studies are being published using the EQ-5D in economic analyses in cancer patients[25–28] and other patient groups. Few of these studies have examined the validity of EQ-5D scores in the cancer population. The only study that has employed the EQ-5D in breast cancer patients[29] used just the visual analog scale. There is an eagerness to employ these tools in economic analyses despite the fact that there are still unresolved measurement issues. Just as the measurement of HRQL arose out of an important gap in the traditional outcome measures of mortality and morbidity, so the development of preference-based measures has arisen out of gaps in traditional HRQL measures.

Costs

The cost of a service is the product of the resources (labor, medicines, equipment, services) that are used to produce it and the monetary price paid for these resources (or the value that the resources would have in their best alternative use, if they are unpaid). Laupacis et al[6] identify several criteria that can be used for the assessment of costs, including the direct measurement of resource use (rather than measures based on professional opinion) and the measurement of costs (resources and their prices) in the setting in which the services are provided. These criteria address internal validity issues. In addition, there are external validity criteria that must be addressed: costs should be measured in settings that are representative of the environments in which care takes place.

Grades of recommendation

The topic of 'grades of recommendation' is related to the interpretation of the results. Assuming that a high-quality study was done, one is then faced with the task of interpreting the results. Cost-effectiveness analysis provides only the numbers. Investigators or policy-makers must develop their own standards in order to evaluate the numbers. For example, assume that we have two drug therapies, A and B: the cost of A is $US 40 000 and the cost of B is $US 50 000 per patient. Therapy A has a 40% chance of a positive response, whereas B has a 70% chance. Referring to our definition of the cost-effectiveness ratio as the ratio of differences in costs and differences in outcomes, the differences in cost between the two interventions is $US 10 000 and the difference in the probability of a response is 0.3. The cost-effectiveness ratio is $US 10 000 for a 0.3 increase in response. For each positive response, the cost would be $US 10 000/0.3 or $US 33 333 per positive response.

Is it worth it? There are some instances in which this answer would be easy. If B cost less and had better outcomes, then B would be the 'dominant' intervention and would be the more acceptable alternative. However, in this case B costs more and is better, and so the policy-maker is faced with a dilemma. The cost-effectiveness analysis in this case tells us how much more we have to spend, and what we get for this additional expenditure. Policy-makers must develop standards to help them interpret these results. Cost-effectiveness analysis, by itself, cannot tell someone whether or not $US 33 000 is worth the additional expense.

Some investigators have devised their own standards for cost–utility analysis.[6] These standards stated that, if an intervention achieved an additional QALY for under $US 20 000, then there was 'strong evidence' for its adoption. Moderate evidence was provided if the cost-effectiveness ratio fell in the range $US 20 000–100 000 per QALY. These standards are useful in setting up some kind of benchmark. However, they are the results of the authors' own valuations, and should be recognized as such.

AN OVERVIEW OF THE LITERATURE

Method

We conducted a review of the cost-effectiveness analysis literature on breast cancer therapy. We searched the MEDLINE and HealthSTAR databases from 1993 to 1999. The searches were restricted to English and human studies only. The subject word used was 'breast neoplasms'; it was searched together with 'cost' or 'costs or economic' or 'economic' in the title. MEDLINE had 105 citations and HealthSTAR had 146 citations using this search strategy. We also searched manually for additional articles using the bibliographies of any articles that we identified. We selected for abstraction five articles. All were decision analyses and were among the highest quality of the studies published.

Results

The results of the five articles that we surveyed are presented in Table 3.1. In this we refer to the indications, the alternative interventions and the cost-effectiveness ratios. All studies were decision analyses, and so the data that were used to put together the studies came from a variety of sources. This will have a bearing on the quality of the studies.

The method used to determine effectiveness was randomized clinical trials (RCTs) in all studies. The outcome measures that were used in the RCTs were usually survival. In two of the studies,[32,33] the authors directly used the survival measures in their cost-effectiveness ratios, deriving a measure of cost per life-year saved. However, in three of the studies,[30,31,34] the investigators

Table 3.1   Summary of results for selected cost-effectiveness studies in breast cancer

Study	Indication	Interventions	Cost-effectiveness ratio
Hillner[30]	Node-negative, estrogen-receptor-negative breast cancer (stage I)	• Adjuvant chemotherapy • No best supportive care	$US 15 400 per QALY for women aged 45 $US 18 800 per QALY for women aged 60
Hillner et al[31]	Metastatic stage IV breast cancer	• Standard chemotherapy (cyclophosphamide + doxorubicin + 5FU) vs High dosage (cyclophosphamide + cisplatin + carmustine) with bone marrow transplantation	$US 96 000 per life-year
Lee et al[32]	High-risk premenopausal breast cancer	• Post-mastectomy radiation therapy vs No post-mastectomy radiation therapy	$US 19 700 per life-year saved
Silber et al[33]	Early stage breast cancer – chemotherapy	• G-CSF prophylactically after cycle 1 • G-CSF after occurrence of a febrile neutropenic event vs no G-CSF	• G-CSF after cycle 1 vs no G-CSF: $US 254 000 per life-year saved • G-CSF after an event vs no G-CSF: $US 21 000 per life-year saved
Silberman et al[34]	Anthracycline- and paclitaxel-resistant, metastatic breast cancer	• Capecitabine • Continuous infusion of 5FU	$US 17 000 per QALY

G-CSF, granulocyte colony-stimulating factor; 5FU, 5-fluorouracil; QALY, quality adjusted life years.

derived estimates of outcomes in terms of QALYs, using preferences obtained from oncology staff, rather than from the patients; the investigators then replaced the life-years, as derived from the RCTs, with the QALYs that they derived. The cost measures were usually obtained from similar patients in a single medical center,[30,31] from the literature,[32,33] or from administrative data.[34]

The results themselves indicate a wide variety of efficiency levels in treatments that are currently being used in breast cancer. The 'best buys' (strong evidence for adoption according to Laupacis et al[6]) included capecitabine (versus 5-FU) ($US 17 000 per QALY saved), adjuvant chemotherapy (versus best supportive care) ($US 15 400 per QALY saved), and post-mastectomy radiation therapy (versus no radiation) ($US 19 700 per life-year saved). At the margin with regard to moderate evidence (again according to Laupacis et al[6]) was high-dose chemotherapy (versus standard chemotherapy), at $US 96 000 per life-year saved.

Evaluation of the quality of the studies

Of the information obtained in these studies, the effectiveness measures all came from high-quality RCTs. Outcome data were not a uniformly high quality. Those studies that used QALYs as a measure of outcome all obtained these measures from providers, rather than from patients. Thus, the QALYs do not reflect the preferences or the health status of people who experienced the conditions. Finally, cost measures, which are based on data collected from a single hospital, may lack external validity. Nevertheless, these studies were the highest quality studies available in the literature.

CONCLUSIONS

Cost-effectiveness is a tool that can serve as an aide to decision-making in setting treatment guidelines for breast cancer. A number of such studies have been conducted in breast cancer. Most of these have been decision analyses, which obtain their data from a variety of sources. We have provided a description of the sources and an overview of how to evaluate the quality of a cost-effectiveness study. We surveyed the literature on cost-effectiveness analysis and selected for review the most recent and high-quality studies in the area. The results indicate that there is a wide range of efficacies among treatments. The results do provide some guidance for groups that wish to set guidelines. In some cases, such as the use of capecitabine and adjuvant therapy, the results appear to be quite conclusive, using any set of values. In other instances (e.g. high-dose chemotherapy), the analysis will provide little guidance.

REFERENCES

1. Drummond M, O'Brien B, Stoddart GI et al, *Methods for the Economic Evaluation of Health Care Programmes*. Toronto: Oxford University Press, 1997.
2. Jefferson T, Demicheli V, Mugford M, *Elementary Economic Evaluation in Health Care*. London: BMJ Publishing Group, 1996.
3. Gold MR, Siegel JE, Russel LB, Weinstein MC, *Cost-effectiveness in Health and Medicine*. New York: Oxford University Press, 1996.
4. Canadian Coordinating Office for Health Technology Assessment, *The Use of G-CSF in the Prevention of Febrile Neutropenia*. Ottawa: Canadian Coordinating Office for Health Technology (CCOHTA), 1997. [Technology overview: pharmaceuticals, issue 9.0, available from: http://www.ccohta.ca]
5. Brown M, Glick HA, Harnell F et al (1998). Integrating economic analysis into cancer

trials: the National Cancer Institute – American Society of Clinical Oncology Economics Workbook. *J Natl Cancer Inst Monogr* 1998; **24**:1–28.

6. Laupacis A, Feeny D, Detsky AS, Tugwell PX, How attractive does a new technology have to be to warrant adoption and utilization? Tentative guidelines for using clinical and economic evaluations. *Cana Med Assoc J* 1992; **146**:473–81.

7. Jovell AJ, Navarro-Rubio MD, Evaluacion de la evidencia cientifica. *Med Clin* 1995; **105**:740–3.

8. Rubenfeld GD, Angus DC, Pinsky MR et al, Outcomes research in critical care. Results of the American Thoracic Society Critical Care Assembly Workshop on Outcomes Research. *Am J Respir Crit Care Med* 1999; **160**:358–67.

9. Connors AF Jr, Speroff T, Dawson NV et al, The effectiveness of right heart catheterization in the initial care of critically ill patients. *JAMA* 1996; **276**:889–97.

10. Patrick DL, Erickson P, *Health Status and Health Policy*. New York: Oxford University Press, 1993.

11. Schipper H, Clinch JJ, Olweny CLM, Quality of life studies: Definitions and conceptual issues. In: Spilker B, ed., *Quality of Life and Pharmacoeconomics in Clinical Trials*, 2nd edn. Philadelphia: Lippincott-Raven, 1996: 11–23.

12. Osoba D, *Effect of Cancer on Quality of Life*. Boca Raton, FL: CRC Press, 1991.

13. Ware JE, Standards for validating health measures: Definition and content. *Journal of Chronic Diseases* 1987; **40**:473–80.

14. Messick S, Validity. In: Linn R, ed., *Educational Measurement*, 3rd edn. New York: Macmillan Publishing Co, 1989: 13–103.

15. Schipper H, Clinch JJ, McMurray A, Levitt M, Measuring the quality of life of cancer patients: the Functional Living Index – Cancer: development and validation. *J Clin Oncol* 1984; **2**:472–3.

16. Aaronson NK, Ahmedzai S, Bergman B et al, The European Organization for Research and Treatment of Cancer QLQ-C30: A quality-of-life instrument for use in international clinical trials in oncology. *J Nat Cancer Instit* 1993; **85**:365–76.

17. Sprangers MAG, Groenvold M, Arraras JI et al, The European Organization for Research and Treatment of Cancer breast-cancer specific quality-of-life questionnaire module: First results from a three-country field study. *J Clin Oncol* 1996; **14**:2756–68.

18. Anonymous, EuroQol – a new facility for the measurement of health-related quality of life. The EruoQol Group. *Health Policy* 1990; **16**:199–208.

19. Wolfe F, Hawley DJ, Measurement of the quality of life in rheumatic disorders using the EuroQol. *Br J Rheumatol* 1997; **36**:786–93.

20. Brazier J, Jones N, Kind P, Testing the validity of the EuroQol and comparing it with the SF-36 health survey questionnaire. *Quality of Life Research* 1993; **2**:169–80.

21. Essink-Bot ML, Krabbe PF, Bonsel GJ, Aaronson NK, An empirical comparison of four generic health status measures. The Nottingham Health Profile, the Medical Outcomes Study 36-item Short-Form Health Survey, the COOP/WONCA charts, and the EuroQol instrument. *Medical Care* 1997; **35**:522–37.

22. Hollingworth W, Mackenzie R, Todd CJ, Dixon AK. Measuring changes in quality of life following magnetic resonance imaging of the knee: SF-36, EuroQol or Rosser index? *Quality of Life Research* 1995; **4**:325–34.

23. Jenkinson C, Stradling J, Petersen S, How should we evaluate health status? A comparison of three methods in patients presenting with obstructive sleep apnoea. *Quality of Life Research* 1998; **7**:95–100.

24. Jenkinson C, Gray A, Doll H, Lawrence K, Keoghane S, Layte R, Evaluation of index and profile measures of health status in a randomized controlled trial. Comparison of the Medical Outcomes Study 36-Item Short Form Health Survey, EuroQol, and disease specific measures. *Medical Care* 1997; **35**:1109–18.

25. Norum J, Vonen B, Olsen JA, Revhaug A, Adjuvant chemotherapy (5-fluorouracil and levamisole) in Dukes' B and C colorectal carcinoma. A cost-effectiveness analysis. *Ann Oncol* 1997; **8**:65–70.

26. Norum J, Angelsen V, Wist E, Olsen JA, Treatment costs in Hodgkin's disease: a cost-utility analysis. *Eur J Cancer* 1996; **32A**:1510–17.

27. Uyl-de Groot CA, Vellenga E, de Vries EGE, Lowenberg B, Stoter GJ, Rutten FFH, Treatment costs and quality of life with granulocyte-macrophage colony-stimulating factor in patients with antineoplastic therapy-related febrile neutropenia: Results of a randomized placebo-controlled trial. *Pharmacoeconomics* 1997; **12**:351–60.

28. Vellenga E, Uyl-de Groot CA, de Wit R et al, Randomized placebo-controlled trial of granulocyte-macrophage colony-stimulating factor in patients with chemotherapy-related febrile neutropenia. *J Clin Oncol* 1996; **14**:619–27.

29. Glick HA, Shpall EJ, LeMaistre CF et al, Empirical criteria for the selection of quality-of-life instruments for the evaluation of peripheral blood progenitor cell transplantation. *Int J Technol Assessment Health Care* 1998; **14**:419–30.

30. Hillner BE, Financial costs, benefits, and patient risk preferences in node-negative breast cancer: insights from a decision analysis model. *Recent Res Cancer Res* 1993; **125**:277–84.

31. Hillner BE, Smith TJ, Desch CE, Efficacy and cost-effectiveness of autologous bone marrow transplantation in metastatic breast cancer: estimates using decision analysis while awaiting clinical trial results. *JAMA* 1992; **267**:2055–61.

32. Lee JH, Solin LJ, Glick HA, A decision-analytic model and cost-effectiveness evaluation of post-mastectomy radiation therapy for high-risk breast cancer. *American Society of Clinical Oncology Annual*, Abstract no. 1621, 1998. [Available from: http://asco.infostreet.com/prof/me/html/98abstracts/hre/m_1621.htm]

33. Silber JH, Fridman M, Shpilsky A et al. Modeling the cost-effectiveness of granulocyte colony-stimulating factor use in early-stage breast cancer. *J Clin Oncol* 1998; **16**:2435–44.

34. Silberman G, Gupta S, Berkowitz N, Leyland-Jones B, Cost-effectiveness of capecitabine, continuous infusion 5FU, gemcitabine and vinorelbine in the treatment of metastatic breast cancer. *American Society of Clinical Oncology (ASCO)* 1999. Abstract no. 1629. [Available from: http://asco.infostreet.com/prof/me/html/99abstracts/hsr/m_1629.htm]

4

RECIST: Response evaluation criteria in solid tumors

Janet Dancey, Patrick Therasse, Susan G Arbuck, Elizabeth A Eisenhauer

All clinical trials should be prospectively planned and conducted under controlled conditions to provide definitive answers to well-defined questions. Yet, despite careful planning and execution, the results of non-randomized trials evaluating the same agent or combination of therapies in the same tumor type can vary widely. Some of this variability is the result of differences in patient characteristics, and reflects the true spectrum of benefit that can be expected from treatment of patients with the disease. It is because of this variability that treatment benefit can be determined definitively only through randomized controlled trials. As a result of the cost, complexity and duration of randomized studies, preliminary evidence of anti-tumor activity is often determined in smaller, single-arm, phase II studies, which use the surrogate end-point of tumor response.

The results of the phase II studies are important for setting the direction of cancer research because they determine whether an agent or regimen is worthy of further evaluation. With an expanding number of agents and combinations for evaluation and a limited number of patients available for clinical trials, the efficient use of these resources is increasingly important. An accurate estimate of drug activity is essential for efficient use of drug development resources; however, the reliability of the estimate depends not only on patient-, disease- and treatment-related factors, but also on the methods of assessing, analyzing and reporting the end-point of interest.

Phase II trials are not designed to be formally compared with the results of other studies; rather, they are designed to identify an absolute level of biologic activity of interest, so that decisions regarding further development can be made. As a result, it is imperative that the methods of evaluating the end-point of interest are consistent across studies. The purpose of this chapter is to describe the limitations of older response criteria and to present the recently revised response criteria in solid tumors (RECIST), which were developed to address these limitations and provide new standards for assessing and reporting response rates.

TUMOR RESPONSE AS AN END-POINT OF CLINICAL TRIALS

The primary goal of phase II trials in oncology is to estimate the anti-tumor activity of either a novel cytotoxic agent or a combined therapeutic regimen against a specific cancer. The end-point of the trial is the objective response rate. There are at least three reasons for using tumor response as an end-point in a phase II study: first, tumor regression implies some degree of anti-tumor activity of the agent being investigated; second, it is an outcome measure that is available early in the trial, so studies require smaller numbers of patients followed for shorter durations than studies assessing survival; and, third, improvements in tumor response rates correlate, to some extent, with improvements in more definitive measures of patient benefit such as palliation of symptoms or prolongation of survival.[1] Although there are many examples of agents, with promising response rates in phase II studies, that were not found to be beneficial in phase III studies, all standard cytotoxic and hormonal treatments currently available were selected for phase III evaluation, based on promising phase II results. Until better methods of assessing anti-tumor activity are available, some measure of change in tumor size will continue to be used as an end-point for phase II studies assessing anti-cancer agents that are likely to induce tumor regression.

Obtaining an accurate estimate of drug activity in phase II studies for the prioritization of agents for phase III evaluation is essential; however, the reported tumor response rate may be influenced by a number of factors. These factors include not only the choice of patients, disease stage and the details of treatment, but also the criteria for the assessment of therapeutic effect and analysis of results. The definition of tumor response, the techniques for assessing tumor size and their associated errors of measurement, the sample size of the trial and the frequency with which treated patients are excluded from analysis all influence the reported response rates obtained from phase II studies.[2–5] In fact, the definition and criteria for determining the objective response affect the response rate, response dura-

tion, progression-free survival and time to treatment failure. Although unknown patient and tumor-related factors may vary from study to study despite careful planning, use of common definitions and criteria can reduce variability in assessing and reporting these clinical outcomes.

Among the criteria that have been published for breast cancer trials are those of the National Cancer Institute (NCI),[6] the Union Internationale Contre le Cancer (UICC),[7] and the British Breast Cancer Group;[8] for solid tumors, are the criteria of those of the World Health Organization (WHO),[9] the Eastern Co-operative Oncology Group (ECOG),[10] the Southwest Oncology Group (SWOG)[11] and the European Organization for Research and Treatment of Cancer (EORTC).[12] These criteria were developed through consensus among experts. Unsurprisingly, as different individuals were involved in the development of these criteria, specific definitions and recommendations vary between them. Which tumor deposits are considered assessable, the number of lesions that should be assessed and the changes in measurable and non-measurable disease, which define significant tumor regression or growth, are some of the areas of discrepancy.

Worldwide, the WHO criteria have been the most commonly used in phase II trials of solid tumors. The WHO criteria classify disease as bi-dimensionally and uni-dimensionally measurable, non-measurable evaluable and unevaluable, stipulate the method for determining tumor burden and define four categories of tumor response: complete response (CR), partial response (PR), stable disease (SD) and progressive disease (PD). Although the WHO criteria include both uni-dimensional and bi-dimensional disease as measurable, over time, various research groups redefined measurable disease to mean measurable in two dimensions because of difficulties in integrating uni- and bi-dimensional lesions into response definitions. Thus, in most trials, tumor burden is calculated by summing, for each measured lesion, the products obtained by multiplying the largest diameter by its largest perpendicular diameter. The definition of complete response is the disappearance of all evidence of disease for a minimum of 4 weeks. Partial response is defined as a 50% or more decrease in total tumor load of the lesions that have been measured for a minimum of 4 weeks without evidence of progression in other sites. The advantages of specifying a minimum duration for CR or PR are thought to be twofold: a response of short duration is unlikely to be of clinical benefit and the requirement for a second assessment before declaring that the response may reduce the likelihood of misclassification as a result of measurement error. Progressive disease is defined as an increase of 25% in the size of one or more measurable lesions or the appearance of new lesion(s). Changes in tumor load that do not fit the definitions for CR, PR or PD are classified as SD.

As the effect of therapy on tumor burden is most probably a continuum from the complete disappearance of all tumor to virtually unimpeded tumor growth, the 'cut-offs' used to create the four response categories are arbitrary. The definitions are based on assumptions about the magnitude of tumor reduction that would be measurable, unlikely to occur spontaneously and likely to provide patient benefit. Similarly, the definition of progression was thought to be the minimum change in tumor growth that should result in discontinuation of a usually toxic and clearly ineffective therapy. The assumptions underlying these definitions – that objective tumor response results in patient benefit and that changes in tumor burden can be accurately and reliably determined – are questionable. A 50% reduction in tumor area represents a cut-off in the spectrum of changes in tumor size that can occur while patients are receiving treatment. There is no reason to believe that clinical outcome will be substantially different for patients with slightly lesser or greater changes in tumor burden. It is not surprising that phase III studies have shown that higher response rates may or may not be associated with improved survival or that the survival of patients with partial responses or stable disease have been found to differ modestly or not at all.[13] Although many studies have shown that responders live longer than non-responders, such comparisons do not prove that the survival of responders was prolonged as a result of treatment, because such an analysis is confounded and biased. Patients with disease sensitive to cytotoxic or hormonal therapy may have been destined to do well anyway because of favorable prognostic factors. Patients who die early, even those who die of treatment-related complications, are included among the non-responders.[1,14]

The classification of response requires repeated measurements of tumor nodules; thus, the accuracy of the results will depend on the method of assessment. The definition of CR – the disappearance of all evidence of disease for a minimum of 4 weeks – is straightforward, although it will be influenced by the sensitivity of the tests used to identify and follow sites of disease. However, PR, PD and SD are defined by 'cut offs' and may therefore be influenced by errors in measurement. Various studies of simulated tumor nodules,[3,5,15] neck nodes[5] and lung metastases on radiograph[5,16] have shown up to an 8% chance of falsely declaring a PR and a 30% chance of falsely declaring progression. The chance of error is higher when lesions are small, physical examination is the method of assessment and different observers make the measurements. As lesions are assessed at multiple intervals during treatment, the chance of a false progression being recorded is likely to be higher during a clinical trial.[15] The measurement of more than one lesion and the requirement for sequential measurements at least 4 weeks apart can reduce the number of false PRs; however, these safeguards are not uniformly applied to the determination of progression. The use of such small changes in tumor area based on a single observation can lead to premature discontinuation of a potentially effective therapy as a result of measurement error.[5]

To provide more reproducible and objective assessments of change in tumor size, response assessment has become more rigorous and technology based. Recent studies have used chest radiograph, computed tomography (CT) and magnetic resonance imaging (MRI) in preference to physical examination, ultrasonography and nuclear medicine studies. Cross-sectional imaging techniques such as computed tomography and MRI allow accurate lesion assessment and independent review at a later date.[17] However, even such sophisticated technologies as computed tomography and MRI vary in quality and interpretation. When performing CT and MRI examinations, such factors as the level of technology, expertise, quantity, timing and method of injecting intravenous contrast material, and the choice of slice thickness and pulse sequences (for MRI), may result in differences between the quality of the generated image and its subsequent interpretation.[18]

As CT and MRI procedures have improved and sophisticated software for calculating tumor volume is becoming more generally available, advocates for using volumetric tumor measurement are becoming more common. This has led to some confusion about how to integrate three-dimensional measures into response assessment. A 50% reduction in tumor volume is not as strict a criterion for response as a 50% reduction in tumor cross-sectional area.[19] In fact, a 65% reduction in volume would be equivalent of a 50% reduction in cross-sectional area. Although these technologies may more accurately assess change in tumor burden, whether this improvement in precision of measurement will translate into more reliable estimates of anti-tumor effect and correlate better with patient-related outcomes is uncertain.

In the ensuing two decades since their development, the WHO criteria have been adapted by different research organizations to integrate measurable and evaluable disease into response evaluation, define the minimum size and number of lesions to be measured, and modify the definition of progression. The lack of standardization in these areas among research organizations, as well as the development of new imaging technologies and other modalities of assessing tumor burden, led researchers to the realization that a revision of existing standards for evaluating tumor response was required.

THE RECIST CRITERIA

Over a period of 5 years, representatives of research organizations, industry and regulatory authorities from North America, Europe and Japan revised the WHO criteria. The result of this international collaboration is the new RECIST criteria, which include new definitions of measurable disease and tumor response as well as recommendations for assessing tumor burden and for reporting results. Although standardization and simplification were priorities, the new criteria were devised to allow results of future studies to be compared with historical data. The following discussion highlights some of the significant elements of the RECIST criteria. For a complete description, readers are referred to the full publication.[20]

Measurable and non-measurable disease

As objective response is determined by comparing overall tumor burden assessed at baseline with subsequent measurements, it follows logically that only patients with at least one measurable lesion should be eligible for studies in which objective tumor response is the primary endpoint. If the measurable disease is restricted to a solitary lesion, its neoplastic nature should be confirmed by cytology/histology. The definitions of measurable and non-measurable disease are the first significant change to be found in the RECIST criteria and the rationale for this change will be discussed in detail.

By RECIST criteria, tumor lesions are categorized as either measurable or non-measurable. Measurable lesions must have a longest diameter of ⩾20 mm or more with conventional techniques or ⩾10 mm or more with spiral CT scan. Measurements should be recorded in metric notation, using a ruler or callipers. Non-measurable lesions include small lesions as well as bone lesions, leptomeningeal disease, ascites, pleural/pericardial effusion, inflammatory breast disease, lymphangitis cutis/pulmonis, abdominal masses that are not confirmed and followed by imaging techniques, and cystic lesions. Non-measurable disease is recorded as present or absent. All baseline evaluations should be performed as close as possible to the start of treatment and never more than 4 weeks before.

All measurable lesions – up to a maximum of five lesions within an organ and ten lesions representative of all involved organs – should be measured and recorded at baseline. These 'target' lesions should be selected on the basis of their size and suitability for accurate repetitive measurements. A sum of the longest diameter (LD) for all target lesions should be calculated and reported as the baseline sum LD. The baseline sum LD will be used to determine objective tumor response of the measurable dimension of the disease. All other lesions or sites of disease should be identified as non-target lesions, recorded at baseline and followed to determine whether they are 'present' or 'absent'.

Clearly, the use of a single measurement, the LD, rather than the product of two measurements, the LD and its largest perpendicular diameter, from each tumor nodule is a significant change from the other published criteria. However, both theoretical and practical considerations, as well as data from clinical trials, support the use of the LD rather than the sum of the products to estimate change in tumor burden. Assuming that a tumor nodule approximates a sphere, there is a fixed mathematical relationship between the diameter, surface area and volume. Thus, a 50% decrease in area is equivalent to a 30% decrease in diameter or a 65% decrease in volume. Alternatively, a 25% increase in area corresponds to a 12% increase in diameter and a 40% increase in volume. As most tumor deposits are spherical, the maximum diameter correlates well with the longest perpendicular diameter, the surface and with tumor perimeter,[15] becoming very inaccurate as an estimate of tumor size only when the length is more than twice its width.[21] For spherical tumors of 1–10 cm in diameter, the relationship between tumor diameter and logarithm of the cell number is more proportional than the product of the longest perpendicular diameters.[22] Thus, changes in diameter are approximately independent of initial tumor size, whereas changes in the sum of the products of larger tumors are the result of smaller log cell reduction compared with changes in smaller lesions. Theoretically, the sum of the diameters may be a better approximation of change in tumor burden because of its more linear relationship to logarithm of cell number;[23] however, the clinical significance of this is uncertain.

Retrospective analyses of clinical trial data to determine response rates using either one-dimensional or two-dimensional measurements yielded remarkably similar results. James et al[23] analyzed tumor response rates by WHO and one-dimensional RECIST criteria from data obtained on 569 patients enrolled on eight clinical trials. With few exceptions, the same patients were considered to be responders by either method and, without exception, the same conclusions were reached about the efficacy of the regimen under study. These results were confirmed in a much larger data set of 4614 patients obtained from industry and American and Canadian cooperative group studies.[20] The best response for each patient was calculated using the WHO and RECIST criteria. As falsely declaring progression as a result of errors in measurement was a concern, a 20% increase in diameter, equivalent to a 44% increase in area and a 73% increase in volume, was chosen to define progression by the RECIST criteria. Whether the calculations were based on the WHO or the RECIST criteria, the response rates and progressive disease rates were essentially identical: 25.6% versus 25.4% and 30.3% versus 29%, respectively. Based on these results, the use of one-dimensional measurements should not result in active drugs being discarded because of perceived inactivity.

By requiring a greater change in tumor size for the classification of PD, the date that PD is declared should be later by RECIST criteria than by WHO criteria. To determine the magnitude of the difference, time to progression as defined by WHO and RECIST criteria were compared, using subset of trials obtained from SWOG. SWOG criteria define progression as a 50% increase in the sum of the products of bi-dimensional measurements – an increase of 10 cm^2 – or the appearance of new lesions. Based on results obtained from 234 patients with breast, colorectal, melanoma and lung cancers, the same date of progression was found for 91.2% of cases. Unsurprisingly, an earlier date of progression with WHO criteria was obtained for 7.3% of patients. For most of these cases, the difference between the dates of progression was unknown, because RECIST criteria were not reached at the time the data were censored. These results suggest that there is no meaningful difference in response and progression categorization by WHO or RECIST criteria.

The similarity of results obtained by either WHO or RECIST criteria supports the simplification of the response evaluation by using the sum of the LDs instead of the sum of the products. There are a number of advantages to requiring only a single measurement of each tumor nodule. Time and effort are saved by not calculating products of individual tumor nodules. Simplification of tumor assessment encourages the measurement of more lesions in an individual patient, reducing the risk of errors.[24] The rate of accrual and completion time of phase II studies may be improved as patients with disease measurable only uni-dimensionally, who would have been excluded from phase II studies using older criteria, would be eligible for studies using RECIST criteria. There is little chance that promising therapies will be missed by allowing patients with only uni-dimensional disease or measuring change in the sum of the LDs to participate in phase II clinical trials.[23,25]

Measurement of lesions

The RECIST document includes a number of recommendations for evaluating disease to minimize measurement error. As a result of the unreliability of repeated physical examinations, clinical lesions should be considered measurable only when they are superficial (e.g. skin nodules, palpable lymph nodes). In the case of skin lesions, documentation by color photography, including a ruler to estimate the size of the lesion, is recommended.

Imaging-based evaluation is preferred to evaluation by clinical examination when both methods have been used to assess the anti-tumor effect of a treatment. Care must be taken because radiographic measurement may also be subject to errors introduced by different techniques in sequential radiographic studies. The same method of assessment and the same technique should be used to characterize each identified and reported lesion at baseline and during follow-up. Chest radiographs are acceptable to assess lesions that are clearly defined and surrounded by aerated lung. However, computed tomography and MRI are the most accurate and reproducible methods to measure target lesions selected for response assessment.[17,18,26] It is important to ensure consistent quality of enhancement and precise matching of lesions and measurements. To evaluate lesions within the chest, abdomen and pelvis, conventional computed tomography and MRI should be performed with cuts of 10 mm or less in slice thickness contiguously and spiral computed tomography should be performed using a 5-mm contiguous reconstruction algorithm. Head and neck and extremities usually require specific protocols. Although it is not necessary for centers participating in studies to standardize their CT and MRI scanning protocols, it is important that, within each center, standards are used to ensure comparability of sequential studies.

Some modalities, such as ultrasonography, nuclear medicine scans, endoscopy and tumor markers, should not be used to estimate changes in tumor burden in clinical trials using objective response as the primary end-point, because they are unreliable or lack validity. As ultrasonography is subjective and highly operator dependent, accurate lesion assessment on subsequent examinations and independent review at a later date are difficult.[17] Ultrasonography can be an alternative to clinical measurements for superficial lymph nodes, subcutaneous lesions and thyroid nodules, and may be used to confirm the complete disappearance of superficial lesions assessed by clinical examination. The utilization of laparoscopy and endoscopy techniques for objective tumor evaluation may be useful to confirm complete pathologic response when biopsies are obtained. However, their use in the assessment of changes in tumor size has not yet been fully validated, and requires sophisticated equipment and a high level of expertise that may be available only in some centers. Therefore, the utilization of such techniques for objective tumor response should be restricted to validation purposes in reference centers. Specific additional criteria for standardized usage of prostate-specific antigen[27,28] and CA-125[29,30] response in support of clinical trials are being developed and can be incorporated into objective response evaluations once fully validated.

Determining best overall response

The best overall response is defined as the best response recorded from the start of the treatment until disease progression/recurrence. The increase in size is based on the smallest measurements recorded since treatment started. In general, the patient's best response assignment will depend on the achievement of both measurement and confirmation criteria.

Complete response is defined as disappearance of all target and non-target lesions and normalization of tumor markers. In some circumstances, it may be difficult to distinguish residual disease from normal tissue. When the evaluation of CR depends on this determination, it is recommended that the residual lesion be investigated by fine-needle aspirate/biopsy to confirm CR status. Partial response is at least a 30% decrease in the sum of baseline LDs of target lesions, without evidence of progression in non-target lesions. Thus, the persistence of one or more non-target lesions and/or maintenance of tumor marker levels above normal limits, even in the presence of a CR of measurable lesions, results in the designation for overall tumor response of PR. Progression is at least a 20% increase over the smallest sum LD recorded or the appearance of one or more new lesions. Changes in sum LD that do not meet criteria for PR or PD are classified as SD.

Occasionally, the patients' physical status worsens without clear documentation of worsening disease. Patients with a global deterioration of health status requiring discontinuation of treatment without objective evidence of disease progression at that time should be reported as 'symptomatic deterioration'. Every effort should be made to document the objective progression even after discontinuation of treatment, to prove that deterioration is the result of worsening disease rather than treatment toxicity or other illness.

The main goal of confirmation of objective response is to minimize the risk of overestimation of the response rate. Designations of PR or CR require that changes in tumor measurements be confirmed by repeat studies performed no less than 4 weeks after the criteria for response are first met. Longer intervals, as determined by the study protocol, may also be appropriate. Repeat studies to confirm changes in tumor size may not always be feasible or may not be part of the standard practice in protocols, where progression-free survival and overall survival are the key end-points. These patients should be reported as having 'unconfirmed responses'. For SD, measurements must have met the SD criteria at least once after study entry, at a minimum interval that is defined in the study protocol. This time interval should take into account the expected clinical benefit that such a status may bring to the population under study.

All patients included in the study must be assessed for response to treatment, even if there are major protocol treatment deviations or if they are ineligible. Each patient should be assigned to one of the following categories: CR, PR, SD, PD, early death whether caused by malignant disease, toxicity or other causes, or 'unknown' resulting from insufficient data. All patients who met the eligibility criteria should be included in the main analysis of the response rate. Those patients removed from treatment early should be considered as treatment failures. Incorrect treatment schedule or drug administration is not a cause of exclusion from the analysis of the response rate. Thus, to determine an objective response rate, the numerator should be composed of the number of patients with confirmed CRs and PRs, and the denominator should include all eligible patients. It is preferable to report the response rate with the 95% confidence limits. Subanalyses may then be done on the basis of a subset of patients, excluding those for whom major protocol deviations have been identified. Reasons for excluding patients from the analysis should be clearly reported. However, these subanalyses should not serve as the basis for drawing conclusions about treatment efficacy; all conclusions should be based on analyses of the outcome of all eligible patients.

For trials in which the response rate is the primary end-point, it is strongly recommended that all responses be reviewed by an expert(s) independent of the study. Consistent application of response criteria by an independent panel may significantly reduce response rates, but they should produce greater consistency and reproducibility of results.[17,26]

As the type and schedule of treatment can dictate the frequency of tumor re-evaluation, RECIST recommendations are limited to stipulating that the frequency of reassessment be specified in the protocol. Follow-up every other cycle (i.e. 6–8 weeks) seems a reasonable norm;

however, smaller or greater time intervals could be justified for specific regimens or circumstances. After completion of treatment, the need for repetitive tumor evaluations depends on whether the phase II trial has as a goal the response rate or 'time to event' (progression/death). If 'time to event' is the main end-point of the study, routine re-evaluation of patients is warranted at frequencies determined by the protocol.

Duration of response

The duration of overall response is measured from the time when measurement criteria are met until the first date that recurrent or progressive disease is objectively documented. The duration of overall CR is measured from the time measurement criteria are first met for CR until the first date that recurrent disease is documented. Stable disease is measured from the start of the treatment until the criteria for progression are met. It is worth reiterating that PD is defined as a 20% increase in sum of LDs over the smallest measurements recorded since the treatment started. The durations of response, SD and progression-free survival are influenced by the frequency of follow-up after baseline evaluation. Any comparisons among trials must take into account the lack of precision of the measured end-point.

Application of RECIST to clinical trials

When the response rate is the primary outcome measure of a trial, rigorous evaluation of tumor response as outlined in the RECIST criteria is justified. However, application of these criteria to evaluation of tumor response in phase III trials, in which objective response is *not* the primary end-point, is not required. For example, in such trials it might not be necessary to measure as many as 10 target lesions, or to confirm response with a follow-up assessment after 4 weeks or more. Methods to evaluate response should be specified in the protocol and these deviations from RECIST criteria should appear in reports of the trial. However, if the response rate is chosen to be the primary end-point of a phase III trial because there is a direct relationship between objective tumor response and a real therapeutic benefit for the population to be studied, the same criteria as those applying to phase II trials should be used.

CONCLUSIONS AND FUTURE DIRECTIONS

Expeditious clinical development and approval of new anti-cancer therapies that are beneficial to patients are matters of high priority. The decision to proceed with definitive phase III trials with their added complexity and intensive use of resources depends on informal comparisons of phase II trial results. Variability in the reporting of response rates for a given set of data, as a result of differences in measurement and reporting criteria, is detrimental because it makes judgments about the relative merits of experimental treatments difficult. To evaluate the results of clinical trials depends on consistent definitions of tumor response and the use of reliable and reproducible methods of tumor measurement. The use of standard assessment criteria is not only desirable but also imperative.

Over the decades since the development of the WHO criteria, our understanding of issues of study design and patient assessment have evolved, and this evolution will undoubtedly continue in the years to come. The RECIST guidelines are meant to resolve discrepancies that have arisen as research organizations have sought to overcome limitations of the WHO criteria, which became apparent over decades of use. These guidelines are not meant to discourage development and validation of new techniques, which may provide more reliable surrogate end-points than objective tumor response to predict therapeutic benefit for cancer patients. Future changes in study design and patient assessment, as well as the drugs under study, may render the current trial methodology equally outmoded. New techniques to establish better objective tumor response will be integrated into these criteria when they are fully validated. In the meantime, these new guidelines advocate a more rigorous and technology-based assessment of tumor response to improve the reliability of phase II trial results and they are the standard against which newer techniques should be compared.

REFERENCES

1. Buyse M, Piedbois P, On the relationship between response to treatment and survival time. *Stat Med* 1996; **15**:2797–812.
2. Davis HL Jr, Multhauf P, Klotz J, Comparisons of Cooperative Group evaluation criteria for multiple-drug therapy for breast cancer. *Cancer Treat Rep* 1980; **64**:507–17.
3. Moertel CG, Hanley JA, The effect of measuring error on the results of therapeutic trials in advanced cancer. *Cancer* 1976; **38**:388–94.
4. Tonkin K, Tritchler D, Tannock I, Criteria of tumor response used in clinical trials of chemotherapy. *J Clin Oncol* 1985; **3**:870–5.
5. Warr D, McKinney S, Tannock I, Influence of measurement error on assessment of response to anticancer chemotherapy: proposal for new criteria of tumor response. *J Clin Oncol* 1984; **2**:1040–6.
6. Breast Cancer Force Treatment Committee, National Cancer Institute, *Report from the Combination Chemotherapy Trials Working Group.* US Department of Health, Education and Welfare. DHEW Publication No. 77–1192, 1977.
7. Anonymous, Assessment of response to treatment in advanced breast cancer. British Breast Group. *Lancet* 1974; **ii**:38–9.
8. Hayward JL, Carbone PP, Heuson JC, Kumaoka S, Segaloff A, Rubens RD, Assessment of response to therapy in advanced breast cancer: a project of the Programme on Clinical Oncology of the International Union Against Cancer, Geneva, Switzerland. *Cancer* 1977; **39**:1289–94.
9. Miller AB, Hoogstraten B, Staquet M, Winkler A, Reporting results of cancer treatment. *Cancer* 1981; **47**:207–14.
10. Oken MM, Creech RH, Tormey DC et al, Toxicity and response criteria of the Eastern Cooperative Oncology Group. *Am J Clin Oncol* 1982; **5**:649–55.
11. Green S, Weiss GR, Southwest Oncology Group standard response criteria, endpoint definitions and toxicity criteria. *Invest New Drugs* 1992; **10**:239–53.
12. van Oosterom AT, Tumor eligibility and response criteria for phase II and phase III studies and (sub)acute toxicity grading (with suggested amendments to the WHO criteria). *EORTC Data Center Manual*, Brussels, 1992: 84–6.
13. Torri V, Simon R, Russek-Cohen E, Midthune D, Friedman M, Statistical model to determine the relationship of response and survival in patients with advanced ovarian cancer treated with chemotherapy. *J Natl Cancer Inst* 1992; **84**:407–14.
14. Anderson JR, Cain KC, Gelber RD, Analysis of survival by tumor response. *J Clin Oncol* 1983; **1**:710–19.
15. Lavin PT, Flowerdew G, Studies in variation associated with the measurement of solid tumors. *Cancer* 1980; **46**:1286–90.
16. Gurland J, Johnson RO, How reliable are tumor measurements? *JAMA* 1965; **194**:973–8.
17. Gwyther S, Bolis G, Gore M et al, Experience with independent radiological review during a topotecan trial in ovarian cancer. *Ann Oncol* 1997; **8**:463–8.
18. Gwyther SJ, Response assessment using radiological methods. *Crit Rev Oncol Hematol* 1999; **30**:45–62.

19. Clamon G, Clamon L, Relationship between tumor area, tumor volume, and criteria of response in clinical trials. *J Clin Oncol* 1993; **11**:1839.

20. Therasse P, Arbuck SG, Eisenhauer EA et al, New guidelines to evaluate the response to treatment in solid tumors. *J Natl Cancer Inst* 2000; in press.

21. Spears CP, Volume doubling measurement of spherical and ellipsoidal tumors. *Med Pediatr Oncol* 1984; **12**:212–17.

22. Collins VP, Loeffler RK, Tivey H, Observations on growth rates of human tumors. *Am J Roentgenol* 1956; **78**:988–1000.

23. James K, Eisenhauer E, Christian M et al, Measuring response in solid tumors: unidimensional versus bidimensional measurement. *J Natl Cancer Inst* 1999; **91**:523–8.

24. James K, Eisenhauer E, Therasse P, Re: Measure once or twice does it really matter? *J Natl Cancer Inst* 1999; **91**:1780.

25. Jett JR, Su JQ, Krook JE, Goldberg RM, Kugler JW, Measurable or assessable disease in lung cancer trials: does it matter? *J Clin Oncol* 1994; **12**:2677–81.

26. Gwyther SJ, Aapro MS, Hatty SR, Postmus PE, Smith IE, Results of an independent oncology review board of pivotal clinical trials of gemcitabine in non-small cell lung cancer. *Anticancer Drugs* 1999; **10**:693–8.

27. Bubley GJ, Carducci M, Dahut W et al, Eligibility and response guidelines for phase II clinical trials in androgen-independent prostate cancer: Recommendations from the Prostate-Specific Antigen Working Group. *J Clin Oncol* 1999; **17**:3461–7.

28. Dawson NA, Response criteria in prostatic carcinoma. *Semin Oncol* 1999; **26**:174–84.

29. Cruickshank DJ, Terry PB, Fullerton WT, CA125-response assessment in epithelial ovarian cancer. *Int J Cancer* 1992; **51**:58–61.

30. Rustin GJ, Nelstrop AE, Bentzen SM, Piccart MJ, Bertelsen K, Use of tumour markers in monitoring the course of ovarian cancer. *Ann Oncol* 1999; **10**(suppl 1):21–7.

5
Definitions of trial design

Jean-Marc Nabholtz, Katia Tonkin

DEFINITIONS

We use reasoning to determine our course of action when faced with a patient and a clinical decision. However, there are different types of reasoning. The first is *clinical reasoning*. In this, we use the case history and make informal generalizations to make inferences on behalf of the individual patient, and thus arrive at a treatment decision.

Statistical reasoning is a way of thinking. It is a formal study of inference in the presence of uncertainty. It provides an objective framework for investigation, placing theory and data on an equal footing. Experimental design produces data in such a way as to quantify systematic and random error. We then use formal methods that combine theory and data to analyze results.

Research reasoning needs clinical and statistical reasoning. Data generated from relatively small experiments are used to make formal generalizations. The development of clinical trials has depended on new medical ideas, which often reject accepted practice. When positive, their results lead to major changes in the everyday practice of medicine.

A *clinical trial* is a planned experiment, which involves patients and is designed to determine the most appropriate treatment for future patients with a given medical condition. The essential characteristic is that the results from a sample of patients are used to make inferences regarding treatment for the general population of patients needing treatment in the future. Clinical trials require groups of patients and large groups often need to be accrued in a short space of time in order to obtain results that can be translated into routine practice in a timely fashion.

All clinical trials attempt to control and quantify factors that are extraneous to the effect of interest, which can be random or systematic (bias) variations. A *randomized clinical trial* (RCT) is often a crucial step in evaluating interventions used in prevention, diagnosis or treatment of a disease. In the presence of the uncertainty of benefit, randomized trials are not only ethical but also an important step, applying evidence to the practice of medicine. Adequate numbers and randomization of patients for treatment assignment avoid both random and systematic errors. Randomization is also a method for balancing known and unknown predictive factors. Stratification controls for specific groups that are expected to influence outcome and later analysis. Concurrent control groups allow for differences in time trends that are particularly relevant with respect to supportive care for cancer patients. In addition, validity of tests for statistical significance can be guaranteed within randomized trials. Examination of many trials leads to new algorithms for patient care and future trial strategy development.

As RCTs provide the most credible outcome data for new therapies, there are appropriate standards to protect the rights and human dignity of subjects. The first step is to ensure that the research protocol has scientific merit and the data obtained are credible. This means that the results will be relevant to the body of scientific information on the particular topic studied. This first step requires the protocol to state clearly the question addressed by the study, the nature of the intervention and the outcome measure. The study needs to address the possibility of systematic error, ethical concerns and feasibility. The defined subject population with clear inclusion and exclusion criteria, along with the data analysis procedures, should then allow for the results to be generalizable. This latter point is always contentious in breast cancer studies, because clinical trials do not enroll more than 5% of all breast cancer patients. The ability to take the results of such a small subpopulation of patients and make rational statements concerning all breast cancer patients is at present an unresolved issue.

The European Union, Japan, the USA and other countries use the published International Conference on Harmonization (ICH) *Guidelines for Good Clinical Practice* (GCP).[1] Many other nations use the World Health Organization's (WHO) *GCP for Trials on Pharmaceutical Products* from 1995.[2] A few nations such as Australia, Brazil and Korea, have written their own GCP guidelines. The purpose of these guidelines is to address quality assurance, auditing practices and ethical standards. They ensure that individuals involved in clinical trials describe scientifically sound trial design within clear written protocols.

A *written study protocol* should contain background details and study objectives. It should contain clear criteria for subject selection, intervention and methods for evaluating outcomes. It should identify the sample size and the statistical analyses planned. It should outline registration, randomization and adverse events, and how to handle protocol violations. Clear statements on data forms and data handling, along with trial monitoring and administrative procedures, are all part of a clinical protocol.

Good trials generally define the question and limit the primary outcome to answer one hypothesis. Secondary outcomes are common and usefully generate new primary hypotheses for future trials and support the primary hypothesis. Multiple comparisons are undesirable, because they are likely to generate positive results by chance. Trial size and duration are crucial because they determine the feasibility of the trial design. A trial that takes too many years to accrue patients is likely to fail because newer therapies become available and researchers move on to answer other questions. A trial of treatment in small subpopulations is also more difficult to undertake for the same reasons and because its results are not easily generalizable. Stopping rules are an important safety issue with new and potentially toxic treatments. This is true in breast cancer therapy where the trend to more intensive treatment has led to use of unproved high-dose regimens with stem cell transplantation before adequate data have been obtained from randomized studies.

Randomization and attention to its detail can limit trial bias. Although blinding of treatment is feasible in studies of new hormone therapies or supportive treatment such as bisphosphonates or new cytokine growth factors, it is often not feasible for new chemotherapy regimens. Well-designed trials allow, within limits, generalizable results that can be applied to a broader population of patients. The caveat is, of course, that only a small population of patients ever participates in breast cancer trials, which makes their results difficult to generalize.

A trial can be successful only with the commitment of all investigators and research staff with no unrealistic expectations. Feasibility is a key element in the successful undertaking of trials. Finally and most importantly, patient safety must be a primary concern. Ethics approval, a letter of information and informed consent are all part of the process that ensures that a patient can freely participate but withdraw at any time without any prejudice to care.

Once a trial is complete, the statistician will make efficient use of all the information in the analysis. The analysis must meet the objectives of the study, making sure that the design meets the scientific objectives. Internal validity assures an appropriate estimate of the treatment effect and necessary steps ensure external validity. There is responsible exploration of the data for unanticipated effects and characterization of strengths and weaknesses of evidence generated as part of the unplanned analyses.

The counting of all eligible patients without post-hoc exclusions gives an unbiased estimate of the probability of benefit. *Intent to treat* (ITT) *analysis* is preferable because it compares the groups as determined by the randomization process. If as-treated analysis is undertaken, the groups compared are based on compliance with treatment. The ITT analysis, however, accounts for the benefits of the randomization process with its ability to rule out bias, and gives confidence that the selection of patients in the two arms is not determined by a process that might give advantage to one arm. There are several reasons why as-treated groups may seem appropriate, including post-randomization ineligibility, unreliable estimates of end-points for patients who withdraw or who are lost to follow-up, and

patients who are not compliant. The reasons for non-compliance are, however, liable to influence the outcome measure when compliance relates to toxicity and patient or physician bias toward treatments. Compliance is a complex phenomenon because it can be a marker for following medical advice and may be influenced by patient status. A patient closest to treatment failure may be most likely to cease taking prescribed medication. In the analysis of as-treated patients, the balance that randomization attempts to introduce is altered and the result becomes a biased comparison of subgroups within the initially randomized trial. The primary analysis should therefore always be ITT even though it includes a dilution effect of individuals who do not take the treatment as originally planned. Many clinical trials look at the ITT result and the analysis of those that complied to some predefined extent. When these results are similar, bias and dilution are unlikely to be major factors. If, however, the results are at variance, investigators are faced with a data credibility issue.

STAGES IN THE DEVELOPMENT OF NEW THERAPY

There are three recognized stages in the evaluation of new anti-cancer therapies.

Early development, phase I

The first phase is required to determine clinical pharmacology and toxicology; it also involves dose-finding designs. The primary purpose is drug safety, not efficacy. All these involve three components. The first is to use biologic knowledge, prior information and clinical judgment about the relationship between dose and toxicity. The second is to specify decision rules for dose escalation, which include decisions on cohort size and rules for stopping because of toxicity. The third is to define the maximum tolerated dose (MTD) or suitable optimal dose for further study. Traditionally, the modified Fibonacci design is used, but continual reassessment methods (CRM) are now felt to be superior with more efficiency and less bias. Typically, phase I studies involve 20–80 patients.

Middle development, phase II

This is the stage of clinical investigation of treatment effect. This phase revolves around safety and efficacy. There needs to be a reference for the effect of standard therapy external to the trial. There is a need for a reference standard to enable comparison with the new treatment. There should be criteria for recommending a comparative study. Most importantly, suitable outcome criteria must be defined. When appropriate, surrogate end-points should be used because these will shorten the trial duration.

The use of staged or sequential designs can permit the early termination of unfavorable treatment and randomization can reduce selection bias when more than one new treatment is being studied. Sample size calculations should take into consideration reporting of results using 95% confidence limits and the chance of toxicities with the new therapy. The design of phase II studies has been made simpler by the use of optimal two-stage design software.

Late development, phase III

This is a full-scale evaluation of the treatment; it occurs when the new drug or regimen is compared with current standards in a large trial. This is the most rigorous and extensive type of scientific investigation of a new treatment. There are three components to its design: the first is randomization, which removes selection bias; the second is to have a definitive clinical outcome; and the third is to have sufficient precision for reliable detection of clinically important differences. Stratification can be used to control for

differences in specific group outcomes and type I errors can be set at 5% or 10%, with limitation of multiple comparisons and end-points to ensure validity of the results. If there is only a small effect, it must be reliably distinguished from random error.

The first step is to define the purpose of the trial with the specific hypothesis stated. Then a written protocol with trial design is completed followed by identification of the trial organization. Once the trial has been undertaken, the data must be analyzed and the results are published in order that conclusions can be drawn. This last step often leads to the next trial to answer further questions raised by the results of the first trial. The difficulty in breast cancer trials is that the next trial must often be designed and undertaken before knowing the results of the first trial or several years would elapse while the study data mature.

EVALUATION OF PATIENT RESPONSE

The fundamental aim of a phase III trial is to compare patient response with different treatment strategies, each of which defines as rigorously as possible the implementation of the drug schedule(s) being evaluated. It is therefore crucial to have, as far as possible, reproducible techniques for evaluating tumor response in advanced disease, with clear documentation of disease progression and definitions for the outcome(s) of interest.

The current evaluations of complete response (CR), partial response (PR), stable disease (SD) and progressive disease (PD) are currently undergoing re-evaluation by the major trial groups on both sides of the Atlantic, to improve reproducibility and simplify documentation (see Chapter 3). The current definitions should be written into all phase III trials.

The documentation of disease progression

toxicities and other outcomes of interest should likewise be clearly stated in all phase III written protocols. It is usual to use the NCI common toxicity criteria and, where these do not exist, grading is done as follows

1 mild (asymptomatic)
2 moderate (symptomatic but not interfering significantly with function)
3 severe (causing significant interference with function)
4 life threatening.

It is also usual to specify that tumor evaluation should be made at specific times such as within 4 weeks of study drug administration and then at each cycle, with formal radiological evaluation after three and six cycles of treatment and at the end of administration of the study drug. Clearly, the same type of study needs to be performed at each time interval, so that the measurements can be compared. Disease measurability is also important. For clinical skin nodules or lymph nodes, a minimum of 10 mm × 10 mm is the standard to ensure that changes in size can feasibly be documented. For radiological lesions on chest radiographs, 10 mm × 10 mm is used and for computed tomography (CT) scans or ultrasonography 20 mm × 10 mm is used. If a lesion is only one-dimensional, the clinical size is 10 mm and on computed tomography or ultrasonography by 20 mm. The following are the standard response criteria.

Complete response: disappearance of all known disease determined by two observations not less than 4 weeks apart. Complete disappearance of all known disease for at least 4 weeks.

Partial response: for two-dimensionally measurable lesions this is at least a 50% decrease in the sum of the products of the largest perpendicular diameters of all measurable lesions by two determinations not less than 4 weeks apart. For one-dimensionally measurable lesions, a PR is a decrease of 50% in the sum of the largest diameters of all lesions, as determined by two measurements not less than 4 weeks apart. No lesion should have progressed and no new lesions should have appeared.

No change (NC): less than a 50% decrease and more than a 25% increase in the sum of the products of the largest perpendicular diameters of all measurable lesions. For one-dimensionally measurable lesions, NC is less than a 50% decrease and more than a 25% increase in the sum of the diameter of all lesions. No new lesions should have appeared. At least 6 weeks must have elapsed (usually two cycles) before NC is assigned.

Progressive disease: an increase of 25% or more in at least one two-dimensionally or one-dimensionally measurable lesion, in comparison with the nadir measurement or the appearance of a new lesion. For new pleural effusions or ascites, there must be cytological proof of disease.

For evaluable disease, the following are the criteria:

CR: complete disappearance of all known disease for at least 4 weeks.
PR: estimated decrease in tumor size of 50% or more for at least 4 weeks.
NC: no significant change after 6 weeks (usually two cycles of treatment). This includes stable disease, estimated decrease of less than 50% and estimated increase of less than 25%.
PD: appearance of any new lesions or estimated increase of 25% or more in existing lesions.

OUTCOME EVALUATION

Duration of response
Complete and partial response will date from the date of randomization until the documentation of progression.

Time to progression

This is from date of randomization to first documentation of progression. If the patient receives other anti-cancer treatment before this date, the patient will be censored at the time of the last available tumor assessment before he or she received the subsequent treatment.

Survival

This is calculated from the date of randomization to the date of death.

Disease-free survival (DFS)

This is the interval from the date of randomization to the date of local, regional or distant relapse, the date of second malignancy or death from any cause, whichever occurs first. In all of these outcome measures, the date of the first event is known for all patients, but the date of the second event may not. This may be because no information is available or the event has not occurred. These patients are said to be censored for survival: the time from diagnosis to the date last known alive is called the censored survival time.

Survival curve estimates are made either using the life-table, also known as the actuarial method, or the Kaplan–Meier modification of the same. These methods assume that the censored patients are similar to the uncensored individuals in their true survival experience and the method causing censored survival times is statistically independent of their true survival times. Deciding which of two treatments is superior with respect to survival may not be easy, even when two true survival curves are known. Treatment A could be associated with a higher early mortality but a lower late mortality than treatment B. Alternatively, treatment A may have better survival at points studied before 5 years, but when restricted to 5 years or more treatment B is superior. In either case, it is difficult to decide which treatment is better. These problems

are exacerbated if the curves are estimated from the data because of sampling variabilities and, in addition, the late part of the curve is always less reliable than the earlier part. This is further exacerbated with large numbers of censored patients.

Two of the most frequently used tests of differences in survival curves are the **log-rank** or Mantel–Haenszel test and the generalized **Wilcoxon** test. The distributions of these follow approximately a χ^2 distribution. The Wilcoxon test is more sensitive to early differences in the survival curve and the log-rank is better for late differences.

Subgroup analysis occurs commonly and is often done to justify a trial when the main analysis is negative. The trials are expensive and, if a certain subgroup can be found to show benefit, the trial can be deemed to have been worthwhile. It is common to use age, estrogen receptor (ER) or progesterone receptor (PR) status, tumor size, node status and nodal groups, within those that are node positive, to identify a group that may have benefited from the therapy. To compare subgroups, one must be able to use categories that define the groups in question. For a continuous variable, this introduces the problem of cut-off points and how these should be validated. There are computer models that use recursive partitioning to achieve the smallest p value, but this means that the p value obtained cannot be interpreted as a probability of the observed difference resulting from chance. The p value obtained in this way is much smaller than the true p value. By examining many cut-offs, there is a greater chance that one will be significant by chance alone. Similarly, the same is true if multiple statistical comparisons are made. In a trial in which subgroup analysis has been made, it may be shown that premenopausal women have a significant improvement with one treatment whereas postmenopausal women do not. This may occur when the two treatments have the same effect, but the postmenopausal group is too small to detect a difference, or too few deaths occurred. In addition, competing causes of death may obscure the effect. One way to overcome this problem is to apply a **test for interaction**. Such tests are usually **quantitative**. In such an interaction, changing from one subgroup to another changes the true magnitude of the difference in treatment effect on outcome. It is possible that the direction of the treatment is changed but this is not necessarily true, because there are several ways to test for interaction using logistic regression, log-linear or additive and multiplicative models. The important issue is to apply the correct model according to the circumstances. A **qualitative interaction**, on the other hand, is one in which switching from one subgroup to another changes the direction of the effect. The mathematical model used affects these tests far less and they are always clinically important, because they imply that difference subgroups should be treated in different ways.

Definitions of populations

All randomized patients are included in the ITT analysis according to the treatment received. Eligible and evaluable patients are also included in the **evaluable population**. To be part of this population, a patient should be eligible and, have received a minimum of two cycles of treatment, unless progression has occurred before this in which case the patient is evaluable–early progression. The patient must also have had all baseline lesions evaluated at least once after the second cycle using the baseline method and have experienced no major protocol violation while on the study, such as concomitant anti-cancer treatment.

Surrogate end-points

To provide a valid substitute for the actual outcome of a trial, a surrogate must be closely associated or correlated with the actual outcome.

Surrogates are chosen because they generally give a result earlier than the actual outcome of interest. They are chosen because the surrogate has been found, in observational studies, to have a correlation to the outcome of interest and the biology of the disease makes it plausible that changes in the surrogate will inevitably lead to changes in the outcome of interest. The strength of the association is measured by the relative risk (RR) or the odds ratio. It is also important that the surrogate has been consistent across studies after adjustment for known confounders. If a surrogate is associated with an outcome after adjusting for confounders, it is called an independent association. We can rely on a surrogate only when it has been proved in large randomized trials. It is easier for the clinician if trials have shown the usefulness of the surrogate when other drugs of the same or similar class were being evaluated. In addition, the clinician will have more confidence in the surrogate if the result shows a large difference with narrow 95% confidence limits, and the effect persists over a long period of time. When deciding whether a particular treatment is appropriate for an individual patient, the use of a surrogate can be difficult. If there are several large randomized trials, all of which show benefit, the decision can be relatively straightforward but in reality these data are rarely available. When comparing drugs of different classes and looking at the surrogate, one can be misled into extrapolating these data to assume that the actual outcome for the new drug would be the same as for the older therapy. This is not necessarily true because the action of the drugs is likely to be different and the magnitude of the effect on the surrogate may not indicate the expected benefit on the eventual outcome.

In the end, clinicians need to consider the adverse effects as well as the benefits of a therapy and the alternative options before recommending a treatment based solely on surrogate end-points.

REFERENCES

1. US Department of Health and Human Services Food and Drug Administration, *Guidance for Industry – E6 Good Clinical Practice: Consolidated Guidance*. April, 1996.

2. World Health Organization, *Guidelines for Good Clinical Practice (GCP) for Trials on Pharmaceutical Products*. WHO Technical Reports Series, No. 850, 1995, Annex 3.

6

The need for large-scale randomized evidence for reliable assessment of moderate benefits

Richard Peto, Colin Baigent

THE NEED TO ASSESS *MODERATE* DIFFERENCES IN OUTCOME

Many interventions produce only moderate effects (i.e. proportional reductions of about 10–20%) on major outcomes such as death or serious disability. But, even a moderate effect of treatment, if demonstrated clearly enough for that treatment to be adopted widely, could prevent substantial numbers of premature deaths. Moreover, if more than one moderately effective treatment can eventually be identified for a particular type of patient, the combination of two or three individually moderate improvements in outcome may collectively result in substantial gains. There is often no reliable alternative to large-scale randomized evidence from meta-analyses of many trials to allow for reliable identification of moderate effects on major outcomes.

TWO FUNDAMENTAL REQUIREMENTS FOR THE RELIABLE ASSESSMENT OF MODERATE TREATMENT EFFECTS: NEGLIGIBLE BIASES AND SMALL RANDOM ERRORS

Any clinical study with the main objective of assessing moderate treatment effects must ensure that any biases and any random errors that are inherent in its design are both substantially smaller than the effect that is to be measured. This limits the range of study designs that can be informative (Table 6.1).[1]

Negligible biases

If moderate differences are to be assessed, the study design must guarantee the exclusion of moderate biases, and this generally requires appropriate analysis of properly randomized evidence. For, if the allocation of treatment is not properly randomized, characteristics of the disease (or of the patient) that affect the prognosis may also affect the choice of treatment. Such pre-existing differences could well bias a non-randomized study. It may well be difficult or impossible to avoid such biases altogether, or to adjust fully for their effects, so even if non-randomized comparisons happen to get the right answer, nobody will really know that they have done so. This is true unless the difference in outcome is extraordinarily large or the outcome is one that could not plausibly be associated with those aspects of the disease that might influence the choice of treatment. Thus, as non-randomized study designs cannot generally be guaranteed to exclude moderate biases, they are

---

Table 6.1 Requirements for reliable assessment of *moderate* treatment effects

---

1. **Negligible biases (i.e. guaranteed avoidance of *moderate* biases)**
   Proper *randomization* (non-randomized methods cannot guarantee the avoidance of moderate biases)
   Analysis by *allocated* treatment (i.e. an 'intention-to-treat' analysis)
   Chief emphasis on *overall* results (with no unduly data-derived subgroup analyses)
   Systematic *meta-analysis* of all the relevant randomized trials (with no unduly data-dependent emphasis on the results from particular studies)

2. **Small random errors (i.e. guaranteed avoidance of *moderate* random errors)**
   Large numbers (with minimal data collection, because detailed statistical analyses of masses of data on prognostic features generally add little to the effective size of a trial)
   Systematic *meta-analysis* of all the relevant randomized trials

---

of little practical value if the primary aim is to assess moderate treatment effects (whether beneficial or adverse), particularly if long-term outcome is of interest.

In the current medical literature (and at many conferences), a particularly important source of bias is unduly data-dependent emphasis on particular trials or on particular subgroups of the randomized patients. Such emphasis is often entirely inadvertent, arising from a perfectly reasonable desire to understand the randomized trial results in terms of exactly who to treat, exactly which treatments to prefer or disease mechanisms. But, whatever its origins, unduly selective emphasis on particular parts of the evidence can often lead to seriously misleading conclusions, because reliable identification of categories of patients for whom treatment is particularly effective (or ineffective) requires surprisingly large quantities of data. Even if the real sizes of the effects of treatment do vary substantially among subgroups of patients, subgroup analyses are so statistically insensitive that they may well fail to demonstrate these differences. On the other hand, if the real proportional risk

reductions are about the same for everybody, subgroup analysis can vary so widely, just by the play of chance, that the results in selected subgroups may be grossly distorted. Even when highly significant 'interactions' are found, they may be a poor guide to the sizes (or even the directions) of any genuine differences in the proportional improvements in particular outcomes among specific categories of patients, as the more extreme results may still owe more to chance than to reality. This is particularly the case when such interactions have emerged after an examination of multiple subgroups.

Despite these difficulties, such subgroup analyses still get widely reported, and widely believed, in ways that may lead to the inappropriate management of hundreds of thousands of patients. For further discussion of this key issue see Collins et al[1] – or see the analyses of the 1988 ISIS-2 report[2] which, if interpreted incautiously, would have indicated that aspirin for patients with acute myocardial infarction works only for those not born under the astrological star signs of Libra or Gemini!

Appropriate meta-analyses help to avoid

unduly data-dependent emphasis on especially striking results within particular trials, and hence help to provide a better guide to the true effects of treatments. Occasionally, when detailed information on individual patients is available within a really large meta-analysis that includes several thousand major outcomes, such as death or cancer recurrence,[3] it may be feasible to identify particular groups of individuals in whom the benefits or hazards of treatment really are especially great. Sometimes, however, even a meta-analysis of all the trials in the world is too small for reliable subgroup analyses – indeed, in many meta-analyses, the total number of randomized patients is too small for even the main analyses to be statistically reliable, let alone the analyses of subgroups.

Small random errors

Although avoidance of moderate biases chiefly requires careful attention both to the randomization process and to the analysis and interpretation of the available trial evidence, the avoidance of moderate random errors chiefly requires large numbers of events, and hence even larger numbers of patients. For many therapeutic questions, the scale of randomized evidence that is necessary for the assessment of major outcomes may well not be available yet, even through a meta-analysis of all the completed randomized trials in the world. In that case, the key need is to find some practicable way of generating new trials that do provide really large-scale evidence.

RANDOMIZED TRIALS CAN BE LARGE IF THEY ARE KEPT SIMPLE

If trials of the effects of treatments on major outcomes are to become substantially larger, as many of the main barriers to rapid recruitment need to be removed as possible. One of the most effective ways to ensure failure to recruit large numbers is to burden busy clinicians with the task of obtaining large amounts of information. The information that really needs to be recorded at entry can often be surprisingly brief (including at most only a few major prognostic factors and only a few variables that are thought likely to influence substantially the benefits or hazards of treatment). Similarly, the information recorded at follow-up can sometimes be limited largely to a few major outcomes and approximate measures of compliance. (Other outcomes that are of interest, but do not need to be studied on such a large scale, may best be assessed in separate smaller studies, or in subsets of these large studies when this is practicable.) Often, less information per patient may mean better science.

THE 'UNCERTAINTY PRINCIPLE': ETHICALITY, HETEROGENEITY AND MAXIMAL SAMPLE SIZE

For ethical reasons, randomization is appropriate only if both the doctor and, to the extent that they are part of the process of determining which treatments to use, the patient feel substantially uncertain as to which trial treatment is best. The 'uncertainty principle' (see box) maximizes the potential for recruitment within this ethical constraint.[1,4]

If many hospitals are collaborating in a trial, wholehearted use of the uncertainty principle encourages clinically appropriate heterogeneity in the resulting trial population and this, in large trials, may add substantially to the practical value of the results. Homogeneity of those randomized may be a serious defect in clinical trial design, whereas heterogeneity may be a scientific strength: after all, trials do need to be relevant to a very heterogeneous collection of future patients.

> **The 'uncertainty principle'**
> A patient can be entered if, and only if, the responsible physician is substantially uncertain about which of the trial treatments would be most appropriate for that particular patient. A patient should not be entered if the responsible physician or the patient are, for any medical or non-medical reasons, reasonably certain that one of the treatments that might be allocated would be inappropriate for this particular individual (either in comparison with no treatment or in comparison with some other treatment that could be offered to the patient in or outside the trial).

The 'uncertainty principle' not only ensures ethicality and clinically useful heterogeneity, but is also easily understood and remembered by busy collaborating clinicians, which in turn helps the randomization of large numbers of patients. There is scope, therefore, for many more trials to adopt this as their eligibility criterion.

CAN ALTERNATIVE STUDY DESIGNS SUBSTITUTE FOR LARGE-SCALE RANDOMIZED EVIDENCE?

Might it be possible to circumvent the need for large trials, either by using routinely collected observational data (sometimes referred to as 'outcomes research') or perhaps by analyzing previously published randomized trials (with meta-analyses)?

Outcomes research

'Outcomes research' means various things to various people, but, as commonly used, the term refers to the use of routinely collected, non-randomized data to compare the effects of various treatments. Even within a carefully designed observational study, where specific arrangements to minimize sources of bias and confounding are planned and monitored, the guaranteed avoidance of biases that would correspond to a moderate increase or decrease in risk may well not be feasible. The effects of uncontrolled, and often uncontrollable, biases or confounding may therefore be at least as big as the sort of moderate effect that is to be assessed. This is because of the so-called 'indication bias' that occurs when there is a tendency to use particular treatments for particular types of patient who are considered to have specific indications. It follows, therefore, that routinely collected data from 'outcomes research' projects are unlikely to be able to assess reliably any moderate effects on outcome, and should generally not be considered as providing credible evidence if attempts are made to use them for this purpose. This is particularly important when non-randomized studies suggest that certain treatments have surprisingly large effects, and such findings may well be refuted when those treatments are assessed in large randomized trials.

Biases and random errors in small-scale meta-analyses

As meta-analyses are appearing in medical journals with increasing frequency, it is important to be able to judge the reliability of such reviews – and, in particular, the extent to which confounding, biases or random errors could lead to mistaken conclusions. (In randomized trials, 'confounding' exists when a comparison of some particular treatment in one group versus a control group involves the routine co-administration in one group, but not the other, of some co-intervention that might affect the outcome.) To avoid any possibility of confounding, and to avoid any flexibility in the question of which trials to include, those who perform or interpret meta-analysis should generally adopt the rule that they will include only unconfounded, properly randomized trials. The main problems that then remain are those of biases and random errors.

Two types of bias could affect the reliability of a meta-analysis: those that occur within individual trials and those that relate to the selection of trials. Such defects have unpredictable consequences for particular trials, however, and no reliable generalizations about the likely size, or even direction, of the resultant biases are possible.

'Selection bias' can arise when some relevant trials are not identified (or are excluded once they have been identified). Unfortunately, the subset of trials that are eventually published (and, hence, are conveniently available) is often a biased sample of the trials that have been done. Trials may well be more likely to be submitted or accepted for publication if their results are strikingly positive than if they are negative or null. Such 'publication bias' can, along with other sources of bias, produce surprisingly impressive-looking evidence of effectiveness for treatments that are actually useless. The particular circumstances in which publication bias has contributed to producing misleading estimates of treatment efficacy are, however, difficult to identify and it is still more difficult to generalize about the likely size of any such bias.

The problem of incomplete ascertainment is likely to be particularly acute within small meta-analyses that contain no more than a few hundred major outcomes, and consist chiefly of small published trials. This is because results from trials with only a limited number of endpoints are subject to large random errors and such trials are, therefore, particularly likely to generate implausibly large effect estimates. If publication bias then results in unduly selective emphasis on the more promising of these small trial results, the resulting meta-analysis will be unreliable. Hence, unless the particular circumstances of a small-scale meta-analysis suggest that publication bias is unlikely, it may be best to treat such results as no more than 'hypothesis generating'. On the other hand, a thoroughly conducted meta-analysis that in aggregate contains sufficient numbers of major outcomes to constitute 'large-scale' randomized evidence[3] is unlikely to be materially affected by publication bias. Provided that there are no serious uncontrolled biases (see above) within the individual component trials, it is likely to be fairly trustworthy, at least in its overall conclusions – although, even then, inappropriate subgroup analyses may generate wrong answers.

CONCLUSION: THE PAST 50 YEARS AND THE NEXT 50 YEARS OF RANDOMIZED EVIDENCE

At present we are still getting importantly wrong answers to many therapeutic questions, chiefly from non-randomized evidence, inappropriately small randomized trials or small meta-analyses. During the past 50 years, the principle of doing randomized trials and, more recently, meta-analyses to avoid moderate bias has been widely accepted. In recent, years, the need for such studies to be large enough to avoid moderate random errors has also begun to be accepted, although there is still far to go. If the trend toward really large-scale randomized evidence can be maintained, then over the next 50 years the true potential of randomization will at last begin to be realized, with substantial patient benefits.

To argue the need for some large, simple, randomized trials is not to argue that all other trials are useless; indeed, small (or complicated) trials will continue to be needed for certain purposes, as will many other types of clinical research. But, for many important questions about moderate therapeutic improvements in the common causes of death or serious disability, there is no reliable alternative to large-scale randomized evidence.

REFERENCES

1. Collins R, Peto R, Gray R, Parish S, Large-scale randomized evidence: trials and overviews. In: Weatherall D, Ledingham JGG, Warrell DA eds. *Oxford Textbook of Medicine*, Vol 1. Oxford: Oxford University Press, 1996: 21–32.
2. Second International Study of Infarct Survival (ISIS-2) Collaborative Group, Randomized trial of intravenous streptokinase, oral aspirin, both, or neither among 17,187 cases of suspected acute myocardial infarction: ISIS-2. *Lancet* 1988; ii:349–60.
3. Early Breast Cancer Trialists' Collaborative Group, Systemic treatment of early breast cancer by hormonal, cytotoxic, or immune therapy: 133 randomized trials involving 31,000 recurrences and 24,000 deaths among 75,000 women. *Lancet* 1992; **339**:1–15 (Part I); 71–85 (Part II).
4. Collins R, Doll R, Peto R, Ethics of clinical trials. In: Williams CJ ed. *Introducing New Treatments for Cancer: Practical, ethical and legal problems*. Chichester: John Wiley & Sons, 1992: 49–65.

7

How to analyze evidence

Jean-Marc Nabholtz, Katia Tonkin

The analysis of evidence can be undertaken in many different ways according to the intent of the author. The analysis of raw data from trials requires statisticians who should, of course, be involved in the design of trials at their inception. This ensures appropriate power and primary and secondary end-points, and that other crucial aspects are taken into consideration before a trial is started, so that once data have been collected analysis proceeds according to the predefined plan. The type of analysis should be decided before trial start-up and, although subgroup analysis and data dredging are done, one should always focus on the primary and secondary end-points because these are the results for which the trial was designed and for which data are secure. Clearly, when primary and secondary end-points are negative, investigators are likely to look for positive results in subgroups, partly to increase chances of publication. Medical journals should be encouraged to publish results of negative trials when these are large, well designed and executed, and reported appropriately because negative results are equally, and sometimes more, important for patient care as positive results.

When this book was in the planning stages, we wanted to focus our attention on evidence that could be applied by clinicians in the everyday setting of the clinic. We did not intend to repeat the laborious details of the evidence-based approach requiring lengthy meta-analysis. We wanted a new pragmatic approach which focused on phase III evidence whenever it was available. However, we wanted the reader to have some kind of benchmark by which the individual could compare one study to another. We therefore sent to each author Table 7.1, giving an outline of one approach to levels of evidence.

These levels of evidence are widely recognized and are promoted by the American Society of Clinical Oncology.[1] The advantages of such a table is that authors can, whenever possible, apply the same criteria to different data sets in order to give recommendations of benefit for treatments. In this way, treatments can be compared across different trials, at least to some extent.

There are, of course, caveats to any system. The five levels do not describe the quality or even the credibility of the evidence. They indicate only the nature of the evidence being reviewed. A randomized trial may be the gold standard with the greatest credibility, but it may have defects in design and these need to be mentioned in any review. It is crucial that evidence

Table 7.1   Type and grading of evidence for recommendations

Level	Type of evidence for recommendation
I	Evidence obtained from meta-analysis of multiple, well-designed, controlled studies; randomized trials with low false-positive and low false-negative errors (high power)
II	Evidence obtained from at least one well-designed experimental study; randomized trials with high false-positive and/or negative errors (low power)
III	Evidence obtained from well-designed quasi-experimental studies, such as non-randomized controlled, single-group pre–post, cohort, time or matched case–control series
IV	Evidence from well-designed, non-experimental studies, such as comparative and correlation descriptive and case studies
V	Evidence from case reports and clinical examples

Category	Grade of evidence
A	There is evidence of type I or consistent findings from multiple studies of types II, III or IV
B	There is evidence of types II, III, or IV, and findings are generally consistent
C	There is evidence of types II, III, or IV, but findings are inconsistent
D	There is little or no systemic evidence
NG	Grade not given

based on too few observations should be assigned to only level II and not level I, even if the trials were randomized because trials with insufficient power would probably have high rates of false-positive and false-negative results. On the other hand, level III results, although less credible than level I trials, are important if there are several with consistent results.

In addition to these basic guidelines, there are several 'user guides to the medical literature' published in series form or in books.[2,3] The starting point for these is, from a clinician's standpoint, when an individual practitioner has limited time and a clinical problem to solve. This is clearly a common problem and one worthy of much time and effort. It is also one that is complex and not easily solved by any one system. Clinical medicine still has a place for the experience of the clinician in assessing the needs of the individual patient, in the light of the evidence that is published for any one particular clinical condition or set of circumstances. This is particularly true in oncology.

This book is not one that attempts to duplicate these efforts. We have assumed that we are reaching out to busy academic clinicians. These individuals are treating women with breast cancer, in either the adjuvant or the metastatic setting. These are also individuals with an opportunity to influence not only current therapy for patients, but future trial design. In other words, their current clinical questions can and should be used as the basis for future clinical trials, whenever feasible. The busy academic will, when possible, offer a patient entry into a clinical trial, because this is often the best choice for optimal patient care. Patients have the opportunity to receive new drugs or regimens that would not otherwise be available outside the clinical trial setting and patients may, to their advantage, be followed more closely than in normal clinical practice. However, patients also risk side-effect profiles, which are often more serious and less well understood, as a trade-off for the opportunity to enter into protocol therapy. This is how clinical medicine progresses and without clinical trials all we would have would be supposition and clinical acumen, which, however valuable, remains flawed.

The globalization of breast cancer clinical trials through the Breast Cancer International Research Group (BCIRG) will enable us to get results from large phase III trials in a much more timely fashion than we have done in the past. We have recently become used to relying upon overviews or meta-analysis of data as the only way to determine whether regimens have a definite, even if only a modest, benefit. Witness the importance of the Oxford overview and the continuing results that emerge at each 5-year cycle. Not every overview of meta-analysis is necessarily a good one, however. There are important technical details that need to be applied and understood, most of which are beyond the scope of this text. We believe that a pragmatic approach is important. A steady flow of US Food and Drug Administration level evidence from large phase III trials in both the metastatic and adjuvant setting is an important advance for patient care. The BCIRG provides a huge opportunity to advance patient management rapidly.

The resolution of a clinical question begins with finding valid data including, where appropriate, overviews and practice guidelines. Optimal clinical care requires optimal use of the medical literature. Clinicians need to approach any text with clear questions about probability of benefit, magnitude of that benefit, and the likelihood of and type of side effects. The decision to apply a particular treatment is then a decision of risk versus benefit for a particular patient in a particular set of circumstances, knowing what the alternative treatment options are, including the option of best supportive care.

Randomized trials are clearly an efficient way to answer clinical questions. A simple two-arm trial with supporting scientific questions provides a wealth of important data with which to guide future clinical management and future trial design. However, trials can be designed with three arms or using a factorial design so that more than one question is answered, thus ensuring flexibility at the cost of some complexity. In factorial designs, one can cease randomization to one dimension, as a result of accumulation of favorable or unfavorable results that arise during the course of data monitoring, while continuing to randomize to other facets of the trial. Even in phase II trials, it is possible to include some randomization. In early phase II trials, there should be single-arm studies to determine activity of a drug or regimen. However, randomization in late phase II trials could be employed to test several promising agents or treatments to find the best. This is especially important at the present time, when we are faced with an ever-expanding list of new and, in particular, novel therapies. One could even combine a phase II and III trial by having standard versus new active (traditional phase III) versus promising new experimental (in late phase II). This provides comparable groups in a situation of uncertainty as to the best option.

In some situations, one can use the concept of large simple trials. This is important, given the heterogeneity even in a disease such as breast cancer and, when one wants reliable estimates of benefit, trials of thousands of patients can prove very useful. In such cases, the design needs to be simple and of course data collection must also be simple otherwise the costs would be untenable. The clearest example of a large simple trial in breast cancer, which is currently open to accrual to patients, is the ATLAS (Adjuvant Tamoxifen Longer Against Shorter) adjuvant tamoxifen trial run by Professor Peto's group in Oxford. The main advantage is that the results are likely to have wide generalizability. Such trials can also have built into them subgroups from which more detailed information is collected to satisfy the desire for detailed information and analysis.

One of the continuing difficulties, especially in adjuvant trials, is that the outcome of interest, which is survival, requires many years of follow-up. Clearly, it would be useful to have some kind of surrogate end-point. A variety of surrogates have been studied, particularly in metastatic disease and AIDS,[3-7] but unfortunately none has been widely accepted or adopted because they are in some way or another unreliable.

In the final analysis there is no single way to analyze evidence. We look at any single trial in the context of other confirmatory data and in the light of our own clinical experience. We apply new drugs and regimens to our patient population, in the hope of obtaining the same results that were obtained in the reported trials. If our own experience differs markedly, particularly with respect to side effects, we are unlikely to pursue any new therapy, however promising. That is human nature and, however scientific we try to be, the human element, usually for the betterment of our patients, will always have an effect on the way we practice oncology.

REFERENCES

1. American Society of Clinical Oncology, Recommended breast cancer surveillance guidelines. *J Clin Oncol* 1997; **15**:2149–56.
2. Oxman AD, Sackett DL, Guyatt GH, User's guide to the medical literature. *JAMA* 1993; 270:2093–7.
3. Greenhalgh T, *How to Read a Paper: The basics of evidence based medicine*. London: BMJ Books, 1997.
4. Prentice RL, Surrogate endpoints in clinical trials: definitions and operational criteria. *Stat Med* 1989; **8**:431–40.
5. Gotzsche OP, Liberati A, Torri V et al, Beware of surrogate outcome measures. *Int J Health Technol Assess* 1996; **12**:238–46.
6. Jacobson MA, Bacchetti P, Kolokathis A et al, Surrogate markers for survival in patients with AIDS and AIDS related complex treated with zidovudine. *BMJ* 1991; **302**:73–8.
7. Tsoukas CM, Bernard NF, Markers predicting progression of HIV-related disease. *Clin Microbiol Rev* 1994; **7**:14–28.

PART II

Treatment Modalities

SECTION 1: Chemotherapy

Section Editors: J-M Nabholtz, MS Aapro

8

Taxanes: paclitaxel and docetaxel

Jean-Marc Nabholtz, Katia Tonkin

This chapter discusses the development of paclitaxel (Taxol) and docetaxel (Taxotere) from preclinical to current and future trials. The two drugs are discussed together and each is compared and contrasted in order to evaluate both the benefits of and the differences between the compounds.

There have been several novel-acting chemotherapeutic drugs introduced in the last decade. The taxanes have emerged as the most powerful compounds in the treatment of breast cancer and available results suggest that they will be remembered as the breast cancer chemotherapy of the 1990s. The two taxanes currently available, paclitaxel and docetaxel, share some characteristics but are also significantly different both in preclinical profile and, most importantly, in clinical characteristics. These relate to different efficacy:toxicity ratios in relation to dose and schedule, and the ability to integrate paclitaxel and docetaxel in anthracycline–taxane-containing regimens, as a result of major differences in pharmacokinetic interactions between each taxane and anthracyclines and potential differences in synergism between the taxanes and Herceptin (trastuzumab).

The taxanes are already standard therapy for metastatic breast cancer after failure of prior chemotherapy, in particular the anthracyclines. Their impact in combination with anthracyclines in first-line therapy of advanced breast cancer is still emerging and will probably have a major impact on their future role in the adjuvant setting. The results of completed and ongoing phase III trials in first-line metastatic and adjuvant patients will no doubt determine whether or not the taxanes will improve the outcome for women with all stages of breast cancer.

THE TAXANES

Paclitaxel (Taxol) was initially extracted from the bark of the Pacific yew, *Taxus brevifolia*, and characterized in 1971 by Wani et al.[1] Its development was impaired by scarce drug supply.[2] Subsequent research showed that paclitaxel had a wide spectrum of antineoplastic activity, including against breast cancer.[2] To provide a renewable source of taxane in 1986, docetaxel (Taxotere), a semisynthetic analog of paclitaxel, was synthesized using a precursor extracted from the needles of the European yew, *Taxus baccata*.[3] Differing from paclitaxel by two minor chemical structural modifications, docetaxel had favorable preclinical characteristics in vitro and in vivo, which prompted its clinical development.[4]

After initial phase I studies[5–18] in 1986–87, the development of paclitaxel was hampered as a result of hypersensitivity reactions that required systematic use of premedication,[19] which also turned out to be necessary, although slightly different, for docetaxel.[20] The first report of clinical activity of paclitaxel in breast cancer was seen in 1991.[21] This was followed by a large number of small, phase II, monochemotherapy trials, which did not define a clear relationship between dose and schedule with respect to the efficacy : toxicity ratio.[19,22–40] It took several large randomized trials to unravel the problem of the dose–schedule relationship for paclitaxel.[41–45] More information became available later in the 1990s with data on paclitaxel monochemotherapy, including the results of several large phase III trials which compared paclitaxel with doxorubicin or polychemotherapy such as CMFP (cyclophosphamide, methotrexate, 5-fluorouracil and prednisone).[46–49] These data also revealed difficulties with respect to combinations of paclitaxel in anthracycline–taxane combinations for metastatic disease,[48,50–61] which led to the current, almost exclusive, sequential strategies of phase III adjuvant trials.[62,63]

Docetaxel's clinical development started with phase I studies in 1992–93.[64–70] The recommended dose for further phase II and III studies of docetaxel monochemotherapy was clearly established as 100 mg/m² by 1-hour infusion every 3 weeks. This fact led to consistent efficacy seen in phase II and III monochemotherapy trials, and quickly established the appropriate dose and schedule for docetaxel. Thus, the first important clinical difference between the two taxanes emerged in relation to dose and schedule

in the definition of the efficacy : toxicity ratio.[71] Further development of docetaxel was extremely swift, with phase II and III monochemotherapy trials being performed in first-line[72–78] or second-line[79–88] metastatic disease and in patients previously exposed to anthracyclines.[89–94] Several phase II and phase III studies based on an anthracycline–docetaxel combination followed. There was no pharmacokinetic problem in combining these two agents, with no added cardiotoxicity above that expected from anthracycline therapy alone.[95–99] These promising results led to further development of docetaxel using both sequential and polychemotherapy strategies in the adjuvant setting.

TAXANES IN METASTATIC BREAST CANCER

Taxane monochemotherapy
Phase I trials
Paclitaxel phase I studies have been performed using several infusion schedules, from short daily infusions over 5 days every 3 weeks,[5,6] infusions of 1–6 hours every 3 weeks,[7–11] to longer infusions every 3 weeks, e.g. 24 hours,[12–16] 96 hours[17] or even 120 hours.[18] Each schedule has different maximum tolerated doses with various toxicity profiles, for which dose and infusion duration were both factors. The main toxicity was neutropenia with some vomiting, alopecia, myalgia and arthralgia, as well as fatigue and skin reactions. Hypersensitivity reactions were apparent except for infusion times of 120 hours, which led to the universal use of premedication. Recent trials have used weekly infusions of paclitaxel given over 1 or 3 hours,[36–40] for which the optimum dose appears to be around 80 mg/m² per week. At this dose or below, the safety profile is very favorable, with, in particular, low incidences of neutropenia and alopecia. With higher doses, severe and early

neurotoxicity appeared to be the limiting factor. The important conclusion from all the phase I trials with paclitaxel was that no particular schedule or dose was recommended for further development in phase II and III studies, thus creating confusion in trying to define the optimal efficacy : toxicity ratio.

Several phase I studies were performed with docetaxel. Schedules ranged from 1-hour infusion every 3 weeks,[64,69] 1-hour infusions 1 week apart every 3 weeks,[68] 5 days in a row every 3 weeks[67] and longer infusions of 2–6 hours[65] or 24 hours.[66] The usual dose-limiting toxicities related to neutropenia and mucositis, whereas neurotoxicity emerged as the limiting toxicity with doses above 120–130 mg/m^2 given over 1 hour every week. Hypersensitivity was underestimated in phase I trials, but was confirmed in subsequent studies, which led to the use of steroid premedication.[100] Docetaxel investigators were in consensus with the recommended doses (85–115 mg/m^2) and schedule (1-hour infusion every 3 weeks), and, subsequently, 1-hour infusion of 100 mg/m^2 every 3 weeks was chosen for further development for docetaxel monochemotherapy.

As for paclitaxel, recent data have been presented on the use of weekly docetaxel[101–104] and have confirmed a threshold of toxicity around 40 mg/m^2 per week. At this level or below, docetaxel appears to be very well tolerated, with limited incidence of neutropenia and alopecia, although fatigue may be a factor with long-term therapy. Above 40 mg/m^2 per week, classic toxicities of docetaxel occur, limiting further dose escalation.[105]

Phase II trials

Initial phase II paclitaxel results are summarized in Tables 8.1 and 8.2. Dose and schedule have defined the efficacy : toxicity ratio for this drug. Most of the short-infusion studies (3-hour infusion) used doses from 135 mg/m^2 to 250 mg/m^2, either in patients previously exposed to or resistant to anthracyclines[22–28] or as first-line therapy of metastatic breast cancer[23,25,27,32,35] (Table 8.1). Response rates were between 6% and 42% for patients with prior anthracycline exposure and between 32% and 60% as first-line chemotherapy. Median time to progression was usually 3–4 months and toxicity was very mild for lower doses.

Several studies investigated longer infusion schedules with doses of 135–250 mg/m^2 for the 24-hour infusion, but 125–140 mg/m^2 using 96- or 120-hour infusions (Table 8.2). A 24-hour infusion confirmed response rates of 32% (135 mg/m^2) to 56% (250 mg/m^2) in first-line metastatic and 24% (175 mg/m^2) to 33% (200–250 mg/m^2) for patients previously exposed to anthracyclines. Median time to progression appeared longer than with the 3-hour infusion (4–6 months), with more significant neutropenia.

The question of the optimal schedule and dose for paclitaxel generated significant debate. Efficacy was claimed at 250 mg/m^2 over 24 hours, but toxicity and feasibility were assessed at 175 mg/m^2 over 3 hours. In the second half of the 1990s, several large-scale randomized trials addressing the issue of schedule and dose have been either published or presented (Table 8.3).[41–45] The registration trial of paclitaxel in breast cancer compared two doses (135 mg/m^2 and 175 mg/m^2), using a 3-hour infusion schedule[41] in the treatment of 471 patients with metastatic breast cancer. Response rates were 29% with paclitaxel given at 175 mg/m^2 (36% for first-line patients and 26% for patients previously exposed to anthracyclines) and 22% with the lower dose ($p =$ NS). The only difference between the two arms was a modestly longer time to progression in favor of the higher dose (median 4.2 months versus 3.0 months,

Table 8.1   Single-agent 3-hour paclitaxel in phase II trials of metastatic breast cancer

Trial	Dose (mg/m^2)	No. of patients (treated/evaluable)	Response rate (%)	Median survival
Initial treatment				
Seidman et al[25]	250	25	Lowest: 32	NA
Mamounas et al[35]	250	82	43	NA
Bonneterre et al[32]	225	101	44	NA
Gianni et al[27]	175 or 225	24	46	NA
Fountizilas et al[26]	175		54	NA
Davidson et al[23]	225	30	Highest: 60	12.8 months
Second-line: prior anthracyclines				
Vermorken et al[28]	250	33	Lowest: 6	NA
Seidman et al[25]	175	41	21	NA
Vici et al[22]	135–175	41	22	
Michael et al[24]	175	24	25	
Gianni et al[27]	175–225	50	38	11 months
Fountzilas et al[26]	175	33	Highest: 42	9.4 months

NA, not available.

$p = 0.02$). As a result of the low response rates and minimal effect on outcome, when compared with phase II studies performed in North America using a 24-hour infusion, the results of this study were reviewed critically. This led to a second randomized trial performed by the same Canadian–European group, comparing 3 hours versus 24 hours of paclitaxel using a dose of 175 mg/m^2.[42] A total of 521 patients were randomized in this study and the results were consistent with those of the registration trial.[41] Response rates were found to be 29% with paclitaxel 175 mg/m^2 over 3 hours (identical to the registration trial with the same dose and schedule) and 31% with the 24-hour arm. Time to progression was not significantly different between the two arms, but the toxicity profile was more favorable in the 3-hour arm. At that time, the recommendation was 175 mg/m^2 over 3 hours as standard therapy.

In 1998, three additional randomized trials were presented.[43–45] The first one addressed the dose question using a 3-hour schedule, comparing 175 mg/m^2 with 210 mg/m^2 and 250 mg/m^2 using mostly patients with second-line metastatic disease.[43] In 475 patients, results showed response rates ranging from 21% to 28% (p = NS), whereas time to progression was significantly longer with 250 mg/m^2 than with 175 mg/m^2 (4.8 months versus 3.8 months, $p = 0.03$). Toxicity analysis favored the lower dose. The last two trials studied long infusion schedules.

The National Surgical Adjuvant Breast and Bowel Project (NSABP) B-26 designed a random-

Table 8.2   Single-agent 24-hour or longer paclitaxel in phase II trials of metastatic breast cancer

Trial	Dose (mg/m^2)	No. of patients (treated/evaluable)	Response rate (%)	Median survival
Initial: 24-h infusion				
Swain et al[34]	135	19	32	NA
Holmes et al[21]	250	14	57	
Reichman et al[33]	250	26	62	NA
After anthracyclines				
24-h infusion				
Abrams et al[30]	175	153	24	NA
Seidman et al[29]	200–250	40	33	NA
Holmes et al[21]	250	6	33	NA
96-h infusion				
Constenla et al[31]	125	20	30	NA
Wilson et al[17]	140	33	48	9.8 months

NA, not available

ized trial of a 3-hour versus a 24-hour schedule using a dose of 250 mg/m^2.[44] A total of 563 patients were randomized between the two arms. The only difference in favor of the 24-hour arm was in terms of response rate (50% versus 40%, $p = 0.02$), whereas time to progression and survival were comparable. However, toxicity was worse in the 24-hour schedule, with significantly more neutropenia and fatigue. The results did not favor use of a 24-hour schedule in clinical practice (with the additional problem of practicality). This important, large, randomized trial confirmed that high response results could be obtained with paclitaxel using high doses (250 mg/m^2) and long schedules (24 hours). Finally, a 96-hour infusion schedule at a dose of 140 mg/m^2 was compared with a 3-hour infusion given at 250 mg/m^2 in 179 patients with advanced breast cancer.[45] Response rates were

identical, respectively 29% and 23%, whereas toxicity and practicality were tested against the long-infusion arm.

Weekly schedules have shown promising efficacy in small phase II trials, with response rates ranging from 29% (80 mg/m^2) to 53% (100 mg/m^2). However, high doses produce significant neurotoxicity. Only one large phase II trial has been completed to date. Results on 200 patients with metastatic breast cancer patients treated either as first- or second-line treatment found response rates between 20% and 30%, warranting a large-scale randomized trial comparing weekly with 3-weekly treatment, in order to finally settle the issue of scheduling.

The question of optimal schedule and dose for paclitaxel has been largely answered, as both schedule and dose play a crucial role in the definition of the efficacy : toxicity ratio. Paclitaxel

Table 8.3   Randomized phase II trials with paclitaxel (P)

Study	Design	No. of patients	ORR (%)	p value	TTF or TTP Median (months)	p value	Overall survival Median (months)	p value
Nabholtz et al[41]	P 135 mg/m^2	471	22		3		10.5	
	R			NS		0.02		NS
	P 175 mg/m^2		29		4.2		11.7	
	Schedule: 3-h infusion							
Peretz et al[42]	P as 3-h infusion	521	29		No difference		NA	
	R			NS				
	P as 24-h infusion		31				NA	
	Dose: 175 mg/m^2							
Winer et al[43]	P 175 mg/m^2	475	21		3.8		9.8	
	R P 210 mg/m^2		28	NS	4.1	0.03	11.8	
	P 250 mg/m^2		22		4.8			
	Schedule: 3-h infusion						11.9	
Mamounas et al[44]	P as 3-h infusion	563	40		NA		No difference	
	R			0.02				
	P as 24-h infusion		50					
	Dose: 250 mg/m^2							
Holmes et al[45]	P as 3-h infusion	179	23		NA		11	
	R			NS				NS
	P as 96-h infusion		29				10	
	Dose: 3-h arm: 250 mg/m^2							
	96-h arm: 140 mg/m^2							

NA, not available; NS, not significant; R, randomization; ORR, objective response rate; TTF, time to treatment failure; TTP, time to progression.

can be very active if given at high doses (250 mg/m^2) over long schedules (24 hours): response rates are, in this context, consistently in the 50% range. However, this occurs along with excessive toxicity such as neutropenia and fatigue and an impractical regimen. Although lower doses (175–200 mg/m^2) given over 3 hours are more feasible, with easy outpatient adminis-

tration, they have consistently less efficacy, with response rates in the range of 25–30%. Consequently, for current clinical practice, the balance of data favors doses of 175–200 mg/m^2 over 3 hours every 3 weeks, with insufficient evidence from phase II data on weekly 1-hour infusion schedules at present.

In contrast, there has been no real controversy

regarding docetaxel schedule and dose. Most phase II studies used docetaxel at 100 mg/m^2 given over 1 hour every 3 weeks,[72,74–77,80–83,89–91] although some researchers studied 75 mg/m^2 [72,73,84,85] and 60 mg/m^2 in Japan.[86–88] The 1-hour schedule and the small difference in doses used in phase II studies probably account for the consistent results observed throughout the various studies. Table 8.4 shows phase II data for patients with metastatic breast cancer treated with docetaxel 100 mg/m^2 as first-line treatment, with response rates ranging from 38% to 68%.[72,74–77] It also shows second-line therapy, with response rates of 34–58%,[74,80–83] including patients previously exposed to anthracyclines with response rates of 29–50%.[89–91] Phase II results with a dose of 75 mg/m^2 every 3 weeks show that activity is maintained, with responses rates between 40% and 52% in first-line[72,73] and between 44% and 48% in second-line metastatic therapy.[84,85] Japanese investigators have reported response rates between 40% and 56% with docetaxel 60 mg/m^2.[86–88] The European Organization for Research and Treatment of Cancer (EORTC) is currently undertaking a randomized trial comparing docetaxel 100 mg/m^2 with 75 mg/m^2. Toxicity consists mainly of neutropenia, alopecia and fatigue, with mild neurotoxicity and rare allergic reactions. Specific toxicities of docetaxel such as nail changes and fluid retention are prevented or controlled with 3-day steroid prophylaxis.[100]

Phase III trials

To date, three phase III trials have reported results of paclitaxel versus monochemotherapy or polychemotherapy in first-line treatment of metastatic breast cancer[46–49] (Table 8.5). EORTC data[46,47] of paclitaxel given over 3 hours at a dose of 200 mg/m^2 suggest that it is not as potent as doxorubicin 75 mg/m^2. Results strongly favor the anthracycline, with doxorubicin response rate of 41% versus 25% ($p = 0.003$) and with signific-

antly longer time to progression (7.5 months versus 4.2 months, $p = 0.001$). There was no survival difference between the two arms, which could be related to the prospective crossover built into the study. Patients failing doxorubicin were systematically treated with paclitaxel, allowing a prospective assessment of the potential non-cross-resistance between the two drugs. In patients with no response to doxorubicin, paclitaxel had a 13% response rate whereas secondary resistant patients (initial response to doxorubicin, but relapse while still on doxorubicin) or non-resistant, previously exposed patients (relapse after completion of successful initial doxorubicin therapy) experienced objective responses in 14% of cases. This challenges any concept of non-cross-resistance between doxorubicin and paclitaxel, which was suggested by earlier limited phase II series and subgroup analysis from larger studies.[25–29,41]

The American Intergroup[48] compared three treatment arms, two of which were monotherapies. The paclitaxel was given over 24 hours at 175 mg/m^2 and compared with doxorubicin 60 mg/m^2 or both drugs given together (paclitaxel 150 mg/m^2 and doxorubicin 50 mg/m^2). Response rates were, respectively, 33%, 34% and 46% ($p = $ NS) and median time to treatment failure was 5.9, 6.2 and 8.0 months, respectively ($p = <0.05$). A crossover was also built into this trial, with a 20% response rate seen in patients treated with 24-hour paclitaxel after failing doxorubicin.

The third trial[49] compared paclitaxel 175 mg/m^2 given over 3 hours with CMFP. Efficacy was comparable, with objective response rates of 29% for paclitaxel and 35% for CMFP ($p = $ NS) and median progression-free survival of 5.3 months for the taxane versus 6.4 months for the polychemotherapy ($p = $ NS). Overall survival was longer for paclitaxel (median 17.3 months versus 13.9 months), but did not reach statistical significance ($p = 0.068$).

Table 8.4   Phase II studies with single-agent docetaxel in metastatic breast cancer

Trial	Dose (mg/m^2)/ Schedule (1 h)	No. of patients evaluable	ORR (%)
Initial treatment			
Ten Bokkel Huinink[74]	100	8	Lowest: 38
Trudeau et al[72]	75	15	40
Dieras et al[73]	75	31	52
Alexopoulos et al[71]	100	43	54
Hudis et al[75]	100	34	56
Trudeau et al[72]	100	32	63
Chevallier et al[76]	100	31	68
Fumoleau et al[77]	100	37	Highest: 68
After prior chemotherapy			
Taguchi et al[87]	60	47	Lowest: 40
Vorobiof et al[82]	100	28	43
Adachi et al[86]	60	72	44
Leonard et al[84]	75–100	287	44
Shapiro et al[85]	75–100	23	48
Terzoli et al[83]	100	18	50
Alexopoulos et al[81]	100	43	54
Taguchi et al[88]	60	64	56
Ten Bokkel Huinink[74]	100	24	Highest: 58
Anthracycline-resistant			
Bonneterre et al[91]	100	51	Lowest: 29
van Oosterom et al[80]	100	94	34
Valero et al[89]	100	41	46
Ravdin et al[90]	100	42	Highest: 50

ORR, overall response rates (complete response + partial response).

Four phase III docetaxel monochemotherapy trials have been published or reported to date[78,92–94] (Table 8.5). In the first trial, 100 mg/m^2 was compared with doxorubicin 75 mg/m^2 in first-line metastatic treatment after failure of alkylating agents.[78] Docetaxel induced more responses than doxorubicin (48% versus 33%, $p = 0.008$), and median time to progression was longer with docetaxel (26 weeks versus 21 weeks, $p = $ NS), although overall survival was identical in both treatment arms. As the risk : benefit ratio appeared to favor docetaxel, the result suggests that doc-

Table 8.5   Metastatic breast cancer: randomized phase III taxane trials

Study	Design	No. of patients	ORR (%)	p value	TTF or TTP Median	p value	Overall survival Median (months)	p value
Paclitaxel: first-line metastatic								
Sledge et al	Paclitaxel 175 mg/m²	739	33		5.9 mos			NS
Intergroup[48a]	R Doxorubicin 60 mg/m²		34	NS	6.2 mos	<0.05		
	Paclitaxel 150 mg/m²		46		8.0 mos			
	+ doxorubicin 50 mg/m²							
	Schedule of paclitaxel: 24-h infusion							
Bishop et al[49]	Paclitaxel 175 mg/m²	209	29		5.3 mos		17.3	
	R			NS		NS		NS
	CMFP		35		6.4 mos		13.9	
	Schedule of paclitaxel: 3-h infusion							
Gamucci et al	Paclitaxel 200 mg/m²	331	25		4.2 mos		NS	
EORTC[46]	R			0.003		0.001		
	Doxorubicin 75 mg/m²		41		7.5 mos			
	Schedule of paclitaxel: 3-h infusion							
Docetaxel: first-line metastatic (prior alkylating agents)								
Chan et al[78]	Docetaxel 100 mg/m²	326	48		26 wks		NS	
	R			0.008		NS		
	Doxorubicin 75 mg/m²		33		21 wks			
Docetaxel: anthracycline failure								
Bonneterre et al[94]	Docetaxel 100 mg/m²	172	43		28 wks		NS	
	R			NS		NS		
	Vinorelbine 25 mg/m²		39		22 wks			
	+CI 5-fluorouracil 750 mg/m²							
Sjostrom et al[93]	Docetaxel 100 mg/m²	283	42		27 wks		NS	
	R			<0.0001		<0.001	(crossover	
	Methotrexate 200 mg/m²		21		13 wks		built-in)	
	+5-fluorouracil 600 mg/m²							
Nabholtz et al[92]	Docetaxel 100 mg/m²	392	30		19 wks		11.4	0.0097
	R			<0.0001		<0.001	8.7	
	Mitomycin C 12 mg/m²		12		11 wks			
	+ vinblastine 6 mg/m²							
Docetaxel: first-line metastatic – polychemotherapy								
Nabholtz et al[106]	AT	426	60		37.1 wks			NA
	R			0.012		0.01		
	AC		47		31.9 wks			
	AT: docetaxel 75 mg/m² + doxorubicin 50 mg/m²							
	AC: doxorubicin 60 mg/m² + cyclophosphamide 600 mg/m²							

[a]Evaluable basis; NA, not available; NS, not significant; R, randomization; ORR, objective response rate; TTF, time to treatment failure; TTP, time to progression; CI, continuous infusion.

etaxel might be more powerful than doxorubicin as first-line therapy of advanced breast cancer.

The three other phase III trials were performed in patients with metastatic breast cancer who had failed anthracyclines. Docetaxel 100 mg/m^2 given over 1 hour was compared with various salvage regimens. The largest study (392 patients) randomized patients between docetaxel and mitomycin C (12 mg/m^2 every 6 weeks) plus vinblastine (6 mg/m^2 every 3 weeks).[92] Docetaxel had a higher overall response rate (30% versus 12%, $p = 0.001$), longer time to treatment failure (19 weeks versus 11 weeks, $p = 0.001$) and, most importantly, longer overall survival (11.4 months versus 8.7 months, $p = 0.0097$). A further study (283 patients) performed by the Scandinavian group compared docetaxel with methotrexate plus 5-fluorouracil (200 mg/m^2 and 600 mg/m^2 on days 1 and 8 every 3 weeks, respectively).[93] This confirmed the previous trial, with better response rates for docetaxel (42% versus 21%, $p = 0.0001$) and longer time to progression (27 weeks versus 13 weeks, $p = 0.0001$). Survival was similar in both arms, possibly related to the built-in crossover. In the last trial[94] of 172 patients, docetaxel was compared with NAF (vinorelbine 25 mg/m^2 on days 1 and 5 every 3 weeks plus continuous-infusion 5-fluorouracil 750 mg/m^2 over days 1–5 every 3 weeks). The docetaxel response rate was 43% versus 39% for NAF ($p = $ NS). Time to progression and overall survival were longer for docetaxel (28 weeks versus 22 weeks and 19.1 months versus 13.9 months, respectively), but did not reach statistical significance.

Accrual to the only randomized trial comparing docetaxel (100 mg/m^2, 1-hour infusion) and paclitaxel (175 mg/m^2, 3-hour infusion) in patients with prior anthracycline exposure is near completion. Data should be available in 2000 and will clarify the relative efficacy : toxicity ratio of these two drugs.

Available results of studies with both paclitaxel and docetaxel provide sufficient evidence to justify the use of single-agent taxanes for patients with both previously treated and untreated metastatic breast cancer.[71]

Conclusion

These data provide level I evidence for superiority of doxorubicin over paclitaxel. There is level I evidence for superiority of doxorubicin over paclitaxel for time to progression. There is level I evidence for superior response and time to progression of docetaxel over doxorubicin and for survival against a salvage regimen in anthracycline failures using mitomycin C and vinblastine.

Taxane polychemotherapy: Taxane–doxorubicin-containing combinations
Phase II trials

As anthracyclines are currently the mainstay of adjuvant programs, there has been a strong emphasis on integrating taxanes into anthracycline strategies in order to develop new adjuvant approaches. Anthracycline–taxane-containing regimens have been developed for both paclitaxel and docetaxel. This has been done with the expectation that both agents would be used in polychemotherapy. There have been two separate trends in the development of phase II trials of paclitaxel–doxorubicin combinations, both related to the schedule of paclitaxel (3 hours versus 24 hours or more) (Table 8.6). With paclitaxel 175–200 mg/m^2 infused over 3 hours plus doxorubicin 50–60 mg/m^2, very high response rates were reported (up to 94%).[50–56] The main toxicities were neutropenia, mucositis and unexpectedly significant cardiotoxicity (around 20% congestive heart failure at the time of therapy). Cardiotoxicity was discovered to occur as a result of a previously unknown pharmacokinetic interaction between paclitaxel and doxorubicin.[107] Paclitaxel given by short infusion decreases the liver clearance of the metabolite of doxorubicin, doxorubicinol, and results in an increase in the area under the curve (AUC) of the anthracycline, resulting in high tumor activity and, unfortunately, high cardiac toxicity. The pharmacokinetic interaction effect was reported to be greater if the paclitaxel was given before the doxorubicin and if there was a short interval between the two drugs (<1 hour).[107] As most cardiac events are seen at a cumulative dose of doxorubicin of over 360 mg/m^2, some authors have introduced the concept of decreasing the usable cumulative dose of doxorubicin to 360 mg/m^2 when using the combination of a paclitaxel 3-hour infusion plus doxorubicin. This limitation could be acceptable in the palliative setting; however, 360 mg/m^2 severely limits adjuvant approaches.

Use of a time interval of 16 hours between paclitaxel and doxorubicin[52] decreases the cardiac side effects. This has resulted in the disappearance of the pharmacokinetic interaction between the two drugs, with acceptable cardiac toxicity profile but lower efficacy and practicality.

The second trend for paclitaxel–doxorubicin combinations relates to the use of long schedules of paclitaxel (≥24 hours), which also incidentally leads to a loss of the pharmacokinetic interaction between paclitaxel and doxorubicin.[57,59,60] The consequence is excellent tolerance in terms of cardiac toxicity, but a decreased efficacy profile. Neutropenia and mucositis have impaired any increase of dose for both agents above paclitaxel 150 mg/m^2 and doxorubicin 50 mg/m^2. Several phase II trials have reported response rates of from 42% to 69% when paclitaxel was given over 24 hours[57,59] and 72% with paclitaxel infused over 72 hours. The American Intergroup has presented the only phase III trial testing a combination of paclitaxel and doxoru-

bicin (Table 8.5).[48] This large three-arm trial (739 patients) compared paclitaxel 175 mg/m^2 by 24-hour infusion versus doxorubicin 60 mg/m^2 versus paclitaxel 150 mg/m^2 over 24 hours plus doxorubicin 50 mg/m^2. The combination resulted in a response rate of 46% versus 33% and 34% for the monochemotherapies ($p < 0.007$), with a median time to treatment failure of 8.0 months versus 5.9 months and 6.2 months for the monochemotherapies ($p < 0.009$). These results were felt to be inadequate to pursue the development of adjuvant programs based on paclitaxel given over 24 hours with doxorubicin, and further fuelled the North American adjuvant sequential strategies based on the AC model (doxorubicin, cyclophosphamide) followed by paclitaxel.

The development of docetaxel–doxorubicin-based combinations appears, in contrast, to have been relatively straightforward. Several docetaxel–doxorubicin-based trials have been completed (Table 8.7). A dose-finding study in advanced breast cancer defined the recommended 3-week dose as docetaxel 75 mg/m^2 plus doxorubicin 50 mg/m^2, or docetaxel 60 mg/m^2 plus doxorubicin 60 mg/m^2.[95] Three multicenter phase II studies have evaluated these doses in first-line metastatic breast cancer (MBC). One trial used doxorubicin (A) 50 mg/m^2 plus docetaxel (T) 75 mg/m^2 (A50/T75),[97] whereas the Eastern Cooperative Oncology Group (ECOG) studied the AT combination with doxorubicin 60 mg/m^2 and docetaxel 60 mg/m^2 (A60/T60).[98] The third trial explored a three-drug TAC combination: docetaxel 75 mg/m^2, doxorubicin 50 mg/m^2 plus cyclophosphamide (C) 500 mg/m^2 (T75A50C500).[96] This was done to define a combination that could be compared with a standard doxorubicin-containing regimen at equivalent doses of doxorubicin (e.g. FAC: 5-fluorouracil, doxorubicin, cyclophosphamide) in both the first-line metastatic and, more importantly, the adjuvant setting. Results showed an overall

Table 8.6   Paclitaxel and doxorubicin combinations

Study	Regimen (mg/m^2)		No. of patients evaluable	Efficacy: ORR (%)	Toxicity (CHF) (%)
	Doxorubicin	Paclitaxel			
3-h infusion					
Colomer et al[55]	50	175	58	Lowest: 43	NA
Cazap et al[56]	60/bolus	200	27	48	0
Sparano et al[54]	60/bolus	200	47	52	4
Latorre et al[53]	50 day 1	130–250 day 2[a]	30	70	NA
Frassineti et al[52]	50/bolus	130–250[a]	19	79	NA
Schwartsmann et al[58]	60/bolus	250	25	80	NA
Gehl et al[51]	50–60/30 min	155/200	29	83	23
Gianni et al[50]	60/bolus	200	47	Highest: 94	21
24-h infusion					
Sledge et al[57]	50–60/bolus	150–175	12	Lowest: 42	NA
Sledge et al[48]	50/bolus	150	238	46	4.5
	75/bolus	200	12	58	NA
Holmes et al[59]	48–60/24 h	125–150	9	Highest: 69	NA
72-h infusion					
Fisherman et al[60]	60–75/72 h	160–200	39	72	NA

ORR, overall response rate; NA, not available; [a]G-CSF, granulocyte colony-stimulating factor used; CHF, congestive heart failure.

response rate from 57% for A60T60 to 74–77% for A75/T50 and T75A50C500, a response duration of 59–62 weeks, a time to progression of 47–59 weeks and a 2-year survival rate of 57–66%. The high response rates were maintained in patients with unfavorable prognostic features, such as multiple metastatic disease sites, visceral metastases, including liver and lung, and prior exposure to adjuvant chemotherapy.

Neutropenia and febrile neutropenia were the most common toxicities, although neutropenia was usually brief in duration and infections infrequent. The non-hematologic toxicities were mild and the docetaxel-specific toxicities such as fluid

Table 8.7   Docetaxel and doxorubicin combinations

Study	Regimen (mg/m²)		No. of patients evaluable	Efficacy: ORR (%)	Toxicity (CHF) (%)
	Docetaxel	Doxorubicin			
Sparano et al[98]	60	60	51	57	4
Dieras et al[95]	85*	50*	42	81	0
Dieras et al[97]	75	50	39	74	0
Nabholtz et al[96]	75	50 (+C500)	48	77	4

C, cyclophosphamide; NA, not available; CHF, congestive heart failure.
Anthracycline administered before docetaxel.
*Used range of doses for both drugs, maximum tolerated dose (MTD) quoted.

retention and nail changes were not a clinical problem. More importantly, with these docetaxel–doxorubicin-based combinations, there was no evidence of significant cardiac toxicity (the incidence of congestive heart failure was between 0% and 4%). Evidence is accumulating that there is no pharmacokinetic interaction between docetaxel and doxorubicin with any effect on the AUC of doxorubicin.[108–110] This is in contrast to the pharmacokinetic interaction between doxorubicin and docetaxel that increases the AUC of docetaxel by 50% to 75%.[108,109]

Thus, the potential for the integration of paclitaxel or docetaxel with anthracyclines is clearly different, largely as a result of the pharmacokinetic interaction of the drugs. This has resulted in paclitaxel's development in the adjuvant setting being largely in sequential strategies, while docetaxel is capable of being developed in both sequential and polychemotherapy regimens.

Phase III trials

Various phase III trials are currently studying the role of taxane–anthracycline-based combinations versus standard anthracycline-containing regimens in first-line metastatic breast cancer. The EORTC is conducting a phase III trial comparing paclitaxel 175 mg/m² by 3-hour infusion plus doxorubicin 60 mg/m² with AC (doxorubicin 60 mg/m² plus cyclophosphamide 600 mg/m²). Results are not yet available. Two pivotal randomized phase III trials of docetaxel–doxorubicin-based combinations have been completed (AT versus AC and TAC versus FAC). Final results of the phase III trial comparing AT with AC as first-line treatment for patients with metastatic breast cancer were recently presented[106] (Table 8.5). A total of 429 patients without prior anthracycline exposure were randomized to a maximum of eight cycles of AT ($n = 215$) or AC ($n = 214$). The overall response rate (independently reviewed by a panel of experts) in patients treated with AT was statistically significantly higher than that of patients treated with AC (60% versus 47%, $p = 0.012$). Of particular note were the response rates obtained with AT versus AC in patients with unfavorable prognostic features: respectively, visceral metastases (50% versus 42%), liver metastases (62% versus 43%), lung metastases (59% versus 36%) and involvement of three or more organs (60% versus 41%). Patients treated with AT also experienced significantly longer time to disease progression ($p = 0.01$) and time to treatment failure ($p = 0.02$) than those treated with AC. This improved efficacy of the AT regimen was accompanied by an increase in neutropenia: 96% of patients in the AT arm experienced grade 3/4 neutropenia versus 82% of patients in the AC arm. The only statistically significant difference seen between the two arms in terms of toxicity was related to the incidence of febrile neutropenia: 33% of patients on AT versus 10% on AC (6% versus 2% of cycles). However, because of the short duration of neutropenia in both arms, the incidence of documented infection and septic death was very low (no septic death on AT, one patient on AC). Most neutropenic events occurred during the first two cycles. The rest of the toxicities were similar in both arms; in particular, the docetaxel-specific toxicities of fluid retention and nail changes were not a clinical problem.

These phase III results show for the first time that a taxane–doxorubicin combination has higher efficacy than anthracycline-containing polychemotherapy in first-line therapy for advanced breast cancer. Such a combination appears to be a new therapeutic option for patients in this setting, in particular if they present with poor prognostic features such as visceral metastases. Further results from this trial, including survival and quality of life, are necessary before being able to draw definitive conclusions. Results from the other phase III trials available soon will help define the ultimate role for these combinations in the initial therapy of advanced breast cancer.

In addition, these results give some idea of the expectations of the impact of this type of taxane–doxorubicin-based combination in the adjuvant setting.

Conclusion

There is level I evidence for superior response rate, time to disease progression and time to treatment failure for AT over AC. Data are immature with respect to survival.

TAXANES IN THE ADJUVANT SETTING

Two current strategies are being pursued with respect to the role of taxanes in the adjuvant setting and have led to the current ongoing large phase III trials.

The first strategy is related to the concept of sequential chemotherapy, for which both paclitaxel and docetaxel are being investigated. This is exemplified by: (1) the CALGB (Cancer and Leukemia Group B) ATC regimen (doxorubicin followed by paclitaxel followed by cyclophosphamide; (2) the AC regimen followed by paclitaxel or docetaxel (CALGB, NSABP); (3) AT (docetaxel) followed by CMF (Breast Adjuvant Study Team and International Breast Cancer Study Group, IBCSG); and (4) FEC (5-fluorouracil, epirubicin, cyclophosphamide) followed by docetaxel (French Cooperative Group).

The alternative strategy follows the classic polychemotherapy concept, for which, quasi-exclusively, docetaxel-based combinations are being studied. Protocols such as TAC (docetaxel) at doses of 75, 50 and 500 mg/m^2 have been compared with FAC (Breast Cancer International Research Group, BCIRG) or AT (docetaxel) at doses of 60 and 60 mg/m^2 has been compared with AC (ECOG).

The only results currently available comparing a taxane-containing regimen with standard chemotherapy as adjuvant therapy in primary breast cancer comes from CALGB Trial 9344 presented in 1998.[63] This trial was criticized for its short follow-up (median of 20 months) and the fact that it compared four cycles of chemotherapy (AC) versus eight cycles (AC followed by paclitaxel). The results suggest that the sequential addition of paclitaxel to AC may offer improved overall survival and disease-free survival in patients with node-positive primary breast cancer. However, longer follow-up is required before being able to draw any reliable conclusions from this trial.

The first adjuvant trials that compare taxane–anthracycline-containing combinations with classic anthracycline-containing polychemotherapy have mostly been completed. The trend in the second generation of adjuvant trials is for both arms to contain taxanes. The American Intergroup is using the sequential approach, comparing AC followed by either paclitaxel or docetaxel (weekly or 3-weekly). NSABP is comparing the sequential strategy with polychemotherapy, with AC followed by docetaxel versus AT ($60/60$ mg/m^2) $\times$ 4 versus TAC ($60/60/600$ mg/m^2) $\times$4 and BCIRG is comparing AC followed by docetaxel vs TAC ($75/50/500$ mg/m^2) $\times$ 6.

Conclusion

Level I evidence is that sequential addition of paclitaxel to AC $\times$ 4 improves disease-free and overall survival in node-positive breast cancer, although the report is at a very early stage (median 20 months) and needs to be reviewed with longer follow-up and confirmed. No other adjuvant data are available as yet for either taxane.

TAXANES AND BIOLOGIC MODIFIERS

The first biologic modifier with clinical evidence of activity in breast cancer is Herceptin (trastuzumab). This compound is undoubtedly the beginning of a new era of targeted therapies, which, it is hoped, will lead to individualized therapies for breast cancer. Herceptin, which is an antibody in the HER2/*neu* protein, is active in

patients whose breast cancer overexpresses the proto-oncogene. This gene is involved in the regulation of normal cell growth, and HER2/*neu* gene amplification or overexpression produces activated HER2 receptors (human epidermal growth factor receptor 2, also known as c-ErbB-2). HER2/*neu* overexpression occurs in 15–25% of patients with breast cancer and has been reported to be linked with poor prognosis and more importantly shortened disease-free and overall survival.[111]

Several trial results in advanced breast cancer have recently been presented, the most important of which is the registration for Herceptin: Trial 648.[112,113] Several fundamental concepts have emerged:

1. Herceptin is largely active in patients with (3+) HER2/*neu* overexpression. These patients with metastatic breast cancer have increased response rates, progression-free survival and overall survival when comparing Herceptin and chemotherapy with chemotherapy alone. In Trial 648, patients previously exposed to anthracyclines (166 patients) were randomized to paclitaxel alone given at a dose of 175 mg/m^2 versus paclitaxel at the same dose and schedule plus Herceptin weekly (initial dose 4 mg/kg followed by 2 mg/kg weekly until relapse). Paclitaxel alone gave a response rate of 16%, in keeping with previous prospective data from EORTC, but paclitaxel plus Herceptin results in a 42% response rate ($p = 0.0001$). In addition, time to progression was significantly longer for the paclitaxel plus Herceptin combination (6.9 months versus 3.0 months, $p = 0.0001$). Survival data were in favor of the combination of either AC or paclitaxel with Herceptin over chemotherapy alone, with combined data showing 25.4 months ($n = 235$) versus 20.9 months ($n = 234$) ($p = 0.045$) with a median follow-

up of 25 months.[113] The relative risk of death was 0.77 (95%CI = 0.60–0.99). The advantage was seen with AC (33.4 versus 24.5 months) and with paclitaxel (22.1 versus 18.4 months). This suggests that the optimal use of Herceptin could be in combination with chemotherapy followed by maintenance Herceptin post-chemotherapy.

2. There remains significant discussion about standardization of available tests for identifying patients who overexpress HER2/*neu*.

3. Cardiac toxicity appears to be a problem when Herceptin is given with anthracyclines. In Trial 648, one group of patients (not previously exposed to anthracyclines) was treated with AC (doxorubicin 60 mg/m^2 plus cyclophosphamide 600 mg/m^2) or AC plus Herceptin. The incidence of cardiac toxicity was 27% with AC plus Herceptin and 7% with AC alone. Grade III/IV cardiac events (according to the New York Heart Association classification) were seen in 16% of patients with the combination and 3% of patients with AC. In the taxane group (paclitaxel versus paclitaxel plus Herceptin), patients had been previously exposed to anthracyclines with a median interval of 20.5 months since anthracycline exposure. Patients treated with paclitaxel plus Herceptin experienced a recall of cardiac toxicity (12% overall incidence and 4% grade III/IV), whereas cardiac events were seen in 1% of patients treated with paclitaxel alone.

Conclusions

There is level I evidence for improved response to Herceptin and chemotherapy compared with chemotherapy alone. There is level I evidence for improved time to progression and for increased survival for the combination compared with chemotherapy alone. Further data are required before definitive conclusions can be made about which chemotherapy regimens are most appro-

priate with Herceptin, for how long they should be used and for how long Herceptin should be continued afterwards.

The results have lead to further Herceptin trials both in North America and in Europe. A number of trials of Herceptin in combination with taxanes are under consideration for patients with metastatic breast cancer. Several cooperative groups have decided to proceed to the adjuvant setting and integrate Herceptin in second-generation taxane phase III trials using a taxane-containing regimen versus a taxane-containing regimen plus Herceptin.

The unexpected cardiac toxicity documented with doxorubicin and Herceptin in metastatic breast cancer patients creates some difficulties for the adjuvant setting when doxorubicin is one of the standard drugs employed. At the present time, two approaches are being considered. The first is based on adding Herceptin to the present anthracycline-containing adjuvant strategies. Despite the risk of using concurrent Herceptin and doxorubicin and the potential risk of recall cardiac toxicity when using short-sequence anthracycline–Herceptin, two American cooperative groups (Intergroup and NSABP) are planning to add Herceptin to sequential chemotherapy in the adjuvant setting. They are planning phase III trials comparing AC followed by paclitaxel (various schedules, weekly or 3-weekly) with or without Herceptin.

The second approach is based on building a combination program around Herceptin following synergism data between Herceptin and chemotherapy, in order to get a regimen that has biologic rationale instead of adding Herceptin to the currently most popular chemotherapies. Following data from D Slamon et al (personal communication, 1999), three main therapeutic interventions are synergistic, in vitro and in vivo with Herceptin, according to the Chou definition:[114] platinum compounds (cisplatin and carboplatin), docetaxel and radiotherapy. The remainder of the chemotherapeutic agents either have an additive effect with Herceptin (paclitaxel, doxorubicin, cyclophosphamide, etc.) or an antagonistic effect (5-fluorouracil), meaning by this definition non-additive.

This has led to the present adjuvant second-generation taxane/Herceptin strategy of the BCIRG:

1. Phase III trial comparing TCH for six courses (docetaxel, platinum compound × 6 and Herceptin for 1 year), with AC × 4 followed by T × 4 and Herceptin for 1 year with AC × 4 followed by T × 4 (docetaxel) in the adjuvant treatment of breast cancer patients overexpressing HER2/*neu*.
2. Validation phase III trial of the control arm TAC × 6 versus AC × 4 followed by T × 4.

OVERALL CONCLUSIONS

Many exciting new chemotherapeutic agents have become available for the treatment of breast cancer in the 1990s. Without doubt, the taxanes have emerged as the most powerful compounds, and results available to date suggest that they will be remembered in the future as the breast cancer chemotherapy of the 1990s.

The two members of the present taxane family (paclitaxel and docetaxel) share some characteristics, but are also significantly different in terms of their preclinical and clinical profiles. Two main clinical differences have emerged. First, there is their different efficacy : toxicity ratio relative to dose and schedule: high and comparable efficacy can be obtained with both agents (paclitaxel 250 mg/m^2 given over 24 hours or docetaxel 100 mg/m^2 over 1 hour), but practicality and toxicity need to be considered. Lower doses and short schedules of paclitaxel (175 mg/m^2 over 3 hours) are well tolerated and practical, but

compromise efficacy. The true value of weekly schedules for both agents is still unclear and is under active investigation.

The second clinical difference is related to the ability to integrate the taxanes in anthracycline–taxane-containing regimens, secondary to different phamacokinetic interactions between them and the anthracyclines. The difficulties of integrating paclitaxel in polychemotherapy regimens have led almost exclusively to sequential adjuvant strategies. In contrast, docetaxel has a favorable pharmacokinetic profile with the anthracyclines, allowing development of both sequential and classic combination adjuvant strategies.

Finally, an additional potential difference relates to the level of synergism between each taxane and Herceptin. More data, which currently favor docetaxel, are needed in this regard. However, the clinical relevance is currently under investigation in the adjuvant setting.

The taxanes should be considered standard therapy in metastatic breast cancer after failure of prior chemotherapy, especially anthracyclines. Their role in combination with anthracyclines in first-line therapy of advanced breast cancer is emerging, with data showing that the clinical benefit of docetaxel–doxorubicin could be superior to that of classic anthracycline-containing polychemotherapy (AC). Although this benefit is probably true for high-risk metastatic patients (with visceral metastases, rapidly progressing advanced disease, etc.), survival data are needed in order to assess whether this type of combination is able to change our philosophy significantly in the treatment of metastatic breast cancer.

It is accepted that classic chemotherapy strategies in advanced disease do not make a significant survival difference, although modest but real advances have been seen with these combinations in the adjuvant setting. The fact that we are starting to see differences occurring with taxanes in the metastatic setting should induce reasonable optimism for the potential role of taxanes in the adjuvant setting.

The impact of the taxanes on the natural history of breast cancer has yet to be defined. Current evidence strongly suggests that these agents will lead to significant advancements in the management of advanced breast cancer and, more importantly, in adjuvant therapy.

Clinical research strategies for taxanes in breast cancer have been appropriately designed to answer the important questions. Only time (1–2 years for metastatic and 1–5 years for adjuvant therapy) will give us the definitive answer to the fundamental question: Are the taxanes going to change the natural history of breast cancer and, if so, by what magnitude?

REFERENCES

1. Wani MC, Taylor HL, Wall ME, Coggon P, McPhail AT, Plant antitumour agents VI. The isolation and structure of Taxol, a novel antileukemic and antitumour agent from *Taxus brevifolia*. *J Am Chem Soc* 1971; **93**:2325–7.

2. Rowinsky EK, Donehower RC, Drug therapy: paclitaxel (Taxol). *N Engl J Med* 1995; **332**:1004–14.

3. Lavelle F, Gueritte-Voegelein F, Guenard D, Le Taxotere: des aiguilles d'if a la clinique. *Bull Cancer* 1993; **80**:326–38.

4. Bissery MC, Nohynek S, Sanderink GJ et al, Docetaxel (Taxotere®): a review of preclinical and clinical experience. Part 1: preclinical experience. *Anti-cancer Drugs* 1995; **6**:339–68.

5. Legha SS, Tenney DM, Krakoff IR, Phase I study of Taxol using a 5 day intermittent schedule. *J Clin Oncol* 1986; **4**:762–6.

6. Grem JL, Tutsch KD, Simon KJ et al, Phase I study of Taxol administered as a short i.v. infusion daily for 5 days. *Cancer Treat Rep* 1986; **71**:1179–84.

7. Donehower RC, Rowinsky EK, Grochow LB et al, Phase I trial of Taxol in patients with advanced cancer. *Cancer Treat Rep* 1987; **71**:1171–7.

8. Wiernik PH, Schwartz EL, Strauman JJ et al, Phase I clinical and pharmacokinetic study of Taxol. *Cancer Res* 1987; **47**:2486–93.

9. Schiller JH, Storer B, Tutsch K et al, Phase I trial of 3-hour infusion of paclitaxel with or without granulocyte colony-stimulating factor in patients with advanced cancer. *J Clin Oncol* 1994; **12**:241–8.

10. Kris MG, O'Connell JP, Gralla RJ et al, Phase I trial of Taxol given as a 3-hour infusion every 21 days. *Cancer Treat Rep* 1986; **70**:605–7.

11. Brown T, Halvin K, Weiss G et al, A phase I trial of Taxol given by a 6-hour intravenous infusion. *J Clin Oncol* 1991; **9**: 1261–7.

12. Wiernik PH, Schwartz EL, Einzig A et al, Phase I trial of Taxol given as a 24-hour infusion every 21 days: Responses observed in metastatic melanoma. *J Clin Oncol* 1987; **5**:1232–9.

13. Ohmura T, Zimet AS, Coffey VA et al, Phase I study of Taxol in a 24-hour infusion schedule. *Proc Am Soc Clin Oncol* 1985; **26**:167.

14. Hurwitz CA, Relling MV, Weitman SD et al, Phase I trial of paclitaxel in children with refractory solid tumors: A Pediatric Oncology Group study. *J Clin Oncol* 1993; **11**:2324–9.

15. Rowinsky EK, Burke PJ, Karp JE et al, Phase I and pharmacodynamic study of Taxol in refractory adult acute leukemias. *Cancer Res* 1989; **49**:4640–7.

16. Sarosy G, Kohn E, Stone DA et al, Phase I study of Taxol and granulocyte colony-stimulating factor in patients with refractory ovarian cancer. *J Clin Oncol* 1992; **10**:1165–70.

17. Wilson WH, Berg S, Bryant G et al, Paclitaxel in doxorubicin-refractory or mitomycin-refractory breast cancer: A phase I/II trial with 96-hour infusion. *J Clin Oncol* 1994; **12**:1621–9.

18. Spriggs DR, Tondini C, Taxol administered as a 120 hour infusion. *Invest New Drugs* 1992; **10**:275–8.

19. Weiss RB, Donehower RC, Wiernik PH et al,

Hypersensitivity reactions from Taxol. *J Clin Oncol* 1990; **12**:1263–8.

20. Trudeau ME, Docetaxel (Taxotere): An overview of first-line monotherapy. *Semin Oncol* 1995; **22**(Suppl 13):17–21.

21. Holmes FA, Walters RS, Theriault RL et al, Phase II trial of Taxol: An active drug in the treatment of metastatic breast cancer. *J Natl Cancer Inst* 1991; **83**:1797–805.

22. Vici P, Di Lauro S, Conti L et al, Paclitaxel activity in anthracycline refractory breast cancer patients. *Tumori* 1997; **83**:661–4.

23. Davidson NG, Single agent paclitaxel as first-line treatment of metastatic breast cancer: The British experience. *Semin Oncol* 1996; **23**(Suppl 11):6–10.

24. Michael M, Bishop JF, Levi JA et al, Australian multicentre phase II trial of paclitaxel in women with metastatic breast cancer and prior chemotherapy. *Med J Aust* 1997; **166**:530–3.

25. Seidman AD, Hudis C, Tiersten A et al, Phase II trial of paclitaxel by 3-hour infusion as initial and salvage chemotherapy for metastatic breast cancer. *J Clin Oncol* 1995; **13**:2575–81.

26. Fountzilas G, Athanassiades A, Giannakakis T et al, A phase II study of paclitaxel in advanced breast cancer resistant to anthracyclines. *Eur J Cancer* 1996; **32A**:47–51.

27. Gianni L, Munzone E, Capri G et al, Paclitaxel in metastatic breast cancer: A trial of two doses by a 3-hour infusion in patients with disease recurrence after prior therapy with anthracyclines. *J Natl Cancer Inst* 1995; **87**:1169–75.

28. Vermorken D, Ten Bokkel Huinink WW, Mandjes IAM et al, High dose paclitaxel with granulocyte colony-stimulating factor in patients with advanced breast cancer refractory to anthracycline therapy: A European Cancer Center trial. *Semin Oncol* 1995; **22**:16–22.

29. Seidman AD, Reichman BS, Crown JP et al, Paclitaxel as a second and subsequent therapy for metastatic breast cancer: Activity independent of prior anthracycline response. *J Clin Oncol* 1995; **15**:1152–9.

30. Abrams JS, Vena DA, Baltz J et al, Paclitaxel activity in heavily pretreated breast cancer: A National Cancer Institute Treatment Referral Center trial. *J Clin Oncol* 1995; **13**:2056–65.

31. Constenla M, Lorenzo I, Garcia-Arroyo FR et al, Phase II trial of paclitaxel 96-hour infusion with G-CSF in anthracycline-resistant metastatic breast cancer. *Proc Am Soc Clin Oncol* 1997; **16**:165a.

32. Bonneterre J, Tubiana-Hulin M, Chollet PH et al, Taxol (paclitaxel) 225 mg/m^2 by 3-hour infusion without G-CSF as first-line therapy in patients with metastatic breast cancer (MBC). *Proc Am Soc Clin Oncol* 1996; **15**:179.

33. Reichman BS, Seidman AD, Crown JPA et al, Paclitaxel and recombinant human granulocyte colony-stimulating factor as initial chemotherapy for metastatic breast cancer. *J Clin Oncol* 1993; **11**:1943–51.

34. Swain S, Hinig S, Walton L et al, Phase II trial of paclitaxel (Taxol) as first-line chemotherapy for metastatic breast cancer (MBC). *Proc Am Soc Clin Oncol* 1995; **14**:132 (Abst 227).

35. Mamounas E, Brown A, Fisher B et al, 3-Hour high-dose Taxol infusion in advanced breast cancer: A NSABP phase II study. *Proc Am Soc Clin Oncol* 1995; **14**:206.

36. Luftner D, Flath B, Printz B et al, Weekly fractionated paclitaxel in metastatic breast cancer – Dose optimizing study. *Eur J Cancer* 1997; **33**:S196 (Abst 694).

37. Breier A, Ledbedinsky C, Pelayes L et al, Phase I/II weekly paclitaxel 80 mg/m^2 in pretreated breast and ovarian cancer. *Proc Am Soc Clin Oncol* 1997; **16**:163a (Abst 568).

38. Chang A, Hui L, Boros R et al, Phase I study of weekly one-hour paclitaxel treatment in advanced malignant diseases. *Proc Am Soc Clin Oncol* 1997; **16**:232a (Abst 817).

39. Seidman AD, Hudis CA, Albanel J et al, Dose-dense therapy with weekly 1-hour paclitaxel infusions in the treatment of metastatic breast cancer. *J Clin Oncol* 1999; **16**:3353–61.

40. Perez EA, Irwin DH, Patel R et al, A large phase II trial of paclitaxel administered as a weekly one hour infusion in patients with metastatic breast cancer. *Proc Am Soc Clin Oncol* 1999; **18**:126a.

41. Nabholtz J-M, Gelmon K, Bontenbal M et al, Multicenter, randomized comparative study of two doses of paclitaxel in patients with metastatic breast cancer. *J Clin Oncol* 1996; **14**:1858–67.

42. Peretz T, Sulkes A, Chollet P et al, A multicenter randomized study of two schedules of paclitaxel (PTX) in patients with advanced breast cancer (ABC). *Eur J Cancer* 1995; **31**(Suppl 5):S75a.

43. Winer E, Berry D, Duggan D et al, Failure of higher dose paclitaxel to improve outcome in patients with metastatic breast cancer – Results from CALGB 9342. *Proc Am Soc Clin Oncol* 1998; **17**:101a (Abst 388).

44. Mamounas E, Rown A, Smith R et al, Effect of Taxol duration of infusion in advanced breast cancer (ABC): Results from NSABP B-26 trial comparing 3- to 24-hour infusion of high-dose Taxol. *Proc Am Soc Clin Oncol* 1998; **17**:101a (Abst 389).

45. Holmes FA, Valero V, Buzdar AU et al, Final results: Randomized phase III trial of paclitaxel by 3-hr versus 96-hr infusion in patient (pt) with metastatic breast cancer (MBC). *Proc Am Soc Clin* 1998; **17**:110a (Abst 426).

46. Gamucci T, Piccart M, Brunning P et al, Single-agent Taxol (T) versus doxorubicin (D) as first- and second-line chemotherapy (CT) in advanced breast cancer (ABC): Final results of an EORTC randomized study with crossover. *Proc Am Soc Clin Oncol* 1998; **17**:111a (Abst 428).

47. Awada A, Paridaens R, Brunning P et al, Doxorubicin or Taxol as first-line chemotherapy for metastatic breast cancer (MBC): Results of an EORTC–IDBBC/ECSG randomized trial with crossover (EORTC 10923). *Breast Cancer Res Treat* 1997; **46**:23 (Abst 2).

48. Sledge GW, Neuberg D, Ingle J et al, Phase III trial of doxorubicin (A) vs paclitaxel (T) vs doxorubicin + paclitaxel (A + T) as first-line therapy for metastatic breast cancer (MBC): an intergroup trial. *Am Soc Clin Oncol* 1997; **16**:1a (Abst 2).

49. Bishop J, Dewar J, Toner G et al, Initial paclitaxel improves outcome compared with CMFP combination chemotherapy as front-line therapy in untreated metastatic breast cancer. *J Clin Oncol* 1999; **17**:2355–64.

50. Gianni L, Munzone E, Capri G et al, Paclitaxel by 3-hour infusion in combination with bolus doxorubicin in women with untreated metastatic breast cancer: High antitumor efficacy and cardiac effects in a dose-sequence-finding study. *J Clin Oncol* 1995; **13**:2688–99.

51. Gehl J, Boesgaard M, Paaske T et al, Combined doxorubicin and paclitaxel in advanced breast cancer: Effective and cardiotoxic. *Ann Oncol* 1996; **7**:687–93.

52. Frassineti GL, Zoli W, Tienghi A et al, Phase I/II study of sequential and combination of paclitaxel and doxorubicin in the treatment of advanced breast cancer. *Proc Am Soc Clin Oncol* 1996; **15**:103.

53. Latorre A, Lorusso V, Guida M et al, Paclitaxel and doxorubicin in the treatment of advanced breast cancer: A phase I/II study. *Proc Am Soc Clin Oncol* 1997; **16**:179a (Abst 627).

54. Sparano JA, Hu P, Rao RM et al, Phase II trial of doxorubicin plus paclitaxel plus G-CSF in metastatic breast cancer: An Eastern Cooperative Oncology Group trial (E4195). *Breast Cancer Res Treat* 1997; **46**:23.

55. Colomer R, Montere A, Lluch A et al, circulating Her-2/neu predicts resistance to Taxol/Adriamycin, in metastatic breast cancer: Preliminary results of a multicentric prospective study. *Proc Am Soc Clin Oncol* 1997; **16**:140a (Abst 492).

56. Cazap E, Ventriglia E, Rubio G et al, Taxol plus doxorubicin in the treatment of metastatic breast cancer. *Proc Am Soc Clin Oncol* 1996; **15**:146 (Abst 248).

57. Sledge GW, Robert B, Sparano JA et al,

Eastern Cooperative Oncology Group study of paclitaxel and doxorubicin in advanced breast cancer. *Semin Oncol* 1995; **22**(Suppl 6):105–8.

58. Schwartsmann G, Menke CH, Caleffi M et al, Phase II trial of Taxol, doxorubicin plus G-CSF in patients with metastatic breast cancer. *Proc Am Soc Clin Oncol* 1996; **15**:126 (Abst 168).

59. Holmes FA, Madden T, Newman RA et al, Sequence-dependent alteration of doxorubicin pharmacokinetics by paclitaxel in a phase I study of paclitaxel and doxorubicin in patients with metastatic breast cancer. *J Clin Oncol* 1996; **14**:2713–21.

60. Fisherman JS, Cowan KH, Noone M et al, Phase I/II study of 72 hours infusional paclitaxel and doxorubicin with granulocyte colony stimulating factor in patients with metastatic breast cancer. *J Clin Oncol* 1996; **14**:774–82.

61. Klein JL, Dansey RD, Karanes C et al, Induction chemotherapy with doxorubicin and paclitaxel for metastatic breast cancer. *Breast Cancer Res Treat* 1997; **46**:94 (Abst 405).

62. Norton L, Evolving concepts in the systemic drug therapy of breast cancer. *Semin Oncol* 1997; **24**(Suppl 10):3–10.

63. Henderson IC, Berry D, Demetri G et al, Improved disease-free (DFS) and overall survival (OS) from the addition of sequential paclitaxel (T) but not from the escalation of doxorubicin (A) dose level in the adjuvant chemotherapy of patients (PTS) with node-positive primary breast cancer (BC). *Proc Am Soc Clin Oncol* 1998; **17**:390a.

64. Extra JM, Rousseau F, Bruno R et al, Phase I and pharmacokinetic study of Taxotere (RP 56976; NSC 628503) given as a short intravenous infusion. *Cancer Res* 1993; **53**: 1037–42.

65. Burris H, Irvin R, Kuhn J et al, Phase I clinical trial of Taxotere administered as either a 2-hour or 6-hour intravenous infusion. *J Clin Oncol* 1993; **11**:950–8.

66. Bissett D, Setanoians A, Cassidy J et al, Phase

I and pharmacokinetic study of Taxotere (RP 56976) administered as a 24-hour infusion. *Cancer Res* 1993; **53**:523–7.

67. Pazdur R, Newman RA, Newman BM et al, Phase I study of Taxotere: Five-day schedule. *J Natl Cancer Inst* 1992; **84**:1781–8.

68. Tomiak E, Piccart MJ, Kerger J et al, Phase I study of docetaxel administered as a 1-hour intravenous infusion on a weekly basis. *J Clin Oncol* 1994; **12**:1458–67.

69. Taguchi T, Furue H, Niitani H et al, Phase I clinical trial of RP 56976 (docetaxel), a new anticancer drug. *Gan To Kagaku Ryoho* 1994; **21**:1997–2005.

70. Van Oosterom AT, Schrivers D, Docetaxel (Taxotere), a review of preclinical and clinical experience. Part II: Clinical experience. *Anticancer Drugs* 1995; **6**:356–68.

71. Nabholtz JM, The role of taxanes in the management of breast cancer. *Semin Oncol* 1999; **26**(Suppl 8):1–3.

72. Trudeau ME, Eisenhauer EA, Higgins BP et al, Docetaxel in patients with metastatic breast cancer: A phase II study of the National Cancer Institute of Canada Clinical Trials Group. *J Clin Oncol* 1996; **14**:422–8.

73. Dieras V, Chevallier B, Kerbrat P et al, A multicentre phase II study of docetaxel 75 mg/m² as first-line chemotherapy for patients with advanced breast cancer: A report of the Clinical Screening Group of the EORTC. *Br J cancer* 1996; **74**:650–6.

74. Ten Bokkel Huinink WW, Prove AM, Piccart M et al, A phase II trial with docetaxel (Taxotere) in second line treatment with chemotherapy for advanced breast cancer. A study of the EORTC–ECTG. *Ann Oncol* 1994; **5**:527–32.

75. Hudis CA, Seidman AD, Crown JPA et al, Phase II pharmacologic study of docetaxel as initial chemotherapy for metastatic breast cancer. *J Clin Oncol* 1996; **14**:58–65.

76. Chevallier B, Fumoleau P, Kerbrat P et al, Docetaxel is a major cytoxic drug for the treatment of advanced breast cancer: A phase II trial of the Clinical Screening Co-operative

Group of the EORTC. *J Clin Oncol* 1995; **13**:314–22.

77. Fumoleau P, Chevallier B, Kerbrat P et al, A multicentre phase II study of the efficacy and safety of docetaxel as first-line treatment of advanced breast cancer: A report of the Clinical Screening Group of the EORTC. *Ann Oncol* 1996; **7**:165–71.

78. Chan S, Friedrichs K, Noel D et al, Prospective randomized trial of docetaxel versus doxorubicin in patients with metastatic breast cancer. *J Clin Oncol* 1999; **17**:2341–54.

79. Ten Bokkel Huinink WW, Prove AM, Piccart M et al, A phase II trial with docetaxel (Taxotere) in second line treatment with chemotherapy for advanced breast cancer: A study of the EORTC Early Clinical Trials Group. *Ann Oncol* 1994; **5**:527–32.

80. Van Oosterom AT, Dieras V, Tubiana-Hulin M et al, Taxotere in previously treated patients with metastatic breast carcinoma (MBC) stratification for anthracycline resistance. *Proc Am Soc Clin Oncol* 1996; **15**:141 (Abst 231).

81. Alexopoulos CG, Rigatos G, Efremidou A et al, Phase II study of Taxotere monotherapy in previously treated patients with advanced breast cancer. *Eur J Cancer* 1997; **33**(Suppl 8):S153 (Abst 680).

82. Vorobiof DA, Chasen MR, Moeken R, Phase II trial of single agent docetaxel in previously treated patients with advanced breast cancer (ABC). *Proc Am Soc Clin Oncol* 1996; **15**:130 (Abst 185).

83. Terzoli E, Nistico C, Garufi C et al, Docetaxel in advanced breast carcinoma (MBC) patients (pts) pretreated with anthracyclines. *Proc Am Soc Clin Oncol* 1998; **17**:177a (Abst 682).

84. Leonard RC, O'Brien M, Barrett-Lee P et al, A prospective analysis of 390 advanced breast cancer patients treated with Taxotere throughout the UK. *Ann Oncol* 1996; **7**(Suppl 5):19 (Abst 810).

85. Shapiro JD, Michael M, Millward MJ et al, Activity and toxicity of docetaxel (Taxotere) in women with previously treated metastatic breast cancer. *Aus NZ J Med* 1997; **27**:40–4.

86. Adachi I, Wantabe T, Takashima S et al, A late phase II study of RP 56976 (docetaxel) in patients with advanced or recurrent breast cancer. *Br J Cancer* 1996; **73**:210–16.

87. Taguchi T, Hirata K, Kuni Y et al, An early phase II study of RP 56976 (docetaxel) in patients with breast cancer. *Gan To Kagaku Ryoho* 1994; **21**:2453–60.

88. Taguchi T, Mori S, Abe R et al, Late phase II clinical study of RP 56976 (docetaxel) in patients with advanced/recurrent breast cancer. *Gan To Jagaku Ryoho* 1994; **21**:2624–32.

89. Valero V, Holmes F, Walters RS et al, Phase II trial of docetaxel: A new, highly effective antineoplastic agent in the management of patients with anthracycline-resistant metastatic breast cancer. *J Clin Oncol* 1995; **13**:2886–94.

90. Ravdin PM, Burris HA, Cook G et al, Phase II trial of docetaxel in advanced anthracycline-resistant or anthracenedione-resistant breast cancer. *J Clin Oncol* 1995; **13**:2879–85.

91. Bonneterre J, Guastalla JP, Fumoleau P et al, A phase II trial of docetaxel in patients with anthracycline resistant metastatic breast cancer. *Breast Cancer Res Treat* 1995; **37**:89 (Abst 305).

92. Nabholtz J-M, Senn HJ, Bezwoda WR et al, Prospective randomized trial of docetaxel versus mitomycin C plus vinblastine in patients with metastatic breast cancer progressing despite previous anthracycline-containing chemotherapy. *J Clin Oncol* 1999; **17**:1413–24.

93. Sjostrom J, Mouridsen H, Pluzanska A et al, Taxotere versus methotrexate 5-fluorouracil in patients with metastatic breast cancer as 2nd line chemotherapy: A phase III study. *Proc Am Soc Clin Oncol* 1998; **17**:111a .

94. Bonneterre J, Monnier A, Roche H et al, Taxotere versus 5-fluorouracil + Navelbine in patients with metastatic breast cancer as 2nd line chemotherapy: A phase III study. *Breast Cancer Res Treat* 1997; **50**:261.

95. Dieras V, Docetaxel in combination with dox-

orubicin: a phase I dose-finding study. *Oncology* 1997; **6**(Suppl 6):17–20.

96. Nabholtz JM, Smylie M, Mackey JR et al, Docetaxel/doxorubicin/cyclophosphamide in the treatment of metastatic breast cancer. *Oncology* 1997; **11**(Suppl 8):37–41.

97. Dieras V, Barthier S, Beuzeboc P et al, Phase II study of docetaxel in combination with doxorubicin as 1st line chemotherapy of metastatic breast cancer. *Breast Cancer Res Treat* 1998; **50**:262.

98. Sparano JA, Ju P, Schadfer PL et al, Phase II trial of doxorubicin and docetaxel plus granulocyte-colony stimulating factor in metastatic breast cancer: An Eastern Cooperative Oncology Group trial (E1196). *Breast Cancer Res Treat* 1998; **50**:27.

99. Nabholtz JM, Docetaxel (Taxotere) plus doxorubicin-based combinations: the evidence of activity in breast cancer. *Semin Oncol* 1999; **26**(Suppl 9):7–13.

100. Riva A, Fumoleau P, Roche H et al, Efficacy and safety of different corticosteroid premedications in breast cancer patients treated with Taxotere®. *Proc Am Soc Clin Oncol* 1997; **16**:188a.

101. Hainsworth JD, Burris HA, Erland JB et al, Phase I trial of docetaxel administered by weekly infusion in patients with advanced refractory cancer. *J Clin Oncol* 1998; **16**:2164–8.

102. Luck HJ, Donne S, Glaubitz M et al, Phase I study of weekly docetaxel in heavily pretreated breast cancer patients. *Eur J Cancer* 1997; **33**:703a.

103. Loffler TM, Freud W, Droge C et al. Activity of weekly Taxotere in patients with metastatic breast cancer. *Proc Am Soc Clin Oncol* 1998; **17**:113a.

104. Burstein HJ, Younger J, Bunnell CA et al, Weekly docetaxel (Taxotere) for metastatic breast cancer: a phase II trial. *Proc Am Soc Clin Oncol* 1999; **18**:127a.

105. Loffler TM, Is there a place for 'dose-dense' weekly schedules of the taxoids? *Semin Oncol* 1998; **25**(Suppl 12):32–4.

106. Nabholtz JM, Falkson G, Campos D et al, A phase III trial comparing doxorubicin (A) and docetaxel (T) (AT) to doxorubicin and cyclophosphamide (AC) as first line chemotherapy for MBC. *Proc Am Soc Clin Oncol* 1999; **18**: 127a (Abst 485).

107. Gianni L, Vigano L, Locatelli A et al, Human pharmacokinetic characterization and in vitro study of the interaction between doxorubicin and paclitaxel in patients with breast cancer. *J Clin Oncol* 1997; **15**:1906–15.

108. Schuller J, Czejka M, Kletzl H et al, Doxorubicin and Taxotere: A pharmacokinetic study of the combination in advanced breast cancer. *Proc Am Soc Clin Oncol* 1998; **17**:205a.

109. Bellot R, Robert J, Dieras V et al, Taxotere does not change the pharmacokinetic profile of doxorubicin and doxorubicinol. *Proc Am Soc Clin Oncol* 1998; **17**:221a.

110. D'Incalci M, Schuller J, Colombo T et al, Taxoids in combination with anthracyclines and other agents: pharmacokinetic considerations. *Semin Oncol* 1998; **25**(Suppl 13): 16–20.

111. Slamon D, Godolphin W, Jones LA et al, Studies of the Her-2/neu proto-oncogene in human breast and ovarian cancer. *Science* 1989; **244**:707–12.

112. Slamon D, Leylan-Jones B, Shak S et al, Addition of herceptin (humanized anti-Her2 antibody) to first line chemotherapy for HER2 overexpressing metastatic breast cancer markedly increases anticancer activity: A randomized, multinational controlled phase III trial. *Proc Am Soc Clin Oncol* 1998; **17**:98a (Abst 377).

113. Norton L, Slamon D, Leyland-Jones B et al, Overall survival (OS) advantage to simultaneous chemotherapy (CRX) plus the humanized anti-HER2 monoclonal antibody Herceptin (H) in HER2-overexpressing (HER2+) metastatic breast cancer (MBC). *Proc Am Soc Clin Oncol* 1999; **18**:127a (Abst 483).

114. Chou TC, Talalay P, Quantitative analysis of dose-effects relationships: the combined effects of multiple drugs or enzyme inhibitors. *Adv Enzyme Regul* 1984; **22**:27–55.

9
Vinorelbine

Marc Spielmann, Laurent Zelek

The original observation that vinca alkaloids produced an anti-leukemic effect in mice prompted intense research, which led to the use of vincristine, vinblastine, vindesine and, later, vinorelbine. Vinorelbine differs chemically from other vinca alkaloids because of an original synthesis that generates substitutions on the catharantine moiety. Its antitumor activity, demonstrated in experimental studies, led to clinical studies that have confirmed its value in a broad spectrum of malignancies, including breast cancer.

As with other vinca alkaloids that exhibit selective activity against mitotic microtubules, vinorelbine binds to tubulin, thereby interfering with microtubule assembly. Differences between neurons and other cell types in their tubulin-associated protein content probably account for the decreased neurotoxicity (peripheral neuropathy) of vinorelbine compared with that of other vinca alkaloids.

Vinorelbine concentration in plasma decays according to a three-compartment model with a long terminal-phase, elimination half-life:

$$t_{\frac{1}{2}\alpha} = 2\text{--}6 \text{ min}, \ t_{\frac{1}{2}\beta} = 1.9 \pm 0.8 \text{ h}, \ t_{\frac{1}{2}\gamma} = 40 \pm 18 \text{ h}.$$

Initial high protein binding (80%) decreases to 50% after 96 hours. The pharmacokinetic profile of vinorelbine is not strikingly different from that of other vinca alkaloids. Its metabolism and elimination have been studied in animals and humans after the administration of radiolabeled vinorelbine. In summary: (1) intense hepatic extraction occurs and less than 60% of the infused dose is recovered in the vascular effluent within the first 2 hours; (2) biliary excretion is active, with a concentration in the bile that is 7000-fold higher than that in the effluent; and (3) less than 12% of vinorelbine is found in urine within 72 hours.[1]

SINGLE-AGENT ACTIVITY

Several phase II studies[2–14] have investigated the activity of single-agent vinorelbine against breast cancer, and these are summarized in Table 9.1. The weekly schedule was chosen more frequently,[2–4] at a starting dose of 30 mg/m² per week. Alternative schedules such as a 5-day continuous infusion have been proposed, but were not demonstrated to be superior to weekly vinorelbine;[5,6] the daily × 3 schedule is not recommended because of hematological toxicity.[7] Response rates ranging from 34%[4] to 50%[3] are consistently reported, with a median time to treatment failure of about 6 months and a median survival exceeding 1 year[2–4] even when vinorelbine is given as second-line therapy after failure with anthracyclines.[4] No other vinca alkaloid has attained this level of activity in breast cancer; only anthracyclines and taxanes exhibit comparable potency in this malignancy.

Excellent tolerance and low toxicity have consistently been reported in all of these trials. The main side effect documented was grade 3–4 neutropenia, which occurred in 75% of patients, although fever did not invariably ensue. Furthermore, analyses of quality of life suggested that patients with advanced breast cancer receiving weekly vinorelbine maintained a satisfactory score and that, in some respects, it could be considered comparable to or even better than other salvage agents.[8]

More recently, single-agent vinorelbine has been evaluated in patients at risk of more severe chemotherapy-induced side effects, i.e. elderly patients with advanced breast cancer and liver metastases. In patients older than 60 years with advanced breast cancer, findings reported are similar to those found in younger patients, especially with regard to tolerance; no pharmacokinetic rationale justifies reducing the dose of vinorelbine in elderly patients.[9,10] In patients with liver metastases, a vinorelbine dose reduction is warranted in the event of severe liver failure, but is not mandatory in patients with moderate hepatic insufficiency.[11]

Of particular interest is the study by Jones et al,[12] which is the only one to have compared single-agent vinorelbine with a more conventional salvage regimen after failure with first-line anthracycline-based therapy. A total of 150 patients were randomized to receive either weekly vinorelbine at a starting dose of 30 g/m[2] per week or intravenous melphalan given every 28 days at a dose of 25 mg/m[2]. Despite the moderate dose intensity delivered (19.3 mg/m[2] per week), essentially limited by delays in hematological recovery, vinorelbine proved to be significantly more effective than melphalan, whatever the endpoints considered:

- the 1-year survival rate was 35.7% versus 21.7% ($p = 0.034$)
- the median time to progression was 12 versus 8 weeks ($p < 0.001$)
- the objective response rate was 16% (complete responses: 5%) versus 9% (complete responses: 2%) ($p = 0.06$).

Although all patients had previously received anthracycline-based chemotherapy, tolerance remained acceptable. In particular, only 10% of patients had to be readmitted for febrile neutropenia, whereas 75% of them experienced grade 3–4 neutropenia. Moreover, it is noteworthy that quality of life was not impaired with vinorelbine. This randomized study is among the few that demonstrate a survival benefit with second-line chemotherapy in metastatic breast cancer; taxanes were in the investigational arm in all the others.

More recent studies[13,14] suggest that single-agent vinorelbine should continue to be included in the most active regimens after failure with taxanes. Dose intensity appears to be a crucial issue, and the suboptimal schedule of the only negative trial[15] probably explains its results. With weekly schedules, however, objective responses have been reported to attain 25% with delivered dose intensities of 27.7 mg/m[2] per week plus granulocyte colony-stimulating factor (G-CSF)[13] and 22.5 mg/m[2] per week without G-CSF.[14] In this population, the limiting toxicity is not only hematological, but also neurological (neuropathy or ileus);[14,15] given this critical adverse effect, caution should be exercised when using G-CSF to maximize dose intensity.

These last studies demonstrate that vinorelbine continues to be one of the most active salvage therapies after failure with gold-standard

Table 9.1   Clinical trials with single-agent vinorelbine

Author	Main selection criterion	Regimen	No. of patients	Main grade 3–4 toxicities[a] (%)	Response rate (%)[b]	Median duration of response
Phase II trials						
Fumoleau[2]	First-line stage IV	Vinorelbine 30 mg/m²/wk	157	Neutropenia (72)	41 (7)	6 mos
Garcia-Conde[3]	First-line stage IV	Vinorelbine 30 mg/m²/wk	54	Neutropenia (71)	50 (2)	9 mos
Weber[4]	First- and second-line stage IV	Vinorelbine 30 mg/m²/wk	107	Neutropenia (80)	34 (11)	34 wks
Toussaint[5]	Stage IV, up to third-line	Vinorelbine 8 mg/m², d1 (bolus) followed by: 5.5–10 mg/m²/d, d1–4 (continuous infusion)	64	Neutropenia (52.2)	36 (3)	6 mos
Ibrahim[6]	Stage IV, salvage therapy	Vinorelbine 8 mg/m², d1 (bolus) followed by: 11 mg/m²/d, d1–4 (continuous infusion)	47	Neutropenic fever Mucositis (36)	16 (2 of 44)	4.3 mos
Sorio[9]	>65 years old, stage IV	Vinorelbine 30 mg/m², d1, 8 (d1 = d21)	25	Neutropenia (37)	30 (0)	5 mos
Vogel[10]	>60 years old, stage IV	Vinorelbine 30 mg/m²/wk	56	Neutropenia (80)	38 (4)	6 mos
Fazeny[15]	Stage IV after failure with taxanes	Vinorelbine 30 mg/m², d1, 5 (then every 21 days after fourth cycle)	14	Neuropathy (4 of 14 patients)	0	–
Livingstone[13]	Stage IV, taxane-refractory	Vinorelbine 30 mg/m²/wk + G-CSF	40	Neutropenia (58)	25	13 wks
Zelek[14]	Stage IV after failure with taxanes	Vinorelbine 30 mg/m²/wk without G-CSF	40	Neutropenia (52.5) Neuropathy (12.5)	25 (0)	6 mos
Randomized trial						
Jones[12]	Stage IV after failure with anthracyclines	Vinorelbine 30 mg/m² weekly vs melphalan 25 mg/m² d1 (every 28 d)	115 / 64	Neutropenia (75) vs Neutropenia (69) Thrombocytopenia (59)	16 (5) vs 9 (2)[c]	35 wks vs 31 wks[c]

G-CSF, granulocyte colony-stimulating factor; TTP, time to progression; NA, data not available; [a]Percentages in parentheses; [b]Complete responses (%) in parentheses; [c]Statistically significant difference.

regimens, including taxanes. The absence of cross-resistance with other agents and a favourable tolerance profile make vinorelbine highly attractive for combination regimens.

MULTI-AGENT REGIMENS INCLUDING VINORELBINE

The results of the first prospective randomized phase III trial comparing a two-drug combination with vinorelbine (vinorelbine 25 mg/m² on days 1 and 8 plus doxorubicin 50 mg/m² on day 1) versus a standard FAC (5-fluorouracil, doxorubicin and cyclophosphamide) regimen were published recently.[16] A total of 177 patients (of whom 170 were evaluable) were randomly assigned to one of these two treatment arms. As response rates (74 and 75%) and median survival (17.3 and 17.8 months) were similar in each arm, the authors concluded that the activity of vinorelbine plus doxorubicin was equivalent to that of a standard three-drug schedule. The fact that only 25% of the patients in the control arm had previously received adjuvant therapy versus 52% in the investigational arm should be underscored because exposure to adjuvant therapy reduces the likelihood of achieving a response to a first-line regimen.[17] Although the authors did not find that previous adjuvant therapy had an adverse effect on response, the study population was too small really to appreciate the impact of prior exposure to anthracyclines. Noteworthy are the improved response rates and survival obtained with vinorelbine plus doxorubicin in patients with liver metastases.

Two other trials with a doxorubicin-based control arm were presented as meeting abstracts:[18,19] the most recent[19] compared vinorelbine plus mitoxantrone versus FAC, and its conclusions do not differ markedly from those of Blajman et al;[16] the National Cancer Institute of Canada trial,[18] comparing vinorelbine versus

doxorubicin versus doxorubicin alone, found no significant difference in response rates or times to failure in the preliminary analysis in 1996, but definitive results are still awaited. The last randomized trial of interest[20] compared vinorelbine 25 mg/m² on days 1 and 5 plus 5-fluorouracil 750 mg/m² per day on days 1–5 versus docetaxel 100 mg/m² every 21 days. The latter regimen can now be regarded as the gold-standard second-line therapy: the objective response rate and the duration of response were 44% and 6 months, and 54% and 8 months, respectively.

A variety of pilot studies have been published in which vinorelbine was combined with various cytotoxic agents: anthracyclines, taxanes, 5-fluorouracil, ifosfamide and mitomycin C.[22–45] They are listed in Table 9.2. They all demonstrated excellent feasibility and encouraging response rates. Whatever the regimen considered, neutropenia was the most frequent limiting toxicity, with grade 3–4 occurring in about 75% of the patients; it chiefly led to deferral of treatment and/or dose reductions rather than to febrile neutropenia, which was observed in no more than 10% of patients.

Few trials use vinorelbine-containing regimens as neoadjuvant therapy.[23,24] The provocative pathological complete response rate of 30% yielded in the series by Chollet et al[24] is among the highest ever reported in the literature at the expense of severe, although not life-threatening, hematological toxicity. Further investigations are needed to corroborate these results.

The most recent trials[39–45] combined taxanes with vinorelbine. A solid biological rationale supports such combinations because it has been suggested that resistance to taxanes could be mediated in vitro by excess depolymerized tubulin, thereby increasing the likelihood of cell death produced by vinca alkaloids.[46] The absence of cross-resistance with taxanes and encouraging response rates after failure with

Table 9.2   Vinorelbine-containing regimens

Author	Main selection criterion	Regimen[a]	No. of patients	Main grade 3–4 toxicities[b]	Response rate (%)[c]	Median duration of response (mos)
Vinorelbine + anthracycline						
Spielmann[21]	First-line stage IV	VNB 50 mg/m^2, d1, 8 DOX 50 mg/m^2, d1	89	Neutropenia (41)	74 (21)	12
Blomqvist[22]	Stage IV, dose-finding study	VNB 15 mg/m^2, d1; 20 mg/m^2, d1; 20 mg/m^2, d1, 8 (three levels) EPI 60 mg/m^2, d1	40	Neutropenia (75)[d]	60 (20)[d]	5.1
Adenis[23]	Neoadjuvant, stage II and III	VNB 25 mg/m^2, d1, 8 MXT 10 mg/m^2, d1	104	Neutropenia (83)	64% of downstaging allowing conservative surgery	–
Chollet[24]	Neoadjuvant, T > 3 cm with adverse prognostic factors	VNB 25 mg/m^2, d1, 4 THP 20 mg/m^2, d1–3 CPM 300 mg/m^2 d1–4 5-FU 400 mg/m^2 d1–4	50	Neutropenia (81) Anaemia (25) Thrombocytopenia (20)	88 (51) including pCR 30%	–
Llombart-Cussac[25]	First-line stage IV	VNB 25 mg/m^2, d1, 8 MXT 10–12 mg/m^2, d1	66	Neutropenia (46)	49 (6)	7
Baldini[26]	First-line stage IV	VNB 25 mg/m^2, d1, 8 EPI 90 mg/m^2, d1	51	Neutropenia (70)	61.7 (8.5)	10
Nistico[27]	First-line stage IV	VNB 25 mg/m^2 weekly EPI 90 mg/m^2 weekly + G-CSF	52	Neutropenia (39)	77 (19)	10
Vinorelbine + 5-fluorouracil						
Dieras[28]	First-line stage IV	VNB 30 mg/m^2, d1, 5 5-FU 750 mg/m^2, d1–5 (inf.)	63	Neutropenia (90) Mucositis (37)	61.6 (12.6)	8.4
Zambetti[29]	Previously treated stage IV	VNB 20 mg/m^2, d1, 6 5-FU 700 mg/m^2, d1–5 (inf.)	28	Neutropenia (20)	61 (14)	8
Nole[30]	First-line stage IV Phase I–II with dose-escalation	VNB 25–30 mg/m^2, d1, 3 5-FU 350 mg/m^2, d1–3 (i.v.) LV 100 mg/m^2, d1–3	45	Neutropenia (77)	62 (18)	10
Kornek[32]	First- and second-line stage IV	VNB 40 mg/m^2, d1, 14 5-FU 400 mg/m^2, d1–5 (i.v.) LLV 100 mg/m^2, d1–5 + G-CSF	53	Neutropenia (36) Mucositis (6)	First-line: 59 (13) Second-line: 19 (0)	First line: 10.5 Second-line 7

Table 9.2   Continued

Author	Main selection criterion	Regimen[a]	No. of patients	Main grade 3–4 toxicities[b]	Response rate (%)[c]	Median duration of response (mos)
Vinorelbine + alkylating agents						
Fabi[33]	Second-line stage IV	VNB 30 mg/m², d1, 8; TTP 12 mg/m², d1, 8	33	Neutropenia (72); Anaemia (48)	28 (6)	9
Campisi[34]	Anthracycline-resistant stage IV (phase I–II)	VNB 25 or 30 mg/m², d1; 25 mg/m², d1, 8; IFM 1500–2000 mg/m², d1–3	42	Neutropenia (33)	36.5 (4.8)	7
Vinorelbine + mitomycin C						
Scheithaur[35]	Second-line stage IV	VNB 30 mg/m², d1; MMC 10 mg/m², d1	34	Neutropenia (12); Thrombocytopenia (15)	35 (6)	6.3
Vici[36]		VNB 25 mg/m², d1, 8; MMC 15 mg/m², d1	60	Neutropenia (17)	40 (5)	7
Vinorelbine + CDDP						
Ray-Coquard[37]	Previously treated stage IV	VNB 6 mg/m², d1 (i.v.), 6 mg/m², d1–5 (inf.); CDDP 20 mg/m², d1–5	58	Neutropenia (78); Thrombocytopenia (12); Neuropathy (5)	41 (3)	9.2
Shamseddine[38]	Previously treated stage IV	VNB 25 mg/m², d1, 8; CDDP 30 mg/m², d1–3	23	Thrombocytopenia (27); Neutropenia (9.2)	61 (26)	4
Vinorelbine + taxanes						
Michelotti[39]	Stage IV anthracycline pre-treated	VNB 25 mg/m², d1 and 8 or 3; TXL 135 mg/m², d1	37	Neutropenia (97)	38	6.5
Fumoleau[40]	First-line stage IV Phase I dose-finding study	VNB 20–22.5 mg/m², d1, 5; TXT 60–100 mg/m², d1	27	Neutropenic fever (3 patients at third dose level)	66 (80 OR at the highest dose level)	NA
Tortoriello[41]	Pre-treated stage IV Phase I–II study	VNB 30 mg/m², d1; TXL 90–210 mg/m², d1 ±G-CSF	34	Neutropenia (2 patients at the fifth dose level); Neuropathy (3 patients at the sixth dose level)	38 (9)	12
Romero Acuna[42]	First-line stage IV	VNB 30 mg/m², d1, 8; TXL 135 mg/m², d1	49	Neutropenia (46 of 49); Neuropathy (grade 1/2: 67%; no grade 3)	60 (7)	7
Ellis[43]	Stage IV anthracycline pre-treated, dose-finding study	VNB 22.5–27.5 mg/m², d8, 15; TXL 26–32 mg/m², d1–4 (inf.) + G-CSF	32	Neutropenia (9); Neuropathy (6)	50 (22)	6.1

Reference	Stage/indication	Regimen	N	Toxicity	Response % (CR %)	Median survival
Budman[44]	Stage IV Phase I dose-finding study	VNB 7–13 mg/m², d1–3 TXL 135–200 mg/m², d3±G-CSF	28	Neutropenia (G-CSF required after first dose level) Myalgia, fatigue (with VNB 13 mg/m²/d + TXL 200 mg/m²)	12 of 25	NA
Randomized trials						
Blajman[15]	First-line stage IV	VNB 25 mg/m², d1, 8 DOX 50 mg/m², d1 vs	85	Neutropenia (7)	75 (6)	17.8
		5-FU 500 mg/m², d1 DOX 50 mg/m², d1 CPM 500 mg/m², d1	85	Neutropenia (7)	74 (13)	17.3
Norris[17]	First- and second-line stage IV	VNB 25 mg/m², d1, 8 DOX 50 mg/m², d1 vs	151	Neutropenia (86)	35 (NA)	6.9
		DOX 70 mg/m² d1	152	Neutropenia (87)	30 (NA)	6.4
Namer[18]	First-line stage IV	VNB 25 mg/m², d1, 8 MXT 12 mg/m², d1 vs	142	Neutropenia (16)	35.5 (NA)	NA
		5-FU 500 mg/m², d1 DOX or EPI 50 mg/m², d1 CPM 500 mg/m², d1	139	Neutropenia (3)	33.3 (NA)	NA[c]
Bonneterre[19]	Stage IV after failure with anthracyclines	NVB 25 mg/m², d1, 5 5-FU 750 mg/m², d1–5 (inf.) vs	45	Neutropenia (65)	44	6
		TXT 100 mg/m², d1	46	Neutropenia (78)	54	8

[a] VNB, vinorelbine; DOX, doxorubicin; EPI, epirubicin; MXT, mitoxantrone; THP, pirarubicin; 5-FU, 5-fluorouracil; LV, leucovorin; LLV, L-leucovorin; TTP, thiotepa; IFM, ifosfamide; MMC, mitomycin C; CDDP, cisplatin; TXL, paclitaxel; TXT, docetaxel; CPM, cyclophosphamide; pCR, pathological complete response; i.v., intravenous bolus; inf., infusional. [b] Percentages in parentheses. [c] Complete responses (%) in parentheses; [d] At highest dose level; [e] No significant difference.

taxanes, observed in two studies,[13,14] should be emphasized. All published trials have demonstrated that the feasibility of taxane–vinorelbine regimens is good despite severe but manageable hematological toxicity; the incidence of neuropathy is below what could have been expected (see Table 9.2). Amid the wide variety of schedules combining taxanes and vinorelbine, no particular one has proved superior in terms of either tolerance or efficiency. This fact contrasts strongly with the results of experimental studies, which demonstrated that the cytotoxicity of such combinations is exceedingly schedule-dependent.[46]

CONCLUSION

An unsolved question is whether vinorelbine should be considered as salvage chemotherapy for metastatic breast cancer or as a component of front-line combinations containing major drugs.

From the results of published trials, the following can be concluded:

- Vinorelbine is one of the most active agents against breast cancer, with a favorable tolerance profile, even in patients at risk of severe side effects such as elderly people or those with massive liver involvement (level I evidence). When used as a single agent, the schedule of choice seems to be weekly administration at a starting dose of 30 mg/m^2 per week. However, this dose does not appear to be feasible in pretreated patients, mainly because of delays in hematological recovery (level II evidence).
- No cross-resistance is observed with other major drugs (i.e. taxanes and anthracyclines) and vinorelbine is valuable as salvage therapy even in taxane-refractory patients (level I evidence), although it is less effective than docetaxel given as second-line therapy after

failure with anthracyclines (level I evidence). These facts, together with its tolerance profile, provide a clinical rationale for first-line combination regimens.
- Regimens combining vinorelbine and other agents are readily feasible and as effective as other standard chemotherapy combinations (level I evidence). In such regimens, vinorelbine was usually given at a dose of 20–30 mg/m^2 on days 1 and 3, 5 or 8 with optional G-CSF support. Whether one combination has an edge over the others remains to be established.

ACKNOWLEDGEMENT

The authors are grateful to Lorna Saint Ange for editorial assistance.

REFERENCES

1. Marty M, Extra JM, Dieras V, Espie M, Ohana-Leandri S, Vinorelbine. In: Cvitkovic E, Droz JP, Armand JP, Khoury S, eds. *Handbook of Chemotherapy in Clinical Oncology*. Jersey: Scientific Communication International, 1993: 317–26.
2. Fumoleau P, Delgado FM, Delozier T et al, Phase II trial of weekly intravenous vinorelbine in first-line advanced breast cancer chemotherapy. *J Clin Oncol* 1993; **11**:1245–52.
3. Garcia-Conde J, Lluch A, Martin M et al, Phase II trial of weekly IV vinorelbine in first-line advanced breast cancer chemotherapy. *Ann Oncol* 1994; **5**:854–7.
4. Weber BL, Vogel C, Jones S et al, Intravenous vinorelbine as first-line and second-line therapy in advanced breast cancer. *J Clin Oncol* 1995; **13**:2722–30.
5. Toussaint C, Izzo J, Spielmann M et al, Phase I/II trial of continuous infusion vinorelbine for advanced breast cancer. *J Clin Oncol* 1994; **12**:2102–12.

6. Ibrahim NK, Rahman Z, Valero V et al, Phase II study of vinorelbine administered by 96-hour infusion in patients with advanced breast carcinoma. *Cancer* 1999; **86**:1251–7.

7. Havlin KA, Ramirez MJ, Legler CM et al, Inability to escalate vinorelbine dose intensity using a daily ×3 schedule with and without filgrastim in patients with metastatic breast cancer. *Cancer Chemother Pharmacol* 1999; **43**:68–72.

8. Bertsch LA, Donaldson G, Quality of life analyses from vinorelbine (Navelbine) clinical trials of women with metastatic breast cancer. *Semin Oncol* 1995; **22**(Suppl 5):45–53; discussion 53–4.

9. Sorio R, Robieux I, Galligoni E et al, Pharmacokinetics and tolerance of vinorelbine in elderly patients with metastatic breast cancer. *Eur J Cancer* 1997; **33**:301–3.

10. Vogel C, O'Rourke M, Winer E et al. Vinorelbine as first-line chemotherapy for advanced breast cancer in women 60 years of age or older. *Ann Oncol* 1999; **10**:397–402.

11. Robieux I, Sorio R, Borsatti E et al, Pharmacokinetics of vinorelbine in patients with liver metastases. *Clin Pharmacol Ther* 1996; **59**: 32–40.

12. Jones S, Winer E, Vogel C et al, Randomized comparison of vinorelbine and melphalan in anthracycline-refractory advanced breast cancer. *J Clin Oncol* 1995; **13**:2567–74.

13. Livingston RB, Ellis GK, Gralow JR et al, Dose-intensive vinorelbine with concurrent granulocyte colony-stimulating factor support in paclitaxel-refractory metastatic breast cancer. *J Clin Oncol* 1997; **15**:1395–400.

14. Zelek L, Barthier S, Delord JP et al, Results of weekly vinorelbine after failure with taxanes in advanced breast cancer. *Breast Cancer Res Treat* 1999; **57**:89.

15. Fazeny B, Zifko U, Meryn S, Huber H, Grisold W, Dittrich C, Vinorelbine-induced neurotoxicity in patients with advanced breast cancer pretreated with paclitaxel – a phase II study. *Cancer Chemother Pharmacol* 1996; **39**:150–6.

16. Blajman C, Balbiani L, Block J et al, A prospective, randomized phase III trial comparing combination chemotherapy with cyclophosphamide, doxorubicin, and 5-fluorouracil with vinorelbine plus doxorubicin in the treatment of advanced breast carcinoma. *Cancer* 1999; **85**:1091–7.

17. Bonadonna G, Valagussa P, Moliterni A, Zambetti M, Brambilla C, Adjuvant cyclophosphamide, methotrexate, and fluorouracil in node-positive breast cancer: the results of 20 years of follow-up. *N Engl J Med* 1995; **332**:901–6.

18. Norris B, Pritchard K, James K et al, A phase III comparative study of vinorelbine (VNB) combined with doxorubicin (DOX) versus doxorubicin alone in metastatic/recurrent breast cancer (MBC): A National Cancer Institute of Canada (NCIC CTG) study. *Proc Am Soc Clin Oncol* 1996; **15**:A59.

19. Namer M, Soler-Michel P, Turpin F et al, Prospective randomized study comparing mitoxantrone (M) and vinorelbine (V) with fluorouracil (F), epirubicin (E) or Adriamycin (A) and cyclophosphamide (C) in patients with metastatic breast cancer). *Proc Am Soc Clin Oncol* 1997; **16**:A520.

20. Bonneterre J, Roche H, Monnier A et al. Taxotere (TXT) versus 5-fluorouracil + Navelbine (FUN) as second-line chemotherapy (CT) in patients (pts) with metastatic breast cancer (MBC) (preliminary results). *Proc Am Soc Clin Oncol* 1997; **16**:A564.

21. Spielmann M, Dorval T, Turpin F et al, Phase II trial of vinorelbine/doxorubicin as first-line therapy of advanced breast cancer. *J Clin Oncol* 1994; **12**:1764–70.

22. Blomqvist C, Hietanen P, Teerenhovi L, Rissanen P, Vinorelbine and epirubicin in metastatic breast cancer. A dose finding study. *Eur J Cancer* 1995; **31A**:2406–8.

23. Adenis A, Vanlemmens L, Fournier C, Hecquet B, Bonneterre J, Does induction chemotherapy with a mitoxantrone/vinorelbine regimen allow a breast-conservative treat-

ment in patients with operable locoregional breast cancer? A French Northern Oncology Group Trial in 105 patients. French Northern Oncology Group. *Breast Cancer Res Treat* 1996; **40**:161–9.

24. Chollet P, Charrier S, Brain E et al, Clinical and pathological response to primary chemotherapy in operable breast cancer. *Eur J Cancer* 1997; **33**:862–6.

25. Llombart-Cussac A, Pivot X, Rhor-Alvarado A et al, First-line vinorelbine–mitoxantrone combination in metastatic breast cancer patients relapsing after an adjuvant anthracycline regimen: results of a phase II study. *Oncology* 1998; **55**:384–90.

26. Baldini E, Tibaldi C, Chiavacci F et al, Epirubicin/vinorelbine as first line therapy in metastatic breast cancer. *Breast Cancer Res Treat* 1998; **49**:129–34.

27. Nistico C, Garufi C, Barni S et al, Phase II study of epirubicin and vinorelbine with granulocyte colony-stimulating factor: a high-activity, dose-dense weekly regimen for advanced breast cancer. *Ann Oncol* 1999; **10**:937–42.

28. Dieras V, Extra JM, Bellissant E et al, Efficacy and tolerance of vinorelbine and fluorouracil combination as first-line chemotherapy of advanced breast cancer: results of a phase II study using a sequential group method. *J Clin Oncol* 1996; **14**:3097–104.

29. Zambetti M, Demicheli R, De Candis D et al, Five-day infusion fluorouracil plus vinorelbine i.v. in metastatic pretreated breast cancer patients. *Breast Cancer Res Treat* 1997; **44**:255–60.

30. Nole F, de Braud F, Aapro M et al, Phase I–II study of vinorelbine in combination with 5-fluorouracil and folinic acid as first-line chemotherapy in metastatic breast cancer: a regimen with a low subjective toxic burden. *Ann Oncol* 1997; **8**:865–70.

31. Goss PE, Fine S, Gelmon K et al, Phase I studies of fluorouracil, doxorubicin and vinorelbine without (FAN) and with (SUPER-FAN) folinic acid in patients with advanced breast cancer. *Cancer Chemother Pharmacol* 1997; **41**:53–60.

32. Kornek GV, Haider K, Kwasny W et al, Effective treatment of advanced breast cancer with vinorelbine, 5-fluorouracil and l-leucovorin plus human granulocyte colony-stimulating factor. *Br J Cancer* 1998; **78**:673–8.

33. Fabi A, Tonachella R, Savarese A et al, A phase II trial of vinorelbine and thiotepa in metastatic breast cancer. *Ann Oncol* 1995; **6**:187–9.

34. Campisi C, Fabi A, Papaldo P et al, Ifosfamide given by continuous-intravenous infusion in association with vinorelbine in patients with anthracycline-resistant metastatic breast cancer: a phase I–II clinical trial. *Ann Oncol* 1998; **9**:565–7.

35. Scheithauer W, Kornek G, Haider K et al, Effective second line chemotherapy of advanced breast cancer with navelbine and mitomycin C. *Breast Cancer Res Treat* 1993; **26**:49–53.

36. Vici P, Di Lauro L, Carpano S et al, Vinorelbine and mitomycin C in anthracycline-pretreated patients with advanced breast cancer. *Oncology* 1996; **53**:16–18.

37. Ray-Coquard I, Biron P, Bachelot T et al, Vinorelbine and cisplatin (CIVIC regimen) for the treatment of metastatic breast carcinoma after failure of anthracycline- and/or paclitaxel-containing regimens. *Cancer* 1998; **82**:134–40.

38. Shamseddine AI, Taher A, Dabaja B, Dandashi A, Salem Z, El Saghir NS, Combination cisplatin–vinorelbine for relapsed and chemotherapy-pretreated metastatic breast cancer. *Am J Clin Oncol* 1999; **22**:298–302.

39. Michelotti A, Gennari A, Salvadori B et al, Paclitaxel and vinorelbine in anthracycline-pretreated breast cancer: a phase II study. *Ann Oncol* 1996; **7**:857–60.

40. Fumoleau P, Fety R, Delecroix V, Perrocheau G, Azli N, Docetaxel combined with vinorelbine: phase I results and new study designs. *Oncology (Huntingt)* 1997; **11**(Suppl 6):29–31.

41. Tortoriello A, Facchini G, Caponigro F et al, Phase I/II study of paclitaxel and vinorelbine in metastatic breast cancer. *Breast Cancer Res Treat* 1998; **47**:91–7.

42. Romero Acuna L, Langhi M et al, Vinorelbine and paclitaxel as first-line chemotherapy in metastatic breast cancer. *J Clin Oncol* 1999; **17**:74–81.

43. Georgiana K, Gralow H, Ellis JR et al, Infusional paclitaxel and weekly vinorelbine chemotherapy with concurrent filgrastim for metastatic breast cancer: high complete response rate in a phase I–II study of doxorubicin-treated patients. *J Clin Oncol* 1999; **17**:1407–12.

44. Budman DR, Weiselberg L, O'Mara V et al, A phase I study of sequential vinorelbine followed by paclitaxel. *Ann Oncol* 1999; **10**: 861–3.

45. Lokich JJ, Anderson N, Bern M, Coco F, Dow E, The multifractionated, twice-weekly dose schedule for a three-drug chemotherapy regimen: a phase I–II study of paclitaxel, cisplatin, and vinorelbine. *Cancer* 1999; **85**: 499–503.

46. Kano Y, Akutsu M, Suzuki K, Ando J, Tsunoda S, Schedule-dependent interactions between vinorelbine and paclitaxel in human carcinoma cell lines in vitro. *Breast Cancer Res Treat* 1999; **56**:79–90.

10

Liposomal doxorubicin in the treatment of metastatic breast cancer

Michael Smylie

Doxorubicin was discovered and introduced into clinical practice in the late 1960s. It remains the most commonly used anthracycline, and one of the most active agents in metastatic breast cancer (MBC).[1] Single-agent response rates vary from 30% to 50% in MBC. When anthracycline and non-anthracycline regimens are compared, the anthracycline-containing regimens have shown greater response rate, duration of response and time to progression, and a significant improvement in survival.[2] The recent overview analyses of randomized clinical trials in adjuvant breast cancer patients have shown that anthracycline-containing regimens produced a greater reduction of recurrence and mortality rates when compared with non-anthracycline-containing regimens.[3]

The antitumor effects of doxorubicin are exerted through a variety of mechanisms, including intercalation with DNA, inhibition of topoisomerases I and II, membrane binding, metal chelation and through the generation of free radicals.[4] Maximal toxicity occurs during the S phase of the cell cycle.

The optimum schedule of doxorubicin has yet to be defined. The drug can be given as an intravenous bolus every 3 weeks, as a weekly bolus or as a prolonged infusion. Theoretically, prolonged infusions of doxorubicin would be most effective; however, response rates in phase II trials have been disappointing. The only randomized trial comparing doxorubicin given as a 3-weekly bolus versus a weekly bolus versus a prolonged infusion was closed as a result of poor accrual.[5] There is a clear dose–response relationship with doxorubicin, albeit at the cost of significant toxicity.[6] Trials of prolonged infusions of doxorubicin (48–96 hours) have been shown to significantly reduce the incidence and severity of cardiac toxicity at equivalent dose levels.[7]

The dose-limiting toxicity with anthracyclines is myelosuppression; however, other acute toxicities include nausea/vomiting, alopecia, mucositis, risk of extravasation injury, and both acute and chronic cardiac toxicity. Acute cardiac toxicity is rare but can manifest as arrythmias, pericarditis/myocarditis and acute heart failure. The most worrisome toxicity is the cumulative dose-dependent cardiomyopathy that can lead to congestive heart failure. The risk can vary from 7% to 42% of patients receiving a total dose of 550 and 900 mg/m^2 by bolus, respectively.[4,8]

The cardiac toxicity is related to peak plasma levels of doxorubicin and, although the exact causal mechanism of the cardiomyopathy is unclear, most of the available evidence suggests that free-radical formation is involved.[9] Once formed, these free radicals interact with iron molecules, causing a multitude of cellular effects such as lipid peroxidation of mitochondrial membranes, and thus myocyte damage. Histologic changes include a variety of subcellular alternatives such as loss of myofibrils, distension of the sarcoplasmic reticulum and vacuolization of myocardial cells.

A variety of approaches have been used in an attempt to reduce cardiac toxicity. As cardiac toxicity is related to peak plasma levels, one approach is to use prolonged infusions, thereby decreasing the peak levels of drug, and this shift in delivery has led to a reduced incidence of cardiac toxicity and allows higher cumulative doses of doxorubicin.

A second approach is to augment normal cellular defences against free radical damage by using exogeneous antioxidants such as α-tocopherol or by using an iron chelator such as ADR-529 or amifostine.[10]

Newer analogs of doxorubicin such as epirubicin, and a related anthracenedione, mitoxantrone, have shown clinical efficacy with less cardiotoxicity.[11] In a randomized trial comparing doxorubicin with mitoxantrone the reported response rate to mitoxantrone was 20.6% versus 29.3% for doxorubicin, although mitoxantrone was less toxic.[12]

A fourth approach is to use a carrier system such as a liposome. Liposomes form spontaneously when phospholipids are placed in water, and can be loaded with a variety of drugs.[13,14] There are three compartments in the liposome in which drugs can be loaded. The first is the aqueous core, which is the desired locus for water-soluble drugs; the second is the lipid-rich membrane, which is the desired locus for fat-soluble drugs; the last is the interface between the lipid-soluble membrane and the adjacent water, in which small molecules, such as peptides and small proteins, can be loaded. A whole spectrum of drug release rates can be engineered into these structures. As an example, selection of highly unsaturated fatty acids increases the rate of drug release, whereas selection of saturated fatty acids and cholesterol slows the rate of drug release. With the advent of the commercial liposome industry in the early 1980s, two major problems were identified. The first was to prepare stable drug-loaded liposomes in a reproducible manner; the second major obstacle was pharmacologic. By virtue of the fact that liposomes are opsonized by plasma proteins, they are recognized as 'foreign' and are rapidly broken down by cells of the reticuloendothelial system (RES), thereby decreasing their plasma half-life. To overcome this problem, investigators began looking for ways to avoid liposome breakdown by cells of the RES. Allen and Chonn[15] demonstrated that coating liposomes with specialized glycolipids (GM1) prolonged circulation time. Scientists at Sequus Pharmaceuticals demonstrated that methoxypolyethylene glycol (MPEG), a hydrophilic polymer, could be engrafted on to the surface of the liposome, and this altered liposome demonstrated prolonged longevity in the circulation.

There are currently two liposomal preparations of doxorubicin, and one liposomal daunorubicin, undergoing clinical development in breast cancer. A pegylated liposomal doxorubicin, Caelyx (Doxil), is approved for Kaposi's sarcoma, and a non-pegylated liposomal doxorubicin, TLC D-99 (Evacet), is being evaluated in MBC.

Preclinical studies with doxorubicin-containing, MPEG-coated liposomes showed more activity on a dose-equivalent basis than either free doxorubicin or non-pegylated doxorubicin-containing liposomes. These new liposomes are remarkably stable in the circulation, and can circulate intact for many days. Ulti-

Table 10.1   Billingham scale for grading anthracycline-induced cardiomyopathy

Biopsy grade	Morphology
0	No evidence of anthracycline-specific damage
0.5	Not completely normal but no evidence of anthracycline-specific damage
1.0	Isolated myocytes affected and/or early myofibrillar loss; damage to 5% of all cells
1.5	Changes similar to grade 1 except with damage to 6–15% of all cells
2.0	Clusters of myocytes affected by myofibrillar loss and/or vacuolization, with damage to 16–25% of all cells
2.5	Many myocytes, 26–35% of all cells, affected by vacuolization and/or myofibrillar loss
3.0	Severe diffuse myocyte damage (>35% of all cells)

mately, the liposomes are removed by macrophages but at a relatively slow rate, and not by the macrophages attached to blood vessels, but by those residing in the tissues. MPEG-coated liposomes are relatively small, with a diameter of approximately 100 nm. This small size allows them to circulate freely and to extravasate through endothelial gaps in the capillary.

In a pilot pharmacokinetics trial using an early version of Caelyx, patients were crossed over from Caelyx 50 mg/m^2 to free doxorubicin. Caelyx showed a prolonged circulation time, with a half-life of approximately 50 hours. In the same study, investigators also showed that doxorubicin was not released from the liposome during the prolonged circulation time into the plasma. The volume of distribution at steady state (V_{ss}, in L/m^2) was only slightly greater than the plasma volume, indicating that the liposomes were clearly confined during their plasma distribution to the central compartment. This is in contrast to conventional doxorubicin, which has a volume of distribution that includes virtually the entire body (approximately 1000 litres in humans). The area under the curve (AUC) for Caelyx is hundreds of times greater than that of equivalent doses of conventional doxorubicin.

Liposomal encapsulation of anthracyclines lowers peak plasma levels of free drug, and a variety of animal models have shown a decrease in cardiac toxicity. Non-invasive methods of monitoring cardiac toxicity, such as left ventricular ejection fraction (LVEF), and clinical examination are used most frequently to monitor for signs of heart failure. However, considerable irreversible heart damage must occur before these tests indicate abnormality. The diagnostic test with the greatest specificity and sensitivity for doxorubicin-induced cardiomyopathy is endomyocardial biopsy. These histologic changes can be graded on a scale of 1–3 to quantify the amount of doxorubicin-induced damage (Table 10.1).

A paper by Berry et al[16] reported a reduced cardiotoxicity with pegylated liposomal doxorubicin. Myocardial biopsies from 10 patients with AIDS-related Kaposi's sarcoma (AIDS-KS) who had received cumulative Caelyx doses (20 mg/m^2 every 2 weeks) of 440–840 mg/m^2 were compared with historical controls assembled from patients who had received cumulative doses of conventional doxorubicin of 174–671 mg/m² in two earlier cardiac biopsy protocols. Two control groups were selected based on both cumulative and peak doxorubicin dose (60 or 20 mg/m², group 1) or peak dose alone (20 mg/m², group 2). Median biopsy scores for the pegylated liposomal doxorubicin and doxorubicin groups, respectively, were 0.3 versus 3.0 ($p = 0.002$, Cochran–Mantel–Haenszel row mean difference test) for group 1 and 1.25 for group 2 ($p < 0.001$, Wilcoxon rank-sum test). MPEG-coated liposomes, because of their small size, can extravasate through capillary endothelial junctions. Tumor capillaries are more leaky than their normal tissue counterparts. Therefore more liposomes should extravasate into tumors, thereby giving increased drug concentration to the tumor tissue. Northfield showed that biopsies of AIDS-KS lesions in patients pretreated with Caelyx had several-fold higher concentrations in the tumor tissue than in the normal skin. The difference was highest 46 hours after dosing.

The results of two phase I trials of Caelyx in solid tumors have recently been reported.[17] Antitumor activity was seen in breast cancer, prostate cancer, non-small cell lung cancer, renal cell carcinoma, head and neck cancer, and ovarian carcinoma. A phase II trial of Caelyx in MBC was recently reported by Ranson et al.[18] Based on the prior phase I studies, a Caelyx dose of 60 mg/m² given every 3 weeks was chosen. The objectives were to define the safety and tolerability of Caelyx and to obtain preliminary data on its antitumor activity in MBC.

Patients enrolled in the study had histologically confirmed MBC. They were also allowed to have had one prior chemotherapy, provided that it did not contain anthracyclines. Seven of the first 13 patients developed palmar–plantar erythrodysthesia of grade ≥3 after multiple cycles of

treatment, and the dose was reduced to 45 mg/m² every 3 weeks. A subsequent detailed analysis of the phase I data suggested that the development of skin toxicity may be particularly influenced by dosing interval; thus, a third cohort of patients was treated at a dose of 45 mg/m² every 4 weeks. Of the patients evaluable for response, 6% obtained a complete response and 25% a partial response, for an overall response rate of 31%. The median overall survival was 7 months, and the median time to disease progression was 9 months in responding patients. Myelosuppression, alopecia, nausea and vomiting were seen but were mild. The most significant toxicities were palmar–plantar erythrodysthesia and mucositis. In all cases, the skin toxicity was reversible.

Although this study was not designed to assess cardiac toxicity, extensive preclinical data support the notion that liposomal preparations are associated with reduced cardiac toxicity. Based on these encouraging results, a phase III trial was designed to compare Caelyx in advanced MBC patients who were refractory to taxanes with a standard comparator such as vinorelbine or mitomycin C/vinblastine. The primary endpoint was to compare progression-free survival, with secondary endpoints to compare overall response rate, response duration, overall survival and tolerability. This study has completed accrual and results are pending.

The pivotal trial to assess the activity of Caelyx in MBC is currently under way. This trial will accrue a total of 400 patients worldwide and will randomize them to either Caelyx 50 mg/m² or single-agent doxorubicin 60 mg/m². Patients will be randomized according to the following parameters: previous anthracycline therapy, WHO performance status (0–1 versus 2) and presence of bone metastases only. The primary objective of this trial will be to compare the time to disease progression of Caelyx versus doxorubicin as first-line treatment of women with MBC. Secondary objectives are to compare response rate, overall survival time, time to treatment failure, toxicity, clinical benefit response, quality of life and health care utilization of Caelyx versus doxorubicin. At the time of writing, the trial is about half-way to accrual.

Several other phase I/II trials are under way to assess Caelyx-containing regimens. Drugs that are currently being evaluated in combination with Caelyx include cyclophosphamide, vinorelbine, paclitaxel and docetaxel.[19–22] The feasibility of combining Caelyx with Herceptin is also being explored.

Two other liposomal preparations of doxorubicin are also undergoing clinical development. TLC D-99 (Evacet), manufactured by the Liposome Company, is a liposomal-encapsulated form of doxorubicin that incorporates doxorubicin loading by generating an electropotential gradient across the liposome membrane. This mechanism for remote loading involves the generation of a pH gradient between the inside of the liposome and the extraliposomal buffer, which acts to pull the doxorubicin into the vesicle. Evacet does not contain a polyethylene coating and has been shown to concentrate in organs rich in reticuloendothelial cells.

A phase I trial of TLC D-99 performed at Roswell Park Memorial Institute demonstrated that the dose-limiting toxicity was myelosuppression.[23] Other toxicities such as gastrointestinal distress (i.e. nausea and vomiting, diarrhea), alopecia, malaise, rigors and fever were mild. No cardiac toxicity was seen. An open-label, non-randomized trial of TLC D-99 75 mg/m^2 to 32 patients resulted in an overall response rate of 56%. Toxicity was tolerable, with 10 patients (31%) having grade 4 leukopenia and 1 (3%) having grade 4 thrombocytopenia. Grade 3 mucositis occurred in 10% of the patients.

A recent phase II trial of TLC D-99 in combination with 5-fluorouracil and cyclophosphamide has been reported;[24] 41 patients were enrolled and were treated with TLC D-99 60 mg/m^2, cyclophosphamide 500 mg/m^2 on day 1 every 21 days, and 5-fluorouracil 500 mg/m^2 on days 1 and 8 every 21 days. The overall objective response rate was 73% and the median overall survival duration was 19.4 months. Myelosuppression was the most common adverse event causing dose delays and dose reductions; in addition, 17 patients developed neutropenic fever. Cardiac toxicity was low despite the high cumulative doxorubicin dose. No cases of congestive heart failure (CHF) were seen during the study, although one patient developed CHF during the follow-up period that was not felt to be anthracycline-induced. Unlike liposomes with an MPEG coating, no cases of palmar–plantar erythrodysthesia were encountered.

A new-drug application for approval of Evacet as first-line treatment of MBC in combination with cyclophosphamide was submitted to the US Food and Drug Administration (FDA).[25] Two multicenter, randomized, parallel, open-label, phase III trials were submitted in support of this application. In study 1 of 297 patients, the combination of Evacet 60 mg/m^2 and cyclophosphamide 600 mg/m^2 was compared with the combination of doxorubicin 60 mg/m^2 and cyclophosphamide 600 mg/m^2. The overall response rate was 44% (62 of 142) for the Evacet arm and 43% (67 of 155) for the doxorubicin arm (relative risk, RR 1.01; 95% confidence interval, 95%CI 0.78–1.34; $p > 0.9$). The median overall survival was 21.2 months for the Evacet arm and 16.4 months for the doxorubicin arm (hazard ratio, HR 1.01; 95%CI 0.71–1.43; $p > 0.9$). The time to progression was 5.6 months for the Evacet arm and 6 months for the doxorubicin arm (HR 1.07; 95%CI 0.81–1.41; log-rank $p = 0.65$). In study 2 in 224 patients, Evacet 75 mg/m^2 was compared with doxorubicin

75 mg/m^2. Dose escalation was allowed in this trial. The response rate was 26% (28 of 108) for the Evacet arm and 26% (30 of 116) for the doxorubicin arm (RR 1.003; 95%CI 0.62–1.68; $p = 0.9$). The median overall survival was 14.6 months for the Evacet arm and 20.1 months for the doxorubicin arm (HR 0.75; 95%CI 0.54–1.03; $p = 0.07$). The time to progression was 3.8 months for the Evacet arm and 4.3 months for the doxorubicin arm (HR 0.91; 95%CI 0.66–1.26; log-rank $p = 0.58$).

In both study 1 and study 2, Evacet showed less cardiac toxicity. In addition, there was less mucositis and diarrhea associated with Evacet than with doxorubicin. The incidence of neutropenic fever, thrombocytopenia and grade 3 or 4 vomiting was similar for both drugs.

The Committee agreed that the clinical studies demonstrated that Evacet is significantly less cardiotoxic than doxorubicin. In addition, the Committee agreed that study 1 demonstrated the efficacy of Evacet in combination with cyclophosphamide in the first-line treatment of MBC. In study 2, although the response rates were similar for Evacet and doxorubicin, the criteria established for formal equivalence were not met. Given that the study also demonstrated a trend towards a more favorable survival in association with doxorubicin, the Committee indicated that it could not rely on response rates alone as a demonstration of the efficacy of Evacet. The Committee voted against recommending the approval of Evacet for the first-line treatment of MBC because of the failure of study 2 to replicate the efficacy of Evacet that was demonstrated in study 1. The Committee was concerned that the data did not allow it to conclude with confidence that the liposomal formulation, although less cardiotoxic, was not also less efficacious in treating breast cancer.

Daunorubicin, a related anthracycline, has also been prepared as a liposomal preparation, DaunoXome.[26] Although daunorubicin is used primarily in hematologic malignancies, DaunoXome has been evaluated in MBC and has shown encouraging activity.[27] Similar to Caelyx and TLC D-99, DaunoXome has shown no significant alopecia or cardiac toxicity. Nausea and vomiting were mild to moderate, as was hematologic toxicity.

In summary, liposome-encapsulated doxorubicin exhibits a very different toxicity profile to free doxorubicin. Whereas the dose-limiting toxicity of free doxorubicin is myelosuppression, that of Caelyx is mucositis and palmar–plantar erythrodysthesia. Other chemotherapy side effects that are distressing to patients, such as alopecia, nausea and vomiting, were also uncommon and when present tended to be mild. More importantly, cardiac toxicity was rarely seen, which was probably the result of minimal free doxorubicin released into the circulation. The phase II study of Caelyx reported by Ranson et al[18] yielded a response rate of 31% in patients with MBC. This response rate is on the low side of response rates reported by other phase II studies for free doxorubicin, but is similar to the recent response rate reported by Chan et al in their phase III study of doxorubicin versus docetaxel.[19] The patient population in Ranson's study also included patients who had received prior non-anthracycline-based chemotherapy for metastatic disease and two or more lines of hormonal therapy, and many patients had three or more sites of disease and a high incidence of visceral metastases. Unfortunately, mucositis and palmar–plantar erythrodysthesia limit the ability to dose-escalate Caelyx and it is not clear whether Caelyx at its present recommended dose is dose-equivalent to free doxorubicin. The current phase III trial comparing Caelyx with free doxorubicin should better define the true activity of Caelyx compared with doxorubicin, and thus its place in our armentarium of breast cancer chemotherapy drugs. If, indeed, Caelyx is dose-equivalent to doxorubicin, then there is the potential for Caelyx to replace doxorubicin. In adjuvant patients, a drug without the potential for cardiac toxicity would be particularly attractive.

Likewise, both TLC D-99 and DaunoXome have shown encouraging results in MBC, with a corresponding decrease in cardiac toxicity, but, as with Caelyx, further studies are warranted to define their activity better.

Liposomes offer a unique carrier system for cytotoxic agents that drastically change their pharmacokinetic parameters and their toxicities. To date, however, their true efficacy is unproven and further studies are warranted in solid tumors such as breast cancer before their routine use can be advocated.

REFERENCES

1. Honing SF, Treatment of metastatic disease, hormonal therapy and chemotherapy. In: Harris JR, Lippman ME, Morrow M, Hellman S, eds. *Breast Diseases*. Philadelphia: JB Lippincott, 1996: 669–734.

2. A'Hern RP, Smith IE, Ebbs SR, Chemotherapy and survival in advanced breast cancer: The inclusion of doxorubicin in Cooper type regimens. *Br J Cancer* 1993; **67**:801–5.

3. Early Breast Cancer Trialists' Collaborative Group, Polychemotherapy for early breast cancer: An overview of the randomised trials. *Lancet* 1998; **352**:930–42.

4. Shan K, Lincoff AM, Young JB, Anthracycline-induced cardiotoxicity. *Ann Intern Med* 1996; **125**:47–58.

5. Lokich J, Auerbach M, Smith L et al, A comparative trial of three schedules for single-agent doxorubicin in advanced breast cancer: An aborted investigation. *J Infus Chemother* 1992; **2**(4):185–92.

6. Jones RB, Holland JF, Bhardwaj S et al, A

7. Ewer MS, Benjamin RS, Cardiac complications. In: Holland JF, Frei III E, Bast RC Jr et al, eds. *Cancer Medicine*, 3rd edn. Baltimore: Williams & Wilkins, 1997; 3197–215.

8. Legha SS, Benjamin RS, Mackay B et al, Reduction of doxorubicin cardiotoxicity by prolonged continuous intravenous infusion. *Ann Intern Med* 1982; **96**:133–9.

9. Singal P, Iliskovic N, Doxorubicin-induced cardiomyopathy. *N Engl J Med* 1998; **13**: 900–5.

10. Hochster H, Wasserheit C, Speyer J, Cardiotoxicity and cardioprotection during chemotherapy. *Curr Opin Oncol* 1995; **7**: 304–9.

11. Von Hoff DD, Layard MW, Basa P et al, Risk factors for doxorubicin-induced congestive heart failure. *Ann Intern Med* 1979; **91**:710–17.

12. Henderson C, Allegra J, Woodcock T et al, Randomized clinical trials comparing mitoxantrone with doxorubicin in previously treated patients with metastatic breast cancer. *J Clin Oncol* 1989; **7**:560–71.

13. Martin FH, STEALTH® Liposome Technology: An Overview. DOXIL Clinical Series 1: 1–11, 1997.

14. Gabizon A, Goren D, Cohen R, Barenholz Y, Development of liposomal anthracyclines: from basics to clinical applications. *J Controlled Release* 1998; **53**:275–9.

15. Allen TM, Chonn A, Large unilamellar liposomes with low uptake by the reticuloendothelial system. *FEBS Lett* 1987; **223**:42–6.

16. Berry G, Billingham M, Alderman E et al, The use of cardiac biopsy to demonstrate reduced cardiotoxicity in AIDS Kaposi's sarcoma patients treated with pegylated liposomal doxorubicin. *Ann Oncol* 1998; **9**:711–16.

17. Uziely B, Jeffers S, Isacson R et al, Liposomal doxorubicin: antitumor activity and unique toxicities during two complementary phase I studies. *J Clin Oncol* 1995; **13**:1777–85.

phase I–II study of intensive-dose Adriamycin for advanced breast cancer. *J Clin Oncol* 1987; **5**:172–7.

18. Ranson MR, Carmichael J, O'Byrne K et al, Treatment of advanced breast cancer with sterically stabilized liposomal doxorubicin: results of a multicenter phase II trial. *J Clin Oncol* 1997; **15**:3185–91.

19. Chan S, Friedrichs K, Noel D et al, Prospective randomized trial of docetaxel versus doxorubicin in patients with metastatic breast cancer. The 303 Study Group. *J Clin Oncol* 1999; **17**:2341–54.

20. Israel VK, Jeffers S, Gernal G et al, Phase I study of Doxil® (liposomal doxorubicin) in combination with paclitaxel. *Proc Am Soc Clin Oncol* 1997; **842**:239a.

21. Burstein HJ, Ramirez MF, Petros WP et al, Phase I study of Doxil and vinorelbine in metastatic breast cancer. *Ann Oncol* 1999; **10**:1113–16.

22. Sparano JA, Wolffe A, Phase I trial of liposomal doxorubicin (Doxil) and docetaxel (Taxotere) in patients (pts) with advanced breast cancer (ABC). *Proc Am Soc Clin Oncol* 1998; **672**:175a.

23. Cowens JW, Creaven PJ, Greco WR et al, Initial clinical (phase I) trial of TLC D-99 (doxorubicin encapsulated in liposomes). *Cancer Res* 1993; **53**:2796–802.

24. Valero V, Buzdar A, Theriault R et al, Phase II trial of liposome-encapsulated doxorubicin, cyclophosphamide and fluorouracil as first-line therapy in patients with metastatic breast cancer. *J Clin Oncol* 1999; **17**:1425–34.

25. Cortazar P, Williams G, Evacet (doxorubicin HCl liposome injection), the Liposome Company. FDA Report: Oncologic Drugs Advisory Committee (ODAC) Meeting, September 1999; 16–17.

26. Gill PS, Espina BM, Cabriales S et al, Phase I/II clinical and pharmacokinetic evaluation of liposomal daunorubicin. *J Clin Oncol* 1995; **13**:996–1003.

27. Darskaia EI, Zubarovskaia LS, Afanas'ev BV, Administration of liposomal preparation of DaunoXome for breast cancer in patients with poor prognosis. *Vopr Onkol* 1999; **45**:440–4.

11

Capecitabine in the treatment of metastatic breast cancer

Joyce A O'Shaughnessy

Approximately 35% of women who develop breast cancer will recur with clinically overt metastatic disease and will generally require continued therapy during their remaining life. Although the median survival for metastatic breast cancer is 2–3 years, the natural history of this disease is highly heterogeneous and about 15% of patients will survive 5 years. As metastatic breast cancer is incurable, careful attention must be paid to sequencing therapies to maximize patients' overall survival, functional status, quality of life and freedom from tumor-related symptoms.

Combination chemotherapy has not been shown to be associated with improved patient outcomes compared with the sequential administration of effective chemotherapy agents.[1,2] Administering effective single agents sequentially has become a common approach to treating metastatic breast cancer because of the balance achieved between tumor control and improvement in tumor-related symptoms, on the one hand, and therapy-related toxicities, on the other.[3]

The anthracyclines and taxanes have historically been considered the most active agents for treating breast cancer. With the increasing use of anthracyclines as adjuvant chemotherapy for early stage breast cancer, single-agent paclitaxel or docetaxel has become a common choice for first-line therapy of metastatic disease. Several studies have shown retained antitumor activity of paclitaxel and docetaxel in patients whose breast cancers have progressed with anthracycline treatment.[4,5] Less clear, however, is what the optimal choice of second- or third-line chemotherapy agent is in a patient whose breast cancer has been previously treated with both an anthracycline and a taxane. Before the approval of capecitabine by the US Food and Drug Administration (FDA) in 1998, no chemotherapy agent had been approved for this situation. This is an important clinical consideration, because metastatic breast cancer patients often require continued therapy for increasing tumor-related symptoms.

High-dose vinorelbine (35 mg/m^2 per week) with continuous granulocyte colony-stimulating factor (G-CSF) has documented antitumor activity in anthracycline- and paclitaxel-pre-treated breast cancer, with an associated response rate (RR) of 25%.[6] Perez et al[7] have shown that weekly paclitaxel is associated with a 20% RR in patients who have been previously treated with paclitaxel or docetaxel on a 3-weekly schedule. Herceptin (trastuzumab) has been demonstrated

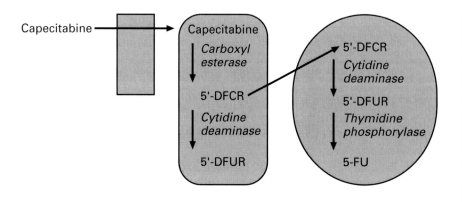

Figure 11.1
Mechanism of action of capecitabine following oral administration, it is activated by a cascade of three enzymatic reactions. The middle box represents the normal liver and the right-hand box represents the tumor. 5'-DFCR, 5'-deoxy-5-fluorocytidine; 5'-DFUR, 5'-deoxy-5-fluorouridine; 5-FU, 5-fluorouracil.

to have a 15% objective RR in women with heavily pre-treated metastatic breast cancer, two-thirds of whom had been previously treated with paclitaxel.[8] Docetaxel administered every 21 days has been shown to have an associated 18% RR in patients who have been previously treated with paclitaxel.[9] Finally, Ragaz et al[10] have shown that continuous-infusion 5-fluorouracil (5-FU) is associated with a 12% RR in metastatic breast cancer patients whose disease has progressed after treatment with an anthracycline and paclitaxel. These studies provide the only available data documenting the anti-tumor activity of third-line chemotherapy after anthracycline and taxane treatment.

Capecitabine is a rationally designed, oral, tumor-activated fluoropyrimidine carbamate, which is converted to 5-FU after a series of three enzymatic reactions (Figure 11.1). After gastrointestinal absorption, capecitabine is hydrolyzed in the liver first by carboxylesterase to produce 5'-deoxy-5-fluorocytidine, which is then deaminated on the pyrimidine ring by cytidine deaminase to produce 5'-deoxy-5-fluorouridine.[11] The final step in capecitabine activation is catalyzed by thymidine phosphory-lase, producing 5-FU at the tumor site. Thymi-dine phosphorylase is expressed at higher levels in most human cancers, including breast cancer, compared with the corresponding normal

tissues.[12] Thymidine phosphorylase is a potent angiogenic factor that is overexpressed in high-grade cancers.[13] Preclinical studies have shown that the ratio of thymidine phosphorylase to dihydropyrimidine dehydrogenase, the enzyme responsible for the catabolism of 5-FU, may be a significant predictor of tumor sensitivity to capecitabine.[14]

Preclinical studies have demonstrated that capecitabine produces greater than 50% tumor inhibition in 75% of various human cancer xenografts compared with 25% and 8% for UFT (tegafur and uracil) and 5-FU, respectively.[15] Pharmacokinetic studies have shown that the gastrointestinal absorption of capecitabine is rapid and extensive (≥70%). Peak plasma con-centrations of capecitabine and its metabolites occur a median of 2 hours after administration and then decline with half-lives in the range 0.7–1.2 hours.[11] The pharmacokinetics of the end-product of capecitabine metabolism, 5-FU, are not significantly affected by food intake or by hepatic dysfunction caused by liver metastases.[16] Elevated tumor-to-normal tissue and tumor-to-plasma 5-FU levels have been demonstrated in colon cancer patients who received capecitabine before tumor resection, demonstrating the rela-tive tumor selectivity of the conversion of capecitabine prodrug to 5-FU.[17]

The intermittent schedule of capecitabine administration, 2500 mg/m^2 per day in two divided doses for 14 days followed by a 7-day rest, was chosen for phase II testing, based on a randomized phase II study of capecitabine in colon cancer patients comparing this intermittent schedule with continuous capecitabine administration and intermittent capecitabine plus calcium folinate (leucovorin). Although the response rates in metastatic colon cancer were similar with the three schedules (22–25%), time to progression was significantly longer with the intermittent schedule (without calcium folinate) and the toxicity profile was more favorable without the addition of calcium folinate.[18]

PHASE II STUDY OF CAPECITABINE IN METASTATIC BREAST CANCER

Capecitabine has been evaluated in four phase II studies in patients with metastatic breast cancer. A large randomized phase III trial evaluating time to disease progression with docetaxel treatment versus docetaxel plus capecitabine has recently completed accrual.

The largest phase II study of capecitabine is the pivotal trial that led to FDA approval for metastatic breast cancer patients whose disease has been pre-treated with both an anthracycline and paclitaxel. In this multicenter study, 162 metastatic breast cancer patients were treated with capecitabine 2500 mg/m^2 per day divided into two daily doses, administered for 14 days, followed by a 7-day rest; 135 patients had bi-dimensionally measurable disease and the remaining 27 had evaluable disease. Patients received capecitabine as either third- or fourth-line therapy; 91% of patients had been previously treated with an anthracycline and all patients had been previously treated with paclitaxel.[19] Of the patients, 82% had been previously treated with 5-FU as part of CMF (cyclophosphamide,

methotrexate, 5-FU) or CAF (cyclophosphamide, doxorubicin, 5-FU) combination regimens. The patients had been treated with a median of 2.5 prior chemotherapy regimens for metastatic disease, and 75% of patients had more than two organ sites involved with metastatic disease. The objective response rate in this phase II study was 20% (95% confidence interval, 95% CI: 14–28%), with a median duration of response of 8 months.[19] In addition, 40% of patients achieved stable disease for a median duration of 3.5 months. Median time to disease progression in the 162 patients was 3.1 months and median overall survival was 12.8 months. Of the patients, 52% were alive 1 year after beginning therapy. In a subgroup of 42 patients whose breast cancer was refractory to both an anthracycline and paclitaxel (metastatic disease progressed while receiving these agents), the objective response rate was 29%.[19]

In this phase II study, clinical benefit response was determined from a composite profile of the patients' pain intensity, analgesic consumption and Karnofsky performance status. Of all treated patients, 20% achieved a significant clinical benefit response. Of the 51 patients who had at least 20 mm of pain as assessed by the Memorial Visual Analog Scale at study entry, 47% achieved at least 50% reduction in their pain with capecitabine treatment.[19]

Adverse events associated with capecitabine included hand–foot syndrome in 56.2% of patients, with 9.9% having severe symptoms (grade 3). Diarrhea occurred in 54.3% of patients, with 11.1% having severe diarrhea (grade 3) and 3.1% life-threatening diarrhea (grade 4). Stomatitis occurred in 9.3% of patients, with 2.5% developing severe symptoms. Myelo-suppression was rare, with 1.8% of patients developing grade 4 neutropenia. No significant alopecia was seen with capecitabine treatment. Six patients developed treatment-related grade 4 adverse events. Seven percent of patients stopped treatment as a result of toxicity and there were no treatment-related deaths.[19]

The investigators in this study concluded that capecitabine had a clinically meaningful objective response rate in heavily pre-treated patients with manageable toxicity that was rarely life-threatening. In view of the strong preference that patients have for oral drugs for palliative treatment, capecitabine represents a significant advance by allowing home-based therapy.

In a second confirmatory phase II study, 74 advanced breast cancer patients whose metastatic disease had been pre-treated with either paclitaxel or docetaxel were treated with capecitabine using the standard intermittent schedule. Similar response rates were seen in paclitaxel- and docetaxel-pre-treated patients: 27% and 21% respectively.[20] The median duration of response was 8 months and the median time to progression was 3.7 months. The median overall survival in all patients was 12.6 months. The most common treatment-related adverse events in this study were hand–foot syndrome, diarrhea, nausea, vomiting and fatigue. In both of these phase II studies, 42% of patients required a dose reduction at some point during their treatment. Loss of therapeutic benefit was not observed with a 25% dose reduction in responding or stable disease patients who required a dose reduction.

Two additional small randomized phase II studies of capecitabine in metastatic breast cancer patients have also been completed. In the first study, patients who had previously been treated with an anthracycline were randomized to receive treatment with either capecitabine or paclitaxel. Capecitabine was administered according to the standard intermittent schedule and paclitaxel 175 mg/m^2 was administered every 3 weeks. In total, 42 patients were randomized: 22 to capecitabine and 20 to paclitaxel. Accrual to this study was closed prematurely because of

difficulty encountered in randomizing patients to an oral versus intravenous therapy. The median age of the patients was 52 years and the median Karnofsky performance status was 80 for both groups. The objective response rates observed were 36% (95%CI: 17–59%) with capecitabine and 21% (95%CI: 6–46%) with paclitaxel.[21] The median time to disease progression was identical at 3 months each. Treatment-related grade 3 or 4 events were reported by 22% of patients on capecitabine and 58% of patients on paclitaxel, with the greater rate with paclitaxel caused by neutropenia. Although limited by sample size, this study suggests that oral capecitabine has comparable antitumor activity to paclitaxel in metastatic breast cancer patients whose disease has progressed on an anthracycline.

In a second randomized phase II study, women who were aged at least 55 years with metastatic breast cancer were randomized to receive first-line chemotherapy with capecitabine versus CMF. The less dose-intensive intravenous CMF regimen was chosen for investigation because of concern that the classic oral CMF regimen would be associated with significant toxicity in this older patient population. Patients underwent a two-to-one randomization to standard capecitabine versus intravenous CMF 600/40/600 mg/m^2 administered every 21 days. Ninety-five patients were randomized: 62 to capecitabine and 33 to CMF. The median age of the patients was 69 years for capecitabine and 70 years for CMF. The objective response rates observed were 30% (95%CI: 19–43%) with capecitabine and 16% (95%CI: 5–33%) with CMF.[22] The median time to disease progression was 4 months with capecitabine and 3 months with CMF, a difference that was not statistically significant. The median overall survival with CMF was 17.5 months, compared with 21.9 months for capecitabine; these results were not statistically significant. Treatment-related grade 3 or 4 adverse events occurred in 44% of patients who received capecitabine and 20% of patients with CMF.[22] The difference was primarily the result of hand–foot syndrome (16% versus 0%), and diarrhea (8% versus 3%) with capecitabine and CMF, respectively; grade 3 or 4 hematologic toxicity was more frequent with CMF (47%) than with capecitabine (20%). Grade 1 or 2 alopecia was more common with CMF (19%) compared with capecitabine (8%). Although limited by sample size, this study demonstrated that oral monotherapy with capecitabine has at least comparable activity to intravenous CMF in older women as first-line therapy for metastatic breast cancer. The Cancer and Leukemia Group B (CALGB) plans to conduct a phase III study of capecitabine compared with classic oral CMF or AC (doxorubicin, cyclophosphamide) as adjuvant therapy for postmenopausal early stage breast cancer patients who are aged at least 65 years.

These phase II studies demonstrate the effectiveness and safety associated with capecitabine in metastatic breast cancer. Capecitabine, docetaxel, weekly paclitaxel, high-dose vinorelbine with G-CSF, and Herceptin (in HER2/*neu*-overexpressing breast cancer) have documented antitumor activity as third-line treatment of metastatic breast cancer after an anthracycline and a taxane. 5-FU is not administered as often as it once was as adjuvant therapy, yet it is active against breast cancer. Oral capecitabine offers patients convenient and titrable therapy, which leads to higher intratumoral levels of 5-FU than intravenous therapy.

CAPECITABINE AND TAXANE COMBINATION THERAPY

Preclinical studies have demonstrated that treatment of nude mice bearing xenografts of the capecitabine-resistant human colon cancer WiDr with either paclitaxel or docetaxel resulted in at least a sixfold increase in tumor expression of thymidine phosphorylase.[23] This increased thymidine phosphorylase activity was noted 4–6 days after taxane treatment and persisted for up to 10 days. In these studies, paclitaxel, docetaxel, capecitabine and 5-FU administered as single agents did not appreciably inhibit tumor growth. In contrast, the combination of capecitabine with either paclitaxel or docetaxel resulted in synergistic antitumor activity.[23] The combination of 5-FU or UFT (a mixture of tegafur and uracil) with paclitaxel resulted in only additive antitumor activity.[23]

These interesting studies have led to the initiation and now completion of phase I studies of capecitabine combined with paclitaxel or docetaxel, and phase II studies of both combinations are currently ongoing. In the phase I study of paclitaxel and capecitabine, the recommended phase II dose for further evaluation was paclitaxel 175 mg/m^2 every 21 days together with capecitabine 1650 mg/m^2 per day for 14 days followed by a 7-day rest, repeated every 21 days.[24] The dose-limiting toxicity of this combination was hand–foot syndrome. The phase I study of this combination was conducted in 19 metastatic breast cancer patients who had been previously treated with an anthracycline but who were paclitaxel-naive. None of the 11 patients who were treated with 175 mg/m^2 and 1650 mg/m^2 of the paclitaxel–capecitabine combination developed a dose-limiting toxicity, and only two patients required a dose reduction. Nine of 16 patients (56%) with measurable disease had an objective response, including two complete responses. Three additional patients with evaluable bone and/or chest wall disease had objective clinical and functional improvement. Four of six patients who had undergone prior bone marrow transplantation experienced major responses. No pharmacokinetic interactions were noted between paclitaxel and capecitabine in this phase

I study.[24] Based on the preclinical models, which demonstrated synergistic antitumor activity, the combination of paclitaxel and capecitabine is expected to be a very active regimen in the treatment of breast cancer. A phase II study of this combination is currently ongoing, as is a phase I study of weekly paclitaxel in combination with capecitabine. Combined paclitaxel and capecitabine will probably prove to be sufficiently promising to evaluate as part of adjuvant therapy for breast cancer.

A phase I study of docetaxel and capecitabine has also been completed. The recommended doses for further evaluation were docetaxel 75 mg/m² every 3 weeks together with capecitabine 2500 mg/m² per day on the intermittent schedule (14 days on, 7 days off).[25] With docetaxel 100 mg/m², dose-limiting toxicities of asthenia and febrile neutropenia were noted. With docetaxel 75 mg/m² and capecitabine 2500 mg/m² per day, no febrile neutropenia was noted, in spite of the occurrence of moderate-to-severe neutropenia in most patients. Significant antitumor responses were seen in patients with breast and colon cancer, as well as a variety of other tumors. A phase I study of weekly docetaxel with capecitabine is currently ongoing. A large phase III study of docetaxel at 100 mg/m² versus docetaxel 75 mg/m² plus capecitabine 2500 mg/m² per day on the intermittent schedule in anthracycline-pre-treated metastatic breast cancer patients has recently completed accrual. The primary endpoint of this large study is time to disease progression, and overall survival will also be evaluated.

At the current time, data from only level of evidence (LOE) II studies are available that define the antitumor activity of capecitabine as treatment for metastatic breast cancer. The preponderance of this evidence demonstrates that capecitabine is associated with an objective response rate of about 20% in patients with anthracycline- and taxane-pre-treated metastatic breast cancer. Two LOE II studies suggest that the response rate of capecitabine in less heavily pre-treated metastatic breast cancer is approximately 30–36%. Capecitabine has been studied and approved by regulatory authorities at a dose and schedule that is associated with toxicity requiring dose adjustment in 42% of patients. As severe diarrhea and hand–foot syndrome can generally be avoided by dose interruptions and adjustments for grade 2 toxicity, education of patient and physician is critical for the successful palliative use of this drug. The ability to titrate the dose of capecitabine on a daily basis leads to significant patient control, and gives women the opportunity to hold their next dose of capecitabine if they develop diarrhea or pain in their hands or feet. Phase II studies of capecitabine at a dose of 2000 mg/m² on two additional schedules – 14 days followed by a 7-day rest and 5 days followed by a 2-day rest each week – are planned. Capecitabine is still early in its clinical development, and additional studies are needed to optimize dose and schedule.

Presently, there are only early LOE II data regarding the effectiveness of capecitabine in combination with paclitaxel or docetaxel. However, both the antitumor activity and the non-overlapping toxicity profiles of these combinations appear promising at present. These combinations are of particular interest for the adjuvant treatment of breast cancer, because the taxanes are playing an increasing role in this setting. LOE I data will soon be available regarding the clinical effectiveness of combined docetaxel and capecitabine compared with docetaxel alone. If improved time to progression and/or overall survival are demonstrated with combination therapy, it will be important to advance this regimen rapidly for testing in the adjuvant setting. In the palliative treatment of metastatic breast cancer, the weekly taxane schedules in combination with capecitabine hold promise for providing significant tumor palliation while avoiding grade 2 alopecia in most patients.

Home-based oral therapy with capecitabine represents a new paradigm in the treatment of breast cancer. The preponderance of evidence suggests that patients readily accept oral chemotherapy in the palliative setting[26] and achieve excellent treatment compliance. Patient education about dose titration to avoid significant toxicity is critical to the successful use of this agent. As the taxanes upregulate the expression of thymidine phosphorylase and are associated with synergistic preclinical antitumor activity in combination with capecitabine, these regimens are of particular interest both as palliative and as adjuvant treatment. Early clinical studies have begun to determine whether higher ratios of thymidine phosphorylase to dihydropyrimidine dehydrogenase levels in patients' breast cancers will predict for a higher likelihood of clinical response with capecitabine. The finding of consistent and significant antitumor activity associated with capecitabine has reopened a chapter in breast cancer treatment: oral, home-based therapy.

REFERENCES

1. Fossati R, Confalonieri C, Torri V et al, Cytotoxic and hormonal treatment for metastatic breast cancer: a systematic review of published randomized trials involving 31,510 women. *J Clin Oncol* 1998; **16**:3439–60.
2. Joensuu H, Holli K, Heikkinen M et al, Combination chemotherapy vs single-agent therapy as first- and second-line treatment in metastatic breast cancer: A prospective randomized trial. *J Clin Oncol* 1998; **16**:3720–30.
3. Sledge GW, Neuberg D, Ingle J et al, Phase III trial of doxorubicin vs paclitaxel vs doxorubicin plus paclitaxel as first-line therapy for metastatic breast cancer. An intergroup trial. *Proc Am Soc Clin Oncol* 1997; **16**:1A.
4. Ravdin PM, Burris HA, Cook G et al, Phase II trial of docetaxel in advanced anthracycline-resistant or anthracenedione-resistant breast cancer. *J Clin Oncol* 1995; **13**:2879–85.
5. Seidman AD, Reichman BS, Crown JPA et al, Paclitaxel as second and subsequent therapy for metastatic breast cancer: Activity independent of prior anthracycline response. *J Clin Oncol* 1995; **13**:1152–9.
6. Livingston RB, Ellis GK, Gralow JR et al, Dose-intensive vinorelbine with concurrent granulocyte colony-stimulating factor support in paclitaxel-refractory metastatic breast cancer. *J Clin Oncol* 1997; **15**:1395–400.
7. Perez EA, Irwin DH, Patel R et al, A large phase II trial of paclitaxel administered as a weekly one hour infusion in patients with metastatic breast cancer. *Proc Am Soc Clin Oncol* 1999; **18**:480A.
8. Cobleigh MA, Vogel CL, Tripathy D et al, Multinational study of the efficacy and safety of humanized anti-HER2 monoclonal antibody in women who have HER2-overexpressing metastatic breast cancer that has progressed after chemotherapy for metastatic disease. *J Clin Oncol* 1999; **17**:2639–48.
9. Valero V, Jones SE, Von Hoff DD et al, A Phase III study of docetaxel in patients with paclitaxel-resistant metastatic breast cancer. *J Clin Oncol* 1998; **16**:3362–8.
10. Ragaz J, Campbell C, Gelman K et al, Can patients with metastatic breast cancer (MBC) pretreated with cyclophosphamide (C), anthracyclines (A) or Taxol (Tax) respond to infusions of 5-FU (FUI)? Rationale for FUI-containing chemotherapy (CT) regimens. *Breast Cancer Res Treat* 1997; **46**:411A.
11. Mackean M, Planting A, Twelves C et al, Phase I and pharmacologic study of intermittent twice-daily oral therapy with capecitabine in patients with advanced and/or metastatic cancer. *J Clin Oncol* 1998; **16**:2977–85.
12. Fox SB, Westwood M, Moghaddam A et al,

The angiogenic factor platelet-derived endothelial growth factor/thymidine phosphorylase is up-regulated in breast cancer epithelium and endothelium. *Br J Cancer* 1996; 73:275–80.

13. Takebayashi Y, Akiyama S, Akiba S et al, Clinicopathologic and prognostic significance of an angiogenic factor, thymidine phosphorylase, in human colorectal carcinoma. *J Natl Cancer Inst* 1996; 88:1110–17.

14. Ishikawa T, Sekiguchi F, Fukase Y et al, Positive correlation between the efficacy of capecitabine and doxifluridine and the ratio of thymidine phosphorylase to dihydropyrimidine dehydrogenase activities in tumours in human cancer xenografts. *Cancer Res* 1998; 58:685–90.

15. Ishikawa T, Utoh M, Sawada N et al, Capecitabine, a new oral fluoropyrimidine carbamate, selectively delivers fluorouracil to tumor tissues in human cancer xenografts. *Biochem Pharmacol* 1998; 55:1091–7.

16. Reigner B, Verweij J, Dirix L et al, Effect of food on the pharmacokinetics of capecitabine and its metabolites following oral administration in cancer patients. *Clin Cancer Res* 1998; 4:941–8.

17. Schuller J, Cassidy J, Reigner BG et al, Tumor selectivity of Xeloda in colorectal cancer patients. *Proc Am Soc Clin Oncol* 1997; 16:797A.

18. Findlay M, Van Cutsem E, Kocha W et al, A randomized phase II study of Xeloda™ (capecitabine) in patients with advanced colorectal cancer. *Proc Am Soc Clin Oncol* 1997; 16:227A.

19. Blum JL, Jones SE, Buzdar AM et al, Multicenter phase II study of capecitabine in paclitaxel-refractory metastatic breast cancer. *J Clin Oncol* 1999; 17:485–93.

20. Blum JL, Buzdar AM, Dieras V et al, Phase II trial of Xeloda (capecitabine) in taxane-refractory metastatic breast cancer. *Proc Am Soc Clin Oncol* 1999; 18:403A.

21. Moiseyenko V, O'Reilly SM, Talbot DC et al, A randomized phase II study of Xeloda™ (capecitabine) vs paclitaxel in breast cancer patients failing previous anthracycline therapy. *Ann Oncol* 1998; 9:62A.

22. O'Shaughnessy J, Moisenyenkio V, Bell D et al, A randomized phase II study of Xeloda (capecitabine) vs CMF as first line chemotherapy of breast cancer in women aged 55 years. *Proc Am Soc Clin Oncol* 1998; 17:398A.

23. Sawada N, Ishikawa T, Fukase Y et al, Induction of thymidine phosphorylase activity and enhancement of capecitabine efficacy by Taxol/Taxotere in human cancer xenografts. *Clin Cancer Res* 1998; 4:1013–19.

24. Khoury P, Villalona-Calero M, Blum J et al, Phase I study of capecitabine in combination with paclitaxel in patients with previously treated metastatic breast cancer. *Proc Am Soc Clin Oncol* 1998; 17:816A.

25. Pronk LC, Vasey P, Sparreboom A et al, A matrix-designed phase I dose finding and pharmacokinetic study of the combination of Xeloda™ plus Taxotere. *Proc Am Soc Clin Oncol* 1998; 17:816A.

26. Liu G, Franssen E, Fitch MI et al, Patient preferences for oral versus intravenous palliative chemotherapy. *J Clin Oncol* 1997; 15:110–15.

SECTION 2: High-Dose Chemotherapy

Section Editor: J Crown

12.1
Role of high-dose chemotherapy as an adjuvant in high-risk early breast cancer

John Crown

BACKGROUND: THEORY OF ADJUVANT CHEMOTHERAPY

Most breast cancer patients are diagnosed with stage I–II disease. Although locoregional therapy will cure many, about 50% of patients with node-positive and 30% with node-negative disease will ultimately die from metastases, and thus must have had occult dissemination. Systemic 'adjuvant' therapy would thus be necessary to effect cure. Support for this approach came from the work of Skipper and Schabel,[1] whose experiments revealed that chemotherapy killed a constant proportion of cells, and that there was an inverse relationship between the size of a tumor and its curability by chemotherapy. Their model appeared to be particularly relevant to breast cancer, in that metastatic disease is partially chemosensitive, but is rarely cured.[2] Adjuvant chemotherapy regimens do produce a benefit in patients with earlier stage disease,[3] but the magnitude is modest, and stage I–II breast cancers frequently remain fatal.

Norton and Simon[4] proposed an explanation for this observation. They hypothesized that tumors grew and regressed according to Gompertzian kinetics, i.e. the growth rate varied inversely with the size of the tumor – large tumors had lower growth fractions than smaller ones, and hence were less sensitive to drugs. Thus, cell kill is directly related to the size of the dose, and to the growth rate of the unperturbed tumor at that point in its growth curve.[4] They proposed that patients should first be treated with 'induction' therapy to reduce their tumor burden, at which point eradication might be attempted with 'intensified' therapy. Several randomized trials that tested this hypothesis,[5,6] using generally modest intensification, have indicated a benefit for the approach.

CHEMOTHERAPY DOSE–RESPONSE EFFECT

Experimental models show that there is a relationship between dose and cell kill.[1,7] The degree of dose escalation that is required to eradicate cancers is in general of a log order of magnitude. The colony-stimulating factors (CSFs) facilitate relatively modest increases in dose and intensity.[8] Moderately dose-intensified regimens (i.e. increases in dose that do not require autograft support) have, not surprisingly, produced marginal and inconsistent results.[9-16]

HEMATOPOIETIC SUPPORT OF HIGH-DOSE CHEMOTHERAPY

Very high-dose chemotherapy with hematopoietic autograft support has been reported to produce exceptionally high rates of complete response in patients with metastatic breast cancer, with some of these remissions remaining durable at 5 years.[17] Treatment-related death was a relatively frequent occurrence.[18,19] The use of hematopoietic CSFs after marrow re-infusion resulted in a dramatic abbreviation of the period of neutropenia, and a consequent fall in mortality.[20] They also mobilize large numbers of hematopoietic progenitors (PBPs) into the peripheral blood,[21] from whence they can be harvested, and used as a substitute for autologous bone marrow (ABM). These PBPs were demonstrated to be superior to growth factors alone or to marrow in prospective random assignment trials.[22,23]

As discussed below, single-arm studies of high-dose chemotherapy produced promising provocative results in early stage, high-risk breast cancer, and in patients with metastatic disease. The possibility of case-selection bias mandated that these results be confirmed in randomized trials.[24] Before analyzing the randomized trials that have been reported, it is necessary to outline the various high-dose chemotherapy strategies that have been developed.

HIGH-DOSE CHEMOTHERAPY STRATEGIES

Primary high-dose chemotherapy

In this strategy, high-dose chemotherapy (HDC) is administered as one (or, uncommonly, two or more), definitive cycles of 'stand alone' treatment to patients with cancer. High rates of usually short-lived responses were reported in several of these studies, especially in metastatic breast cancer.[25] Primary high-dose chemotherapy has had rather little investigation, primarily because late intensification rapidly became the dominant strategy for HDC.

Late intensification

This model is an adaptation of the work of Norton and Simon.[4] Obviously, autografting allowed a substantial degree of dose escalation, and, during the 1980s, late intensification became the most widespread application of HDC. In addition to the kinetic rationale, several other clinical arguments were advanced in support of using HDC as a form of late intensification. It was proposed that the cytoreduction that was achieved by conventional chemotherapy might increase the ability of the subsequent high-dose cycle to eradicate the cancer, by presenting it with a smaller tumor burden. Conventional chemotherapy might also improve the performance status of patients with advanced cancer before they are subjected to high-dose treatment. However, a historical comparison using identical HDC regimens, either with or without conventional induction, did not suggest a major benefit for the induction component of a late-intensification regimen.[17,26]

Peters and colleagues[17] treated patients with breast cancer involving at least 10 axillary lymph nodes with an aggressive doxorubicin-based adjuvant regimen, followed by a single cycle of high-dose late-intensification chemotherapy supported by an autograft of bone marrow or peripheral blood, and reported a 70% rate of long-term remission.[27]

There have now been seven randomized trials in which late-intensification, autograft-supported HDC has been compared with non-high-dose approaches in the therapy of either high-risk early stage or metastatic breast cancer. These are discussed in detail later, but it is salutary to note, at this stage, that all have been either negative or ambiguous.

High-dose sequential

The high-dose sequential (HDS) approach devised by Gianni and colleagues[28] in Milan enables very high doses of drugs to be delivered in a fashion that does not predispose to overlapping toxicity, and that also attempts to deal with the clonal heterogeneity predicted by Goldie and Coldman. In this approach, patients are treated with a number of different drugs and regimens given at, or close to, maximum dose. Gianni and colleagues[28] studied HDS (see below) in patients with stage II breast cancer involving 10 or more axillary lymph modes. In their study, 65% of patients remained free of relapse.[28]

Multi-cycle high-dose chemotherapy

The multicycle high-dose chemotherapy (MCHDC) model has its origins both in a critical analysis of the general development of clinical chemotherapy theory and practice and in an alternative interpretation of the Norton–Simon model.[29]

Curative chemotherapy has generally involved the identification of highly active regimens and, then, the application of a sufficient number of cycles of those regimens to achieve tumor eradication. Thus, in the early MOPP (mustine, vincristine, procarbazine, prednisone) program of chemotherapy for Hodgkin's disease, patients achieved remission after an average of three cycles of therapy. Another observation that

emerged in early studies in Hodgkin's disease was that the initial use of non-curative therapy compromised the ability of subsequent potentially curative therapy to effect cure.

Investigators in New York demonstrated the feasibility of accelerated, progenitor-supported MCHDC in breast cancer. In one small study that employed four cycles of high-dose alkylating agents as a treatment for metastatic breast cancer, a high rate of remission was achieved, but with a high rate of fatal pulmonary drug toxicity.[30]

RANDOMIZED TRIALS OF HDC IN BREAST CANCER

The results of five randomized trials of high-dose chemotherapy as a treatment for high-risk early stage breast cancer have been reported. As discussed below, one has been called into question. The other four studies, which all studied late intensification,[31–34] have been reported as being negative. In the Scandinavian study, patients received either standard FEC (5-fluorouracil (5-FU), epirubicin, cyclophosphamide) chemotherapy followed by a single high-dose cycle, or individually escalated doses of FEC. Patients on the 'low-dose' arm received higher doses of anthracycline, cyclophosphamide and 5-FU than patients on the 'high-dose' arm.[32] The study was negative, but in fact compared two high-dose strategies. It is also interesting that the patients who received the tailored FEC chemotherapy had an excess of treatment-related leukaemia.

Peters et al[33] randomized patients to receive either high-dose cisplatin, carmustine (BCNU) and cyclophosphamide with an autograft, or lower doses of the same drugs with filgrastim support after induction therapy. At a very early follow-up, no advantage was seen for the high-dose treatment. Patients on the high-dose arm of this study, however, had an unusually high (8%) rate of treatment-related mortality. It seems quite possible that this trial may yet become positive in favor of high doses, because the total number of relapses appears to be smaller on the high-dose arm. Two other very small studies (each with fewer than 90 patients) in which late-intensification HDC was compared with conventionally dosed chemotherapy (CDC) were also negative. One was conducted by investigators in the MD Anderson Cancer Center in Houston, and involved a randomization between standard FAC (5-FU, doxorubicin, cyclophosphamide) chemotherapy with or without tandem cycles of a regimen that is somewhat less intensive than other high-dose programmes.[34] In the other, conducted by Rodenhuis and colleagues, a substantial minority of patients who were randomized to receive high-dose treatment did not in fact receive it.[31]

The fifth trial, conducted by Bezwoda et al,[35] has recently been the subject of an international audit, which found that the results were not reliable as the result of serious departures from ethical clinical research practice. This study, which purported to compare conventional FAC chemotherapy with a primary multi-cycle approach, was found to have in fact used a control arm other than the one delineated in the original report. Thus, there are no verifiable results from any trials other than those that used the late-intensification approach.

Four randomized trials comparing HDC with CDC have also been carried out in patients with metastases. Three used the late-intensification approach and were all either negative or ambiguous.[36–38] The sole study of primary multi-cycle HDC, which showed striking advantages for high-dose treatment, was conducted by the same investigator whose adjuvant high-dose trial was called into question.[39] The results of this metastatic trial have not as yet been verified in audit. The trial was, in any event, relatively small and confirmatory studies would have been required

even if this approach is to be regarded as evidence-based.

Single-cycle late-intensification cannot be regarded as an evidence-based approach for patients with metastatic or multi-node-positive breast cancer.

RESEARCH PRIORITIES AND FUTURE DIRECTIONS

Two broad strategies will need to be addressed in successor trials:

1. Improving the results of treatment: the impact of new high-dose regimens, engineered autograft products,[40,41] adjuvant immunotherapy,[42] gene therapy,[43] anti-angiogenics,[44] allogeneic transplantation,[45] multiple high-dose cycles and late intensification versus HDS and primary HDC strategies should all be studied.
2. There have also been substantial advances in CDC in recent years. Control groups will therefore also have to be optimized.[51]

Thus, the current literature does not invalidate high-dose therapy, but rather suggests a possible route for future investigations. At this point in time, however, HDC with autograft support cannot be considered a standard, evidence-based therapy for either metastatic or high-risk early stage cancer.

REFERENCES

1. Skipper HE, Schabel FM, Quantitative and cytokinetic studies in experimental tumor systems. In: Holland J, Frei FE, eds. *Cancer Medicine.* Philadelphia: Lea & Febiger, 1988: 663–84.
2. Greenberg PAC, Hortobagyi GN, Smith TL et al, Long-term follow-up of patients with complete remission following combination chemotherapy for metastatic breast cancer. *J Clin Oncol* 1996; **14**:2197–205.

3. Early Breast Cancer Trialists' Collaborative Group, Systemic treatment of early breast cancer by hormonal, cytotoxic or immune therapy: 133 randomized trials involving 31,000 recurrences and 24,000 deaths among 75,000 women. *Lancet* 1992; **339**:1–15.

4. Norton L, Simon R, Brereton HD et al, Predicting the course of Gompertzian growth. *Nature* 1976; **264**:542–45.

5. Perloff M, Norton L, Korzun AH et al, Post surgical adjuvant chemotherapy of stage II breast carcinoma with or without crossover to a non-cross-resistant regimen: A Cancer and Leukemia Group B study. *J Clin Oncol* 1996; **14**:1589–98.

6. Cocconi G, Bisagni G, Bacchi M et al, A comparison of continuation versus late intensification followed by discontinuation of chemotherapy in advanced breast cancer. A prospective randomized trial of the Italian Oncology Group for Clinical Research (G.O.I.R.C.). *Ann Oncol* 1990; **1**:36–44.

7. Teicher BA, Holden SA, Cucchi CA et al, Combination thiotepa and cyclophosphamide in vivo and in vitro. *Cancer Res* 1988; **48**:94–100.

8. O'Dwyer PJ, LaCreta FP, Schilder R et al, Phase I trial of thiotepa in combination with recombinant human granulocyte–macrophage colony-stimulating factor. *J Clin Oncol* 1992; **10**:1352–8.

9. Bastholt L, Dalmark M, Gjedde S, Dose–response relationship of epirubicin in the treatment of postmenopausal patients with metastatic breast cancer: a randomized study of epirubicin at four different dose levels performed by the Danish Breast Cancer Cooperative Group. *J Clin Oncol* 1996; **14**:1146–55.

10. Hortobagyi GN, Buzdar AU, Bodey GP et al, High-dose induction chemotherapy of metastatic breast cancer in protected environment units: a prospective randomized study. *J Clin Oncol* 1987; **5**:178–84.

11. Ardizzoni A, Venturini M, Sertoli MR et al, Granulocyte–macrophage colony-stimulating factor (GM-CSF) allows acceleration and dose-intensity increase of CEF chemotherapy: A randomized study in patients with advanced breast cancer. *Br J Cancer* 1994; **69**:385–91.

12. Henderson IC, Berry D, Demetri G et al, Improved disease-free survival and overall survival from the addition of sequential paclitaxel but not from the escalation of doxorubicin dose in the adjuvant chemotherapy of patients with node-positive primary breast cancer. *Proc Am Soc Clin Oncol* 1998; **17**:101a.

13. Fisher B, Anderson S, Wickerham DL et al, Increased intensification and total dose of cyclophosphamide in a doxorubicin–cyclophosphamide regimen for the treatment of primary breast cancer: Findings from National Surgical Adjuvant Breast and Bowel Project B-22. *J Clin Oncol* 1997; **15**:1858–69.

14. Levine MN, Gent M, Hryniuk WM et al, A randomized trial comparing 12 weeks versus 36 weeks of adjuvant chemotherapy in stage II breast cancer. *J Clin Oncol* 1990; **8**:1217–25.

15. Bonneterre J, Roché H, Bremond A et al, Results of a randomized trial of adjuvant chemotherapy with FEC 50 vs FEC 100 in high-risk node positive breast cancer patients. *Proc Am Soc Clin Oncol* 1998; **17**: 124a.

16. Tannock IF, Boyd NF, Deborer G et al, A randomized trial of two dose levels of CMF chemotherapy for patients with metastatic breast cancer. *J Clin Oncol* 1988; **6**:1377–87.

17. Peters WP, Shpall EJ, Jones RB et al, High-dose combination alkylating agents with bone marrow support as initial treatment for metastatic breast cancer. *J Clin Oncol* 1988; **6**:1368–76.

18. Eder JP, Antman K, Peters WP et al, High-dose combination alkylating agent chemotherapy with autologous marrow support for metastatic breast cancer. *J Clin Oncol* 1986; **4**:1592–7.

19. Lazarus H, Reed MD, Spitzer TR et al, High-dose iv thiotepa and cryopreserved autologous bone marrow transplantation for therapy of refractory cancer. *Cancer Treat Rep* 1987; **71**:689–95.

20. Peters WP, Rosner G, Ross M et al, Com-

parative effects of granulocyte–macrophage colony-stimulating factor (GM-CSF) and granulocyte colony-stimulating factor (G-CSF) on priming peripheral blood progenitor cells for use with autologous bone marrow after high-dose chemotherapy. *Blood* 1993; **81**:1709–19.

21. Socinski MA, Elias A, Schnipper L et al, Granulocyte–macrophage colony-stimulating factor expands the circulating haemopoietic progenitor cell compartment in man. *Lancet* 1988; **i**:194–8.

22. Beyer J, Schwella N, Zingsem J et al, Bone marrow versus peripheral blood stem cells as rescue after high-dose chemotherapy. *Blood* 1993; **82**(Suppl 1):454a.

23. Kritz A, Crown J, Motzer R, Beneficial impact of peripheral blood progenitor cells in patients with metastatic breast cancer treated with high-dose chemotherapy plus GM-CSF: A randomized trial. *Cancer* 1993; **71**:2515–21.

24. Rahman ZU, Frye DK, Buzdar AU, Impact of selection process on response rate and long-term survival of potential high-dose chemotherapy candidates treated with standard-dose doxorubicin-containing chemotherapy in patients with metastatic breast cancer. *J Clin Oncol* 1997; **15**:3171–7.

25. Eder JP, Antman K, Peters WP et al, High-dose combination alkylating agent chemotherapy with autologous marrow support for metastatic breast cancer. *J Clin Oncol* 1986; **4**:1592–7.

26. Jones RB, Shpall EJ, Ross M et al, AFM induction chemotherapy followed by intensive agent consolidation with autologous bone marrow support for advanced breast cancer. Current results. *Proc Am Soc Clin Oncol* 1990

27. Peters WP, Ross M, Vredenburgh JJ et al, High-dose chemotherapy and autologous bone marrow support as consolidation after standard-dose adjuvant therapy for high-risk primary breast cancer. *J Clin Oncol* 1993; **11**:1132–44.

28. Gianni AM, Siena S, Bregni M et al, Growth factor supported high-dose sequential adjuvant chemotherapy in breast cancer with >10

positive nodes. *Proc Am Soc Clin Oncol* 1992; **11**:60.

29. Crown J, Norton L, Potential strategies for improving the results of high-dose chemotherapy in patients with metastatic breast cancer. *Ann Oncol* 1995; **6**(Suppl 4):s21–s26.

30. Crown J, Raptis G, Vahdat L et al, Rapid administration of sequential high-dose cyclophosphamide, melphalan, thiotepa supported by filgrastim and peripheral blood progenitors in patients with metastatic breast cancer: A novel and very active treatment strategy. *Proc Am Soc Clin Oncol* 1994; **13**:110.

31. Rodenhuis S, Richel DJ, van der Wall E et al, Randomised trial of high-dose chemotherapy and haemopoietic progenitor-cell support in operable breast cancer with extensive axillary lymph-node involvement. *Lancet* 1998; **352**:515–21.

32. Scandinavian Breast Cancer Study Group, Results from a randomized adjuvant breast cancer study with high dose chemotherapy with CTCb supported by autologous bone marrow stem cell versus dose escalated and tailored FEC therapy. *Proc Am Soc Clin Oncol* 1999; **18**:2a.

33. Peters W, Rosner G, Vredenburgh J et al, for CALGB, SWOG and NCIC, A prospective, randomized comparison of two doses of combination alkylating agents as consolidation after CAF in high-risk primary breast cancer involving ten or more axillary lymph nodes: Preliminary results of CALGB 9082/SWOG 9114/NCIC MA-13. *Proc Am Soc Clin Oncol* 1999; **18**:1a.

34. Hortobagyi GN, Buzdar AU, Champlin R, Lack of efficacy of adjuvant high-dose tandem combination chemotherapy for high-risk primary breast cancer: A randomised trial. *Proc Am Soc Clin Oncol* 1998; **17**:123a.

35. Bezwoda WR, Randomised, controlled trial of high dose chemotherapy (HD-CNVp) vs. standard dose (CAF) chemotherapy for high risk, surgically treated, primary breast cancer. *Proc Am Soc Clin Oncol* 1999; **18**:2a.

36. Stadtmauer EA, O'Neill A, Goldstein LJ et al,

Phase III randomized trial of high-dose chemotherapy (HDC) and stem cell support (SCT) shows no difference in overall survival or severe toxicity compared to maintenance chemotherapy with cyclophosphamide, methotrexate and 5-fluorouracil (CMF) for women with metastatic breast cancer who are responding to conventional induction chemotherapy: The Philadelphia Intergroup Study (PBT-01). *Proc Am Soc Clin Oncol* 1999; **18**:1a.

37. Lotz J-P, Cure H, Janvier M et al, and the PEGASE Group, High-dose chemotherapy (HD-CT) with hematopoietic stem cells transplantation (HSCT) for metastatic breast cancer: results of the French Protocol Pegase 04. *Proc Am Soc Clin Oncol* 1999; **18**:43a.

38. Peters WP, Jones RB, Vredenburgh J et al, A large, prospective, randomized trial of high-dose combination alkylating agents (CBP) with autologous cellular support as consolidation for patients with metastatic breast cancer achieving complete remission after intensive doxorubicin-based induction therapy (AFM). *Proc Am Soc Clin Oncol* 1996; **15**:121.

39. Bezwoda WR, Seymour L, Dansey RD, High-dose chemotherapy with hematopoietic rescue as primary treatment for metastatic breast cancer: a randomised trial. *J Clin Oncol* 1995; **13**:2483–9.

40. Brugger W, Heimfeld S, Berenson RJ et al, Reconstitution of hematopoiesis after high-dose chemotherapy by autologous progenitor cells generated ex vivo. *N Engl J Med* 1995; **333**:283–7.

41. Shpall EJ, Jones RB, Bearman SI et al, Transplantation of enriched CD34-positive autologous marrow into breast cancer patients following high-dose chemotherapy: Influence of CD34-positive peripheral-blood progenitors and growth factors on engraftment. *J Clin Oncol* 1994; **12**:28–36.

42. Kennedy MJ, Vogelzang G, Beveridge R et al, Phase I trial of intravenous cyclosporine to induce graft versus host disease in women undergoing autologous bone marrow transplantation for breast cancer. *J Clin Oncol* 1993; **11**:478–84.

43. Hesdorffer C, Ayello J, Ward M et al, Phase I trial of retroviral-mediated transfer of the human MDR1 gene as marrow chemoprotection in patients undergoing high-dose chemotherapy and autologous stem-cell transplantation. *J Clin Oncol* **16**:

44. O'Reilly MS, Holmgren L, Chen C, Folkman J, Angiostatin induces and sustains dormancy of human primary tumors in mice. *Nature Med* 1996; **2**:689–92.

45. Ueno N, Rondón G, Mirza NQ, Allogeneic peripheral-blood progenitor-cell transplantation for poor-risk patients with metastatic breast cancer. *J Clin Oncol* 1998; **16**:986–93.

46. Chan S, Friedrichs K, Noel D et al, Prospective randomized trial of docetaxel versus doxorubicin in patients with metastatic breast cancer. *J Clin Oncol* 2000; in press.

12.2

High-dose adjuvant therapy for breast cancer: The argument against

Clifford A Hudis, Pamela N Munster

STUDIES OF DOSE ESCALATION

Preclinical data clearly support the conclusion that selected drugs, such as alkylating agents, have a steep dose–response relationship in some cell systems (e.g. MCF-7).[1] Clinically useful drugs with a steep dose–response relationship seen in the laboratory include most alkylating agents and anthracyclines, and their proven efficacy at standard doses makes them excellent candidates for study in this context. In addition, there are ample data for many other drugs, suggesting that increases in dose can successfully overcome cellular resistance. Hence, a large number of drugs have been tested and incorporated into high-dose regimens. The most challenging issue, however, remains identifying which, if any, patients truly benefit from this approach even as we continue to refine and improve the technique.

The exact meaning of 'high-dose therapy' can be vague. Does it include only those regimens that result in myeloablation? Does it include those that require growth factor support? At what point should we group a regimen with others called high-dose? Is there even a reason to consider high-dose therapy as a group or is this really a shared trait among some otherwise quite different regimens? Given the multitude of drugs, specific dose levels, types of support and variations in timing and approach, it is probably inappropriate to consider all high-dose regimens together. On the other hand, the *principle* under scrutiny – that dose escalation improves outcome – can be explored on both a regimen-specific and a setting-specific basis.

Our clinical use of dose-escalated chemotherapy is based on laboratory studies. In addition to demonstrating a dose–response relationship, some experiments specifically suggest that the application of high-dose alkylating agents after optional cytoreduction could eradicate viable tumor even when the same treatment applied earlier was not curative.[2] In other words, maximally effective treatment applied after cytoreduction could be curative because of the kinetic advantage of treating only a small tumor volume. These experiments led to the 'conventional' treatment strategy in which induction or 'run-up' chemotherapy precedes the delivery of a single cycle of high-dose chemotherapy. In addition to the models supporting this approach, the theoretical basis for induction treatment can be traced to the log-kill model of Skipper et al.[3] The assumption is that several cycles of effective chemotherapy will reduce the total tumor burden and that the subsequent application of high-dose treatment will 'mop-up' any remaining sensitive cells. This approach is further supported by the Gompertzian model of tumor growth, which predicts that the smaller volume of tumor cells remaining after effective initial therapy will have a relatively increased growth fraction and therefore greater sensitivity to cell-cycle-specific agents.[4] Although this broadly accepted hypothesis is the basis of most, but not all, high-dose therapy regimens, it is increasingly being challenged as discussed below.

Although modestly sized, one of the earliest reports of high-dose therapy supported by autologous stem cells demonstrated activity and feasibility using an alkylating agent.[5] Dozens of uncontrolled phase II trials have since explored the feasibility of using escalated doses of cyclophosphamide, carmustine (BCNU), cisplatin, etoposide, carboplatin, thiotepa, melphalan, mitoxantrone and ifosfamide, along with other drugs, in various combinations. These regimens have been supported by various growth factors and either harvested autologous bone marrow or peripheral blood stem cells. Review of these reports almost uniformly suggests that the tested regimen is feasible, the results are 'promising' and further study is warranted. As a result, there was widespread consideration of high-dose chemotherapy for patients with metastatic or high-risk early stage disease even before prospective randomized data were available.

The most typical treatment plan is based on the animal models described above. Patients are therefore first treated with two to six cycles of 'conventional', 'induction' or 'run-up' chemotherapy. After completing this treatment in the adjuvant setting or achieving a partial or complete response when measurable or evaluable advanced disease is present, a single cycle of high-dose therapy is delivered. In a few trials, several cycles of high-dose therapy have been used, and there are other schemas with potential superiority. Examples of the latter include initial high-dose treatment, multiple cycles and sequential cycles, and these are increasingly the subject of prospective studies.

PRELIMINARY RESULTS IN METASTATIC DISEASE

Despite a number of clinical trials involving hundreds of patients, as well as many more treated in similar fashion outside formal studies, there is still no clear answer to the questions of efficacy and patient selection for high-dose therapy. The varying eligibility criteria used to select patients for individual studies, the differences in induction and high-dose therapy, and the well-known clinical heterogeneity of breast cancer all contribute to this confusion.

Selection bias is a major concern, particularly when attempting to interpret the results of phase I and II trials. This problem is heightened by comparisons with historical data sets, which frequently include patients who would have been excluded from the trial under consideration. An example of the impact of selection was provided by an analysis of patients at the MD Anderson Cancer Center who did not undergo high-dose therapy. Over 1500 patients treated in a series of 18 clinical trials of conventional-dose chemotherapy were examined, and a subset who would have been eligible for contemporaneous trials of high-dose therapy was identified.[6] This group had been treated with standard-dose doxorubicin-containing regimens. Interestingly, the candidates for high-dose therapy had a significantly higher complete response proportion (27%) than the non-candidates (7%). Not being a prospective randomized study, this is not definitive, but clearly suggests that the subset of patients chosen for high-dose therapy may be more likely to respond in general compared with those not selected. Similar differences were seen in the median time for progression-free survival (16 versus 8 months) and the median overall survival (30 versus 17 months). At 5 years, there was a 15% advantage (21% versus 6%) in survival for high-dose candidates and at 10 years the advantage was 5% (7% versus 2%). Hence, the promising results of non-randomized trials of high-dose therapy could result partially from careful patient selection, and similar bias has been suggested for adjuvant therapy trials. In the latter circumstance, the increased pre-treatment screening required for enrollment clearly eliminates patients otherwise thought to be free of disease and who would have qualified for less intensive treatment protocols, based on more limited pre-treatment evaluations.[7]

Despite the limited interpretations of uncontrolled trials, attempts at drawing at least preliminary conclusions about efficacy have been made. An overview of most of the phase I and II trials of induction therapy followed by high-dose consolidation in metastatic disease shows a complete response proportion of 29–59% and a 3-year progression-free survival rate of 5–30%.[8] It is impossible to determine the 'best' approach from this collection of trials because only prospective randomized trials can properly determine their relative value. Furthermore, although the approach of induction followed by consolidation appears promising, there may be superior strategies to consider. The broadest overview of non-randomized high-dose chemotherapy is that of the North American Autologous Blood and Marrow Transplant Registry. Up to June 1995, they had recorded almost 20 000 autotransplants, including 5886 for breast cancer. In general, the registry shows that mortality and morbidity decreased significantly from 1989 to 1995 and that patients with early stage disease do better than those with established metastases. Among the latter, those with no response to

induction chemotherapy have a very low probability of progression-free survival. It seems fair to conclude that patients selected for and receiving treatment with high-dose chemotherapy are more likely to have responded and to have achieved complete response, and likely to have a more durable response, than the broader group of patients treated historically with conventional-dose chemotherapy. This neither supports nor denies a role for high-dose therapy in metastatic disease.

Bezwoda[9] reported the first prospective randomized trial of high-dose chemotherapy in metastatic disease, but this trial was small, the use of tamoxifen unbalanced, and subsequent revelations concerning his later adjuvant trial make this study exceedingly difficult to interpret.[10] By report, 90 patients with measurable previously untreated metastatic breast cancer were randomly assigned to receive CNV (cyclophosphamide, mitoxantrone and vincristine) for six to eight cycles at conventional dose levels or two cycles of high-dose CNV (substituting etoposide for the vincristine), supported by growth factor and autologous stem cells. Patients on the higher-dose arm had a higher response proportion, increased CR proportion (51% versus 5%) and increased duration of response, as well as improved overall and median survivals. This suggests that, for these drugs (only the cyclophosphamide would be considered standard as initial chemotherapy for metastatic disease by most oncologists), previously untreated patients may benefit from higher doses. If these data are substantiated, larger confirmatory trials testing this approach could be justified.

Other trials in the metastatic setting are even more confusing. Peters and colleagues treated over 400 patients with metastatic disease using AFM (doxorubicin, 5-fluorouracil (5-FU) and methotrexate) as induction. About 100 achieved a complete response, and were randomly assigned to immediate high-dose therapy or to observation, with high-dose treatment reserved only for demonstrated disease recurrence.[11] This last arm delayed the high-dose therapy significantly, violating the principle that treatment should be given when the tumor burden is minimal and that it should be delivered when the tumor is rapidly growing. Instead, these patients were allowed to experience relapse before beginning high-dose therapy, and treatment was delivered when the tumor growth rate, based on Gompertzian kinetics, would be slowing. Finally, the delayed high-dose therapy was delivered without an immediately preceding course of cytoreductive therapy and therefore without a second assessment of chemotherapy sensitivity. Yet, contrary to predictions, the delayed-transplantation arm was associated with a longer median survival and some patients did not experience progression. Hence, this study confirms the early suggestion that a few patients can obtain significant benefit from standard chemotherapy. It also, contrary to the implication of the report from South Africa, suggests that there is no need to rush patients into earlier high-dose therapy. On the other hand, and consistent with the hypothesis that early treatment could be superior, minimal tumor burden was not a prerequisite for improved outcome, nor was an immediate demonstration of chemotherapy sensitivity. Together, these trials most clearly question the adequacy of the 'conventional' high-dose approach because neither relied upon induction and immediate consolidation. Unfortunately, both trials are modest in size and need confirmation.

A clean comparison of 'standard' therapy with or without high-dose consolidation is provided by the Philadelphia Bone Marrow Transplant Trial. Patients with metastatic disease were treated with CAF (cyclophosphamide, doxorubicin, 5-FU) or CMF (cyclophosphamide, methotrexate, 5-FU) and then randomized to receive high-dose therapy or further CMF.[12] As this approach most closely follows standard practice when using high-dose therapy, it could be the most relevant for practicing oncologists. At the time of the 1999 Annual Meeting of the American Society of Clinical Oncology, the trial had failed to show an advantage for one approach over the other overall or in subsets. Longer follow-up or different patient selection might affect these results, but standard CAF followed by STAMP I (cyclophosphamide, cisplatin, carmustine (BCNU)) does not appear, among patients with responding metastatic disease, to offer any significant benefit compared with CMF. On the other hand, equivalent benefit with less time on treatment, particularly if the toxicity is limited, could be a worthwhile improvement for some patients.

EARLY STAGE DISEASE (ADJUVANT THERAPY)

Adjuvant high-dose therapy is especially appealing because of the high performance status of the patients, the possibility of apparent cure and the kinetic advantage of treatment of small-volume disease. For some oncologists, it was even considered standard for all high-risk patients, variously identified as those with ten or more positive nodes, four or more positive nodes, 5 cm maximal tumor diameter or inflammatory disease presentations.

As in metastatic disease, a large number of promising phase I and II trials have been conducted. One of the most widely cited is from Duke University, where patients with 10 or more involved axillary lymph nodes were treated with CAF followed by STAMP I with autologous stem cell and growth factor support.[13] Subsequently, several large prospective randomized studies were conducted, and some have been reported over the past 2 years. The Cancer and Leukemia Group B (CALGB)-led Intergroup Trial (CALGB 9082) compared the Duke regimen of CAF followed by STAMP I against a similar but non-standard approach consisting of CAF followed by a lower-dose version of the components of STAMP I.[14] The drug doses for STAMP I on the latter arm required growth factor support but not autologous stem cell harvesting and infusion. This study is critical because the outcome for the pilot trial at Duke University was so extremely promising, but, as described above for the treatment of patients with metastatic disease, selection and other treatment factors may have contributed. On the pilot trial and the CALGB randomized study, eligibility included a normal contrast-enhanced computed tomography (CT) scan of the head, chest, abdomen and pelvis, along with normal bilateral bone marrow aspiration and biopsies. The identification of patients with detectable metastatic disease using these techniques clearly leads to significant stage migration.[7] In one study, the intensive screening of patients with 10 or more involved nodes, using CT scans and bone marrow aspirates and biopsies, uncovered distant metastatic disease in an additional 23% even after patients were selected for normal serum studies, plain chest radiographs and nuclear bone scans. Another confounder for the pilot trial was the routine addition of radiotherapy after mastectomy. In this regard, two randomized trials recently demonstrated that the addition of chest wall radiotherapy improves not only local control but also distant disease-free and overall survival in patients with node-positive disease.[15,16] Of course, these factors do not mean that the high-dose treatment using STAMP I is not beneficial, but they make comparisons with historical data sets strained at best and underscore the tremendous need for large, prospective, randomized trials. Indeed, one of the interesting observations

on the subsequent randomized trial was that these high-risk patients had, on both arms, a far superior outcome to what had been expected. This may reflect the impact of all of the factors described above. At any rate, when reported orally at ASCO in 1999, the CALGB study, although very preliminary, failed to show a significant benefit for higher- compared with moderate-dose therapy. As a result of the relatively short follow-up of about 3 years, this study should be allowed to mature before definitive conclusions are drawn. At the same time, the lack of a dramatic early difference does not support the routine use of high-dose therapy outside strict research settings.

Mirroring his report in metastatic disease, Bezwoda[17] presented a study with positive results for initial high-dose therapy compared with a CAF control arm among patients with high-risk early stage disease. Unfortunately, this investigator later confessed that CAF was not administered, and significant alleged deviations from standard research practice are currently under investigation.[10] Hence, despite the promise that the South African study first suggested, it must be disregarded in its entirety at present.

Two small, but properly randomized, adjuvant trials were reported in 1998, and, although too under-powered to provide definitive answers, neither suggested a significant advantage for high-dose chemotherapy in high-risk early stage patients. One, from the Netherlands, compared three courses of neoadjuvant FEC (5-FU, epirubicin, cyclophosphamide) followed by surgery and then either a fourth course or the same plus high-dose peripheral-stem-cell-supported therapy consisting of cyclophosphamide 6 g/m², thiotepa 480 mg/m² and carboplatin 1600 mg/m².[18] Radiotherapy and tamoxifen were given postoperatively to all patients. Toxicity was modest on both arms, but there was no difference between the high-dose and the conventional-dose treatment groups after 4 years of follow-up. A second and similarly small trial from the MD Anderson also found no advantage for a high-dose regimen, in comparison with standard combination chemotherapy, for high-risk early stage disease.[19] Another very important adjuvant therapy trial has been performed within the Intergroup under the leadership of the Eastern Cooperative Oncology Group (ECOG), enrolling women similar to those on the CALGB 9082 trial: those with 10 or more positive nodes. Treatment consisted of either six cycles of CAF or the same followed by high-dose chemotherapy. In many ways, this is the purest test of the concept, because half of the patients received truly standard treatment and half the experimental one; unlike the trials in metastatic disease, there was no other prolonged chemotherapy to confound the result. Although completed, the results have not been reported.

Regardless of the longer-term results of these and other, mostly negative, trials,[19] moving forward, we want to continue to improve chemotherapy for breast cancer. In the most optimistic case, if a benefit for 'conventional' high-dose therapy is seen, we will need to consider how to improve outcomes and decrease toxicity further. Purged stem cell products and other multiple-cycle regimens are two possible approaches.

The use of multiple cycles of chemotherapy is based on the same kinetic arguments used to support high-dose treatment in the first place. Assuming that chemotherapy causes log-order or fractional cell kill, a fixed number of sensitive cells should be eliminated with each application. Note that even 99% effective treatment leaves 1% of the original number of sensitive cells surviving, and this can be a significant absolute number. The key is that this model does not predict complete cure after only a single application of even our most effective treatments. Instead, it predicts that multiple, tandem or sequential regimens,

whether high- or standard-dose, could be superior and studies testing this approach are under way. The positive Bezwoda trials could be seen as supporting this concept as well, because they too rely on multiple cycles of relatively closely spaced treatment.

This issue of treatment frequency, as opposed to dose, could be even more important because of the modest impact of dose escalation on outcome in the adjuvant setting. In fact, despite preclinical predictions, clear evidence of a steep dose–response relationship has not emerged for several critical drugs, including both cyclophosphamide and doxorubicin. This is a particularly troubling observation for cyclophosphamide because virtually every high-dose regimen includes alkylating agents, usually cyclophosphamide at high dose. Three clinical trials conducted in node-positive resected breast cancer have examined dose size for cyclophosphamide. The first CALGB trial compared CAF given at low dosage (300/30/300 mg/m^2) every 28 days for four cycles, moderate doses (400/40/400 mg/m^2) for six cycles or high doses (600/60/600 mg/m^2) for four cycles.[20] The high- and moderate-dose arms were superior to the low-dose arm, and a non-significant trend favored the highest dose version, particularly for patients whose tumors overexpressed HER2/neu.[21] Two studies explored the dose and dose intensity of cyclophosphamide among patients with positive nodes, but controlled the dose of doxorubicin at 60 mg/m^2 for four courses throughout.[22,23] In the National Surgical Adjuvant Breast and Bowel Project (NSABP) B-22, cyclophosphamide was administered at standard (600 mg/m^2 × 4) or increased (1200 mg/m^2 × 2) dose intensity or increased dose and dose intensity (1200 mg/m^2 × 4). NSABP B-25 continued by doubling the dose intensity to 2400 mg/m^2 × 2 or both dose and dose intensity by giving 2400 mg/m^2 × 4. Both trials are negative, strongly suggesting that, outside clinical trials, 600 mg/m^2 is a very appropriate dose for cyclophosphamide. The CALGB 9344 trial yields similar information for doxorubicin at 60–90 mg/m^2 administered with a fixed dose of cyclophosphamide.[24] As with cyclophosphamide in the NSABP studies, this trial suggests no advantage for doxorubicin doses above the usual levels (60 mg/m^2) for average node-positive patients outside clinical trials.

If these results are true, and the dose–response relationship reaches a plateau at modest dose levels, we must then consider whether there are any alternative means of increasing the effectiveness of chemotherapy. An approach based on the kinetic models already described includes selecting optimal (rather than maximal) doses of drugs and administering them more frequently. This is called dose-dense therapy and represents not only an alternative to dose-escalated therapy but also a potentially superior overall strategy. Pilot trials were performed in high-risk patient groups at the Memorial Sloan–Kettering Cancer Center in the early 1990s, demonstrating feasibility and promise. However, we must remember this was exactly as was seen for the original studies of high-dose treatment![25] In one study, patients were treated with single-agent doxorubicin at 75 mg/m^2 followed by three cycles every other week of chemotherapy using cyclophosphamide at 3000 mg/m^2. A subsequent South-West Oncology Group (SWOG)-led Intergroup trial (9313) compared this approach with more conventional concurrent therapy with AC (doxorubicin and cyclophosphamide) but the results have not been reported yet.

Building on this pilot trial, paclitaxel was next incorporated along with further increases in dose and dose density for doxorubicin. This regimen, called ATC, consisted of nine cycles of chemotherapy delivered over 18 weeks.[26] Three cycles each of doxorubicin, paclitaxel and cyclophosphamide were administered, and feas-ibility was demonstrated. As a result, the Inter-group designed a trial of particular relevance in the context of high-dose therapy for breast cancer. This SWOG-led Intergroup trial (S9623) is now open to patients with four or more involved axillary lymph nodes. On one experimental arm of this trial, patients receive AC × 4 followed by either STAMP I or STAMP V (cyclophosphamide, carboplatin and thiotepa), whereas the other consists of dose-dense therapy (ATC) as above. This trial could be very helpful in clarifying the relative efficacy and toxicity of these two very different approaches. In the meantime, another trial testing the value of administering standard-dose chemotherapy every other week or every third week is completed.

CONCLUSION

High-dose therapy is a technical triumph made possible because of impressive advances in the areas of stem-cell harvesting and support, growth-factor production, antibiotic use and other supportive care techniques. Appropriate explorations of high-dose therapy in almost all stages of breast cancer have more than amply demonstrated tolerability and feasibility, but raised more questions. Two immediate ones concern the definition of the optimal approach and the unequivocal demonstration of benefit. The former requires continued developmental work whereas the latter requires large, well-planned and rapidly accruing clinical trials. Until these questions are answered with consistent results obtained in more than one center, high-dose therapy should remain an investigational approach, and we should continue to strive to develop more effective and less toxic treatment options. Dose-dense treatment options could be an alternative or complementary approach, but they too require rigorous prospective confirmation of worth.

REFERENCES

1. Frei IE, Canellos G, Dose: a critical factor in cancer chemotherapy. *Am J Med* 1980; **69**:585–94.

2. Skipper HE, Laboratory models: the historical perspective. *Cancer Treatment Rep* 1986; **70**:3–7.

3. Skipper H, Schabel FJ, Wilcox W, Experimental evaluation of potential anticancer agents XIII: On the criteria and kinetics associated with 'curability' of experimental leukemia. *Cancer Chemotherapy Rep* 1964; **35**:1.

4. Norton L, Simon R, Brereton J et al, Predicting the course of Gompertzian growth. *Nature* 1976; **264**:542–5.

5. Redon H, Dupas M, Fasano J et al, Intensive regional chemotherapy of certain cancers under protection of autologous bone marrow transfusion. *Presse Med* 1966; **74**:2619–20.

6. Rahman Z, Frye D, Buzdar A et al, Impact of selection process on response rate and long-term survival of potential high-dose chemotherapy candidates treated with standard-dose doxorubicin-containing chemotherapy in patients with metastatic breast cancer. *J Clin Oncol* 1997; **15**:3171–7.

7. Crump M, Goss PE, Prince M et al, Outcome of extensive evaluation before adjuvant therapy in women with breast cancer and 10 or more positive axillary lymph nodes. *J Clin Oncol* 1996; **14**:66–9.

8. Antman K, Rowlings P, Vaughan W et al, High-dose chemotherapy with autologous hematopoietic stem-cell support for breast cancer in North America. *J Clin Oncol* 1997; **15**:1870–9.

9. Bezwoda W, Seymour L, Dansey R, High-dose chemotherapy with hematopoietic rescue as primary treatment for metastatic breast cancer: A randomized trial. *J Clin Oncol* 1995; **13**:2483–9.

10. Weiss RB, Rifkin RM, Stewart FM et al, High-dose chemotherapy for high-risk primary breast cancer: An on-site review of the Bezwoda study. *Lancet* 2000; **355**:999–1003.

11. Peters W, Jones R, Vredenburgh J et al, A large prospective randomized trial of high-dose combination alkylating agents (CPB) with autologous cellular support (ABMS) as consolidation for patients with metastatic breast cancer achieving complete remission after intensive doxorubicin-based induction therapy (AFM). *Proc Am Soc Clin Oncol* 1996; **15**:121.

12. Stadtmauer E, O'Neill A, Goldstein L et al, Phase III randomized trial of high-dose chemotherapy (HDC) and stem cell support (SCT) shows no difference in overall survival or severe toxicity compared to maintenance chemotherapy with cyclophosphamide, methotrexate and 5-fluorouracil (CMF) for women with metastatic breast cancer who are responding to conventional induction chemotherapy: The 'Philadelphia' Intergroup Study (PBT-1). *Proc Am Soc Clin Oncol* 1999; **18**:Abst 1.

13. Peters WP, Ross M, Vredenburgh JJ et al, High-dose chemotherapy and autologous bone marrow support as consolidation after standard-dose adjuvant therapy for high-risk primary breast cancer. *J Clin Oncol* 1993; **11**:1132–43.

14. Peters W, Rosner G, Vredenburgh J et al, A prospective, randomized comparison of two doses of combination alkylating agents (AA) as consolidation after CAF in high-risk primary breast cancer involving ten or more axillary lymph nodes (LN): Preliminary results of CALGB 9082/SWOG 9114/NCIC MA-13. *Proc Am Soc Clin Oncol* 1999; **18**:Abst 2.

15. Overgaard M, Hansen P, Overgaard J et al, Postoperative radiotherapy in high-risk premenopausal women with breast cancer who receive adjuvant chemotherapy. *N Engl J Med* 1997; **337**:949–55.

16. Ragaz J, Jackson S, Le N et al, Adjuvant radiotherapy and chemotherapy in node-positive premenopausal women with breast cancer. *N Engl J Med* 1997; **337**:956–62.

17. Bezwoda W, Randomised, controlled trials of high dose chemotherapy (HD-CNVp) versus standard dose (CAF) chemotherapy for high-risk, surgically treated, primary breast cancer. *Proc Am Soc Clin Oncol* 1999; **18**:Abst 4.

18. Rodenhuis S, Richel D, van der Wall E et al, Randomised trial of high-dose chemotherapy and haematopoietic progenitor-cell support in operable breast cancer with extensive axillary lymph node involvement. *Lancet* 1998; **352**:515–21.

19. Hortobagyi G, Buzdar A, Champlin R et al, Lack of efficacy of adjuvant high-dose (hd) tandem combination chemotherapy (ct) for high-risk primary breast cancer (hrpbc) – a randomized trial. *Proc Am Soc Clin Oncol* 1998; **18**:Abst 47.

20. Budman D, Berry D, Cirrincione C et al, Dose and dose intensity as determinants of outcome in the adjuvant treatment of breast cancer. *J Natl Cancer Inst* 1998; **90**:1205–11.

21. Thor A, Bery D, Budman D et al, erbB-2, p53 and efficacy of adjuvant therapy in lymph node-positive breast cancer. *J Natl Cancer Inst* 1998; **90**:1346–60.

22. Fisher B, Anderson S, Wickerham D et al, Increased intensification and total dose of cyclophosphamide in a doxorubicin– cyclo-phosphamide regimen for the treatment of primary breast cancer: findings from National Surgical Adjuvant Breast and Bowel Project B-22. *J Clin Oncol* 1997; **15**:1858–69.

23. Fisher B, Anderson S, DeCillis A et al, Further evaluation of intensified and increased total dose of cyclophosphamide for the treatment of primary breast cancer: Findings from National Surgical Adjuvant Breast and Bowel Project B-25. *J Clin Oncol* 1999; **17**:3374–88.

24. Henderson I, Berry D, Demetri G et al, Improved disease-free (dfs) and overall survival (os) from the addition of sequential paclitaxel (t) but not from the escalation of doxorubicin (a) dose level in the adjuvant chemotherapy of patients (pts) with node-positive primary breast cancer (bc). *Proc Am Soc Clin Oncol* 1998; **17**:390a.

25. Hudis C, Fornier M, Riccio L et al, Five-year results of dose-intensive sequential adjuvant chemotherapy for women with high risk node-positive breast cancer: a phase II study. *J Clin Oncol* 1999; **17**:1118–26.

26. Hudis C, Seidman A, Baselga J et al, Sequential dose-dense doxorubicin, paclitaxel, and cyclophosphamide for resectable high-risk breast cancer: feasibility and efficacy. *J Clin Oncol* 1999; **17**:93–100.

13

High-dose chemotherapy and autologous stem cell transplantation for metastatic breast cancer

Edward A Stadtmauer

INTRODUCTION

During the early 1980s, phase I and phase II trials of single-agent and combination chemotherapy for patients with relapsed and refractory metastatic breast cancer were performed.[1-15] Response rates of approximately 70% were observed, with 20–30% of the patients achieving complete remission. The average duration of response was approximately six months, with an average median survival of approximately eight months, with few, if any, long-term relapse-free survivors. This response rate was higher than what would be expected from conventional-dose chemotherapy; however, the median duration of response was similar to that achieved with conventional-dose therapy.

Because of the high frequency of response in patients with relapsed and refractory breast cancer, Peters and colleagues explored the use of a single course of high-dose therapy with stem cell transplantation as the initial therapy of first relapse from primary disease.[1] Patients in this series were generally young, pre-menopausal, and estrogen-receptor-negative, with measurable visceral disease. This trial suggested that a single course of high-dose chemotherapy produces up to 80% response rate and up to 40% complete

response rate in metastatic breast cancer. The updated report from Peters et al showed that with a minimum follow-up of 11 years, 3 of 22 (14%) patients remained continuously disease-free.

By its very nature, a trial of high-dose chemotherapy and stem cell rescue as the initial therapy of metastatic disease would include a very heavily selected patient population. These patients would have to be well enough to undergo high-dose therapy and have adequate bone marrow for stem cell selection. Most trials have therefore utilized a course of conventional-dose induction chemotherapy to reduce tumor burden, improve performance status, and decrease the chance of stem cell tumor contamination. A number of trials of this design suggested an approximately 80% response rate, with 10–30% of patients relapse free at two years (Table 13.1). The mortality rate in these early trials was substantial, however, ranging from 3% to 30% within the first 100 days of transplantation, although the survival benefits were perceived to be superior to historical controls. Registry data as reported to the Autologous Bone Marrow Registry corroborated these results.[16]

Interest in high-dose therapy and stem cell rescue increased and demands on insurers for

Table 13.1   Early pilot trials of high-dose chemotherapy and stem cell transplantation in metastatic breast cancer

Authors	Year	No. of patients	HDC[a]	RR[b] (%)	OS[c] (months)	PFS[d] (%)	Toxic death[e] (%)
Peters et al[1]	1988	22	CBP	73	10.1	14	23
Williams et al[2,4]	1989	27	CT	86	15.1	7	14
Kennedy et al[6]	1991	30	CT	100	22	10	0
Antman et al[3]	1992	29	CTCb	100	24	17	3

[a]High-dose chemotherapy: CBP, cyclophosphamide, carmustine, and cisplatin; CT, cyclophosphamide and thiotepa; CTCb, cyclophosphamide, thiotepa, and carboplatin.
[b]Response rate. [c]Overall survival. [d]Progression-free survival rate. [e]Rate of death within 100 days of stem cell infusion.

coverage increased rapidly. The most common high-dose chemotherapy treatment scenario had become the use of a course of four to six cycles of conventional-dose induction chemotherapy, usually cyclophosphamide, doxorubicin, and 5-fluorouracil (5-FU) (CAF), doxorubicin and cyclophosphamide (AC), or doxorubicin, 5-FU, and methotrexate (AFM), and then assessing for response. Patients achieving complete or partial response then proceeded to stem cell collection followed by a single course of high-dose chemotherapy utilizing primarily one of three regimens – CBP (cyclophosphamide, carmustine, and cisplatin), CTCb (cyclophosphamide, thiotepa, and carboplatin), or CT (cyclophosphamide and thiotepa) – and stem cell rescue. Trials comparing high-dose therapy and stem cell transplant with conventional-dose therapy were developed and initiated in the early 1990s. The results of a number of these trials have recently been reported.

COMPARISON TRIALS OF INDUCTION THERAPY FOLLOWED BY A SINGLE COURSE OF HIGH-DOSE CHEMOTHERAPY

In 1990, the Philadelphia Bone Marrow Transplant Group (Fox Chase, Hahnemann, Temple, and University of Pennsylvania) developed a randomized trial for chemotherapy-untreated metastatic breast cancer. NCCTG, ECOG, and SWOG joined the trial, and it was designated a high-priority trial by the National Cancer Institute. The trial, PBT-1, met its accrual goal, and was closed in December 1998, and the results were reported in May 1999.[17]

PBT-1 was designed to compare the time to progression and overall survival and toxicity of high-dose chemotherapy and stem cell transplantation with those of a prolonged course of maintenance chemotherapy for women with metastatic breast cancer responding to first-line chemotherapy. Eligibility required locally recurrent or distant metastatic disease, pre- or postmenopausal status, age less than or equal to 60 years, no prior chemotherapy for metastatic disease, prior adjuvant chemotherapy greater than six months prior to entry, at least one prior hormonal treatment if estrogen-receptor-positive unless life-threatening visceral disease present, and performance status of zero or one. Patients then received induction chemotherapy with CAF for four to six cycles or CMF (cyclophosphamide, methotrexate, and 5-FU) with optional prednisone if the prior doxorubicin dose was greater than or equal to $400 \, mg/m^2$. Patients achieving stable disease or progressive disease were taken off study, and patients achieving complete or partial response went on to further therapy. To be eligible for randomization, patients could not have had bone marrow involvement with tumor, and required normal hematopoietic, cardiac, pulmonary, and hepatic function. Additionally, the therapy was to begin within eight weeks of the last chemotherapy.

Eligible patients were randomized to autologous stem cell transplantation or to CMF maintenance chemotherapy for up to two years. Patients discontinued CMF early at time of progressive disease, or toxicity, or removal of informed consent. Patients undergoing stem cell transplant underwent bone marrow harvest and granulocyte–macrophage colony-stimulating factor (GM-CSF)-stimulated peripheral stem cell harvest followed by high-dose CTCb therapy with stem cell transplant and GM-CSF-stimulated marrow recovery. In 1995, the trial was amended to allow for granulocyte colony-stimulating factor (G-CSF)-stimulated stem cell harvest as the sole source of stem cells.

Five hundred and fifty-three patients were enrolled in the trial, with 296 achieving response (and therefore potentially eligible for randomization) and 199 proceeding to randomization. Of the 97 patients who responded but did not proceed with randomization, the majority withdrew consent and did not wish to proceed with

randomization or had bone marrow biopsies positive for tumor contamination. This group of patients was similar in demographics and number to the group that proceeded to transplantation.

Of the 199 patients, 110 were assigned to transplantation and 89 to maintenance therapy, and, of these, 15 (7.5%) were ineligible (9 transplantation and 6 CMF), leaving 184 eligible randomized patients (101 transplantation and 83 CMF). With a median follow-up of the entire group of 37 months, there was no difference in median survival between transplant and maintenance therapy (24 months versus 26 months) or three-year survival rate (32% versus 38%) ($p = 0.23$). Patients in complete remission at the time of randomization fared better in both overall survival and time to progression than patients in partial response. There was also no difference in time to progression between transplantation and maintenance chemotherapy, with a median time to progression of 9.6 months versus 9.0 months and a three-year progression-free survival rate of 6% versus 12% ($p = 0.31$). No significant benefit for transplantation was observed in any stratified subgroup, including response, hormone-receptor status, age less than or equal to 42 years versus greater than 42 years, or dominant metastatic site visceral or other.

A surprising finding was the low conversion rate of patients in partial response at the time of randomization to complete response with high-dose chemotherapy. One hundred and thirty-nine patients were in partial response at the time of randomization and 11 (8%) were converted to complete remission after consolidation therapy; 5 were converted by transplantation and 6 by CMF. Another surprising finding was the low lethal toxicity of transplantation in this trial. No lethal toxicity was observed on the CMF arm, and only one patient died (of veno-occlusive disease) on the transplantation arm. Non-lethal severe toxicities, however, were increased on the transplantation arm – including hematologic toxicity, infection, nausea, vomiting and diarrhea, and cardiac, pulmonary and hepatic toxicities – although mucositis was not substantially increased. Overall, of the 184 eligible patients randomized, 20 refused randomized assignment, and this was well balanced in both groups. This study demonstrated that high-dose chemotherapy with stem cell rescue did not confer incremental improvement in overall survival or time to progression to CMF, and there was no substantial difference in lethal toxicity, although non-lethal grade serious toxicities were greater in the transplantation arm. Alternatively, one could conclude that one cycle of high-dose therapy was equivalent to up to 24 months of CMF.

A similar but smaller trial has been conducted in France.[18] Patients with chemotherapy-naive metastatic breast cancer were treated with induction chemotherapy for six cycles, and a partial or complete response was required. patients then went on to two to four additional cycles of induction chemotherapy, or cyclophosphamide plus G-CSF-stimulated stem cell harvest followed by high-dose CMA (cyclophosphamide, melphalan and mitoxantrone) with stem cell transplantation. Thirty-two patients were assigned to transplantation and 29 to conventional-dose therapy. At two years, there was a trend toward improved survival in the transplantation arm, but by five years no significant difference in the two arms was observed. These trials suggests that the use of cyclophosphamide-containing induction chemotherapy followed by high-dose chemotherapy and stem cell transplantation for responding patients has not substantially improved survival in metastatic breast cancer.

Few patients in complete remission were transplanted on these comparative trials. Peters et al[19] have given a preliminary report of a randomized trial examining the use of high-dose chemotherapy and stem cell transplantation as consolidation treatment in patients who achieved a complete remission after intensive induction therapy. Four hundred and twenty-three patients with hormone-insensitive measurable metastatic breast cancer who had not received any prior chemotherapy received two to four cycles of AFM induction therapy. One hundred and six patients (25%) achieved complete remission, and 98 of these patients were randomized to either immediate consolidation with STAMP I (cisplatin, carmustine, and cyclophosphamide) versus observation. The randomization was balanced both for pretreatment patient characteristics and for site and extent of disease. The disease-free survival was significantly improved in the patients who received high dose chemotherapy up front, and, with a median follow-up of 3.9 years, the event-free survival rate at five years is 24% for the high-dose arm versus 8% for the observation arm.

As a second part of this trial, patients assigned to the observation arm went on to high-dose chemotherapy and stem cell transplantation at the time of progression. Patients receiving transplantation at the time of first progression have superior overall survival to patients transplanted initially, with a median overall survival of 2.25 years versus 3.56 years. These results suggest that induction chemotherapy just prior to transplantation may not be the optimal treatment design.

UP-FRONT TRANSPLANTATION AND TANDEM TRANSPLANTATION

The only randomized comparison trial of up-front high-dose chemotherapy versus conventional-dose chemotherapy was reported by Bezwoda et al[20] from South Africa in 1995. This prospective randomized trial enrolled patients who were 50 years of age or younger with histologically confirmed metastatic breast cancer. Patients had to have had no prior chemotherapy for metastatic disease and to have normal organ function. Patients who relapsed or did not respond to prior hormonal therapy were eligible. Patients were randomized to a control arm of CMV (cyclophosphamide 600 mg/m^2, mitoxantrone 12 mg/m^2, and vincristine 1.4 mg/m^2) every three weeks for six to eight cycles versus an experimental arm of tandem high-dose CMV chemotherapy (cyclophosphamide 2.4 g/m^2, mitoxantrone 35–45 mg/m^2, and etoposide 2.5 g/m^2), with cycle 2 given approximately 42 days from cycle 1. Stem cells were collected prior to each transplant using variably marrow alone, cyclophosphamide-mobilized stem cells, and cyclophosphamide- and G-CSF-mobilized stem cells. Following chemotherapy, all patients who were classified as responders received maintenance therapy with tamoxifen 20 mg daily.

Ninety patients were enrolled and 45 were assigned to tandem transplantation and 45 to conventional-dose therapy. Tandem transplantation was superior in inducing a response: a 95% response rate with 51% complete response versus 53% response rate with 4% complete response rate for conventional-dose therapy. Tandem transplantation also resulted in a doubling of the median response duration from 34 weeks to 80 weeks, and a doubling of median survival from 45 weeks to 90 weeks. These promising results have held up with five years of follow-up. One potential confounding factor here is that hormonal therapy was used for 95% of the patients treated with high-dose therapy but for only 53% of patients treated with conventional-dose therapy as per design of the study. This study is now under review as part of a misconduct investigation.[21]

A number of trials utilizing cycles of high-dose chemotherapy in metastatic breast cancer have now been reported.[22] Investigators from the Dana-Farber Cancer institute have reported on 67 women with metastatic breast cancer receiving the sequence of high-dose melphalan followed by STAMP V (carboplatin, thiotepa, and cyclophosphamide). Patients initially received three or four cycles of doxorubicin and 5-FU, followed by G-CSF-stimulated peripheral stem cell harvest. Patients received melphalan 140–180 mg/m^2 with stem cell support followed by STAMP V and then went on to radiotherapy, surgery, and hormonal therapy if estrogen-receptor-positive. Forty-four percent were progression-free a median of 16 months after STAMP V, and the median progression-free and overall survivals were 11 and 20 months respectively. These were not substantially improved from a historical cohort of single stem cell transplant.

The authors considered possible reasons for this outcome in this group of patients. Acquired drug resistance is likely to have played a role in the failure of high-dose chemotherapy. One could conceive how induction chemotherapy could produce enough tumor cytoreduction to result in clinical response, but the minimal residual tumor may have been induced into a state of drug resistance. This is suggested by the failure to significantly convert patients in partial remission into complete remission after the high-dose therapy (approximately 15% in this series). Additionally, the sequence of dose-intensive therapy may play a role. Tumor cells surviving high-dose melphalan may be particularly resistant to the agents in STAMP V, and therefore that sequence of events may not lead to an optimal outcome. This group of investigators[23] has recently reported on 58 patients receiving two courses of induction chemotherapy with doxorubicin 90 mg/m^2 followed by tandem transplantation in the opposite sequence, with STAMP V initially and then a melphalan and paclitoxel combination. Preliminary results show that 78% achieve complete or near-complete response, with 60% event-free survival at two years.

A multi-institutional trial sought to investigate the role of induction chemotherapy as part of tandem sequential high-dose chemotherapy for metastatic breast cancer.[24] Sixty-three patients were treated with four cycles of doxorubicin 50 mg/m^2 and docetaxel 75 mg/m^2, followed by a course of cyclophosphamide 5 g/m^2, etoposide 1.5 g/m^2, and cisplatin 120 mg/m^2, with G-CSF-stimulated stem cell harvesting and followed by a STAMP V transplant. Patients went on to long-term anastrozole. Additionally, a group of 36 patients received the same sequential high-dose chemotherapy without the four cycles of induction therapy. A comparison of these two groups demonstrated a significantly greater complete response rate in the induction-therapy group (42% versus 11%), as well as an improved progression-free survival. There was a 2.3-fold increase in risk of disease progression in the non-induction-therapy group. This one study at least suggests a benefit for induction chemotherapy for metastatic breast cancer.

RESULTS FROM LARGE-REGISTRY RETROSPECTIVE ANALYSIS

The CALGB has conducted a retrospective database comparison utilizing historical data from CALGB metastatic breast cancer trials, and has compared this database with high-dose chemotherapy with stem cell transplantation for metastatic breast cancer as reported to the ABMTR.[25] To be eligible, patients on the CALGB trials had to receive CAF induction chemotherapy, and while the induction chemotherapy was not reported in the ABMTR trials, a response was required. On the CALGB trials, the control arm was further courses of CAF with or without other chemotherapy regimens, while the experimental arm contained all transplants for metastatic breast cancer from 1989 to 1995 that had been reported to the ABMTR. Most patients had received a cyclophosphamide and thiotepa regimen with or without carboplatin. All patients were aged less than 65 years. The overall survival curves of these two groups were not significantly different.

Most recently, a report from the Autologous Bone Marrow Transplant Registry analyzed the factors associated with disease progression or death in a total of 1188 consecutive women aged 18–70 years receiving autologous transplantation for metastatic locally recurrent breast cancer, with a median follow-up of $29\frac{1}{2}$ months.[26] Nine factors were associated with a significantly increased risk of treatment failure: age greater than 45 years, Karnofsky performance score less than 90%, hormone-receptor negativity, prior use of adjuvant chemotherapy, initial disease-free interval after adjuvant chemotherapy less than 18 months, liver metastases, central nervous system metastases, three or more sites of metastatic disease, and less than complete response to standard-dose chemotherapy. Receipt of tamoxifen post-transplantation was associated with a reduced risk of treatment failure in women with hormone-receptor-positive tumors. Women with no risk factors had a three-year probability of progression-free survival of 43%, while this probability was 4% for women with more than three risk factors. The three-year probability of progression-free survival for the entire group was 13%. The group of patients with no risk factors (38 patients) accounted for only 3% of the entire population that was reported, while 84% of the patients registered had two or more risk factors, and experienced outcomes similar to those seen in phase II and phase III trials.

CONCLUSIONS AND FUTURE DIRECTIONS

After almost two decades of clinical research investigating high-dose therapy and stem cell transplantation for metastatic breast cancer, the body of data, particularly in comparative trials

Table 13.2 Randomized trials of high-dose chemotherapy (HDC) in metastatic breast cancer

Study	Total/Total randomized (% randomized of total)	Treatment	Randomized	Toxic death	PR → CR rate (%)	EFS rate (%)		OS rate (%)		Best
						3-yr	5-yr	3-yr	5-yr	
Philadelphia	553/199 (36%)	HDC	110	1	8	6	–	32	–	Same
		Control	89	0		12	–	38	–	
Duke (CR)	425/98 (25%)	HDC	49	7.5%	–	–	24	–	–	HDC
		Control	49	0		–	8	–	(40)[b]	(EFS not OS)
South African	90/90 (100%)	HDC	45	0	–	–	18	–	18	HDC
		Control	45	0		–	4	–	4	
French	–[a]/61	HDC	32	0	11	49	9	55	30	Same
		Control	29	0		21	9	28	18.5	
Philadelphia (CR)	553/45 (8%)	HDC	26	1	–	16	–	42	–	Same
		Control	19	0		25	–	49	–	

[a]Referral at time of CR or PR; [b]Combined group.

and large-registry analyses, has reached the critical mass to aid in clinical decision-making. So what can we conclude from this data (Table 13.2). Unfortunately, there is no evidence as of yet that induction chemotherapy followed by a single course of high-dose chemotherapy with stem cell transplantation improves the outcome for women with metastatic breast cancer – in particular, relapse-free survival and overall survival. Toxicity, however, has been reduced substantially over the last decade, and a single course of high-dose therapy is at least equivalent to cycles of conventional-dose chemotherapy. Quality of life and economic analyses and endpoints remain to be determined, but these must be considered secondary to survival. A phase III trial in Canada is still ongoing, and may add to this information. Additionally, the randomized trials so far presented emphasize the treatment of patients with a number of risk factors for treatment failure, and perhaps a trial for younger patients in complete remission with few sites of metastatic disease may be indicated. However, the preponderance of evidence suggests that high-dose chemotherapy and stem cell transplantation, in the way that this has been utilized over the last two decades, has not made a substantial impact on treatment for metastatic breast cancer.

There are clues, however, in the data to suggest the possibility of improved design of treatment protocols (Table 13.3):

1. Cycles of high-dose therapy appear to be superior to single courses of high-dose therapy.
2. Induction chemotherapy may induce chemotherapy resistance, and improved forms of induction therapy designed to prevent resistance may result in superior outcomes.
3. The role of infusion of contaminated tumor cells in the relapse of patients after high-dose chemotherapy and stem cell infusion remains to be determined, and improved processing

Table 13.3   Future directions
• Cycles of high-dose therapy
• Better induction therapy
• Stem cell processing and purging
• Post-transplantation minimal disease therapy

and purging techniques may have a small but positive impact on outcome.
4. Post-transplantation therapy with tamoxifen for hormone-receptor-positive patients is clearly a benefit after transplant, and other post-transplantation therapies such as cycles of conventional-dose chemotherapy, immunotherapies, anti-angiogenesis therapies, and others, when combined with the maximal cytoreduction of high-dose therapy, may also improve these results.

Collaboration between physicians, patients, and insurers to design and quickly complete phase I and phase II trials to investigate these newer approaches, followed by the sincere use of the data derived from these trials to design phase III randomized comparison trials, if the data are compelling enough to warrant it, will assure the optimal care for our patients with metastatic breast cancer.

REFERENCES

1. Peters WP et al, High-dose combination alkylating agents with bone marrow support as initial treatment for metastatic breast cancer. *J Clin Oncol* 1988; 6:1368–76.
2. Williams SF et al, High dose consolidation therapy with autologous stem cell rescue in stage IV breast cancer. *J Clin Oncol* 1989; 7:1824–30.
3. Antman K et al, A phase II study of high dose cyclophosphamide, thiotepa, and carboplatin

with autologous marrow support in women with measurable advanced breast cancer responding to standard-dose therapy. *J Clin Oncol* 1992; **10**:102–10.

4. Williams SF et al, High-dose consolidation therapy with autologous stem cell rescue in stage IV breast cancer: follow-up report. *J Clin Oncol* 1992; **10**:1743–7.

5. Moonneier JA et al, High dose trialkylator chemotherapy with autologous stem cell rescue in patients with refractory malignancies. *J Natl Cancer Inst* 1990; **82**:29–34.

6. Kennedy MJ et al, High-dose chemotherapy with reinfusion of purged autologous bone marrow following dose intense induction as initial therapy for metastatic breast cancer. *J Natl Cancer Inst* 1991; **83**:920–6.

7. Eddy DM, Review article. High-dose chemotherapy with autologous bone marrow transplantation for the treatment of metastatic breast cancer. *J Clin Oncol* 1992; **10**:657–70.

8. Klumpp TR et al, Phase II pilot study of high-dose busulfan and CY followed by autologous BM or peripheral blood stem cell transplantation in patients with advanced chemosensitive breast cancer. *Bone Marrow Transplant* 1993; **11**:337–9.

9. Lazarus HM et al, A phase I trial of high-dose melphalan, high-dose etoposide, and autologous bone marrow reinfusion in solid tumors: an Eastern Cooperative Oncology Group (ECOG) study. *Bone Marrow Transplant* 1994; **14**:443–8.

10. Weaver CH et al, Phase I study of high-dose busulfan, melphalan, and thiotepa with autologous stem cell support in patients with refractory malignancies. *Bone Marrow Transplant* 1994; **14**:813–19.

11. Vaughan WP et al, High-dose cyclophosphamide, thiotepa and hydroxyurea with autologous hematopoietic stem cell rescue: an effective consolidation chemotherapy regimen for early metastatic breast cancer. *Bone Marrow Transplant* 1994; **13**:619–24.

12. Fields KK et al, Maximum tolerated doses of ifosfamide, carboplatin, and etoposide given over six days followed by autologous stem cell rescue: toxicity profile. *J Clin Oncol* 1995; **13**:323–32.

13. Spitzer TR et al, Phase I–II trial of high-dose cyclophosphamide, carboplatin and autologous bone marrow or peripheral blood stem cell rescue. *Bone Marrow Transplant* 1995; **15**:537–42.

14. Gisselbrecht C et al, Cyclophosphamide/mitoxantrone/melphalan (CMA) regimen prior to autologous bone marrow transplantation (ABMT) in metastatic breast cancer. *Bone Marrow Transplant* 1996; **18**:857–63.

15. Stemmer SM et al, High-dose paclitaxel, cyclophosphamide, and cisplatin with autologous hematopoietic progenitor-cell support: A phase I trial. *J Clin Oncol* 1996; **14**:1463–72.

16. *ABMTR Newsletter* 1998; **5**:5.

17. Stadtmauer EA et al, Conventional-dose chemotherapy compared with high-dose chemotherapy plus autologous hematopoietic stem cell transplantation for metastatic breast cancer. *N Engl J Med* 2000; **342**:1069–76

18. Lotz JP et al, High-dose chemotherapy with hematopoietic stem cells transplantation for metastatic breast cancer: results of the French protocol Pegase 04. *Proc Am Soc Clin Oncol* 1999; **18**:43a.

19. Peters W et al, A large prospective randomized trial of high-dose combination alkylating agents (CPB) with autologous cellular support as consolidation for patients with metastatic breast cancer achieving complete remission after intensive doxorubicin-based induction therapy (AFM). *Proc Am Soc Clin Oncol* 1996; **15**:121.

20. Bezwoda W et al, High-dose chemotherapy with hematopoietic rescue as primary treatment for metastatic breast cancer: a randomized trial. *J Clin Oncol* 1995; **13**:2483–9.

21. Weiss RB, Rifkin RM, Stewart FM et al, High-dose chemotherapy for high-risk primary breast cancer: an on-site review of the Bezwoda study. Lancet 2000; **355**:999–1003.

22. Ayash LJ et al, Double dose-intensive chemotherapy with autologous stem-cell support for metastatic breast cancer: no improvement in progression-free survival by the sequence of high-dose melphalan followed by cyclophosphamide, thiotepa and carboplatin. *J Clin Oncol* 1996; **14**:2984–92.

23. Elias AD et al, Phase I development of double cycle stem cell supported high dose chemotherapy (HDC) for metastatic breast cancer (BC): the DFCI/BIDMC experience. *Proc Am Soc Clin Oncol* 1999; **18**:123a.

24. Pecora A et al, Induction chemotherapy prior to sequential high dose chemotherapy compared to no induction increases the rate of complete response and duration of progression free survival in women with metastatic breast cancer. *Proc Am Soc Clin Oncol* 1999; **18**:123a.

25. Berry DA et al, Conventional vs high-dose therapy for metastatic breast cancer: comparison of Cancer and Leukemia Group B (CALGB) and Blood and Marrow Transplant Registry (ABMTR) patients. *Proc Am Soc Clin Oncol* 1999; **18**:128a.

26. Rowlings PA et al, Factors correlated with progression-free survival after high-dose chemotherapy and hematopoietic stem cell transplantation for metastatic breast cancer. *JAMA* 1999; **282**:1335–43.

SECTION 3: Hormone Therapy

Section Editors: A U Buzdar, A Howell

14

New antiestrogens: Modulators of estrogen action

Anthony Howell

Breast cancer remains the most common cancer and a leading cause of cancer death in women in the USA and Europe.[1] A substantial body of experimental, clinical and epidemiological evidence indicates that steroid hormones play a major role in the etiology of breast cancer. Not only do endogenous estrogens support the development and growth of the breast and breast tumor cells, they also have profound beneficial and carefully regulated effects on other tissues such as the endometrium, vagina, bone, liver and vessels of the cardiovascular system, as summarized in Table 14.1.

The clinical responsiveness of the breast to estrogen deprivation was first demonstrated over 100 years ago.[2] Pharmacologic inhibition of the tumor stimulatory effects of physiologic estrogen concentrations was first reported using high-dose stilbestrol, triphenylchloroethylene and triphenylbromoethylene.[3,4] Antiestrogen therapy since the 1940s, and tamoxifen in particular, has revolutionized the treatment of breast cancer. Today, tamoxifen (Nolvadex, ICI 147,741) is the antiestrogen of choice for adjuvant therapy after surgery and for recurrent breast cancer. Coupled

to this, however, are the general issues surrounding the health of peri- and postmenopausal women associated with changes in their estrogen levels. Breast cancer occurs predominantly in postmenopausal women in whom reduced estrogen levels are associated with skeletal problems resulting from reduced bone density (osteoporosis) and increased cardiovascular risk. Many of the modulators of estrogen action such as tamoxifen have a beneficial effect on bone density and serum lipids, but have adverse effects on the uterus. Thus, an antiestrogen breast cancer therapy, which safely eliminates the negative effects of the menopause on women's health in the absence of toxicity, is the challenge for the new millennium.

The term 'antiestrogen' refers to agents that block the effects of physiologic concentrations of estrogen at the estrogen receptor (ER). 'Selective estrogen receptor modulator' (SERM) was a term coined to describe the phenomenon of apparent blocking of the ER at one site (e.g. the tumor) and stimulatory activity at another (e.g. bone). Thus, a single drug could have both agonist and antagonist activity depending on the cell type.

Table 14.1   Summary of the effects of estrogen (estradiol, 17β-estradiol) on target tissues

Target organ/tissue	Pharmacologic and physiologic effects of estrogen
Breast	Promotes breast epithelial cell proliferation, development and growth of the breast, together with other growth-stimulating factors, progesterone, corticosteroids, prolactin, insulin. Associated with poor clinical outcome in ER-positive breast cancer patients
Endometrium and vagina	Stimulates proliferation of epithelial cells and regulates cyclical changes. Unopposed it is associated with malignancy. Cornification of vaginal epithelium
Cardiovascular system	Reduces risk factors associated with CVD, predominantly serum lipid and lipoprotein composition. Arterial smooth muscle relaxation via ER- and non-ER-mediated pathways
Bone	ER found on both osteoclasts and osteoblasts. Regulates expression of bone cytokines. Increases bone density
CNS (brain)	Feedback actions on the hypothalamus and limbic system. Controls mood swings and cognitive function, possibly delaying the onset and progression of Alzheimer's disease
Liver	Influences liver-derived coagulation factors and plasma proteins and regulation of lipids. (See also cardiovascular system)

ER, estrogen receptor; CVD, cardiovascular disease.

SERMs were then divided into SERM 1 (tamoxifen), SERM 2 (raloxifene) and SERM 3 (a compound with no other common name closely related structurally to raloxifene). However, almost all estrogens may have agonist or antagonist activity depending on drug dose and target cell type. For example, the high doses of estrogens used to inhibit breast tumors have agonist activity in normal tissues.[4] They may also become agonists to the tumor with the passage of time, as demonstrated by the phenomenon of a withdrawal response.[5] An exception to the combined agonist/antagonist activity of most estrogens and antiestrogens may be the so-called steroidal 'pure' antiestrogens, which are apparently devoid of agonist activity. The lack of agonist activity may be related to the fact that they appear to have a different mechanism of action with respect to their effect on ER. Levels of ERs in tumors decline markedly on treatment so that this group of compounds has been called selective estrogen receptor downregulators. The acronym SERM may have some uses, but we have used the term 'antiestrogen' throughout this chapter for the sake of clarity.

Tamoxifen: advantages and disadvantages

Tamoxifen, a non-steroidal, triphenylethylene-based antiestrogen (Figure 14.1) with tissue-specific estrogenic (agonist) and antiestrogenic (antagonist) activity, has been the antiestrogen of choice in the clinic for over 25 years.[6] Its biologic

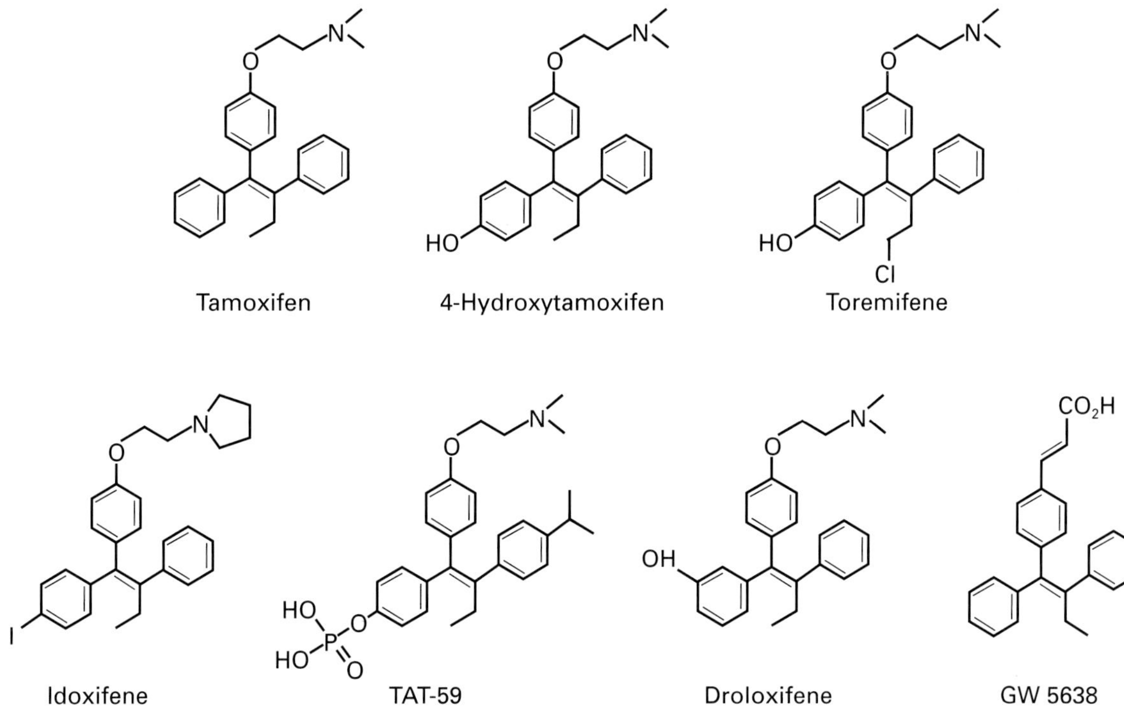

Figure 14.1
Triphenylethylene antiestrogens.

effects are mediated primarily by inhibiting the actions of estrogen through its binding to the ER. The differential actions of tamoxifen occur by selective ER modulation according to the cell and gene promoter type.

The antiestrogenic activity of tamoxifen in the breast has established it as the 'gold standard' for the treatment of all stages of breast cancer. Tamoxifen given for different durations in an adjuvant setting has been associated with a reduction in the risk of both contralateral breast cancer and metastatic cancer.[7] These data supported the prospective evaluation of tamoxifen in the prevention of cancer in women at high risk of the disease.[8] As a result, the US Food and Drug Administration (FDA) has approved tamoxifen for breast cancer prevention.[9]

The estrogenic activity of long-term tamoxifen treatment is associated with at least two other clinical benefits normally associated with premenopausal physiologic estrogen concentrations (Table 14.1). Tamoxifen therapy helps to maintain bone density[10] and lowers circulating low-density lipoprotein cholesterol,[11] effects of importance to perimenopausal and postmenopausal women.

The most frequent side effect associated with tamoxifen therapy is the occurrence of 'hot flushes' which is thought to be related to the antagonistic action of tamoxifen on the hypothalamic–pituitary axis. However, the side effect that causes the most concern is the increased risk of endometrial cancer related to the estrogen agonist activity of tamoxifen on the uterus.[8,12,13]

Table 14.2   Preclinical and clinical assessment of new antiestrogens

Preclinical in vitro and in vivo assessments
- ERα and ERβ receptor binding
- ERα and ERβ transcriptional activation
- Antiestrogenic activity in breast and uterus
- Tumor antagonism in animal models
- Activity in cell lines
- Estrogenic activity on bone and serum lipids
- Mechanism of ER activation (co-activators, co-repressors and ligand-independent activity)

Clinical assessment
- Activity as first-line therapy in metastatic breast cancer
- Activity in tamoxifen-resistant tumors
- Activity as neoadjuvant and adjuvant therapy
- Activity in prevention
- Side-effect profile
- Effects on women's health

In addition, tamoxifen can have more frequent but less serious side effects on the uterus, in the form of endometrial polyps, and simple and complex hyperplasia. Antiestrogen therapy is also associated with an increased incidence of thromboembolic phenomena, including deep vein thrombosis, pulmonary embolism and possibly cerebrovascular events.[8] Finally, tamoxifen therapy is associated with the acquisition by tumors of 'tamoxifen resistance', where tamoxifen no longer inhibits tumor growth but may actually promote it.[5]

Despite these negative aspects of tamoxifen therapy, the benefits for the treatment and prevention of breast cancer are thought to outweigh the risks substantially. The success of tamoxifen in the treatment of breast cancer has proved invaluable in the search for, and development of, new antiestrogens that selectively retain the favorable estrogenic and antiestrogenic properties of tamoxifen. It is the standard against which all new therapies will be measured in well-established preclinical and clinical settings (Table 14.2). Although tamoxifen has revolutionized the treatment of breast cancer, the search continues for new agents that will confer increased response rates and durations of response in patients with advanced disease, increase cure rates and times to relapse in the adjuvant setting, reduce tumor burden in the neoadjuvant setting, play a clearly defined role in disease prevention, and improve the general health of postmenopausal women.[14]

NEW ANTIESTROGENS

Since the publication of a previous review in 1996,[14] there has been a marked increase in the preclinical and clinical information available on the new antiestrogens and in our understanding of their mechanisms of action via the ER.

Three main avenues have been followed in an

Table 14.3   Antiestrogens with past or potential clinical value

Triphenylethylenes (tamoxifen derivatives)
Toremifene
Droloxifene
Idoxifene
TAT-59
GW 5638

Fixed ring compounds
Benzothiophenes
– Raloxifene (LY 156,758)
– SERM 3 (LY 353,381)
Naphthalenes
– Lasofoxifene (CP-336,156)
– LY 326,315
Benzopyrans
– EM 800 (SCH 57050)
– EM 652 (SCH 57068)

Steroidal compounds
ICI 182,780
RU 58608
SR 16234

attempt to improve on tamoxifen. One has been to produce analogs of tamoxifen by chemically altering the triphenylethylene structure in an attempt to block the metabolic hydroxylation at the 4-position and to reduce metabolic inactivation by altering the side chain. Second, new, non-steroidal, fixed-ring structures derived from the stilbene structure of stilbestrol have been synthesized. The aim of these syntheses was to prevent the isomerization that occurs around the double bond in the triphenylethylenes (hence the term 'fixed-ring'). These structures include benzothiophenes,[15,16] naphthalenes[17] and benzopyrans.[18,19] The third approach has been to

synthesize steroidal analogues of estrogen with growth inhibitory activity.[20–23]

These three classes of antiestrogens (triphenylethylenes, fixed-ring and steroidal) (Table 14.3) are known to differ in their affinities for the ER, their mechanisms of action in relation to the ER, and their effects on the key issues as assessed in a whole range of in vitro and in vivo, preclinical, assay systems (see Table 14.2). Clarification of the clinical potential of these and future agents will, however, depend on an improvement in our understanding of the various mechanisms and molecular determinants of ER-mediated response, not only in the breast, but especially at other sites of action such as bone and the cardiovascular system.

The newer triphenylethylenes include tamoxifen analogues toremifene,[24] idoxifene,[25] droloxifene (3-hydroxytamoxifen),[26] TAT-59[27] and GW 5638[28] (see Figure 14.1). The newer fixed-ring compounds include benzothiophenes (raloxifene [LY 156,758] and SERM 3 [LY 353,381]),[15,16] naphthalenes (lasofoxifene [CP-336,156] and LY 326,315):[17,18] and benzopyrans (EM 800 [SCH 58050] and its metabolite EM 600 [SCH 58068])[19] (Figure 14.2). All these agents competitively inhibit estrogen binding to the ER and have mixed agonist/antagonist activity mediated by the ER.

The steroidal antiestrogens (Figure 14.3) include ICI 164,384 and ICI 182,780, in which the addition of a side chain at the 7α position of estradiol leads to the complete abrogation of the trophic/agonist action of estradiol on the uterus and also blocks the uterotrophic action of tamoxifen.[20] Another steroidal pure antiestrogen devoid of any partial agonist activity is RU 58668.[23] It differs from ICI 182,780 in that its bulky side chain extends from the 11β carbon atom of estradiol, rather than from the 7α carbon. The orally active steroidal antiestrogen SR 16234 has a methyl group at the 7α position and a bulky side chain at the 17β position (Figure 14.3).

a. Benzothiophenes

Figure 14.2
Fixed-ring antiestrogens.

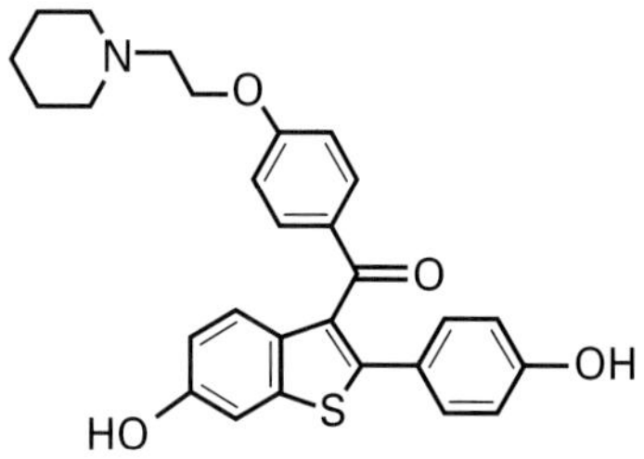

Raloxifene (LY 156,758)

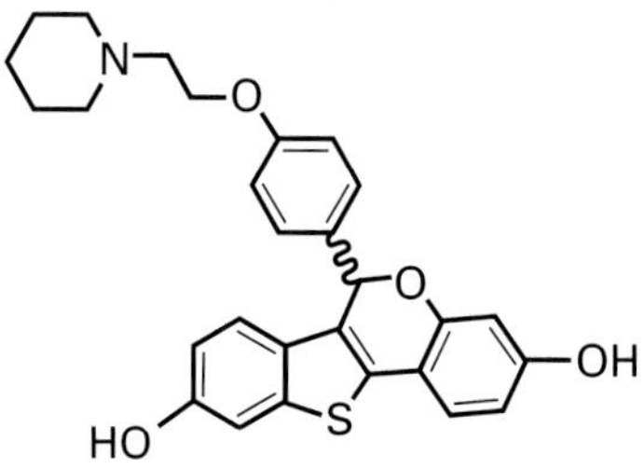

SERM 3 (LY 353,381)

b. Napthalenes

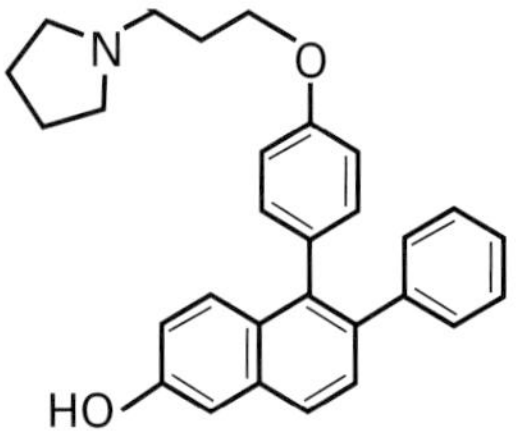

Lasofoxifene (CP 336,156)

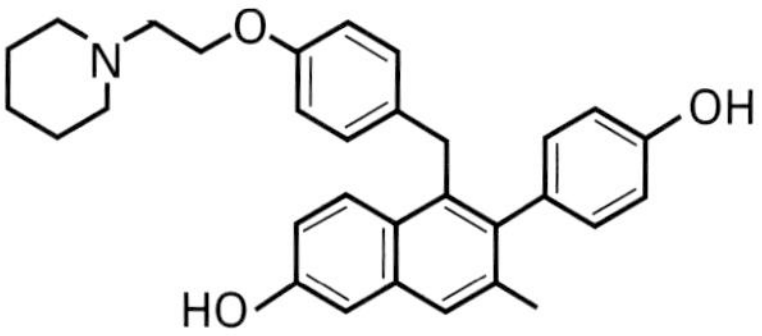

LY (326,315)

c. Benzopyrans

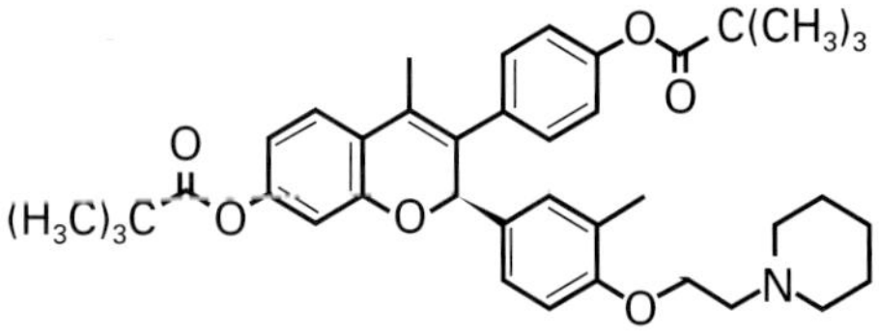

EM 800 (SCH 57050)

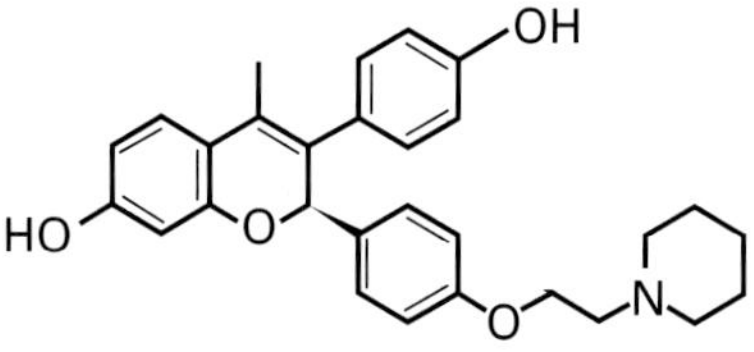

EM 652 (SCH 57068)

Some of the agents outlined above have already been withdrawn from clinical development (particularly many of the triphenylethylenes) for breast cancer treatment because they offer no advantage over tamoxifen. Their preclinical and clinical characteristics are briefly reviewed in the following section, however, in an attempt to provide an insight into the properties that might contribute to the development of optimally clinically effective antiestrogens.

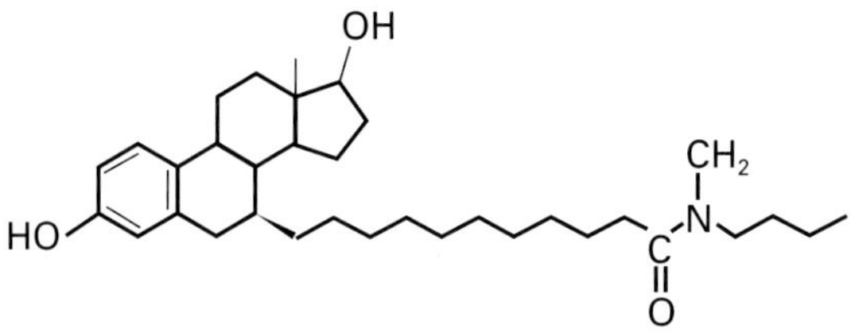

Figure 14.3
Steroidal antiestrogens.

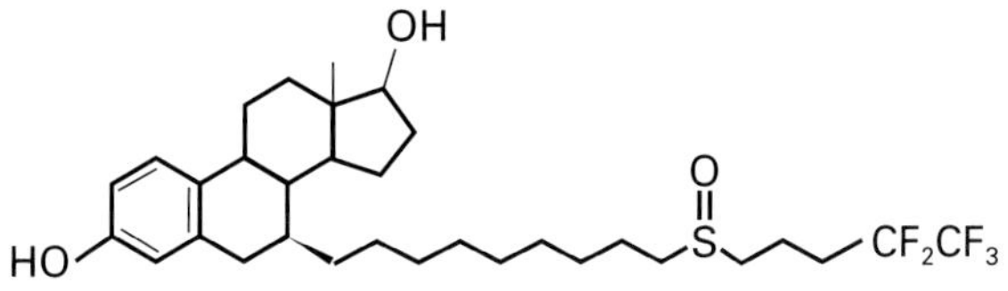

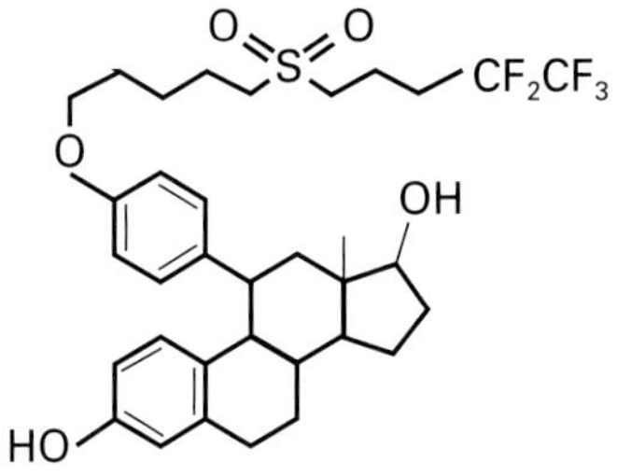

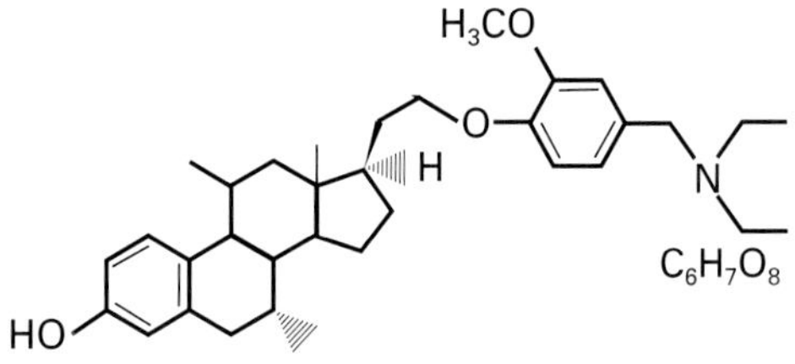

Triphenylethylenes

These are the most extensively studied of all the ER modulators and include the early antiestrogen triphenylchloro- and bromoethylenes, chlomiphene and tamoxifen. It was the concern over the effects of tamoxifen on the uterus and the desire for more active compounds that led to the development of the tamoxifen analogs described below.

Toremifene

Toremifene is a chlorinated analog of tamoxifen (see Figure 14.1), with similar site-specific estrogenic and antiestrogenic activity.[24] It has been shown in preclinical studies to have similar ER binding and anti-tumor activity to tamoxifen,[20] but less DNA adduct formation in the endometrium.[29] Toremifene has similar stimula-

tory effects to tamoxifen on the endometrium in athymic mice[24] and in postmenopausal patients receiving toremifene therapy for 12 months,[30] which suggests that toremifene, like tamoxifen, might be associated with an increased risk of endometrial cancer. Phase III trials[31–33] have demonstrated that toremifene is as effective as tamoxifen in the first-line treatment of metastatic breast cancer (MBC), with a similar side-effect profile. As a result, toremifene has been approved for the first-line treatment of MBC in patients with ER-positive and ER-unknown disease. Use of toremifene in an adjuvant setting also shows no difference in recurrence rates between it and tamoxifen,[34] again with similar side-effect profile. Low response rates in phase II studies in patients previously treated with tamoxifen suggest cross-resistance with tamoxifen.[14,35] Meta-analysis of all clinical trial data comparing toremifene and tamoxifen showed both agents to be equally effective in the treatment of advanced breast cancer in postmenopausal women.[36] Thus, to date, toremifene shows no advantages over tamoxifen.

Idoxifene, droloxifene and TAT-59

Unlike toremifene, all three agents bind to the ER more effectively than tamoxifen.[14,25,27] Idoxifene has an iodine atom at the 4-position of tamoxifen (see Figure 14.1) which is associated with reduced carcinogenic potential.[37] Preclinical[38] and phase I–II studies[25] were moderately encouraging, although idoxifene showed little activity when used after tamoxifen failure.[39] However, idoxifene has been withdrawn from development as a breast cancer therapy and for the treatment of osteoporosis because of uterine effects similar to those seen with tamoxifen.

Droloxifene

The preclinical[26,40] and phase II data[41–44] for droloxifene (3-hydroxytamoxifen) (see Figure 14.1) were also encouraging. However, droloxifene did not appear to offer any advantages over tamoxifen for the treatment of breast cancer patients. As a result droloxifene has also been taken off the market for the treatment of breast cancer and is currently being developed for the prevention of osteoporosis.

TAT-59

This is a prodrug, developed in Japan, that requires dephosphorylation to become the active metabolite of tamoxifen, 4-hydroxytamoxifen (see Figure 14.1). This agent has a high affinity for the ER.[27,45] A phase III trial comparing TAT-59 with tamoxifen in the first-line treatment of MBC has been reported.[46] The overall response rate was 30% in the TAT-59 arm and 26.5% in the tamoxifen arm. The side-effect profile was

mild, and again was similar to that of tamoxifen. There are no details of the effects of TAT-59 on bone density or serum lipid profile. TAT-59 is no longer in clinical development.

GW 5638

This is an acidic triphenylethylene in which the amino side chain has been replaced by a carboxylic acid moiety (see Figure 14.1). When assayed in vitro, it functions as an ER antagonist in a manner that is distinct from that of other known ER modulators.[28] However, quite unexpectedly it has the properties of a bone-selective antiestrogen and exhibits decreased uterotrophic activity relative to tamoxifen in preclinical studies.[28] GW 5638 is currently in clinical development but no data with respect to its effectiveness are available.

Fixed-ring compounds
Benzothiophenes

These were developed in an attempt to avoid the agonist problems associated with the triphenylethylenes on the uterus and to be more selective in their action on specific target tissues, namely breast and bone. Detailed structure activity studies[47] identified raloxifene (see Figure 14.2) as having a unique profile of biological activity. Currently, raloxifene and its derivative SERM 3 are undergoing clinical trials. Raloxifene is effective for the treatment of osteoporosis and prevents breast cancer. SERM 3 is being developed for the treatment of early and advanced breast cancer.

Raloxifene

Raloxifene (formerly called keoxifene) is a nonsteroidal benzothiophene derivative that binds to the ER with high affinity. It has been shown in preclinical studies to have antiestrogen effects on both the breast and the uterus, and estrogenic effects on the bone, cholesterol levels and vascu-

Table 14.4   Response to new antiestrogens as first- or second-line treatments for metastatic breast cancer compared with tamoxifen (as first line)

Drug	Response to SERMs and SERDs in advanced breast cancer			
	n	CR + PR (%)	SD	Total (%)
Tamoxifen	500+	27	25	52
Raloxifene	18	17	28	45
SERM 3	88	32	19	51
SCH 57050[a] (EM 800)	43	14	23	37
ICI 182,780[a] (Faslodex)	19	37	32	69

[a]Denotes previous treatment with tamoxifen for advanced disease.
CR, complete remission; PR, partial remission; SD, standard deviation; MBC, metastatic breast cancer; SERM, selective estrogen receptor modulator; SERD, selective estrogen receptor downregulator.

lar smooth muscle cells.[15,48–50] In fact raloxifene was developed for, and most of its clinical evaluation has been for, the treatment of osteoporosis in postmenopausal women.[51–53] Preliminary clinical studies showed raloxifene to decrease bone turnover and lower serum cholesterol levels without increasing serum triglyceride concentrations or causing endometrial proliferation.[51] These observations were confirmed by Delmas et al,[53] in a 2-year osteoporosis prevention trial, and raloxifene has been approved in the USA for the prevention of osteoporosis in postmenopausal women.

Evidence of the potential of raloxifene as a breast cancer therapy came from the Multiple Outcomes of Raloxifene Evaluation (MORE) trial[54] which showed that the incidence of ER-positive breast cancer was 74% lower in the raloxifene group than in the placebo group. As in the tamoxifen breast cancer prevention trial,[8] the effect was seen exclusively in patients who developed ER-positive breast cancers. Significantly, the incidence of endometrial cancer was not increased, and was in fact slightly lower, in the raloxifene treatment groups when compared with placebo.

There have been two clinical reports involving a total of 32 postmenopausal women. In the first study,[55] no objective tumor response was observed in 14 patients with tamoxifen-resistant disease. In the second, more recent study, three objective responses were reported in 18 patients with ER-positive breast cancer[56] (Table 14.4). The evidence-based technology assessment of the American Society for Clinical Oncology (ASCO), to determine whether tamoxifen and raloxifene were appropriate as breast cancer risk-reduction therapies in clinical practice, suggested that raloxifene use should currently be reserved for its approved indication, i.e. to prevent bone loss in postmenopausal women.[19] A Study of Tamoxifen Against Raloxifene (STAR) is ongoing in

Table 14.5   Phase I and phase II studies with SERM 3

Dose (mg)	Phase I			Phase II		
	Patients	CR/PR/SD	Response (%)	Patients	CR/PR/SD	Response (%)
10	8	0/0/3	38	–	–	–
20	8	0/0/0	0	44	0/14/8	50
50	8	0/0/1	13	44	0/14/9	52
100	8	0/0/2	25	–	–	–
Total	32	0/0/6	19	88	1/27/17	51

CR, complete response; PR, partial response; SD, standard deviation.

postmenopausal women at high risk of developing breast cancer,[57,58] and the results are awaited with interest.

SERM 3

Modification of the carbonyl hinge that attaches the side chain of raloxifene to the ER-binding benzothiophene nucleus (see Figure 14.2) resulted in the production of LY 353,381 or SERM 3. This is one of the most potent oral estrogen antagonists produced to date when assayed in preclinical models of breast cancer.[59] Estrogen antagonist effects were also observed in the uterus. Estrogen agonist effects were observed in assays evaluating effects on bone, lipids and the central nervous system (CNS). Overall SERM 3 is a more potent estrogen antagonist than raloxifene and has better bone- preserving properties.[16,60] Results have been reported from a phase I dose-finding study[61] and a phase II study in which first-line SERM 3 was administered to patients with MBC[62] (Tables 14.4 and 14.5). From the phase I study, two doses of SERM 3 for phase II evaluation were chosen and patients randomized between 20 and 50 mg. Only a small number (approximately 9%) were previously treated with endocrine therapy (all

tamoxifen). Of the patients 39% had locally advanced disease. The preliminary results of this study are shown in Table 14.5. The complete and partial remission rates were 32%, rising to 51% when stable disease for more than 6 months was included. Thus, SERM 3 shows response rates equivalent or possibly superior to tamoxifen. More data are required to be certain of the appropriate dose. There are several ongoing phase II–III studies of SERM 3 in patients with tumors of the breast, ovary and endometrium. In breast cancer, there are ongoing phase III studies versus tamoxifen for the first-line treatment of MBC and an adjuvant trial is planned.

Naphthalenes

The naphthalene nucleus has provided a structural template for several ER modulators including the anti-fertility agent, nafoxidene.[63] Nafoxidene was shown to be equivalent to ethinylestradiol for the treatment of advanced breast cancer, but was withdrawn because of severe skin phototoxicity. A reduced nafoxidene derivative CP 336,156 (see Figure 14.2) has been shown, in preclinical evaluations, to have potent tissue-selective estrogen action when administered orally.[17] Recently, a hydroxynaphthalene ER modulator, LY 326,315, which exhibits fully differentiated agonist/antagonist activity in reproductive and non-reproductive tissues in preclinical assays and has good oral bioavailability, has been reported.[18]

Benzopyrans

Historically, several ER modulators have been based on a benzopyran molecule, including the contraceptive agent centrochroman[64,65] and the osteoporosis/hormone replacement therapy (HRT) agent levormeloxifene.[66]

EM 800 (SCH 57050)

EM 800 is a derivative of centchroman and was originally developed as an orally active 'pure' antiestrogen. EM 800 is a prodrug that requires the removal of two carboxylic acids to produce its active metabolite EM 652 (SCH 57068)[19] (see Figure 14.2). Comparison of the structure of EM 800 with that of centchroman shows that the antiestrogenic component of the centchroman molecule is moved to a position in the non-steriodal skeleton equivalent to the 7α position of the steroidal antiestrogen ICI 182,780 (see Figure 14.3). Both EM 800 and its active metabolite, EM 652, are potent antagonists of the ER subtypes α and β.[67] Preclinical, in vitro data showed EM 800 and EM 652 to be the most potent antiestrogens know to date when tested in breast cancer cell lines. They were also devoid of any estrogen agonist activity, e.g. stimulation of cell growth in ZR 75-1 and MCF-7 cell lines in the absence of estrogen.[68] Mice treated with EM 800 developed uterine and vaginal atrophy that was greater than seen in ovarectomized animals. Also there was complete inhibition of mammary gland development.[69,70] These studies confirmed the 'pure' antiestrogenic effect of EM 800 on the mammary gland, uterus, vagina and hypothalamic–pituitary–gonadal axis.[70] Recent data con-

cerning its activity on bone have led to the reclassification of EM 800 as an antiestrogen with both antagonist and agonist activities.

EM 800 was assessed in a phase II study in patients who had failed tamoxifen treatment as an adjuvant or for advanced disease (see Table 14.4). Of 43 evaluable patients treated, 14% had a complete or partial remission and 23% had stable disease for more than 6 months. Encouraged by these results, a phase III second-line trial of EM 800 versus anastrozole (Arimidex) was initiated, but it was abandoned when the first interim analysis showed inferiority of the antiestrogen to Arimidex. EM 800 has been withdrawn from the clinic for the treatment of MBC. It continues to be developed for breast cancer prevention.

Steroidal antiestrogens

These compounds include the 'pure' antiestrogens ICI 164,384, ICI 182,780 and RU 58668 and the oral agent SR 16234.[23,71] The most advanced of these in terms of both preclinical and clinical evaluation is ICI 182,780.[72,73]

ICI 182,780 and its predecessor ICI 164,383 were developed as pure antiestrogens.[72] ICI 164,383 has been studied extensively in a preclinical setting, but it is the more potent ICI 182,780 that is being actively studied in clinical trials in patients with advanced breast cancer.[21,22,74]

The preclinical characteristics of ICI 182,780, which define this compound as a 'pure' antiestrogen devoid of estrogen-like activity, have been extensively reviewed.[72,75,76] These include affinity for the ER that is approximately 100 times that of tamoxifen, the specific absence of estrogen-like activity on the uterus and the capacity to block completely the stimulatory activities of estrogens and antiestrogens with partial agonist activity, like tamoxifen. Moreover, ICI 182,780 has been shown not to block the uptake of [³H]estradiol in the brain, suggesting that ICI 182,780 does not cross the blood–brain barrier[77] and therefore may not cause hot flushes. The preclinical animal data on the effects of ICI 182,780 on bone density conflict with reports of reduced cancellous bone volume in one study[78] and no effect on overall density in another.[79] The absence of estrogenic activity has important consequences for the development of resistance, which is of major concern during tamoxifen therapy. In vitro studies have demonstrated that tamoxifen-resistant cell lines remain sensitive to growth inhibition by ICI 182,780,[80,81] and that tamoxifen-resistant tumors remain sensitive to ICI 182,780 in vivo.[82] Preclinical studies in nude mice showed that ICI 182,780 suppresses the growth of established MCF-7 xenografts for twice as long as tamoxifen and delays the onset of tumor growth for longer than tamoxifen.[82] Preclinical animal studies have also confirmed the complete absence of uterine stimulatory activity and shown that ICI 182,780 blocks the uterotrophic action of tamoxifen.[72] In ovariec-tomized, estrogen-treated monkeys, the extent of involution of the endometrium was similar in animals treated with ICI 182,780 and in those in which estrogen treatment was withdrawn.[75] Overall, these data indicate that the mode of action and the preclinical effects of ICI 182,780 are distinct from those of tamoxifen and the newer non-steroidal antiestrogens cited above.

The limited data surrounding the clinical potential of ICI 182,780 in patients with metastatic breast cancer are also encouraging. A phase I investigation of the effects of ICI 182,780, on primary ER-positive and -negative breast tumors in postmenopausal patients and comparison with tamoxifen,[21,83,84] showed that ICI 182,780, administered for the short period of time (7 days) between the first clinic appointment and surgery, causes a significant decrease in tumor proliferation as assessed by the Ki67 labeling index (LI). Tamoxifen caused a similar reduction in the Ki67 LI after a median of 21 days of treatment. In ER-positive tumors, ICI 182,780 caused a profound decrease in immunocytochemically detectable ER protein, whereas tamoxifen had no effect, leading to the suggestion that this type of drug be called a 'selective estrogen receptor'. ICI 182,780 also significantly reduced the expression of two estrogen-regulated genes, progesterone receptor and pS2, whereas again tamoxifen had no effect.

One small phase II trial in 19 patients with tamoxifen refractory disease demonstrated a partial response rate of 37% and a stable disease of 32% with a median duration of 25 months[22,27] (see Table 14.4), confirming the lack of cross-resistance with tamoxifen predicted by the animal studies. This trial also suggested that ICI 182,780 might have fewer side effects in terms of menopausal symptoms than tamoxifen.

RU 58668

This is another steroidal antiestrogen believed to be devoid of any estrogen agonist activity.[23] RU 58668 is active in cell culture and possesses all the properties of a 'pure' antiestrogen in animal models.[85,86] Structural comparison with ICI 182,780 (see Figure 14.3) shows that the long hydrophobic side chain is attached at the 11β-position. At present, there are no clinical data available for this antiestrogen, although the preclinical data suggest that RU 58668 may be used for the treatment of ER-positive patients who are resistant to or have escaped from tamoxifen treatment. Also, its inhibition of tumor growth in animals suggests a role in breast cancer prevention.[85,86]

SR 16234

SR 16234 is an orally active steroidal antiestrogen developed in Japan. It has a binding affinity for the ERs similar to that of estradiol and in preclinical studies has been shown to have a potent anti-proliferative activity in vitro and potent anti-tumor activity in vivo, even against tumors generated from a tamoxifen-resistant cell line. It showed potent agonist activity with regard to bone density and serum cholesterol, but little uterotrophic activity. The evidence so far suggests that this compound could be effective in the treatment of patients who have failed on tamoxifen therapy.[87,88] However, to date no clinical data are available, although phase I studies may begin in 2000.

There are therefore several antiestrogens in pre-clinical and clinical development. A major question is which will be the most useful clinically? Clinical utility may be decided by a trade-off between the anti-tumor activity of the antiestrogen and its beneficial effects on normal tissues. To decide and determine how to develop even more selective agents, it is important to understand the mechanism(s) of interaction of antiestrogens with the ER. We need to know whether we can group antiestrogens into particular classes and the molecular determinants of their antagonist and/or agonist activity in specific tissues. The first step in this process is to understand the interaction of the natural ligand estrogen with the ER and the factors that influence its site-specific activity.

ESTROGEN AND THE ESTROGEN RECEPTOR

The direct effects of estrogens on estrogen-responsive tissues are mediated via the ER, which is found in hormone-responsive tissues, in low levels in normal breast tissue and in higher concentrations in about two-thirds of all human breast cancers.[87] The ER mediates most of the biological effects of estrogen on the breast and all the compounds discussed above were designed to interfere with this process. It should be remembered that the ER can be activated in the absence of ligand by growth factors that increase intracellular second messengers.[88] It is only by understanding the complex interactions of estrogen with the ER, and the regulation of its downstream effectors, that we can hope to gain a meaningful insight into the mechanism of action of the antiestrogens.

Structure

The human ER is a member of the steroid hormone receptor superfamily that functions as ligand-inducible DNA transcription factors.[87] In the absence of hormone, the ER is sequestered within the nuclei of the target cell, and maintained in an inactive or repressed state by associated with heat shock proteins (hsp) and/or co-repressors in a multi-protein inhibitory complex.[89] Estrogen signal transduction is now known to be mediated by at least two different ERs: ERα and the recently discovered ERβ.[90–93] The two ERs (ERα and ERβ) have similar overall structures, exhibiting a high degree of amino acid conservation within the DNA-binding domain (DBD), moderate amino acid conservation in the C-terminal, ligand-binding domain (LBD) and considerable divergence at the amino terminus (Figure 14.4). Estrogen binding induces an activating conformational change within the ER; the receptors dissociated from the hsp-inhibitory complex and the ER is phosphorylated.[94] There are at least five phosphorylation sites in the ER, four serines at amino acids 104, 106, 118 and 167 of the AB domain (Figure 14.5), and another at tyrosine 537 in the LBD. Phosphorylation of tyrosine 537 is constitutive and is mediated by Src kinases. Serine phosphorylation occurs in response to estrogen binding. The ligand-bound, phosphorylated ER then undergoes dimerization and binds as homodimers or heterodimers[95,96] to a specific DNA estrogen-responsive element (ERE). From

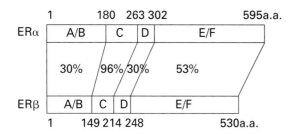

Figure 14.4
Domain structure of the two estrogen receptors ERα
and ERβ. ERα comprises 595 amino acids and ERβ 530.
Percentages refer to the degree of amino acid
homology between the two receptors. C is the
DNA-binding domain where there is a high degree of
homology, whereas elsewhere in the molecules
homology is low.

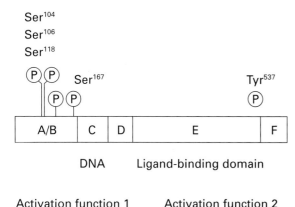

Figure 14.5
Phosphorylation sites and sites for ligand and DNA
binding in ERα. Activation function 1 is in the A/B
domain and activation function 2 in the E domain.

this location on the DNA, the receptor enhances
transcription from the nearby promoter.

Transcriptional activation

Although the precise mechanism by which the
ER regulates transcription remains to be determined, it is known that transcriptional activation
by the ER is mediated by at least two different

activating functions (AFs): AF-1 and AF-2
(Figure 14.5). AF-1 is a weak constitutive AF
that lies in the ER N-terminal (AB) domain and
AF-2 is a stronger estrogen-dependent AF that
lies within the ER C-terminal LBD. Together,
AF-1 and AF-2 synergize strongly to give the
final overall level of estrogen activation. These
transactivating functions are thought to act by
binding co-activators and bringing them to the
promoter.[97–100] The surface of AF-2 consists of
helices 3, 5 and 12 of the estrogen receptor,[101,102]
which form a hydrophobic patch when estrogen
binds to its specific site.[103] This hydrophobic
'patch' binds to a family of proteins, the
p160s,[104–111] which include the glucocorticoid
receptor-interacting protein (GRIP) and its
human homolog TIF2[104–106] and the steroid
receptor co-activator (SRC), SRC-1.[107] In each
case, AF-2 recognizes a specific sequence, LXXLL
(where L is leucine and X is any other amino
acid), termed the 'NR (nuclear receptor) box',
conserved across p160 co-activators and within
the proteins that act as AF-2 repressors (co-
repressors) such as RIP 140.[112–114] The p160s in
turn interact with other co-activator proteins,
and together this large co-activator complex is
responsible for the ability of AF-2 to stimulate
gene expression.

The activity of AF-1 is less well understood.
AF-1 shows little independent activity and is
responsible for the synergy with AF-2. The
amino acid residues responsible for AF-1 activity
lie between amino acids 41 and 120–150,
dependent on cell type.[101,115,116] Within this
region, amino acid sequences that contribute to
AF-1 independent activity (amino acids 41–64)
and synergism with the LBD (amino acids
87–108) have been identified[117] (see Figure
14.5). AF-1 is also regulated by growth factors
acting through the MAP kinase pathway.[118–121]
Several serine residues that are phosphorylated
by MAP kinases or cyclin-dependent kinases

Table 14.6   Distribution of ERα and ERβ in different tissues

Tissue	ERα	ERβ
Breast (normal)	+	+++
Breast (tumor)	+++	++
Uterus	+++	+
Bone	+	+
Cardiovascular system	+	+
CNS	+	+
Gastrointestinal tract	−	++
Liver	++	−
Urogenital tract	+	+++

+, expression; −, no expression.

have been identified.[118,119,122] Each phosphorylated serine contributes to AF-1 activity.[118,119] Although the AF-1 co-activator complex is poorly defined, there is evidence that it shares features with the AF-2 co-activator complex. Webb et al[89] provided evidence that the p160s are direct targets for both AF-1 and AF-2, and that the choice between AF-1/AF-2 synergism and independent AF-1 activity may be regulated by p160s. They demonstrated that the p160, GRIP1, enhances the independent activity of AF-1, and provided a hypothesis for why AF-1 synergizes with AF-2 in some cells, but works independently in others. They proposed that the ordinary weak AF-1/p160 contacts supported the stronger interaction of the ER LBD with the p160s and that this forms the basis of the synergy between AF-1 and AF-2. At increased p160 levels, however, AF-1/p160 contacts become sufficient to recruit p160s independently. The levels of p160s could therefore regulate the balance between AF-1/AF-2 synergy and AF-1 independent activity.

Interactions between ERα and ERβ

ERα and ERβ interact with the same DNA response elements[92] and exhibit similar but non-identical ligand-binding characteristics. ERα and ERβ can also form heterodimers with each other. However, the experimental data clearly indicate that ERβ has biological functions that are distinct from those of ERα. Localization studies have indicated that there are several types of tissue that express both types of receptor[88,123] (Table 14.6), and recent evidence suggests that the relative levels of ERα and ERβ within a tissue are important determinants of cellular sensitivity to estrogens.

Although ERα is a strong transcriptional activator, at physiologic concentrations of estrogen, co-expression of ERβ results in suppression of both the potency and the efficacy of the hormone-stimulated response.[88] In ERα, the activating functions AF-1 and AF-2 act synergistically, whereas the AF-1 of ERβ is masked or replaced by an amino-terminal suppressor domain. The absence of AF-1 in ERβ will clearly

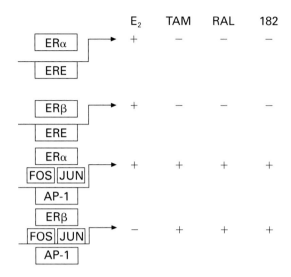

Figure 14.6
Differential effects of estradiol (E_2) and antiestrogens (tam = tamoxifen; ral = raloxifene; 182 = ICI 182,780) on ERα and ERβ, according to whether the receptors bind directly to the estrogen response element (ERE) or to an AP-1 site via the transcription factors fos and jun.

influence its ligand responsiveness, because the AF-1 of ERα is know to be essential for maximal transcriptional activation.[117] Moreover, the AF-2 domain of ERβ functions as an independent activator domain, making it likely that ERα and ERβ will display differences in their preferences for co-activators and co-repressors within their target cells. Furthermore, the α and β ERs signal in opposite ways from their AP-1 site in the presence of the transcription factors *fos* and *jun*[124] (Figure 14.6). When bound to ERα, estrogen activates transcription, whereas when bound to ERβ it inhibits transcription when the receptors act via AP-1 sites.

Thus, one can predict that knowledge of the patterns of co-localization and concentrations of both receptors within different tissues will provide an insight into the biological responses induced by them to estrogen. The observation

that ERβ can act as a transcriptional activator or inhibitor dependent on agonist concentration suggests that it must play a significant role in the mechanism of estrogen action in the many tissues (breast, uterus, bone and cardiovascular) in which it is expressed. It is becoming increasingly obvious that our understanding of the tissue distribution of these receptors will be crucial to the development of new antiestrogen anticancer therapies, and to the development of non-cancerous HRT for postmenopausal women. The known distributions are shown in Table 14.6. The receptors are co-expressed in most tissues (although not necessarily in the same cell), with the exception that ERα is not found in the gastrointestinal tract and ERβ is not found in the liver.

INTERACTION OF NEW ANTIESTROGENS WITH THE ESTROGEN RECEPTOR

Until very recently, all the studies on the elucidation of the molecular mechanisms of ER activity have involved ERα,[125–127] although increasingly data are becoming available for ERβ.

Conformational changes induced by ligand binding

The binding of agonists triggers AF-2 activity by directly affecting the structure of the LBD. Only the binding of agonists triggers the AF-2 activity, whereas the binding of antagonists does not.[128]

Comparison of the structure of the LBD of ERα complexed with estradiol and raloxifene shows that, although both ligands bind at the same site within the core of the LBD,[129] each ligand induces a different conformation of helix 12, the most C-terminal helix of the LBD. Helix 12 in the raloxifene–LBD complex is bound in a hydrophobic groove composed of residues from helices 3 and 5. This alternative orientation of helix 12 partially buries residues in the groove that are necessary for AF-2 activity, suggesting that raloxifene and possibly other antagonists block AF-2 functioning through the disruption of the topography of the AF-2 surface.

Differences in secondary structure between the agonist complexes with estrogen and diethylstibestrol and 4-hydroxytamoxifen also arise from distinct arrangements of the packing interactions induced by the different ligands. 4-Hydroxytamoxifen binds to the AF-2 complex without directly interacting with helix 12 and occludes the co-activator recognition site.[130–132] The binding mode of 4-hydroxytamoxifen has two distinct effects on the positioning of helix 12: firstly, helix 12 is prevented from positioning itself over the ligand-binding pocket by the 4-hydroxytamoxifen side chain and, second, the alternative packing arrangement of ligand-binding residues around 4-hydroxytamoxifen stabilizes a conformation of the LBD that mimics bound co-activator.[130] Raloxifene also sterically hinders the agonist-bound conformation of helix 12,[129] inducing a distinct ER conformation,[133,134] which is dependent on amino acid 351.[135] The differences in the effects on the uterus between tamoxifen and raloxifene have been attributed to distinct ligand conformations.[47]

The ER antagonist ICI 182,780 is also known to induce a distinct ER conformation,[133,134] and specific peptide probes have demonstrated that ER ligands known to produce distinct biologic effects induce distinct conformational changes in the receptors. This provides evidence of a strong correlation between ER conformation and biologic activity.[136] Furthermore, these ER modulators are able to induce distinct conformational changes in ERα and ERβ, suggesting that the biological effects of ER agonists and antagonists operating through these receptors are likely to be different.[136]

Transcriptional activation

Both pure antagonists and partial agonists deliver the ER to its DNA target within the cell, however, the ability of the DNA-bound receptor to activate transcription is dependent on the cell and promoter context.[133] As stated previously, ERα and ERβ share high sequence homology, especially in the regions responsible for specific binding to DNA and in their LBDs.[90,91,137] Moreover, antiestrogen agonism via the ER is for the most part mediated by the AB domain of ERα and is not supported by the AF-1 (AB domain) of ERβ.[138] The domain of ERα made up of 24 amino acids, required for antiestrogen agonism, but not estradiol-stimulated transcription, is not found in ERβ.[117] This suggests that the differences in sequence between the N-terminal domains of ERα and ERβ contribute to the cell- and promoter-specific transcriptional activity of these receptors and their ability to respond to different ligands.

Dose-dependent inhibition studies of estradiol-induced ERα and ERβ activity show that the active metabolite of EM 800, EM 652, was more potent at inhibiting ERα activity than the pure steroidal antiestrogen ICI 182,780, and that both antiestrogens were more potent inhibitors of ERβ than ERα. The inhibitory properties of the various antiestrogens with regard to the activating factors AF-1 and AF-2 are summarized in Table 14.7. EM 652 and ICI 182,780 both inhibit the AF-1 and AF-2 functions of both ERα and ERβ, acting as pure estrogen antagonists on ERα and ERβ transcriptional activities. 4-Hydroxytamoxifen, however, blocks only the AF-2 activity of both ERs[137] which, coupled with the information about antiestrogen agonism being mediated by the AB domain of ERα,[138] might explain the agonist activity of tamoxifen. SRC-1 has been shown to stimulate ERα and ERβ activity in the absence of ligand. The ligand-independent activation of AF-1 is

Table 14.7   Effects of the three different types of antiestrogen

	Triphenylethylene	Fixed ring	Steroidal
Anti-tumor	+	++	+++
Tamoxifen-resistant growth	−	?	++
Bone density	+	++	?
Uterus	+	−	−
Hot flushes	+	+	−
Clotting factors	+	+	−
Serum lipids	+	+	−
Cardiovascular	?	?	?
Brain	?	?	?

presumed to be closely linked to phosphorylation of the steroid receptors by cellular protein kinases.[139] Enhancement of ERβ activation in the absence of ligand was found to be independent of AF-2. Significantly, 4-hydroxytamoxifen had no appreciable effect on SRC-1-induced unliganded activity, whereas EM 652 completely abolished this effect. The absence of the inhibition of the ligand-independent, AF-2-independent, SRC-1 co-activator activity by 4-hydroxytamoxifen could explain why the benefits of tamoxifen are lost after 5 years and why resistance develops.

Biologic effects

Estrogen, the natural ligand for the ER, acts as an agonist in all environments regardless of whether or not AF-1 or AF-2 is the dominant activator. The steroidal pure antiestrogen ICI 182,780, which inhibits the activity of both AF-1 and AF-2, completely blocks the ability of ERα to activate transcription through the classic ERE-mediated pathways. Unlike ICI 182,780, however, the relative agonist/antagonist activities of the other new antiestrogens are determined by the cell and promoter context, and not solely by their ability to regulate AF-1 and AF-2 differentially. For example, the antiestrogens raloxifene and GW 5638 function as estrogens on bone and the cardiovascular system, but do not appear to act as AF-1 or AF-2 agonists. This suggests that the current theories of ER modulation are incomplete and increasingly the role of ERβ has to be considered. Tamoxifen, for example, is a more potent competitive antagonist of ERβ[92] and does not display ERβ agonist activity. This raises the question of whether there is a better response to tamoxfien in ERβ-positive tumors?[140]

Estrogens and antiestrogens are also known to induce differential activation of ERα and ERβ to control the transcription of genes that are under the control of an AP-1 element.[124] The ligand-bound ER binds to EREs as a homodimer, but the ER also mediates gene transcription from an AP-1 enhancer element that requires ligand and the AP-1 transcription factors Fos and Jun.[124] ERα and ERβ were found to signal in opposite ways from the AP-1 site, depending on the ligand (see Figure 14.6). This adds another potential control mechanism for the transcriptional regulation of estrogen-responsive genes. Recently, an

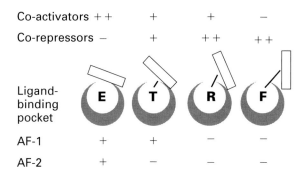

Co-activators + +   +   +   –

Co-repressors –   +   + +   + +

Ligand-
binding
pocket   E   T   R   F

AF-1   +   +   –   –

AF-2   +   –   –   –

Figure 14.7
Cartoon of the potential differences in mechanism of action of three classes of antiestrogen (T = triphenylethylene [tamoxifen]; R = cyclic/fixed-ring structures [raloxifene]; F = steroidal antiestrogens [ICI 182,780, faslodex]). The ligand-binding pocket of ERα is shown with helix 12 as a box. When estrogen occupies the binding site, helix 12 covers the pocket, whereas it is likely that the three classes of antiestrogen sterically hinder the action of helix 12 to differing degrees. Thus, because of their bulky side chain, the steroidal antiestrogens may maximally inhibit binding of co-activators, resulting in inactivation of both activating functions 1 and 2 (AF-1, AF-2).

isoform of human ERβ has been cloned that has the potential to inhibit human ERα-mediated estrogen activity, adding yet another layer of complexity to our attempts to understand the diverse biologic effects of estrogens and antie-strogens.[141]

Clinical relevance of knowledge of ER structure and function

It is clear that the interaction of an ER with a ligand is a highly complex event. The ER may be regarded as an integrator of the functions of a mammary cell – even down to regulating the effects of growth factors such as epidermal growth factor, EGF-1, and insulin-like growth factor, IGF-1, through phosphorylation of the receptor. In the future, more knowledge about the complexity of the ER may allow the development of specific regulators of ERβ or inhibitors

of specific co-activators. At present the most appropriate synthesis of a complex area may be to consider that there are three classes of antie-strogen that affect ERα (at least) in distinctive ways. This is illustrated in Figure 14.7 with respect to binding of estrogen or antiestrogen to the ligand-binding domain of ERα. Estrogen binding allows helix 12 to cover the binding site and for co-activators to bind, whereas the three classes of antiestrogen with progressively larger side chains may block helix 12 movement to different degrees. Steroidal antiestrogens with the largest side chain may block all movement of helix 12 and thus co-activator binding, so that AF-1 and AF-2 are not activated. Such a model would account for the intermediate activity of raloxifene and SERM 3, which have less partial agonist activity on the uterus than tamoxifen. It would also account for the lack of effect of ICI 182,780 on lipid concentrations or bone. It is of interest that mutations of a single amino acid (aspartate 351) in the LBD prevents binding of the side chains of raloxifene and EM 800, making them into estrogens, whereas this mutation does not affect the antiestrogenicity of ICI 182,780, suggesting a different mechanism of binding to the LBD of the ER.[142]

Many antiestrogens have been withdrawn from development. None of the triphenylethyl-enes has been shown to have superior clinical activity to tamoxifen, whereas all have uterotrophic effects that also limit their clinical utility. Thus, we are left in the clinic with two equally active compounds tamoxifen and toremifene.

At present the sole fixed-ring structure being developed for the treatment of breast cancer is SERM 3. Raloxifene and EM 652, which appear to have lower anti-tumor activity, are being used for prevention only.

There is also only one steroidal compound in the clinic. ICI 182,780 appears highly active, but we await phase III trial results to see whether it is superior to anastrozole and tamoxifen. It will be some time before we know whether the newer compounds in each of the three classes of antiestrogen (GW 5638, LY 325,315 and SR 16234) will have superior activities to the agents already available.

We still lack knowledge about many of the potential beneficial activities of the three groups of antiestrogens (see Table 14.7). For example, there are few data on the effects of triphenylethylenes on the cardiovascular system (as opposed to clotting or lipids) and brain, and similar considerations apply to the fixed-ring and the steroidal compounds. In addition, we do not know whether the fixed ring or the steroidal compounds will have greater anti-tumor activity than the triphenylethylenes, although these data should be available in 2001–2002.

REFERENCES

1. Landis SH, Murray T, Bolden S, Wingo PA, Cancer statistics. *CA Cancer J Clin* 1998; 48:6–29.
2. Beatson G, On the treatment of inoperable cases of carcinoma of the mamma: with suggestions for a new method of treatment, with illustrative cases. *Lancet* 1896; ii:104–7.
3. Haddow A, Watkinson JM, Patterson E, Influence of synthetic estrogens upon advanced malignant disease. *BMJ* 1944; ii:393–8.
4. Walpole AL, Patterson E, Synthetic estrogens in mammary cancer. *Lancet* 1949; ii:783–6.
5. Howell A, De Friend D, Anderson E, Clues to the mechanisms of endocrine resistance from clinical studies in advanced breast cancer. *Endocrin-Rel Cancer* 1995; 2:131–9.
6. Cole MP, Jones CTA, Todd IDH, A new antiestrogenic agent in late breast cancer: an early clinical appraisal of ICI 146474. *Br J Cancer* 1971; 25:270–5.
7. Early Breast Cancer Trialists' Collaborative Group, Tamoxifen for early breast cancer: an overview of the randomised trials. *Lancet* 1998; 351:1451–67.
8. Fisher B, Constantino JP, Wickerham DL et al, Tamoxifen for prevention of breast cancer: report of the National Surgical Adjuvant Breast and Bowel Project P-1 Study. *J Natl Cancer Inst* 1998; 90:1371–88.
9. Chlebowski R, Collyar DE, Somerfield MR et al, American Society of Clinical Oncology Technology. Assessment of breast cancer risk reduction strategies: tamoxifen and raloxifene. *J Clin Oncol* 1999; 17:1939–55.
10. Love RR, Mazess RB, Barden HS et al, Effects of tamoxifen on bone mineral density in postmenopausal women with breast cancer. *N Engl J Med* 1992; 326:852–6.
11. Love RR, Newcomb PA, Wiebe DA et al, Effects of tamoxifen therapy on lipid and lipoprotein levels in postmenopausal patients with node-negative breast cancer. *J Natl Cancer Inst* 1990; 82:1327–32.
12. Fisher B, Constantino JP, Redmond CK et al, Endometrial cancer in tamoxifen treated breast cancer patients: finding from the National Surgical Adjuvant Breast and Bowel Project (NASBP) B-14 Study. *J Natl Cancer Inst* 1994; 86:527.
13. Assikis VJ, Neven P, Jordan VC, Vergote I, A realistic clinical perspective of tamoxifen and endometrial carcinogenesis. *Eur J Cancer* 1996; 32A:1464–76.
14. Howell A, Downey S, Anderson E, New endocrine therapies for breast cancer. *Eur J Cancer* 1996; 32A:576–88.
15. Clemens JA, Bennet DR, Black IJ, Jones CD, Effects of a new antiestrogen keoxifene (LY156758), on growth of carcinogen-induced mammary tumors and on LH and prolactin levels. *Life Sci* 1983; 32:2869–75.
16. Palkowitz AD, Glasebrook AL, Thresher KJ et al, Discovery and synthesis of [6-hydroxy-3[4-[2-(piperidinyl)ethoxy]phenoxy)-2-(4-hydroxyphenyl)]benzo[β]thiophene: a novel highly

potent selective estrogen receptor modulator. *J Med Chem* 1997; **40**:1407–16.

17. Ke HZ, Paralkar VM, Grasser WA et al, Effects of CP-336,156, a new, non steroidal estrogen agonist/antagonist, on bone serum cholesterol, uterus and body composition in rat models. *Endocrinology* 1998; **139**: 2068–76.

18. Grese TA, Dodge JA, Selective estrogen receptor modulators (SERMS). *Current Pharmaceutical Design* 1998; **4**:71–92.

19. Gauthier S, Caron B, Cloutier J et al, (S)-(+)-4-[7-(2,2-dimethyl-1-oxopropoxy)-4-methyl-2-[4-[2-(1-piperidinyl)-ethoxy]phenyl]-2H-1-benzopyran-3-yl]-phenyl 2,2-dimethyl-propanoate (EM-800): a highly potent, specific and orally active nonsteroidal antiestrogen. *J Med Chem* 1997; **40**:2117–22.

20. Wakeling AE, Pharmacology of antiestrogens. In, eds. Oettle M, Schillinger E *Estrogens and Anti-estrogens II*, Vol 135. Berlin: Springer, 1999: 179–94.

21. De Friend DJ, Howell A, Nicholson RT et al, Investigation of a new pure antiestrogen (ICI 182780) in women with primary breast cancer. *Cancer Res* 1994; **54**:408–14.

22. Howell A, De Friend DJ, Robertson JFR et al, Pharmacokinetics, pharmacological and anti-tumor effects of the specific antiestrogen ICI 182780 in women with advanced breast cancer. *Br J Cancer* 1996; **74**:300–8.

23. Van De Velde P, Nique F, Planchon P et al, RU 58668: Further in vitro and in vivo pharmacoligical data related to its antitumoral activity. *J Steroid Biochem Mol Biol* 1996; **59**:449–57.

24. Kangas L, Nieminen A-L, Blanco G et al, A new triphenylethylene compound Fc-1157a II. Antitumor effects. *Cancer Chemother Pharmacol* 1986; **17**:109–13.

25. Chander SK, McCague R, Luqmani Y et al, Pyrrolidino-4-iodotamoxifen and 4-iodotamoxifen, new analogues of the anti-estrogen tamoxifen for the treatment of breast cancer. *Cancer Res* 1991; **51**:5851–8.

26. Loser R, Seibel K, Roos W, Eppenberger U, In vivo and in vitro antiestrogenic action of 3-OH-tamoxifen, tamoxifen and 4-OH-tamoxifen. *Eur J Cancer Clin Oncol* 1985; **21**: 985–90.

27. Toko T, Sugimoto Y, Matsuo E et al, TAT-59, a new triphenylethylene derivative with anti-tumor activity against hormone-dependent tumors. *Eur J Cancer* 1990; **26**:397–404.

28. Willson TM, Norris JD, Wagner BL et al, Dissection of the molecular mechanism of action of GW 5638, a novel estrogen receptor ligand, provides an insight into the role of the estrogen receptor in bone. *Endocrinology* 1997; **138**:3901–11.

29. Hemminki K, Rajaniemi H, Lindahl B et al, Tamoxifen-induced DNA adducts in endometrial samples from breast cancer patients. *Cancer Res* 1996; **56**:4374–7.

30. Tomas E, Kauppila A, Blanco et al, Comparison between effects of tamoxifen, toremifene and ICI 182780 on the uterus in postmenopausal breast cancer patients. *Gynecol Oncol* 1995; **59**:261–6.

31. Gershanovich M, Garin A, Baltina D et al, A phase III comparison of two toremifene doses to tamoxifen in post menopausal women with advanced breast cancer. Eastern European Study Group. *Breast Cancer Res Treat* 1997; **45**:251–62.

32. Pyrhonen S, Valavaara R, Modig H et al, Comparison of toremifene and tamoxifen in postmenopausal patients with advanced breast cancer: a randomised double-blind trial, the 'Nordic' phase III study. *Br J Cancer* 1997; **76**:270–7.

33. Hayes DE, Van Zyl JA, Hacking A et al, Randomised comparison of tamoxifen and two separate doses of toremifene in postmenopausal patients with metastatic breast cancer. *J Clin Oncol* 1995; **13**:2556–66.

34. Holli K, Joensun H, Valavaara R et al, Interim results of the Finnish toremifene versus tamoxifen adjuvant trial. *Breast Cancer Res Treat* 1998; **50**:283.

35. Pyrhonen S, Valavaara R, Vuorinen J et al, High dose toremifene in advanced breast cancer resistant to or relapsed during tamoxifen treatment. *Breast Cancer Res Treat* 1994; 29:223–8.

36. Pyrohnen S, Ellmen J, Vuorinen M et al, Meta-analysis of trials comparing toremifene with tamoxifen and factors predicting outcome of antiestrogen therapy in post-menopausal women with breast cancer. *Breast Cancer Res Treat* 1999; 56:133–43.

37. McCague R, Parr IB, Haynes BP, Metabolism of the 4-iodo-derivative of tamoxifen by isolated rat hepatocytes. Demonstration that the iodine atom reduces metabolic conversion and identification of four metabolites. *Biochem Pharmacol* 1990; 40:2277–83.

38. Nuttall ME, Bradbeer JN, Strorp GB et al, Idoxifene a novel selective estrogen receptor modulator prevents bone loss and lowers cholesterol levels in ovariectomised rats and reduces uterine weight in intact rats. *Endocrinology* 1998; 139:5224–34.

39. Johnston SRD, Gumbrell L, Evans TRJ et al, A phase II randomised double blind study of idoxifene (40 mg/d) vs tamoxifen (40 mg/d) in patients with locally advanced metastatic breast cancer resistant to tamoxifen (920 mg/d). *Proc Am Soc Clin Oncol* 1999; 18A:413.

40. Ke HZ, Simmons HA, Pirie CM et al, Droloxifene a new estrogen antagonist/agonist prevents bone loss in ovariectomised rats. *Endocrinology* 1995; 136:2435–41.

41. Abe O, Japanese early phase II study of droloxifene in the treatment of advanced breast cancer. Preliminary dose-finding study. *Am J Clin Oncol* 1991; 14:S40–5.

42. Bellmunt J, Sole L, European early phase II dose-finding study of droloxifene in advanced breast cancer. *Am J Clin Oncol* 1991; 14:S36–9.

43. Haarstad H, Gundersen S, Wist E et al, Droloxifene a new antiestrogen phase II study in advanced breast cancer. *Acta Oncol* 1992; 31:425–8.

44. Rauschning W, Pritchard KI, Droloxifene a new antiestrogen its role in metastatic breast cancer. *Breast Cancer Res Treat* 1994; 31: 83–94.

45. Koh JR, Kubota T, Asanuma F et al, Antitumor effect of triphenylethylene derivative (TAT-59) against human breast carcinoma xenografts in nude mice. *J Surg Oncol* 1992; 51:254–8.

46. Noguchi S, Koyama H, Nomura Y et al, Late phase II study of TAT-59 (new antiestrogen) in advanced or recurrent breast cancer patients: a double-blind comparative study with tamoxifen citrate. *Breast Cancer Res Treat* 1998; 50:307.

47. Grese TA, Sluka JP, Bryant HU et al, Molecular determinants of tissue selectivity in estrogen receptor modulators. *Proc Natl Acad Sci USA* 1997; 94:14105-10.

48. Anzano MA, Peer CW, Smith JM et al, Chemoprevention of mammary carcinogenesis in the rat: combined use of raloxifene and 9-cis-retinoic acid. *J Natl Cancer Inst* 1996; 88:123–5.

49. Black IJ, Sato M, Rowley ER et al, Raloxifene (LY 139481-HCl) prevents bone loss and reduces serum cholesterol without causing uterine hypertrophy in ovariectomised rats. *J Clin Invest* 1994; 93:63–9.

50. Turner CH, Sato M, Rowley ER et al, Raloxifene preserves bone strength and bone mass in ovariectomised rats. *Endocrinology* 1994; 135:2001–5.

51. Draper MW, Flowers DE, Hustler WJ et al, A controlled trial of raloxifene (LY 39481) HCl: impact on bone turnover and serum lipid profile in healthy post-menopausal women. *J Bone Miner Res* 1996; 11:835–42.

52. Walsh BW, Kuller LH, Wild RA et al, Effects of raloxifene on serum lipids and coagulation factors in healthy post menopausal women. *JAMA* 1998; 279:1445–51.

53. Delmas PD, Bjarnason NH, Mitlak BH et al, Effects of raloxifene on bone mineral density, serum cholesterol concentrations and uterine

endometrium in post menopausal women. *N Engl J Med* 1997; **337**:1641–7.

54. Cummings SR, Norton L, Eckert S et al, Raloxifene reduces the risk of cancer and may decrease the risk of endometrial cancer in post menopausal women: two year findings from the Multiple Outcomes of Raloxifene Evaluation (MORE) trial. *Proc Am Soc Clin Oncol* 1998; **17**:2a.

55. Buzdar AV, Marcus C, Holmes F et al, Phase II evaluation of LY 156758 in metastatic breast cancer. *Oncology* 1988; **45**:344–5.

56. Gradishar WJ, Glusman JE, Vogel CH et al, Raloxifene HCl a new endocrine agent is active in estrogen receptor positive (ER+) metastatic breast cancer. *Breast Cancer Res Treat* 1997; **209**:53.

57. Jordon VC, Development of a new prevention maintenance therapy for postmenopausal women. *Rec Results Cancer Res* 1999; **151**:96–109.

58. Jordon VC, Morrow M, Raloxifene as a multi-functional medicine? *BMJ* 1999; **319**:331–2.

59. Sato M, Turner CH, Wang T et al, LY 353381.HCl: a novel raloxifene analog with improved SERM potency and efficacy in vivo. *J Pharmacol Exp Ther* 1998; **287**:1–7.

60. Sato M, Glasebrook AL, Bryant HU, Raloxifene: a selective estrogen receptor modulator. *J Bone Miner Met* 1994; **12**:S9–20.

61. Hudis C, Buzdar A, Munster P et al, Phase I study of a third generation selective estrogen receptor modulator (SERM 3, LY 353381.HCl) in refractory metastatic breast cancer. *Breast Cancer Res Treat* 1998; **50**:306 (Abstract 442).

62. Baselga J, Llombart-Cussac A, Bellet M et al, Randomized double-blind phase 2 study of a selective estrogen receptor modulator SERM (LY 353381) in patients (pts) with locally advanced or metastatic breast cancer. *Breast Cancer Res Treat* 1999; **57**:31 (Abstract 35).

63. Tagnon HJ, Antiestrogens in treatment of breast cancer. *Cancer* 1977; **39**:2959–64.

64. Ray S, Groves P, Kamboj VP et al, Antifertility agent 12. Structure-activity relationship of 3,4-diphenyl-chromenes and chromans. *J Med Chem* 1976; **19**:276–9.

65. Kamboj VP, Ray S, Dhawan RB, Centchroman. *Drugs Today* 1992; **28**:227–32.

66. Holm P, Shalmi M, Korsgaard N et al, A partial oestrogen receptor antagonist with strong anti atherogenic properties without noticeable effect on reproductive tissue in cholesterol-fed female and male rabbits. *Arterioscler Thromb Vasc Biol* 1997; **17**:2264–72.

67. Martel C, Provencher I, Li X et al, Binding characteristics of novel nonsteroidal antiestrogens to the rat uterine estrogen receptors. *J Steroid Biochem Mol Biol* 1998; **64**:199–205.

68. Simard J, Labrie C, Bélanger A et al, Characterisation of the effects of the novel nonsteroidal antiestrogen EM-800 on basal and estrogen-induced proliferation on T-47-D, 2R-75-1 and MCF-7 human cancer cells in vitro. *Int J Cancer* 1997; **73**:104–12.

69. Sourla A, Luo S, Labrie C et al, Morphological changes induced by six month treatment of intact and ovariectomised mice with tamoxifen and the pure antiestrogen EM-800. *Endocrinology* 1997; **138**:5605–17.

70. Luo S, Sourla A, Gauthier S et al, Effect of 24 week treatment with the antiestrogen EM-800 on estrogen-sensitive parameters in intact and ovariectomised mice. *Endocrinology* 1998; **139**:2645–56.

71. Tanabe M, Peters RH, Chao W-R et al, SR 16234, a novel steroidal selective estrogen receptor modulator (SERM). *Breast Cancer Res Treat* 1999; **57**:52 (Abstract 172).

72. Wakeling AE, Dukes M, Bowler J, A potent specific pure antiestrogen with clinical potential. *Cancer Res* 1991; **51**:3867–73.

73. Howell A, De Friend D, Robertson J et al, Response to a specific antiestrogen (ICI 182780) in tamoxifen resistant breast cancer. *Lancet* 1995; **345**:29–30.

74. Howell A, Osborne K, Morris C, Wakeling A, Faslodex (ICI 182, 780). Development of a novel 'pure' antiestrogen. *Cancer* 2000; in press.

75. Dukes M, Miller D, Wakeling AE, Waterton JC, Antiuterotrophic effects of a pure antiestrogen, ICI 182780; magnetic resonance imaging of the uterus in ovariectomised monkeys. *J Endocrinol* 1992; **135**:239–47.

76. Dukes M, Waterton JC, Wakeling AE, Antiuterotrophic effects of the pure antiestrogen ICI 182780 in adult female monkeys (*Macaca nemestrina*): quantitative magnetic resonance imaging. *J Endocrinol* 1993; **138**:203–9.

77. Wade GN, Blaustein JD, Gray JM, Meredith JM, ICI 182780: a pure antiestrogen that affects behaviour and energy balance in rats without acting in the brain. *Am J Physiol* 1993; **34**:R1932–8.

78. Gallagher A, Chambers TJ, Tobias JH, The estrogen antagonist ICI 182780 reduces cancellous bone in female rats. *Endocrinology* 1993; **133**:2787–91.

79. Wakeling AE, The future of pure antiestrogens in clinical breast cancer. *Breast Cancer Res Treat* 1993; **25**:1–9.

80. Coopman P, Garcia M, Brunner N et al, Antiproliferative and anti-estrogenic effects of ICI 164, 384 and ICI 182780 in 4-OH-tamoxifen resistant human breast cancer cells. *Int J Cancer* 1994; **56**:295–300.

81. Hu XF, Veroni M, De Luise M et al, Circumvention of tamoxifen resistance by the pure anti-estrogen ICI 182780. *Int J Cancer* 1993; **55**:873–6.

82. Osborne CK, Coronado-Heinsohn ER, Hilsenbeck SG et al, Comparison of the effects of a pure steroidal antiestrogen with those of tamoxifen in a model of human breast cancer. *J Natl Cancer Inst* 1995; **87**:746–50.

83. Anderson E, Nicholson R, Dowsett M, Howell A, Models of new antiestrogen action in vivo: primary tumors. *Breast* 1996; **5**:186–91.

84. Robertson JFR, Dixon M, Bundred N et al, A partially-blind, randomised, multi-centre study comparing the anti-tumor effects of single doses (50, 125, 250 mg) of long-acting (LA) 'Faslodex' (ICI 182780) with tamoxifen in postmenopausal women with primary breast cancer prior to surgery. *Breast Cancer Res Treat* 1999; **57**:31 (Abstract 28).

85. Van De Velde P, Nique F, Brémaud M-C et al, Exploration of the therapeutic potential of the antiestrogen RU 58668 in breast cancer treatment. *Ann N Y Acad Sci* 1995; **761**:164–75.

86. Van de Velde P, Nique F, Bouchoux J et al, RU 58668, a new pure antiestrogen inducing a regression of human mammary carcinoma implanted in nude mice. *J Steroid Biochem Mol Biol* 1994; **48**:187–96.

87. Evans RM, The steroid and thyroid hormone receptor super family. *Science* 1988; **240**: 889–95.

88. Hall JM, McDonnell DP, The estrogen receptor β-isoform (ERβ) of the human estrogen receptor modulates Era transcriptional activity and is a key regulator of the cellular response to estrogens and antiestrogens. *Endocrinology* 1999; **140**:5566–78.

89. Webb P, Nguyen P, Shinsako J et al, Estrogen receptor activation function 1 works by binding p160 coactivator proteins. *Mol Endocrinol* 1998; **12**:1605–18.

90. Kuiper GGJM, Enmark E, Pelto-Huikko M et al, Cloning of a novel estrogen receptor expressed in rat prostate and ovary. *Proc Natl Acad Sci USA* 1996; **93**:5925–30.

91. Mosselman S, Polman J, Dijkema R, ERβ identification and characterisation of a novel human estrogen receptor. *FEBS Lett* 1996; **392**:49–53.

92. Kuiper GGJM, Carlsson B, Grandien J et al, A comparison of ligand binding specificity and transcript tissue distribution of estrogen receptors α and β. *Endocrinology* 1997; **138**:863–70.

93. Katzenellenbogen BS, Korach KS, Editorial – a new actor in the estrogen receptor drama – enter ERβ. *Endocrinology* 1997; **138**:861–2.

94. Lieberman BA, Estrogen receptor activity cycle: dependence on multiple protein-protein interactions. *Crit Rev Eukaryot Gene Expr* 1997; **7**:43–9.

95. Petersson K, Grandien K, Kuiper GG et al,

Mouse estrogen receptor beta forms estrogen response element binding heterodimers with estrogen receptor alpha. *Mol Endocrinol* 1997; **11**: 1486–96.

96. Cowley SM, Hoare S, Mosselman S, Parker MG, Estrogen receptors alpha and β form heterodimers on DNA. *J Biol Chem* 1997; **272**:19858–62.

97. Le Douarin B, Vom Baur E, Zechel C et al, Ligand-dependent interaction of nuclear receptors with potential transcriptional intermediary factors (mediators). *Philos Trans R Soc Lond Biol Sci* 1996; **351**:569–78.

98. Horowitz KB, Jackson TA, Bain DL et al, Nuclear receptor co-activators and co-repressors. *Mol Endocrinol* 1996; **10**:1167–77.

99. Glass CK, Rose DW, Rosenfeld MG, Nuclear receptor co-activators. *Curr Opin Cell Biol* 1997; **9**:222–32.

100. Shibata H, Spencer TE, Onate SA et al, Role of co-activators and co-repressors in the mechanism of steroid/thyroid receptor action. *Recent Prog Horm Res* 1997; **52**:141–64.

101. Danielian PS, White R, Lees JA et al, Identification of a conserved region required for hormone dependent transcriptional activation by steroid hormone receptors. *EMBO J* 1992; **11**:1025–33.

102. Henttu PM, Kalkhoven E, Parker MG, AF-2 activity and recruitment of steroid receptor coactivator 1 to the estrogen receptor depend on a lysine residue conserved in nuclear receptors. *Mol Cell Biol* 1997; **17**: 1832–9.

103. Feng WJ, Ribeiro RCJ, Wagner RL et al, Hormone-dependent coactivator binding to a hydrophobic cleft on nuclear receptors. *Science* 1998; **280**:1747–9.

104. Hong H, Kohli K, Trivedi A et al, GRIP1, a novel mouse protein that serves as a transcriptional coactivator in yeast for the hormone binding domains of steroid receptors. *Proc Natl Acad Sci USA* 1996; **93**: 4948–52.

105. Hong H, Kohli K, Garabedian MJ, Stallcup MR, GRIP1, a transcriptional coactivator for the AF-2 transcriptional activation domain of steroid, thyroid, retinoid and vitamin D receptors. *Mol Cell Biol* 1997; **17**:2735–44.

106. Voegel JJ, Heine MJS, Tini M et al, The coactivator TIF2 contains three nuclear receptor-binding motifs and mediates transactivation through CBP binding dependent and independent pathways. *EMBO J* 1998; **17**: 507–19.

107. Onate SA, Tsai SY, Tsai MJ, O'Malley BW, Sequence and characterisation of a co-activator for the steroid hormone receptor superfamily. *Science* 1995; **270**:1354–7.

108. Li H, Gomes PJ, Chen JD, RAC3, a steroid/nuclear receptor-associated coactivator that is related to SRC-1 and TIF2. *Proc Natl Acad Sci USA* 1997; **94**:8479–84.

109. Torchia J, Rose DW, Inostroza J et al, The transcriptional co-activator p/CIP binds CBP and mediates nuclear receptor function. *Nature* 1997; **387**:677–84.

110. Chen H, Lin RJ, Schiltz RL et al, Nuclear receptor coactivator ACTR is a novel histone acetyltransferase and forms a multimeric activation complex with P/CAF and CBP/p300. *Cell* 1997; **90**:569–80.

111. Anzick SL, Koonen J, Walker RL et al, AIB1, a steroid receptor co-activator amplified in breast and ovarian cancer. *Science* 1997; **277**:965–8.

112. Heery DM, Kalkhoven E, Hoare S, Parker MG, A signature motif in transcriptional co-activators mediates binding to nuclear receptors. *Nature* 1997; **387**:733–6.

113. L'Horset F, Dauvois S, Heery DM et al, RIP-140 interacts with multiple nuclear receptors by means of two distinct sites. *Mol Cell Biol* 1996; **16**:6029–36.

114. Vom Baur E, Zechel C, Heery D et al, Differential ligand dependent interaction between the AF-2 activating domain of nuclear receptors and the putative transcriptional intermediary factors MSUG1 and TIF1. *EMBO J* 1996; **15**:110–24.

115. Imakado S, Koike S, Kondo S et al, The N-terminal transactivation domain of rat estrogen receptor is localized in a hydrophobic domain of eighty amino acids. *J Biochem (Tokyo)* 1991; **109**:684–9.

116. Metzger D, Ali S, Bornet JM, Chambon P, Characterization of the amino-terminal transcriptional activation function of the human estrogen receptor in animal and yeast cells. *J Biol Chem* 1995; **270**:9535–42.

117. McInerney EM, Katzenellenbogen BS, Different regions in activation function 1 of the human estrogen receptor required for antiestrogen and estradiol dependent transcription activation. *J Biol Chem* 1996; **271**:24172–8.

118. Ali S, Metzger D, Bornert JM, Chambon P, Modulation of transcriptional activation by ligand-dependent phosphorylation of the human estrogen receptor A/B region. *EMBO J* 1993; **12**:1153–60.

119. Le Goff P, Montano MM, Schodin DJ, Katzenellenbogen BS, Phosphorylation of the human estrogen receptor. Identification of hormone regulated sites and examination of their influence on transcriptional activity. *J Biol Chem* 1994; **269**:4458–66.

120. Kato S, Endoh H, Masuhiro Y et al, Activation of the estrogen receptor through phosphorylation by mitogen-activated protein kinase. *Science* 1995; **270**:1491–4.

121. Bunone G, Briand PA, Miksicek RJ, Picard D, Activation of the unliganded receptor by EGF involves the MAP kinase pathway and direct phosphorylation. *EMBO J* 1996; **15**:2174–83.

122. Lahooti H, White R, Danielian PS, Parker MG, Characterization of the ligand-dependent phosphorylation of the estrogen receptor. *Mol Endocrinol* 1994; **8**:182–8.

123. Gustafsson JA, Estrogen receptor α – a new dimension in estrogen mechanism of action. *J Endocrinology* 1999; **163**:379–83.

124. Paech K, Webb P, Kuiper GGJM et al, Differential ligand activation of estrogen receptors ERα and ERβ at AP1 sites. *Science* 1997; **277**:1508–10.

125. Green S, Walter P, Kumar V et al, Human estrogen receptor cDNA sequence expression and homology to v-erb-A. *Nature* 1986; **320**:134–9.

126. Greene GL, Gilna P, Waterfield M et al, Sequence and expression of human estrogen receptor complimentary DNA. *Science* 1986; **231**:1150–4.

127. White R, Lees JA, Needham M et al, Structural organisation and expression of mouse estrogen receptor. *Mol Endocrinol* 1987; **1**: 735–44.

128. Berry M, Metzger D, Chambon P, Role of the two activating domains of the estrogen receptor in the cell type and promoter-context-dependent against activity of the antiestrogen 4-OH-tamoxifen. *EMBO J* 1990; **9**:2811–18.

129. Brzozowski A, Pike A, Dauker Z et al, Molecular basis of agonism and antagonism in the estrogen receptor. *Nature* 1997; **389**:753–8.

130. Shiau AK, Barstad D, Loria PM et al, The structural basis of estrogen receptor/coactivator recognition and the antagonism of this interaction by tamoxifen. *Cell* 1998; **95**:927–37.

131. Jordan VC, Gosden B, Importance of the alkylamino-ethoxy-sidechain for the estrogenic and antiestrogenic actions of tamoxifen and trioxifene in immature rat uterus. *Mol Cell Endocrinol* 1982; **27**:291–306.

132. Robertson DW, Katzenellenbogen JA, Hayes JR, Katzenellenbogen BS, Antiestrogen basicity activity relationships of a comparison of the estrogen receptor binding and antiuterotrophic potencies of several analogues of (Z)1-2-diphenyl-1-[4-[2-dimethylamino)ethoxy]phenyl]-1-butene(tamoxifen, Noluadex) having altered basicity. *J Med Chem* 1982; **25**:167–71.

133. McDonnell DP, Clemm DL, Hermann T et al, Investigation of estrogen receptor function in vitro reveals three distinct classes of antiestrogens. *Mol Endocrinol* 1995; **9**:659–69.

134. Beekman JM, Allan GF, Tsai SY et al, Transcriptional activation by the estrogen receptor requires a conformational change in the

ligand binding domain. *Mol Endocrinol* 1993; 1:1266–74.

135. Levenson AS, Jordan VC, The key to the antiestrogenic mechanism of raloxifene is amino acid 351 (Aspartate) in the estrogen receptor. *Cancer Res* 1998; **58**:1872–5.

136. Paige LA, Christensen DJ, Grøn H et al, Estrogen receptor (ER) modulators each induce distinct conformational changes in ERα and ERβ. *Proc Natl Acad Sci USA* 1999; **96**:3999–4004.

137. Tremblay GB, Tremblay A, Copeland NG et al, Cloning localisation and functional analysis of the murine estrogen receptor β. *Mol Endocrinol* 1997; **11**:353–65.

138. McInerney EM, Weis KE, Sun J et al, Transcription activation by the human estrogen receptor subtype β (ERβ) studied with ERβ and ERα receptor chimeras. *Endocrinology* 1998; **139**:4513–22.

139. Weigel NL, Steroid hormone receptors and their regulation by phosphorylation. *Biochem J* 1996; **319**:657–67.

140. Speirs V, Malone C, Walton DS et al, Increased expression of estrogen receptor β in tamoxifen resistant breast cancer patients. *Cancer Res* 1999; **59**:5421–4.

141. Ogawa S, Inoue S, Watanabe T et al, Molecular cloning and characterisation of human estrogen receptor βcx: a potential inhibitor of estrogen action in human. *Nucl Acid Res* 1998; **26**:3505–12.

142. Levinson AS, Jordan VC, Selective estrogen receptor modulation: molecular pharmacology for the millennium. *Eur J Cancer* 1999; **35**:1628–39.

15

Aromatase inhibitors in the treatment of breast cancer

Aman U Buzdar, Gabriel N Hortobagyi

Hormone or endocrine therapy is an effective treatment option for patients with breast cancer who have estrogen-receptor (ER)- and/or progesterone-receptor (PgR)-positive disease. Several treatment options are available for patients with hormonally sensitive disease. Such treatments are effective in palliating the disease in 25–30% of unselected patients. However, in patients with ER-positive disease, more than half of the patients receive clinical benefit from these treatments.[1–3]

Hormone therapies are directed at reducing the synthesis of estrogen or blocking estrogen action at the receptor level in the tumor. Hormone control of estrogen production is exerted through a complex series of feedback mechanisms involving the hypothalamus, pituitary, ovary, adrenal glands and the breast. These control mechanisms are exerted through the various hormones produced by these glands. In premenopausal patients, the control mechanism is exerted through luteinizing-hormone-releasing hormone (LHRH) produced by the hypothalamus, which acts on the anterior pituitary controlling the production of gonadotropins (follicle-stimulating hormone (FSH) and luteinizing hormone (LH)), which, in turn, act on the ovaries. The anterior pituitary also produces adrenocorticotropic hormone (ACTH), which

acts on the adrenal gland, and prolactin and growth hormones, which act on breast tissue. The adrenal glands produce androgens and corticosteroids; estrogens are produced by aromatization of the adrenal androgens in postmenopausal women.[4]

In this chapter, we discuss the treatment options for postmenopausal women using aromatase inhibitors.

Steroid synthesis and the production of estrogens through adrenal biosynthesis pathways are shown in Figure 15.1. These pathways involve a series of reactions, starting with cholesterol as a common precursor; depending on the biosynthestic pathways followed, cholesterol can be converted into progesterone, aldosterone, cortisol, 11-deoxycortisol, androstenedione, testosterone, estrone and estradiol. A series of related cytochrome P450 enzymes control these reactions. Many cytochrome P450 enzymes involved in steroid synthesis are closely related. Aromatase, the enzyme that controls the conversion of androstenedione or testosterone to estrone and estradiol, respectively, differs from other cytochrome P450 enzymes, in that aromatase contains the usual cytochrome P450 hemoprotein and flavoprotein components – only the hemoprotein is specific for the aromatase

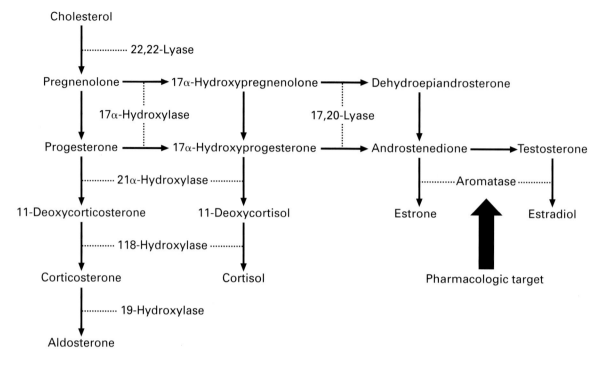

Figure 15.1
Steroids and estrogen biosynthesis pathways

reaction – whereas the cytochrome P450 NADPH reductase is similar to that contained in the other cytochrome P450 enzymes. Aromatization reactions take place in muscle and adipose tissue and the breast tumor itself. About two-thirds of malignant breast tumors contain the aromatase enzyme, potentially leading to in situ production of estrogen and growth stimulation of the tumor.[5,6] The amount of estrogen produced by peripheral aromatization is significantly lower than that produced by the ovary before the menopause; however, it is sufficient to support the growth of estrogen-dependent tumors in women who are postmenopausal. Approximately 100 ng estrone is produced by this pathway. This results in plasma estradiol levels in the range of 10–20 pg/ml.

AROMATASE INHIBITORS

A wide range of aromatase inhibitors have been evaluated in the treatment of breast cancer (Table 15.1). In the development of these agents, the objective was to develop drugs that were selective for the aromatase enzyme and had minimal side effects, while retaining clinical efficacy. A number of candidate compounds have been evaluated, and currently five drugs are available for clinical use: anastrozole, letrozole, exemestane, fadrozole and formestane. A number of non-selective aromatase inhibitors are also available, and these include aminoglutethimide, testolactone and trilostane. Aromatase inhibitors can be divided into two subtypes: type I (suicide or non-competitive inhibitors) and type II (competitive inhibitors). Type I inhibitors are all

Table 15.1   Aromatase inhibitors

	Type	Selectivity	Potency
Non-selective			
Aminoglutethimide	Competitive	Low	Moderate
Testolactone	Non-competitive	Low	Moderate
Trilostane	Competitive	Moderate	Moderate
Selective			
Anastrozole	Competitive	High	High
Fadrozole	Competitive	Moderate	Moderate
Letrozole	Competitive	High	High
Vorozole	Competitive	High	High
Formestane	Non-competitive	High	High
Exemestane	Non-competitive	High	High

steroidal compounds; type II inhibitors can be either steroidal or non-steroidal. Both types mimic normal substrates (androgens), competing with substrate for binding to the normal site on the enzyme.

After initial binding, the next step differs for the two types. Once a non-competitive inhibitor has bound, the enzyme initiates its typical sequence of hydroxylation, but hydroxylation produces an unbreakable covalent bond between the inhibitor and the enzyme protein. Enzyme activity is thus permanently blocked; even if all unattached inhibitor is removed, enzyme activity can be restored only by new enzyme synthesis. Competitive inhibitors reversibly bind to the active enzyme site and either no enzyme activity is triggered or it is without effect. The inhibitors remain and can be disassociated from the binding site, allowing renewed competition between the inhibitor and substrate for binding to the active enzyme site. As a result, the effectiveness of competitive inhibitors depends on the relative concentration and affinity of the

inhibitor and substrate. Continued activity requires a constant presence of the drug. To compete for binding to the active site, both competitive and non-competitive inhibitors must necessarily share important structural features with the natural substrates. Non-competitive inhibitors must also share with androgenic structures a feature allowing them to interact with catalytic residues on the enzyme protein. This renders them inherently selective. By contrast, most competitive inhibitors interact with heme iron, a common feature of all cytochrome P450 enzymes. Some may also bind to the highly conserved oxygen-binding site in addition to the substrate-binding site. The specificity of a competitive inhibitor is reinforced through other structural features. It may block the activity of a wide variety of cytochrome P450 enzymes, as does aminoglutethimide.

Aromatase inhibitors can only be used in women with no ovarian function. In women with intact ovarian function, aromatase inhibition results in increased estrogen production by increasing the gonadotropin-releasing hormone levels. Increases in FSH levels increase aromatase production; increases in LH levels increase ovarian steroidogenesis, particularly androstenedione, the substrate for aromatase.

NON-SELECTIVE AROMATASE INHIBITORS

Non-selective aromatase inhibitors were the first agents of this class available for treatment of metastatic disease. Even though these agents had a number of side effects, these treatments could be offered to patients who would otherwise be poor candidates for surgical ablative procedures, i.e. adrenalectomy or hypophysectomy.[7,8]

Testolactone
The first agent to become available was testolactone.[9,10] Initially it was thought to be an androgen, even though virilizing effects were almost completely absent.[11]

Aminoglutethimide
Aminoglutethimide was more extensively evaluated, and became an alternative to surgical ablative procedures. This drug was initially introduced as an anticonvulsant, but later was withdrawn because of its substantial morbidity as a result of adrenal insufficiency. Aminoglutethimide competitively inhibits aromatization, and decreases circulating estrogen levels by 60–70%. Aminoglutethimide blocks the cholesterol side-chain cleavage, inhibiting steroidal synthesis and leading to a significant reduction in glucocorticoid levels; therefore, hydrocortisone supplementation is needed.

The initial half-life of aminoglutethimide is 12.3 ± 2.6 hours; as the drug induces the enzyme that catalyzes its own elimination, the half-life decreases to 7.3 ± 2.4 hours with prolonged use.[12]

Two major studies evaluated aminoglutethimide in comparison to hypophysectomy

and adrenalectomy in advanced breast cancer, and there were no significant differences in response rate compared with these ablative procedures.[5,7,8]

Aminoglutethimide was also compared with tamoxifen as an initial therapy of patients with metastatic disease; it had a similar response rate and duration of remission.[13–16] Aminoglutethimide was also compared with progestins, and the results suggested that the two treatments had similar efficacy.[17]

Four randomized studies compared aminoglutethimide doses of 500 and 1000 mg/day, both with hydrocortisone replacement. Response rates in the studies varied from 15% to 35%, but the differences were small and not statistically significant.[17–20] Lower doses (as low as 250 mg/day), with or without hydrocortisone, have been evaluated and have antitumor activity in phase II trials.[21,22]

Trilostane
Trilostane is an aromatase inhibitor, and also inhibits 3β-hydroxysteroid dehydrogenase, decreasing the conversion of Δ^5-steroids to the estrogen precursor Δ^4-steroid. Cortisone synthesis is depressed, requiring supplemental replacement therapy. In a phase II study, this compound showed a 26% response rate. Trilostane is associated with significant side effects: nausea, vomiting, lethargy, postural hypotension, rash, hot flushes, facial and tongue pain, cushingoid features, and epigastric discomfort and diarrhea.[4]

STEROIDAL AROMATASE INHIBITORS

4-Hydroxyandrostenedione
4-Hydroxyandrostenedione (formestane, a non-competitive or suicide aromatase inhibitor) was one of the first selective aromatase inhibitors to be developed and was widely investigated. 4-Hydroxyandrostenedione is an irreversible

inhibitor of both peripheral and breast tissue aromatase and has no estrogenic activity. The studies with this agent have shown that formestane is highly selective for aromatase, and there is no effect on serum levels of androstenedione, testosterone, dihydrotestosterone, aldosterone, cortisol or 17-hydroxyprogesterone.[23,24]

After oral administration, formestane does have some weak androgenic activity, as reflected in a 15% fall in serum levels of sex-hormone-binding globulin (SHBG), but there is lack of androgen activity after intramuscular injection, probably reflecting a reduction of hepatic exposure to the drug by this route.[23,25,26]

Formestane needs to be given as an intramuscular injection, and a few patients experience pain and inflammation at the injection site. Other side effects after intramuscular injection include weakness, lethargy, hot flashes, spotting, and mild nausea and vomiting.[27] The drug is well tolerated and 90% of the patients experience no side effects.[28] Studies with different doses of this drug by intramuscular injection have shown no differences in response rates at various dose levels. However, side effects were less frequent at 250 mg every 2 weeks. About 29% of the patients showed clinical benefit, and, at a higher dose, 46%. In one study, 500–1000 mg was given intramuscularly, producing a 27% response rate.[4]

Exemestane

Exemestane is a type I steroidal inactivator and is a derivative of steroidal androgens. As a result of the androgen-like structure of the type I compounds, there is the potential for androgenic side effects after treatment, and patients in early clinical trials with higher doses (up to 200 mg/day) reported androgenic symptoms, including alopecia in 10% and hoarseness in 5% of patients ($n = 78$).[29] The plasma level of SHBG is a sensitive indicator of the androgenic side effect of an orally administered agent. At a drug dose of 25 mg/day, there was minimal change in SHBG levels, suggesting that it is associated with few androgenic side effects.[30] This drug suppresses estradiol levels by 97.9%, which is comparable to anastrozole and letrozole in similar assays.[30]

In two prospective trials, this drug was evaluated as third-line therapy in women previously treated with aminoglutethimide and formestane.[31,32] Approximately 20% of patients in each trial had a major response. In two studies, this drug was evaluated after therapy with non-steroidal aromatase inhibitors.[29,33] A fraction of patients had an objective response and a significant additional fraction of patients had stable disease. These data suggest a partial lack of cross-resistance between these agents. In a large phase III study, this drug has been evaluated in post-menopausal women after tamoxifen therapy.[34] The study design was similar to the phase III studies of anastrozole and letrozole. The control arm was a progestin (megestrol acetate). These data demonstrated that this drug has similar activity to anastrozole in this subset of women (Table 15.2). Partial lack of cross-resistance between this drug and non-steroidal aromatase inhibitors would make this drug appropriate as third-line therapy after progression of disease on one of those agents.

NON-STEROIDAL AROMATASE INHIBITORS

Fadrozole

Fadrozole is a competitive aromatase inhibitor and is more selective than aminoglutethimide, but less than anastrozole. Fadrozole appears to have little or no effect on the enzyme desmolase; however, it does partially inhibit 11-hydroxylase and 18-hydroxylase enzymes. The half-life of fadrozole is 10.5 hours and maximum effects are seen with daily doses of 2–4 mg. Two double-blind, prospective studies compared fadrozole and megestrol acetate in postmenopausal

Table 15.2   Clinical efficacy data of randomized trials (indirect comparisons)

Objective response	Anastrozole 1 mg (n = 263)	Megestrol acetate (n = 253)	Letrozole 2.5 mg (n = 174)	Megestrol acetate (n = 189)	Exemestane 25 mg (n = 366)	Megestrol acetate (n = 403)
CR + PR (%)	12.6	12.2	23.6	16.4	15.0	12.4
CR + PR + SD ≥ 24 weeks (%)	42.2	40.3	34.5	31.7	37.4	34.6
Median TTP (months)	4.8	4.6	5.6	5.5	4.7	3.9[a]
Median survival (months)	26.7	22.5[a]	25.3	21.5	NR	26.7[a]

[a]Statistical significance.
CR, complete response; PR, partial response; SD, stable disease; TTP, time to progression; NR, not reported.

patients who had failed tamoxifen. There were no significant differences in treatment and time to progression, duration of response, objective response and survival observed between the two arms of either study.[35] Overall, among 345 fadrozole-treated patients, 4 (1.2%) had complete response (CR), 34 (10%) had partial response (PR) and 84 (24%) had stable disease for 8 weeks or longer. Results were similar in the progestin-treated population (total patients, 332; 4% CR; 10% PR and 24% stable disease).[35] In a small randomized study in postmenopausal women, this drug was compared with tamoxifen as initial therapy. Response rates were similar to those for tamoxifen, but the safety profile of this drug was favorable compared with tamoxifen (with fewer thromboembolic complications).[29]

Vorozole

Vorozole is the active isomer of R-76713. In vitro, this drug has 10 000-fold selectivity for aromatase compared with any other cytochrome P450 enzyme. In experimental animal models, this drug had no effect on the production of adrenal gluco- or mineralocorticoids even at 200

times the doses needed for estrogen suppression. In phase II studies, the results were encouraging,[4] but subsequent phase III studies failed to demonstrate the superiority of this drug. Further development of this drug has been stopped.

Anastrozole

Anastrozole became available for clinical use in the USA in early 1996. It is a competitive non-steroidal and highly selective aromatase inhibitor. Experimental animal studies show that anastrozole has no significant effect against desmolase or any other enzyme involved in steroid biosynthesis. The average plasma half-life is approximately 50 hours in postmenopausal women, with no significant difference between breast cancer patients and healthy post-menopausal women.[4] Anastrozole 10 mg for 14 days did not alter the plasma cortisol or aldosterone levels or the response to ACTH stimulation.

The antitumor activity and safety of anastrozole were compared with those of megestrol acetate in two large randomized phase III trials in

Table 15.3   Common adverse events of aromatase inhibitors

Adverse event	Anastrozole 1 mg (n = 263)	Letrozole 2.5 mg (n = 174)	Fadrozole		Exemestane	
			Trial 1 (n = 196)	Trial 2 (n = 152)	Trial 1 (n = 91)	Trial 2 (n = 87)
Headache (%)	14	13	7.7	15.1	7	6
Hot flashes (%)	13	6	11.7	14.5	20	16
Nausea (%)	18	11	21.9	36.2	20	26
Vomiting (%)	10	8	9.2	18.4	–	7
Rash (%)	6	6	5.6	11.8	–	6
Fatigue (asthenia) (%)	16	11	16.3	20.4	7	10

postmenopausal women.[36–38] These patients had metastatic disease and their disease had progressed after tamoxifen therapy. Both studies had identical designs and eligibility criteria. The results are summarized in Table 15.2. Initial results, at median follow-up of 6 months, showed no differences in time to progression or survival, but anastrozole was associated with substantially fewer side effects. However, with additional follow-up (31 months), there was a significant improvement in survival for patients treated with 1 mg anastrozole (in the overview of combined data).[38] This drug was well tolerated and its safety profile is summarized in Table 15.3.

Anastrozole was recently evaluated as initial therapy of metastatic disease, in postmenopausal patients in two double-blind placebo-controlled trials.[39,40] The control arm of both studies was tamoxifen. In both studies, anastrozole had comparable antitumor activity to tamoxifen, and in patients with ER-positive tumors, anastrozole was superior to tamoxifen. A higher fraction of patients with ER-positive tumors had clinical benefit with anastrozole therapy, and also the

time to treatment failure was longer in both studies, in favor of anastrozole, in this subset of patients. The safety profile of anastrozole was more favorable compared with tamoxifen (fewer thromboembolic and vaginal bleeding episodes).

Letrozole

Letrozole is a more potent and more selective non-steroidal competitive inhibitor of the aromatase enzyme system. There are no clinically relevant changes in the plasma levels of cortisol, aldosterone, 11-dexycortisol, 17-hydroxyprogesterone, ACTH or plasma renin activity in postmenopausal patients treated with daily doses ranging from 0.1 to 5.0 mg. Letrozole suppresses plasma levels of estradiol, estrone and estrone sulfate by more than 95% within 2 weeks of initiation of treatment at doses of 1 mg/day. In one large European study, the safety and efficacy of letrozole were compared against aminoglutethimide in postmenopausal women.[41] Time to progression, time to treatment failure and overall survival were superior in the letrozole-treated patients compared with the aminoglutethimide subgroup. In another European study, letrozole was compared with progestin (megestrol acetate). In this study, the patients treated with letrozole had a significantly higher response rate compared with the patients treated with progestin.[42] The indirect comparison of these data with data from studies of anastrozole in similar patients suggests that overall clinical benefits (CR, PR and stable disease) were similar, if anything favoring anastrozole. Prospective randomized studies are needed to compare the safety and antitumor activity of these two agents. Anastrozole and letrozole have been evaluated as neoadjuvant therapy in postmenopausal patients, and have shown encouraging results. The sizes of these studies are too small for a true determination of their value, and larger studies are ongoing. Letrozole is currently being evaluated as initial therapy of metastatic disease.

With the availability of phase III data of second-line therapy after progression on tamoxifen, letrozole and anastrozole have become the current therapies of choice for treatment of metastatic disease. With the availability of new data on anastrozole as the initial therapy, compared with tamoxifen, anastrozole can now be offered as initial treatment for postmenopausal women with ER-positive tumors. In this subset of patients, anastrozole resulted in higher response rates, longer control of disease and fewer side effects.

Aromatase inhibitors are being evaluated in adjuvant and neoadjuvant therapy, and the results of these trials should become available in the near future. These drugs are being evaluated in various study designs either concomitantly or sequentially with tamoxifen therapy.

REFERENCES

1. Jensen EV, Block GE, Smith Seal, Estrogen receptors and breast cancer response to adrenalectomy. In: *Prediction of Response in Cancer Therapy*. Washington, DC: US Department of Health, Education and Welfare, 1971: 55–70.

2. Sedlacek SM, Horowitz KB, The role of progestins and progesterone receptors in the treatment of breast cancer. *Steroids* 1984; 44:467–84.

3. Beck WW, *Obstetrics and Gynecology*. Baltimore: Williams & Wilkins, 1989: 126.

4. Buzdar AU, Hortobagyi GN, Update on endocrine therapy for breast cancer. *Clin Cancer Res* 1998; 4:527–34.

5. Longcope C, Pratt JH, Schneider SH, Fineberg SE, Aromatization of androgens by muscle and adipose tissue in vivo. *J Clin Endocrinol Metab* 1978; 46:146–52.

6. Reed MJ, The role of aromatase in breast tumors. *Breast Cancer Res Treat* 1994; 30:7–17.

7. Harvey HA, Santen RJ, Osterman J et al, A comparative trial of transsphenoidal hypophysectomy with aminoglutethimide plus hydrocortisone in women with advanced breast cancer. *Cancer* 1979; 43:2207–14.

8. Santen RJ, Worgul TJ, Samojlik E et al, A randomized trial comparing surgical adrenalectomy with aminoglutethimide plus hydrocortisone in women with advanced breast cancer. *N Engl J Med* 1981; 305:545–51.

9. Segaloff A, Weeth JB, Meyer KK et al, Hormonal therapy in cancer of the breast, XIX, Effect of oral administration of delta[1]-testololactone on clinical course and hormonal excretion. *Cancer* 1962; 15:633–5.

10. Van Rymenant M, Coune A, Tagnon HJ, Somon S, Le traitement hormonal du cancer de sein en phase avancee. Methodes d'etudes – comparaison de la delta-1-testololactone avec le propionate de tetosterone. *Acta Clin Belg* 1963; 18:469–79.

11. Volk H, Deupree RH, Goldenberg IS et al, A dose response evaluation of delta-1-testololactone in advanced breast cancer. *Cancer* 1974; 33:9–13.

12. Swain SM, Lippman ME, Endocrine therapies of cancer. In: Chabner BA, Collins JM, eds.

Cancer Chemotherapy: Principles and Practice. Philadelphia: JB Lippincott, 1990: 59–109.

13. Lipton A, Harvey HA, Santen RJ et al, A randomized trial of aminoglutethimide versus tamoxifen in metastatic breast cancer. Cancer 1982; 50:2265–8.

14. Smith IE, Harris AL, Morgan M et al, Tamoxifen versus aminoglutethimide in advanced breast carcinoma: A randomized cross-over trial. BMJ 1981; 283:1432–4.

15. Alonso-Munoz MC, Ojeda-Gonzalez MB, Beltran-Fabregat M et al, Randomized trial of tamoxifen versus aminoglutethimide and versus combined tamoxifen and aminoglutethimide in advanced postmenopausal breast cancer. Oncology 1988; 45:350–3.

16. Gale KE, Anderson JW, Tormey DC et al, Hormonal treatment for metastatic breast cancer. An Eastern Co-operative Oncology Group Phase III trial comparing aminoglutethimide to tamoxifen. Cancer 1994; 73:354–61.

17. Robustelli DCG, 500 mg versus 1000 mg aminoglutethimide in advanced breast cancer: 3 year results of an Italian multicentric trial. Eur J Cancer 1991; 2:569.

18. Upright C, Ragaz J, Basco V, Grafton C, Double blind randomized trial of conventional versus low dose aminoglutethimide and hydrocortisone in patients with metastatic hormone responsive breast cancer. Proc Am Soc Clin Oncol 1991; 9:45.

19. Illiger HJ, Caffier H, Carterier B et al, Aminoglutethimide in advanced breast cancer low dose vs standard dose. J Cancer Res Clin Oncol 1986; 3:S69.

20. Bonneterre J, Pion JM, Demaille A, Low-dose aminoglutethimide (500 mg/day) and hydrocortisone (30 mg/day) in advanced cancer of breast. Bulletin du Cancer 1987; 74:241–7 (in French).

21. Harris AL, Cantwell BM, Carmichael J et al, Phase II study of low dose aminoglutethimide 250 mg/day plus hydrocortisone in advanced postmenopausal breast cancer. Eur J Cancer 1989; 25:1105–11.

22. Willard EM, Carpenter JT, Low dose aminoglutethimide is active in metastatic breast cancer. Proc Am Soc Clin Oncol 1991; 10:55.

23. Dowsett M, Cunningham DC, Stein RC et al, Dose-related endocrine effects and pharmacokinetics of oral and intramuscular 4-hydroxyandrostenedione in postmenopausal breast cancer patients. Cancer Res 1989; 49:1306–12.

24. Dowsett M, Mehta A, King N et al, An endocrine and pharmacokinetic study of four oral doses of formestane in postmenopausal breast cancer patients. Eur J Cancer 1992; 28:415–20.

25. Brodie AM, Garrett WM, Hendrickson JR, Tsai-Morris CH, Effects of aromatase inhibitor 4-hydroxyandrostenedione and other compounds in the 7,12-dimethylbenz(a)anthracene-induced breast carcinoma model. Cancer Res 1982; 42:3360s–4s.

26. Brodie AM, Banks PK, Inkster SE et al, Aromatase inhibitors and hormone-dependent cancers. J Steroid Biochem Mol Biol 1990; 37:327–33.

27. Dowsett M, Smithers D, Moore J et al, Endocrine changes with the aromatase inhibitor fadrozole hydrochloride in breast cancer. Eur J Cancer 1994; 30A:1453–8.

28. Cunningham DC, Powels TJ, Dowsett M et al, Oral 4-hydroxyandrostenedione, a new endocrine treatment for disseminated breast cancer. Cancer Chemother Pharmacol 1987; 20:253–5.

29. Thuerlimann B, Paridaens R, Serin D et al, Third-line hormonal treatment with exemestane in postmenopausal patients with advanced breast cancer progressing on aminoglutethimide: A phase II multicentre multinational study. Exemestane Study Group. Eur J Cancer 1997; 33:1767–73.

30. Johannessen DC, Engan T, di Salle E et al, Endocrine and clinical effects of exemstane (PNU 155971), a novel steroidal aromatase inhibitor, in postmenopausal breast cancer patients: a phase I study. Clin Cancer Res 1997; 3:1101–8.

31. Murray R, Pitt P, Aromatase inhibition with

4-OH androstenedione after prior aromatase inhibition with aminoglutethimide in women with advanced breast cancer. *Breast Cancer Res Treat* 1995; 35:249–53.

32. Lonning PE, Johannessen DC, Thorsen T, Alterations in the production rate and the metabolism of oesterone and oesterone sulphate in breast cancer patients treated with aminoglutethimide. *Br J Cancer* 1989; 60:107–11.

33. Lonning PE, Bajetta E, Murray R et al, A phase II study of exemestane in metastatic breast cancer patients failing non-steroidal aromatase inhibitors. *Breast Cancer Res Treat* 1998; 50:304.

34. Kaufmann M, Bajetta E, Dirix LY et al, Survival advantage of exemestane (EXE, Aromasin®) over megestrol acetate (MA) in postmenopausal women with advanced breast cancer (ABC) refractory to tamoxifen (TAM): Results of a phase III randomized double-blind study. *Proc Am Soc Clin Oncol* 1999; **18**: (Abst).

35. Buzdar AU, Smith R, Vogel C et al, Fadrozole HCL (CGS-16949A) versus megestrol acetate treatment of postmenopausal patients with metastatic breast carcinoma: Results of two randomized double blind controlled multiinstitutional trials. *Cancer* 1996; 77:2503–13.

36. Jonat W, Howell A, Blomqvist C et al, A randomized trial comparing two doses of the new selective aromatase inhibitor anastrozole (Arimidex) with megestrol acetate in postmenopausal patients with advanced breast cancer. *Eur J Cancer* 1996; **32A**:404–12.

37. Buzdar A, Jonat W, Howell A et al, Anastro-zole, a potent and selective aromatase inhibitor, versus megestrol acetate in postmenopausal women with advanced breast cancer: Results of overview analysis of two phase III trials. *J Clin Oncol* 1996; **14**:2000–11.

38. Buzdar AU, Jones SE, Vogel CL et al, A phase III trial comparing anastrozole (1 and 10 milligrams), a potent and selective aromatase inhibitor, with megestrol acetate in postmenopausal women with advanced breast cancer. *Cancer* 1997; **79**:730–9.

39. Bonneterre J, Thuerlimann BJK, Robertson JFR, Preliminary results of a large comparative multi-centre clinical trial comparing the efficacy and tolerability of Arimidex (anastrozole) and tamoxifen in postmenopausal women with advanced breast cancer. *Eur J Cancer* 1999; **35**:S313.

40. Nabboltz JM, Bonneterre J, Buzdar AU et al, Results of a North American, first-line trial comparing Arimidex with tamoxifen in postmenopausal women with advanced breast cancer. *Breast Cancer Res Treat* 1999; 57:31.

41. Gershanovich M, Chaudri HA, Campos D et al, Letrozole, a new oral aromatase inhibitor: Randomised trial comparing 2.5 mg daily, 0.5 mg daily and aminoglutethimide in postmenopausal women with advanced breast cancer. *Ann Oncol* 1998; 9:639–45.

42. Dombernowsky P, Smith I, Falkson G et al, Letrozole, a new oral aromatase inhibitor for advanced breast cancer: Double-blind randomized trial showing a dose effect and improved efficacy and tolerability compared with megestrol acetate. *J Clin Oncol* 1999; **16**:453–61.

16

Other hormone treatments

Gershon Y Locker

OVARIAN ABLATION

Surgical castration is the oldest form of systemic therapy of advanced breast cancer.[1] Many institutions reported tumor regression and survival prolongation with ovariectomy in large series and made ovarian ablation the standard therapy of premenopausal metastatic breast cancer for decades.[2–6] In the pre-hormone-receptor era, empiric clinical criteria were used to predict which women were most likely to be helped by estrogen deprivation; benefit was often loosely defined. Jensen's isolation of the estrogen receptor (ER) in breast carcinomas in the late 1960s transformed prediction of response into a rational and scientific process.[7,8] At the same time, the difficulty in determining objective response and the appreciation of the survival advantage of tumor stability for more than 6 months[9,10] rendered time to progression (TTP) and overall survival (OS) the important objective criteria in the evaluation of palliative therapies of incurable mammary carcinoma. Unfortunately, even in the modern era, many studies evaluating therapeutic castration for advanced breast cancer include patients whose tumor receptor status is unknown and do not differentiate these women from those with receptor-positive tumors.[11–13] Data are available for premenopausal women with receptor-rich tumors randomized to castration in three prospective phase III trials, from the Mayo Clinic ($n = 22$),[14] the National Cancer Institute of Canada (NCIC) ($n = 19$)[15] and the American Intergroup ($n = 67$).[16] These studies found that ovariectomy benefited (rate of response plus stable disease) 32–52% of premenopausal women with hormone-responsive metastatic breast cancer. They found identical times to progression of 4 months and overall survivals of 24–33 months (level II evidence). These trials and the anecdotal reports that preceded them (level III) consistently support the use of surgical ablation in the treatment of advanced ER-rich (ER-positive) breast carcinoma in premenopausal women (grade A).

Radiation-induced ovarian ablation was introduced 75 years ago.[17] In most reports, it had similar efficacy to that of ovariectomy against advanced breast cancer.[2–4,6] The meta-analysis of adjuvant ovarian ablation (see below) reviewed trials of both surgical and radiation castration.[18] It also found an equivalent effect of the two approaches, but the small numbers and non-randomization between the modalities compromise the finding's reliability.[18] Although the evidence is limited (level III and IV), it does suggest that the two approaches to castration can be considered acceptable alternatives (grade B). The delay in radiation effect on the ovaries and the potential for incompleteness of ablation are potential drawbacks to its use.[19]

Tamoxifen is active against metastatic breast cancer in premenopausal women.[20] Three published[12,14,15] and one unpublished[21] prospective randomized trials compared tamoxifen (T) and ovariectomy (O) as first therapy of advanced mammary cancer in this group of patients. An overview of the four studies obtained individual patient data.[21] Two hundred and twenty eligible patients (T = 109, O = 111) had measurable disease and were menstruating or were less than 1 year from cessation of menses. Criteria for response were similar in the four studies and all had provision for crossover between the treatments. Analysis was by intent to treat. Ten percent of the patients were receptor-negative, and 37% unknown. The two therapies had the same response rates (T 22.9% versus O 22.5%, $p = 0.94$) and rates of stable disease (T 26.6% versus O 26.1%).[21] There was a trend toward longer time to progression for tamoxifen, but it was not statistically significant (odds reduction 14%±12% SD (standard deviation); two-sided $p = 0.32$). There was no significant difference in overall survival between the two (odds reduction 6%±13% SD in favor of T: two-sided $p = 0.72$).

All four trials called for crossover to the alternative treatment after failure of initial therapy, but this was done only in a small number of women. Six of 26 evaluable patients initially treated with tamoxifen responded to ovariectomy (23%). Four of 47 evaluable patients initially treated with ovariectomy responded to tamoxifen (9%). Although there was a trend favoring the sequence tamoxifen to ovariectomy in terms of response ($p = 0.15$), no comparison of survival was given. For the sequence of tamoxifen to ovariectomy, there was a significant corre-lation between objective response to tamoxifen and subsequent response to castration ($p < 0.05$). This is in contrast to the results of a phase II trial of the Southwest Oncology Group (SWOG), which found that response to tamoxifen in 38 premenopausal women with advanced disease (ER-positive or unknown) did not predict for subsequent response to ovariectomy.[22] In the SWOG study, however, the patients were continued on tamoxifen after surgery.

Although the relatively small number of patients evaluated suggests caution, the meta-analysis (level I) supports the equivalence of tamoxifen and ovariectomy as the first therapy of receptor-containing advanced breast cancer in premenopausal women (grade A).[21]

Despite ovariectomy or natural menopause, low levels of estrogen persist in the body with the potential to stimulate receptor-containing breast cancers. A possible approach to the treatment of metastatic breast cancer in premenopausal women with advanced disease would be total estrogen blockade, combining ovarian ablation and antiestrogen, analogous to the total androgen blockade used to treat prostate cancer. There are extremely limited data comparing ovariectomy with ovariectomy plus tamoxifen. Although one randomized study ($n = 37$) reported no significant difference in time to progression or survival between the two, the small numbers make conclusions problematic.[13]

The combination of ovariectomy and chemotherapy in the treatment of premenopausal metastatic breast cancer has been evaluated in several prospective trials. Two studies randomized patients to chemotherapy with or without ovariectomy.[23–25] A Swiss group assigned 42 premenopausal women (receptor unknown) to either CMFVP (cyclophosphamide, methotrexate, 5-fluorouracil, vincristine and prednisone) or ovariectomy plus CMFVP.[25] There was no significant difference in objective response rates, duration of response or survival. The Eastern Cooperative Oncology Group (ECOG) randomized 89 premenopausal women with advanced cancer to CAF (cyclophosphamide, doxorubicin and 5-fluorouracil) or ovariectomy (O) + CAF;[23,24] 50 women were ER-positive. In that group, the response rates (CAF 71%; O + CAF 73%),[23] time to treatment failure (CAF 9.1 months; O + CAF 15.5 months; $p = 0.41$)[23] and survival (CAF 26 months; O + CAF 59 months; $p = 0.66$)[24] were not significantly different between the two arms. A meta-analysis of the Swiss and ECOG studies found a non-significant trend toward survival benefit for the combined chemotherapy plus ovariectomy approach, with a hazard ratio of 0.88 (0.60–1.31).[26] The small numbers of patients randomized (particularly with known receptor positivity) make definitive conclusions problematic, but, based on the available studies (level II), the addition of ovariectomy to chemotherapy in the treatment of advanced breast cancer in premenopausal women is not supported (grade B).

Two studies addressed the role of chemotherapy added to ovariectomy.[27] SWOG assigned 143 premenopausal women with receptor-unknown advanced disease to ovariectomy (O) or O + cyclophosphamide (C) or O + CMFVP. There was a benefit for the combined arms compared with ovariectomy alone (followed by chemotherapy at relapse) for response rate (18% versus 62% and 75%; $p < 0.0001$) and time to treatment failure (TTF) (3 versus 12 and 14 months). There was no survival advantage (O 32 months, O + C 26 months, O + CMFVP 30 months). An ECOG study treated 40 ER-positive or receptor-unknown women with ovariectomy and, if there was no progression after 3 months, randomized them to CMF chemotherapy or no chemotherapy until subsequent progression. Although there was difference between the arms in TTF (O 5.4 months; O to CMF 16.3 months;

$p = 0.004$), there was no significant difference ($p = $ NS) in response rates (O 44%; O to CMF 55%) or survival (O 29 months; O to CMF 41 months). The absence of survival advantages to the addition of chemotherapy to ovariectomy in either study (level II evidence) argues against the combined approach, but again this must be tempered with the small numbers of women treated with known receptor positivity (grade B).[27]

The activity of ovariectomy against metastatic breast cancer in younger women led to trials of the modality as an adjuvant to local therapy of early breast cancer. Schinzinger[28] suggested such an adjuvant therapy years before an attempt was made to use it to treat advanced disease.[1] Although non-randomized series as long as 60 years ago have claimed benefits of the approach,[29] it was only in the era of the prospective randomized trial that its value was demonstrated. The Early Breast Cancer Trialists Collaborative Group (EBCTCG) in 1995 analyzed individual data on 2100 women under the age of 50 with early breast cancer, randomized in 12 trials to local therapy with or without ovarian ablation (surgical or radiation).[18] Seven trials compared ablation with no adjuvant therapy; four evaluated chemotherapy with or without ablation. One study had both types of randomization.[18] Primary data from one published randomized trial were not available and therefore not included.[30] Four studies of adjuvant ablation via gonadotropin-hormone-releasing hormone analogs were also not included.

At the time of analysis, 1130 of 2102 women aged under 50 years had died in the 12 studies reviewed. With 15 years of follow-up, recurrence-free survival (RFS) was significantly improved in women randomized to receive ovarian ablation compared with those not so randomized (45.0% versus 39.0%; two-sided log-rank $p = 0.0007$). The proportional risk of recurrence was decreased by 18.5%. OS was also significantly improved (52.4% versus 46.1%; two-sided $p = 0.001$). The proportional risk of death was decreased by 18.4%. There was no difference in rates of non-breast-cancer deaths in either group.[18] The EBCTCG also evaluated ovarian ablation in women aged over 50. Of 1354 older women randomized to ovarian ablation or no ablation, 1018 had died at the time of analysis. At 15 years of follow-up, there was no difference in RFS with or without ovarian ablation (32.0% versus 28.9%; $p = NS$) or in OS (36.9% versus 34.5%; $p = NS$).

The absolute survival improvement from adjuvant ovarian ablation in all women aged under 50 was 6.3% at 15 years. Only a small minority of patients benefit from an irreversible procedure, with many medical and social consequences. It would be preferable if subset analyses could identify those women most likely to benefit. Unfortunately, most subsets were too small to do more than identify non-statistically significant trends. As chemotherapy may induce the menopause, it is possible that ovariectomy/radiation might not be advantageous when added to cytotoxic therapy. The meta-analysis found the absolute decrease of death from the addition of ovariectomy in the absence of chemotherapy to be 9.4% ($p = 0.006$), but only 2.8% ($p > 0.1$) in the presence of cytotoxic agents.[18] Comparison of the two groups, however, showed no statistically significant difference in the advantage derived from ovarian ablation.[18] Furthermore, it is unclear from the data whether the benefit, if any, from the addition of ovarian ablation to chemotherapy was related to whether or not the cytotoxic agents induced menopause. Confounding the analysis is the observation that most of the women in the chemotherapy trials had involvement of axillary nodes (904 of 933). Could the apparent differences be related to nodal status?

Only in the ablation-without-chemotherapy studies were there enough patients aged under 50 in the node-negative and node-positive groups to make indirect comparisons between them. The proportional decrease in death at 15 years associated with adding castration to local therapy was similar in the two nodal groups: 19.2% for node-negative women and 17.3% in those with involved axillary nodes.[18] The absolute decrease in death was 5.6% with negative nodes (two-sided $p = 0.01$ versus no ovarian ablation) and 12.5% with positive nodes (two-sided $p = 0.0007$). This difference in benefit between the nodal groups was not statistically significant.[18]

Another potential discriminant in determining the value of adjuvant ovarian ablation in younger women is the presence or absence of ER in the breast cancer. There were insufficient receptor data available in the trials of ovariectomy without chemotherapy. Data were available in four of the chemotherapy studies; 194 women aged under 50 had receptor-poor tumors, and there was no difference in survival in that group with or without the addition of ablation to chemotherapy (1.9% difference in survival, $p = NS$).[18] In 550 women with hormone-receptor-containing cancers, the addition of ovarian ablation to chemotherapy decreased death by an absolute 9.2% (relative decrease 17%), but this difference was also not statistically significant.[18]

The EBCTCG 1995 overview is level I evidence, supporting the conclusion that women aged under 50 with operable breast cancer benefit from adjuvant ovariectomy and that older women do not benefit (grade A).[18] Unfortunately, the small subset numbers make other findings from the meta-analysis less secure. It is likely that the RFS and OS advantages are proportionally the same whether a woman's tumor did or did not involve lymph nodes, with a trend favoring a greater absolute benefit in node-positive patients (level II evidence, grade B). Although the data were only from chemotherapy trials, ovarian ablation appears to be more effective, in women with hormone-receptor-containing tumors, than those who are receptor-negative (level II, grade B). Ovarian ablation seems less beneficial when added to adjuvant chemotherapy than when used as the only adjuvant treatment (level II evidence, grade B). This conclusion should be viewed with caution without data on the effect of ovariectomy in the presence or absence of chemotherapy-induced menopause.

The benefit of adjuvant ovarian ablation in women aged under 50 with operable breast cancer is similar to that associated with adjuvant chemotherapy.[31] Only one published study, the Scottish trial, directly compared the two.[32] It randomized 332 premenopausal women with axillary node-positive disease to ovariectomy (with or without prednisolone) or CMF (with or without prednisolone) after local therapy. The CMF was given intravenously every 3 weeks for eight doses, a regimen less effective than the standard CMF developed by Bonadonna.[32–34] There was no difference in event-free survival (EFS) and OS between ovariectomy and CMF (the hazard ratios, HR, with 95% confidence intervals, 95%CI, in square brackets, were as follows: EFS 1.08 [0.77–1.51]; OS 1.12 [0.76–1.63]). ER data were available in 238 patients who received their assigned treatment. There was a trend in EFS favoring chemotherapy for women with receptor-poor tumors and ovariectomy for women with receptor-rich cancers (ER $\geq$ 20 fmol/mg protein). This effect of the receptor reached statistical significance ($p = 0.018$) using the test for interaction in a Cox's survival model.[32] The trial is level II evidence to support the equivalence of low-dose chemotherapy and ovariectomy in unselected premenopausal women with nodal disease (grade B). Its reliability is affected by the small number of patients, the chemotherapy used and its limited power (80% power to detect a 15% dif-

ference in 5-year EFS). The relationship between receptor status and relative efficacy of the two modalities is suggested (level III), but is not sufficient to come to a graded conclusion by itself.

GONADOTROPIN-HORMONE-RELEASING HORMONE ANALOGS

Ovarian secretion of estrogen is controlled by pituitary gonadotropins. Pituitary secretion of gonadotropins is stimulated by the intermittent action of gonadotropin-hormone-releasing hormone (GnRH); constant stimulation of the pituitary by GnRH or its analogs leads to eventual suppression of gonadotropin release and a decline in serum estrogen levels to postmenopausal levels.[35–37] This is the basis for the use of the GnRH analogs, goserelin, buserelin or leuprolide, to achieve a medical ovariectomy. Shortly after their availability, GnRH analogs were reported to cause tumor shrinkage in 32–45% of premenopausal patients with advanced breast cancer; an additional 20–25% had stable disease.[35–39] Response was more common in ER-containing tumors.[38,39] Hot flashes were a common side effect, with nausea and flare of tumor-related pain rarely described.[16,35,36,38] Although it is assumed that the mechanism of the antitumor effect of the GnRH analogs is via estrogen deprivation, there are GnRH receptors in some breast cancer cells[40,41] and rare reports of GnRH-induced shrinkage of ER-negative breast cancers[36] and breast cancers in postmenopausal women.[42] Nevertheless, the use of the GnRH analogs has been restricted almost entirely to premenopausal women with ER- or progesterone-receptor (PgR)-containing advanced mammary carcinomas.

The early reports suggested that the efficacy of GnRH analogs is comparable to that of surgical or radiation ablation, but these studies contained a mixture of patients with receptor-positive and unknown tumors, and did not always use time to progression and survival as endpoints for objective assessment of activity. Three randomized trials were undertaken to compare the activity of surgical or radiation ovarian ablation with that achieved with drug. Unfortunately, all three trials suffered from poor patient accrual.

A multicenter European trial was begun in 1988 comparing ovariectomy with goserelin, but was suspended because of low enrollment of patients.[13] An Italian study of ovarian ablation (with or without tamoxifen) versus goserelin (with or without tamoxifen) in pre/perimenopausal advanced breast cancer was stopped after only 85 patients had been randomized. It found no significant difference in response rates, time to progression or survival between ovarian ablation and goserelin, but it too was under-powered to draw firm conclusions.[13] Even the largest study, that of the American Intergroup, was halted prematurely because of insufficient accrual. It randomized 138 women with ER- or PgR-positive metastatic breast cancer to goserelin or ovariectomy. In patients evaluable for response ($n = 59$), there was no significant difference in objective response rate between ovariectomy and GnRH (31% versus 27%) or in rate of stable disease (28% versus 26%).[16] In all 138 patients, there was no difference in failure-free survival comparing goserelin with ovariectomy (HR 0.73, 95%CI 0.51–1.04) or in overall survival (HR 0.80, 95%CI 0.53–1.20). Although the study was designed to have an 80% power to detect a 50% difference in survival favoring ovariectomy, the low enrollment made that impossible and gave it no better than a power of 60% to detect equal survival (level II evidence).[16] The available evidence (level II) does suggest that ovariectomy and GnRH analog therapies are equivalent in the treatment of receptor-containing advanced breast cancer in premenopausal women (grade B).

Total estrogen blockade combining a GnRH analog and tamoxifen was evaluated in four randomized trials.[13,43–45] Three trials randomized premenopausal women with advanced breast cancer to goserelin with or without tamoxifen, the fourth to buserelin with or without tamoxifen. A meta-analysis collected individual data from the 506 patients in the four studies and was reported in abstract form.[43] The primary endpoint was overall survival and analysis was by intent to treat. At the time of the report, 70% of the patients had died. The GnRH and GnRH-plus-tamoxifen groups were balanced for patient and tumor characteristics. The objective response rate was superior for the combined therapy (39% versus 30%, $p = 0.03$). Progression-free survival was 8.7 months with GnRH plus tamoxifen versus 5.4 months with GnRH (HR 0.7, $p < 0.001$). Overall survival was significantly improved with the combined therapy: 2.9 years versus 2.5 years with a GnRH analog alone (HR 0.78, $p = 0.02$). Subset analysis of receptor status, site of metastases and disease-free interval all showed a trend favoring GnRH plus tamoxifen, but the numbers were small. The data have not yet appeared in a peer-reviewed journal, but, if it is confirmed in a future publication, the overview is level I evidence supporting the superiority of combined GnRH analog plus tamoxifen compared with GnRH alone in the treatment of premenopausal, hormone-responsive, advanced breast cancer (grade A).

The activity of GnRH analogs against advanced disease led to multiple randomized studies evaluating their efficacy as adjuvant therapy for early stage breast cancer. The EBCTCG 2000 overview meta-analysis will review these studies. There are nine phase III trials looking at the role of adjuvant GnRH analogs in premenopausal women with operable and, in most studies, receptor-positive breast cancer (Table 16.1). The GROCTA (Italian Adjuvant Chemo-hormone Therapy Breast Cancer

Study Group)[46,47], ABCSG (Austrian Breast Cancer Study Group),[48,49] ZEBRA (Zoladex Early Breast Cancer Research Association)[50] and GABG (German Adjuvant Breast Study Group)[51] studies compared CMF chemotherapy with goserelin alone (ZEBRA, GABG) or with goserelin plus tamoxifen (GROCTA, ABCSG) (Table 16.1). The European Table-Study Group randomized to CMF or leuprolide.[52] The ZIPP trial (incorporating trials of the CRC (Cancer Research Campaign), southeast Sweden, Stockholm and GIVIO (Groupo Interdisciplinare Valutazione Interventi in Oncologia) groups) allowed previous chemotherapy and randomized to no further therapy, goserelin, tamoxifen or goserelin plus tamoxifen.[53,54] The FNCLCC (Federation of French Cancer Centers) study treated all patients with anthracycline-based chemotherapy then randomized to no further therapy or goserelin (or triptorelin).[18] The International Breast Cancer Study Group (IBCSG) study randomized among goserelin alone, CMF or CMF followed by goserelin.[50] The American Intergroup (ECOG/ SWOG) randomized among CAF, CAF plus goserelin and CAF plus goserelin plus tamoxifen.[55] Approximately 9000 women are enrolled on these nine studies (Table 16.1).

These trials address three issues in premenopausal women with operable breast cancer. Is adjuvant treatment with GnRH analogs better than no treatment with GnRH analogs? Is adjuvant GnRH therapy as effective as chemotherapy? Is there benefit to the combination of GnRH analogs and chemotherapy compared with single-modality therapy? (Table 16.1). Preliminary results for the GROCTA[46,47], ABCSG[48,49], CRC/ZIPP[53,54] and Intergroup trials[55] have been reported in abstract form. Although it is premature to draw any firm conclusions as to the role of adjuvant GnRH analogs based on abstract reports, some trends are apparent. The ZIPP trials ($n = 2631$) analyzed the goserelin versus

no goserelin arms.[54] With 591 events recorded, it found a significant increase in disease-free survival for the goserelin-treated patients (HR 0.77 [95%CI 0.66–0.90], $p = 0.001$).[54] There was a non-significant trend toward improved survival with GnRH (HR 0.84 [95%CI 0.67–1.05], $p = 0.12$).[54] The GROCTA trial ($n = 244$)[46,47] found, with a median follow-up of 76 months, that goserelin plus tamoxifen was equivalent to CMF adjuvant therapy in rate of relapse and overall survival (HR 0.69 [95%CI 0.36–1.33], $p = 0.3$). The trial included some patients who received ovarian ablation rather than GnRH. They were included in the analysis of the hormonal arm. The ABCSG study ($n = 1045$),[48,49] with a 48-month median follow-up, found RFS to be better with goserelin plus tamoxifen compared with CMF ($p < 0.02$), but there was no significant difference in OS. Finally, the Intergroup ($n = 1504$)[55] found no difference in RFS or OS between CAF and CAF plus goserelin, although an analysis of efficacy based on age and menopausal status after chemotherapy is underway. Even with such preliminary reports, it is clear that there are data (level II) to support the use of GnRH analogs as adjuvant therapy in premenopausal women with receptor-containing operable breast cancer (grade B). With the publication of the EBCTCG 2000 overview, there will be level I evidence to make more definitive, higher-grade recommendations.

PROGESTINS

Progestin therapy is among the oldest treatments of advanced breast cancer in postmenopausal women.[56] Its mechanism of action is still controversial. Biologic effects of progestational agents on mammary carcinomas in vitro include downregulation of hormone receptors,[57,58] effects on growth factor receptors,[59–61] interference with estrogen metabolism,[62] decreased

Table 16.1 Adjuvant trials of GnRH analogs

Institution	Patients	Other treatment	n	A	versus	B	versus	C	versus	D
GABG A93[51]	Prem N−/receptor+		561+	CMF ×		3 Gos × 2 y				
ZEBRA[50]	Prem/perim N+ ER+ or unknown		1640	CMF × 6		Gos × 2 y				
GROCTA 02[46,47]	Prem/perim N+/ER+		244	CMF × 6		Gos × 2 y + Tam × 5 y[a]				
ABCSG 05[48,49]	Prem N+/− receptor+		1045	CMF × 6		Gos × 3 y + Tam × 5 y				
ZIPP[53,54]	<50 y N+/− 53% ER+	43% prior chemotherapy	2631	No Rx		Gos × 2 y		Gos × 2 y + Tam × 2 y		Tam × 2 y
IBCGSG VIII[50]	Prem/perim N−		983+	CMF × 6		Gos × 2 y		CMF × 6 Gos × 1.5 y		
FNCLCC[18]	<50 y	All chemotherapy FAC or FEC	746+	No Rx		Gos or triptorelin				
European Table-Study Group[52]	Prem/perim N+ receptor+		133+	CMF × 6		Leuprolide × 2 y				
ECOG/SWOG (INT 0101)[55]	Prem N+ receptor+		1504	CAF × 6		CAF × 6 + Gos × 5 y		CAF × 6 + Gos × 5 y + Tam × 5 y		

[a]30% of patients had ovarian ablation rather than goserelin.
y, years; N, node; Prem, premenopausal; perim, perimenopausal; Gos, goserelin; Rx, treatment.

cyclin-dependent kinase activity,[63] promotion of differentiation,[64] and apoptosis.[65] In patients, progestins suppress pituitary secretion of gonadotropin[66,67] and increase plasma clearance of estrogen.[67] The net effect is to lower serum levels of estrogen in postmenopausal women to the same extent as aromatase inhibitors.[67]

The most commonly used progestational agents for treating breast cancer are medroxy-progesterone acetate (MPA) and megesterol acetate (MA). Early case reports found that about 20% of older women with metastatic breast cancer had an objective response when treated with 17-hydroxyprogesterone derivatives (MPA or MA).[56] For many years, this was the standard alternative to high-dose estrogen in the treatment of advanced disease. With the introduction of tamoxifen, a much less toxic therapy, the issue of the relative efficacy of the two hormonal approaches was addressed.

Seven randomized trials have been reported comparing tamoxifen (T) with MA in about 900 postmenopausal women with advanced breast cancer and no prior additive hormonal therapy.[68–74] The studies were heterogeneous as to receptor status and prognostic features; however, in none of them was there a significant difference between the therapies in objective response rate or rate of response plus stable disease.[68–74] In the seven trials, 129 of 428 patients had an objective response to MA (30%) and 154 of 428 to T (36%). The rates of response plus stable disease were 68% for MA and 69% for T. Survival data are available for six of the seven trials.[69–74] In none of the studies was there a significant survival advantage for either agent by log-rank analysis. Fossati,[26] using the published reports, systematically reviewed the survival data. Although not a true overview meta-analysis using individual patient data, it should be considered level I evidence. In the review, after 469 deaths in 708 patients, there was a marginal, but

not statistically significant, trend to improved survival for tamoxifen relative to MA (HR 1.09; 95%CI 0.91–1.30).[26] In those studies reporting toxicity data, hot flashes and nausea were more common with tamoxifen, and weight gain and fluid retention with MA, but no statistical comparisons were done.[69,70,72,74] Excess cardiovascular toxicity has been described in other randomized trials of MA and MPA.[26] In the five studies in which crossover to the alternative therapy was done after failure of first treatment, 22 of 156 (14%) of patients treated with second-line megesterol had objective shrinkage of tumor and 26 of 160 (16%) of patients treated with tamoxifen.[68,70,71,73,74] Response and stability rates were also similar. There is no significant difference in the efficacy of tamoxifen and MA hormonal therapy for advanced postmenopausal breast cancer (grade A).

There are eight randomized studies encompassing about 900 patients comparing MPA with tamoxifen in the treatment of advanced post-menopausal breast cancer.[75–82] Only four report survival data[76,78,79,82] and are included in the Fossati systemic review.[26] The other four trials contain only information on poorly defined response rates[77,80] or are in preliminary/abstract form.[75,81] Although there are claims that MPA leads to a significantly greater response rate than tamoxifen as the first therapy of metastatic disease,[83] the unclear definition of response, the absence of data on stable disease and the limited information in several of the reports make conclusions about relative response rate questionable (grade C). The Fossati paper reviews survival in 531 patients in the four reports with adequate information.[26] With 373 deaths recorded, there was no difference in survival between women treated with tamoxifen and those treated with MPA (MPA versus T: HR 0.97, 95%CI 0.8–1.1). As with MA, there was a suggestion that weight gain and edema were more common side effects of MPA than of tamoxifen.[76,78,82] Given the more limited data, conclusions on the relative efficacy of tamoxifen and MPA have less support than those related to MA. Nevertheless, there is level II evidence that MPA and tamoxifen are equally effective in the treatment of advanced breast cancer in postmenopausal patients (grade B).

Several studies have addressed whether combined progestin and tamoxifen are more effective than tamoxifen alone in the palliation of advanced postmenopausal breast cancer. Four studies randomized a total of 408 patients to tamoxifen alone or to tamoxifen plus MPA.[84-87] There was no significant difference in response in three of them, but in one there was a trend toward increased objective response with the combination ($p = 0.02$).[85] Survival data are available for three of the studies ($n = 300$).[85-87] With 133 deaths, the Fossati review of the three found no survival difference (T + MPA versus T: HR 0.96; 95%CI 0.69–1.38).[26] Two studies compared tamoxifen with tamoxifen plus MA in 381 women.[73,88] There was no difference in objective response rate in either trial, but in both there was a trend toward better survival in the combination arm.[26,73,88] The overview analysis, after 300 deaths, found a survival benefit for tamoxifen plus MA, with an HR of 0.73 (95%CI 0.57–0.93).[26] It is unclear what the relative toxicities were in the two trials, but they may limit the use of the combination even if it is truly superior. The available data (level II) are not sufficient to support the use of combined tamoxifen plus progestin in the treatment of advanced postmenopausal breast cancer (grade C).

There are anecdotal reports of the response of advanced breast cancer to MPA in premenopausal women.[89,90] One study randomized 40 women to high-dose MPA or ovariectomy.[91] It found no difference in rate of tumor response (MPA 55% versus O 33%, $p = 0.17$) and overall survival.

Despite the limited data (levels II and III), there is evidence to support the activity of MPA in premenopausal advanced breast cancer (grade B).

Multiple studies have compared progestins with aromatase inhibitors as second hormonal therapy of advanced postmenopausal breast cancer.[92-98] They are reviewed in Chapter 15.

Three multi-institutional groups addressed the role of progestins as adjuvant therapy of early breast cancer. The Belgium Adjuvant Breast Project randomized 246 women with node-negative disease to no treatment after local therapy or 6 months of high-dose MPA.[99] Thirty-seven percent ($n = 91$) of the patients were under the age of 50 and 38% of all patients randomized were known to be ER-positive (22% ER-negative). With 13 years of follow-up, overall survival was not improved in women over the age of 50, but was marginally better in women aged under 50 ($p = 0.06$).[99] The small size of the study and the inclusion of receptor-negative patients make interpretation of the results problematic (level II).

The Belgian group also randomized 270 women with node-positive disease to CMF chemotherapy or CMF plus 6 months of high-dose MPA. Thirty-eight percent of the women were aged under 50, 47% were ER-positive and 21% ER-negative. In women aged under 50, survival was significantly worse with CMF plus MPA ($p = 0.01$) than with CMF alone. In older women, there was no difference in survival.[99] An Italian study randomized 151 premenopausal women with node-positive breast cancer to CMF or CMF plus 6 months of MPA.[100] With a short median follow-up (36 months), there was no difference in rates of recurrence, disease-free or overall survival between the two arms. In a second trial, 138 postmenopausal, node-positive, ER-positive or -negative women were randomized to MPA or no further therapy.[100] With a median follow-up of 37 months, there was a decrease in recurrences in the MPA group but no difference in survival.[100] The short follow-up and the inclusion of patients with ER-unknown or ER-negative tumors make interpretation of the trial difficult (level III). A Dutch group randomized 409 women aged under 71 with node-positive, ER-positive or -negative breast cancer to FAC (5-fluorouracil, doxorubicin, cyclophosphamide) chemotherapy or FAC plus 6 months of high-dose MPA.[101] With 218 deaths recorded, there was no difference in disease-free or overall survival (level III). The available evidence, although contradictory and not fully reported (level II/III), does not support the use of MPA by itself or in combination with chemotherapy as adjuvant therapy of early breast cancer (grade B).

REFERENCES

1. Beatson GT, On the treatment of inoperable cases of carcinoma of the mamma: Suggestion for a new method of treatment with illustrative cases. *Lancet* 1896; ii:104–7.

2. Lee YT, Therapeutic castration for advanced breast cancer. *Am J Surg* 1971; **122**:42–9.

3. Fracchia AA, Farrow JH, DePalo AJ et al, Castration for primary inoperable or recurrent breast carcinoma. *Surg Gynecol Obstet* 1969; **128**:1226–34.

4. Lees AW, Giuffre C, Burns PE, Jenkins HJ, Oophorectomy versus radiation ablation of ovarian function in patients with metastatic carcinoma of the breast. *Surg Gynecol Obstet* 1980; **151**:721–4.

5. Veronesi U, Pizzocaro G, Rossi A, Oophorectomy for advanced carcinoma of the breast. *Surg Gynecol Obstet* 1975; **141**:569–70.

6. Block GE, Lampe I, Vial B, Coller FA, Therapeutic castration for advanced mammary cancer. *Surgery* 1960; **47**:877–84.

7. Jensen EV, DeSombre ER, Jungblut PW, Estrogen receptors in hormone-responsive tissues and tumors. In: Wissler RW, Dao TL, Wood S Jr, eds. *Endogenous Factors Influencing Host–Tumor Balance.* Chicago: University of Chicago Press, 1967: 15–30.

8. Desombre ER, Carbone PP, Jensen EV et al, Special Report. Steroid receptors in breast cancer. *N Engl J Med* 1979; **301**:1011–12.

9. Howell A, Mackintosh J, Jones M et al, The definition of the 'no change' category in patients treated with endocrine therapy and chemotherapy for advanced carcinoma of the breast. *Eur J Cancer Clin Oncol* 1988; **24**:1567–72.

10. Robertson JFR, Willsher P, Cheung KL, Blamey RW, The clinical relevance of static disease (no change) category for 6 months on endocrine therapy in patients with breast cancer. *Breast Cancer Res Treat* 1996; **41**:288 (abst).

11. Martoni A, Longhi A, Canova N, Pannuti F, High-dose medroxyprogesterone acetate versus oophorectomy as first line therapy of advanced breast cancer in premenopausal women. *Oncology* 1991; **48**:1–6.

12. Buchanan BR, Blamey RW, Durrant KR et al, A randomized comparison of tamoxifen with surgical oophorectomy in premenopausal patients with advanced breast cancer. *J Clin Oncol* 1986; **4**:1326–30.

13. Boccardo F, Rubagotti A, Perrotta A et al, Ovarian ablation versus goserelin with or without tamoxifen in pre–perimenopausal patients with advanced breast cancer: Results of a multicentre Italian study. *Ann Oncol* 1994; **5**:337–42.

14. Ingle JN, Krook JE, Green SJ et al, Randomized trial of bilateral oophorectomy versus tamoxifen in premenopausal women with metastatic breast cancer. *J Clin Oncol* 1986; **4**:178–85.

15. Sawka CA, Pritchard KI, Shelley W et al, A randomized crossover trial of tamoxifen versus ovarian ablation for metastatic breast cancer: A report of the National Cancer Institute of Canada Clinical Trials Group (NCIC CTG) trial MA.1. *Breast Cancer Res Treat* 1997; **44**:211–15.

16. Taylor CW, Green S, Dalton WS et al, Multi-center randomized clinical trial of goserelin versus surgical ovariectomy in premenopausal patients with receptor-positive metastatic breast cancer: An Intergroup study. *J Clin Oncol* 1998; **16**:994–9.

17. deCourmelles F, La radiothérapie combinée du sein et des ovaires contre les tumeurs du sein. *C R Acad Sci [III]* 1922; **174**:503.

18. Early Breast Cancer Trialists' Collaborative Group, Ovarian ablation in early breast cancer: An overview of randomized trials. *Lancet* 1996; **348**:1189–96.

19. Davidson NE, Ovarian ablation as treatment for young women with breast cancer. *J Natl Cancer Inst Monogr* 1994; **16**:95–9.

20. Sunderland MC, Osborne CK, Tamoxifen in premenopausal patients with metastatic breast cancer: a review. *J Clin Oncol* 1991; **9**:1283–97.

21. Crump M, Sawka CA, DeBoer G et al, An individual patient-based meta-analysis of tamoxifen versus ovarian ablation as first line endocrine therapy for premenopausal women with metastatic breast cancer. *Breast Cancer Res Treat* 1997; **44**:201–10.

22. Hoogstraten B, Fletcher WS, Gad-el-Mawla N et al, Tamoxifen and oophorectomy in the treatment of recurrent breast cancer. *Cancer Res* 1982; **42**:4788–91.

23. Falkson G, Gelman RS, Tormey DC et al, Treatment of metastatic breast cancer in pre-menopausal women using CAF with or without oophorectomy: An Eastern Cooperative Oncology Group study. *J Clin Oncol* 1987; **5**:881–9.

24. Falkson G, Holcroft C, Gelman RS et al, Ten-year follow-up study of premenopausal women with metastatic breast cancer: An Eastern Cooperative Oncology Group study. *J Clin Oncol* 1995; **13**:1453–8.

25. Brunner KW, Sonntag RW, Alberto P et al, Combined chemo- and hormonal therapy in advanced breast cancer. *Cancer* 1977; **39**:2923–33.

26. Fossati R, Confalonieri C, Torri E et al, Cytotoxic and hormonal treatment for metastatic breast cancer: A systematic review of published randomized trials involving 31,510 women. *J Clin Oncol* 1998; **16**:3439–60.

27. Falkson G, Gelman RS, Leone L, Falkson CI, Survival of premenopausal women with metastatic breast cancer. Long term follow-up of Eastern Cooperative Group and Cancer and Leukemia B studies. *Cancer* 1990; **66**:1621–9.

28. Schinzinger A, Ueber carcinoma mammae. *Verh Dtsch Ges Chir* 1889; **18**:28–9.

29. Horsley JS, Bilateral oophorectomy with radical operation for cancer of the breast. *Surgery* 1944; **15**:590–601.

30. Nevinny HB, Nevinny D, Roscoff CB et al, Prophylactic oophorectomy in breast cancer therapy. *Am J Surg* 1969; **117**:531–6.

31. Early Breast Cancer Trialists' Collaborative Group, Polychemotherapy for early breast cancer: An overview of the randomized trials. *Lancet* 1998; **352**:930–42.

32. Scottish Cancer Trials Breast Group and ICRF Breast Unit, Adjuvant ovarian ablation versus CMF chemotherapy in premenopausal women with pathological stage II breast carcinoma: The Scottish trial. *Lancet* 1993; **341**:1293–8.

33. Engelsman E, Rubens RD, Klijn JGM, Comparison of the classical CMF with a three weekly intravenous CMF schedule in post-menopausal patients with advanced breast cancer: an EORTC study. In: *Proceedings of the 4th EORTC Breast Cancer Working Conference* 1987; **Vol 1**:1.

34. Goldhirsch A, Colleoni M, Coates AS et al, Adding adjuvant CMF chemotherapy to either radiography or tamoxifen: Are all CMFs alike? The International Breast Cancer Study Group (IBCSG). *Ann Oncol* 1998; **9**:489–93.

35. Williams MR, Walker KJ, Turkes A, Blamey RW, The use of an LH-RH agonist (ICI 118630, Zoladex) in advanced premenopausal breast cancer. *Br J Cancer* 1986; **53**:629–36.

36. Harvey HA, Lipton A, Max DT et al, Medical castration produced by the GnRH analogue leuprolide to treat metastatic breast cancer. *J Clin Oncol* 1985; **3**:1068–72.

37. Brambilla C, Escobedo A, Aertioli R et al, Medical castration with Zoladex; a conservative approach to premenopausal breast cancer. *Tumori* 1991; **77**:145–50.

38. Kaufmann M, Jonat W, Kleeberg U et al, Goserelin, a depot gonadotropin-releasing hormone agonist in the treatment of premenopausal patients with metastatic breast cancer. *J Clin Oncol* 1989; **7**:1113–19.

39. Dixon AR, Robertson JF, Jackson L et al, Goserelin (Zoladex) in premenopausal advanced breast cancer: Duration of response and survival. *Br J Cancer* 1990; **62**:868–70.

40. Eidne KA, Flanagan CA, Millar RP, Gonadotropin-releasing hormone binding sites in human breast carcinoma. *Science* 1985; **229**:989–91.

41. Miller WR, Scott WN, Morris R et al, Growth of human breast cancer cells inhibited by a luteinizing hormone-releasing hormone agonist. *Nature* 1985; **313**:231–3.

42. Saphner T, Troxel AB, Tormey DC et al, Phase II study of goserelin for patients with postmenopausal metastatic breast cancer. *J Clin Oncol* 1993; **11**:1529–35.

43. Boccardo F, Blamey RW, Klijn JGM et al, LHRH-agonist(LHRH-A) + tamoxifen (TAM) versus LHRH-A alone in premenopausal women with advanced breast cancer (ABC): results of a meta-analysis of four trials. *Proc Am Soc Clin Oncol* 1999; **18**:110a.

44. Klijn JGM, Seynaeve C, Beex L et al, Combined treatment with buserelin (LHRH-A) and tamoxifen vs single treatment with each drug alone in premenopausal metastatic breast cancer: preliminary results of EORTC Study 10881. *Proc Am Soc Clin Oncol* 1996; **15**:117.

45. Jonat W, Kaufmann M, Blamey RW et al, A randomized study to compare the effect of the luteinizing hormone releasing hormone (LHRH) analogue goserelin with or without tamoxifen in pre- and perimenopausal patients with advanced breast cancer. *Eur J Cancer* 1995; **31A**:137–42.

46. Boccardo F, Rubagotti A, Amoroso D et al, Italian Cancer Adjuvant Chemo-Hormone Therapy Cooperative Group Trials. GROCTA trials. *Rec Results Cancer Res* 1998; **152**:453–70.

47. Boccardo F, Rubagotti A, Amoroso D et al, CMF vs tamoxifen (TAM) plus ovarian suppression (OS) as adjuvant treatment of ER positive (ER+) pre–perimenopausal breast cancer. *Breast Cancer Res Treat* 1999; **57**:47 (abst).

48. Jakesz R, Gnant M, Hausmaninger H et al, Combination goserelin and tamoxifen is more effective than CMF in premenopausal patients with hormone responsive tumors in a multicenter trial of the Austrian Breast Cancer Study Group (ABCSG). *Breast Cancer Res Treat* 1999; **57**:25 (abst).

49. Jakesz R, Hausmaninger H, Samonigg H et al, Comparison of adjuvant therapy with tamoxifen and goserelin vs CMF in premenopausal stage I and II hormone-responsive breast cancer patients: Four-year results of Austrian Breast Cancer Study Group (ABCSG) trial 5. *Proc Am Soc Clin Oncol* 1999; **18**:67a.

50. Kaufmann M, Luteinizing hormone-releasing hormone analogues in early breast cancer: updated status of ongoing clinical trials. *Br J Cancer* 1998; **78**(Suppl 4):9–11.

51. von Minckwitz G, Conrad B, Diehl AC et al, Medical ovarian ablation versus polychemotherapy in premenopausal patients with node-negative, receptor positive breast cancer. The ongoing trial A-93 of the German Adjuvant Breast Cancer Study Group (GABG). *Proc Am Soc Clin Oncol* 1999; **18**:105a.

52. Untch M, Possinger K, Vasilijew L, The European table-study group: baseline and first safety data of an ongoing adjuvant study in premenopausal breast cancer comparing

leuprorelin acetate and CMF. *Breast Cancer Res Treat* 1998; **50**:285 (abst).

53. Rutqvist LE, Zoladex and tamoxifen as adjuvant therapy in premenopausal breast cancer: A randomized trial by the Cancer Research Campaign (CRC) Breast Cancers Trials Group, the Stockholm Breast Cancer Study Group, the South-East Sweden Breast Cancer Group & the Gruppo Interdisciplinare Valutazione Interventi in Oncologia (G.I.V.I.O.). *Proc Am Soc Clin Oncol* 1999; **18**:67a.

54. Baum M, Adjuvant treatment of premenopausal breast cancer with Zoladex and tamoxifen. *Breast Cancer Res Treat* 1999; **57**:30 (abst).

55. Davidson N, O'Neill A, Vukov A et al, Effect of chemohormonal therapy in premenopausal, node (+), receptor (+) breast cancer: An Eastern Cooperative Oncology Group phase III Intergroup Trial (E5188, INT-0101). *Proc Am Soc Clin Oncol* 1999; **18**:67a.

56. Stoll BA, Progestin therapy of breast cancer: comparison of agents. *BMJ* 1967; **3**:338–41.

57. Hackenberg R, Hofmann J, Wolff G et al, Down regulation of androgen receptor by progestins and interference with estrogenic or androgenic stimulation of mammary carcinoma cell growth. *J Cancer Res Clin Oncol* 1990; **116**:492–8.

58. Alexander IE, Shine J, Sutherland RI, Progestin regulation of estrogen receptor messenger RNA in human breast cancer cells. *Mol Endocrinol* 1990; **4**:821–8.

59. Goldfine ID, Papa V, Vignieri R et al, Progestin regulation of insulin and insulin-like growth factor receptors in cultured human breast cancer cells. *Breast Cancer Res Treat* 1992; **22**:69–79.

60. Horwitz KB, Wei LL, Sedlacek SM, D'Arville CN, Progestin action and progesterone receptor structure in human breast cancer: A review. *Recent Prog Hormone Res* 1985; **41**:249–316.

61. Murphy LJ, Sutherland RL, Stead B et al, Progestin regulation of epidermal growth factor receptor in human mammary carcinoma cells. *Cancer Res* 1986; **46**:728–34.

62. Pasqualini JR, Paris J, Sitruk-Ware R et al, Progestins and breast cancer. *J Steroid Biochem Mol Biol* 1998; **65**:225–35.

63. Musgrove EA, Swabrick A, Lee CS et al, Mechanism of cyclin-dependent kinase inactivation by progestins. *Mol Cell Biol* 1998; **18**:1812–25.

64. Kester HA, van der Leede BM, van der Burg B, Novel progesterone target genes identified by an improved differential display technique suggest that progestin-induced growth inhibition of breast cancer cells coincides with enhancement of differentiation. *J Biol Chem* 1997; **272**:16637–43.

65. Kandouz M, Lombet A, Perrot JY et al, Proapoptotic effects of antiestrogens, progestins and androgen in breast cancer cells. *J Steroid Biochem Mol Biol* 1999; **69**:463–71.

66. Loprinzi CL, Jensen MD, Jiang N, Schaid DJ, Effects of megesterol acetate on the human pituitary–adrenal axis. *Mayo Clin Proc* 1992; **67**:1160–2.

67. Lundgren S, Helle SI, Lønning PE, Profound suppression of plasma estrogens by megesterol acetate in postmenopausal breast cancer patients. *Clin Cancer Res* 1996; **2**:1515–21.

68. Ettinger DS, Allegra J, Bertino J et al, Megesterol acetate v tamoxifen in advanced breast cancer: Correlation of hormone receptors and response. *Semin Oncol* 1986; **13**(Suppl 4): 9–14.

69. Ingle JN, Ahman DL, Green SJ et al, Randomized clinical trial of megesterol acetate versus tamoxifen in paramenopausal or castrated women with advanced breast cancer. *Am J Clin Oncol* 1982; **5**:155–60.

70. Morgan LR, Megesterol acetate v tamoxifen in advanced breast cancer in postmenopausal patients. *Semin Oncol* 1985; **12**(Suppl 1): 43–7.

71. Muss HB, Wells B, Paschold EH et al, Megesterol acetate versus tamoxifen in advanced

breast cancer: 5 year analysis – A phase III trial of the Piedmont Oncology Association. *J Clin Oncol* 1988; **6**:1098–106.

72. Paterson AHG, Hanson J, Pritchard KI et al, Comparison of antiestrogens and progestagen therapy for initial treatment and consequences of their combination for second-line treatment of recurrent breast cancer. *Semin Oncol* 1990; **17**(Suppl 9):52–62.

73. Gill PG, Gebski V, Snyder R et al, Randomized comparison of the effects of tamoxifen, megesterol acetate or tamoxifen plus megesterol acetate on treatment response and survival in patients with metastatic breast cancer. *Ann Oncol* 1993; **4**:741–4.

74. Stuart NSA, Warwick J, Blackledge GRP et al, A randomized phase III cross-over study of tamoxifen versus megesterol acetate in advanced and recurrent breast cancer. *Eur J Cancer* 1996; **32A**:1888–92.

75. Silva A, Tonato M, Bono S, Medroxyprogesterone acetate versus tamoxifen in advanced breast cancer. *Cancer Chemother Pharmacol* 1985; **14**(Suppl):233 (abst).

76. van Veelen H, Willemse PHB, Tjabbes T et al, Oral high dose medroxyprogesterone acetate versus tamoxifen: A randomized crossover trial in postmenopausal patients with advanced breast cancer. *Cancer* 1986; **58**:7–13.

77. Pannuti F, Martoni A, Fruet F et al, Hormone therapy in advanced breast cancer: High dose medroxyprogesterone acetate vs tamoxifen. Preliminary results. *Eur J Cancer* 1980; (Suppl 1):93–8.

78. Muss H, Case D, Atkins JN et al, Tamoxifen versus high-dose oral medroxyprogesterone acetate as initial endocrine therapy for patients with metastatic breast cancer: A Piedmont Oncology Association study. *J Clin Oncol* 1994; **12**:1630–8.

79. Mattsson W, von Eyben P, Hallster L, A trial of tamoxifen versus high dose medroxyprogesterone acetate in advanced postmenopausal breast cancer. A final report. In: Cavalli F, ed. *International Symposium on Medroxyproges-*

terone Acetate. Amsterdam: Excerpta Medical, 1982: 276.

80. Lorenz I, Medroxyprogesterone acetate versus tamoxifen in the therapy of advanced breast cancer. *Neoplasma* 1985; **32**:119–24.

81. Beretta G, Clerici M, Tedeschi L, Tamoxifen versus oral medroxyprogesterone in advanced breast cancer: updated results. *Current Chemotherapy and Immunotherapy*: In: *Proceedings of 12th International Congress Chemotherapy, Florence, Italy, 1981*.

82. Castiglione-Gertsch M, Pampallona S, Varini M et al, Primary endocrine therapy for advanced breast cancer: To start with tamoxifen or with medroxyprogesterone acetate? *Ann Oncol* 1993; **4**:735–40.

83. Parazzini F, Colli E, Scatigna M, Tozzi L, Treatment with tamoxifen and progestins for metastatic breast cancer in postmenopausal women: A quantitive review of published randomized clinical trials. *Oncology* 1993; **50**:483–9.

84. Mouridsen HT, Ellemann K, Mattsson W et al, Therapeutic effect of tamoxifen versus tamoxifen combined with medroxyprogesterone acetate in advanced breast cancer in postmenopausal women. *Cancer Treat Rep* 1979; **63**:171–5.

85. Giralt E, Jouve M, Palangie T et al, Cancer du sein métastate: étude comparé de l'efficacité du tamoxifène et d'une administration séquentielle de tamoxifène et d'acétate de medroxyprogesterone. *Bulletin du Cancer* 1984; **71**:22–9.

86. Gunderson S, Kvinnsland S, Lundgren S et al, Cyclical use of tamoxifen and high-dose medroxyprogesterone acetate in advanced estrogen receptor positive breast cancer. *Breast Cancer Res Treat* 1990; **17**:45–50.

87. De Lena M, Tommasi S, Schittulli F et al, Sequential alternate administration of tamoxifen and medroxyprogesterone acetate in advanced breast cancer: Clinical–biological randomized trial. *Tumori* 1990; **76**:190–5.

88. Crawford DJ, George WD, Smith DC et al,

Cyclic sequential endocrine therapy for advanced breast cancer using a combination of tamoxifen and megesterol acetate. *Oncology* 1994; **51**(Suppl 1):13–18.

89. Gallagher CJ, Cairndruff F, Smith IE, High dose versus low dose medroxyprogesterone acetate: a randomized trial in advanced breast cancer. *Eur J Cancer Clin Oncol* 1987; **23**:1895–900.

90. Becher R, Miller AA, Hoffken K et al, High-dose medroxyprogesterone acetate in advanced breast cancer. Clinical and pharmacokinetic study with a combined oral and intramuscular regimen. *Cancer* 1989; **63**:1938–43.

91. Martoni A, Longhi A, Canova N, Pannuti F, High-dose medroxyprogesterone acetate versus oophorectomy as first therapy of advanced breast cancer in premenopausal women. *Oncology* 1991; **48**:1–6.

92. Dombernowski P, Smith I, Falkson G, Letrozole, a new oral aromatase inhibitor for advanced breast cancer: double randomized trial showing a dose effect and improved efficacy and tolerability compared with megesterol acetate. *J Clin Oncol* 1998; **16**:453–61.

93. Buzdar A, Jonat W, Howell A, Lee D, Significant improved survival with Arimidex® (anastrazole) versus megesterol acetate in postmenopausal advanced breast cancer: updated results of two randomized trials. *Proc Am Soc Clin Oncol* 1997; **16**:A545.

94. Buzdar AU, Smith R, Vogel C et al, Fadrazole HCL versus megesterol acetate treatment of postmenopausal patients with metastatic breast carcinoma: results of two randomized double blind controlled multiinstitutional trials. *Cancer* 1996; **77**:2503–13.

95. Canney PA, Priestman TJ, Griffiths T et al, Randomized trial comparing aminoglutethimide with high dose medroxyprogesterone acetate in therapy for breast carcinoma. *J Natl Cancer Inst* 1988; **80**:1147–51.

96. Lundgren S, Gundersen S, Klepp R et al, Megesterol acetate verus aminoglutethimide for metastatic breast cancer. *Breast Cancer Res Treat* 1989; **14**:202–6.

97. Kaufmann M, Bajetta E, Dirix LY et al, Survival advantage of exemestane over megesterol acetate in premenopausal women with advanced breast cancer refractory to tamoxifen: results of a randomized double-blind study. *Proc Am Soc Clin Oncol* 1999; **18**:109a.

98. Thurlimann B, Castiglione M, Hsu-Schmitz SE, Formestane versus megesterol acetate in postmenopausal breast cancer patients after failure of tamoxifen: A phase III prospective randomized cross-over trial of second line hormonal therapy. Swiss Group for Clinical Cancer Research. *Eur J Cancer* 1997; **33**:1017–24.

99. Focan C, Beaudin M, Salamon E, Adjuvant high dose medroxyprogesterone for early breast cancer: 13 years update of multicenter randomized trial. *Eur J Cancer* 1998; **34**(Suppl 1):102.

100. Pannuti F, Martoni A, Cilenti G et al, Adjuvant therapy for operable breast cancer with medroxyprogesterone acetate alone in postmenopausal patients or in combination with CMF in premenopausal patients. *Eur J Cancer Clin Oncol* 1988; **24**:423–9.

101. Hupperets P, Blijham G, Wils J et al, Adjuvant therapy with high dose medroxyprogesterone acetate if added to chemotherapy in patients with node-positive operable breast cancer. *Breast Cancer Res Treat* 1998; **50**:285 (abst).

SECTION 4: Biological Response Modifiers

Section Editor: DJ Slamon

17

HER2/*neu* and the clinical development of Herceptin[*]

Mark D Pegram, Gottfried E Konecny, Dennis J Slamon

INTRODUCTION

The HER2/*neu* protein is a member of the type I receptor tyrosine kinase (RTK) family. It is a 185 kDa surface membrane protein that is encoded by the HER2/*neu* gene (also known as the c-*erb*B-2 gene), which has been localized to chromosome 17q21.[1] This protein is expressed in a wide variety of tissues, including the breast, ovary, endometrium, lung, liver, gastrointestinal tract, kidney, and the central nervous system.[2,3] The normal physiological role of the HER2/*neu* protein in these tissues is not completely understood, but it is believed to play an important signaling role in cellular proliferation and differentiation processes. It forms heterooligomers with other members of the RTK family (such as HER1, HER3, and HER4) in response to specific ligands called neuregulins/heregulins.[4–6] Ligand activation of HER2/*neu* protein results in an increase in HER2/*neu* kinase activity, which in turn initiates signal transduction, resulting in cell proliferation or differentiation or both, depending on the experimental conditions.[7–12] In breast cancers, the HER2/*neu* gene is amplified in 25–30% of all cases such that, instead of having two copies of the gene per cell (one on each

chromosome 17), there may be as many as 50–100 gene copies per cell.[13–15] This gene amplification results in overexpression of HER2/*neu* at both the transcript and protein levels, such that there can be of the order of 2 000 000 HER2/*neu* molecules per cell in malignant tissues, instead of the usual 20 000–50 000 molecules per cell. This alteration is a result of a non-inherited event occurring sometime in the life of the patient. The mechanisms by which the amplification/overexpression occurs are completely unknown. When HER2/*neu* is overexpressed at these abnormally high levels, however, the kinase activity becomes constitutively activated, possibly due to autoactivation caused by crowding of adjacent HER2/*neu* receptor molecules within the cell membrane.[7] The net result is ligand-independent activation of HER2/*neu* protein, resulting in an increase in mitogenic cell signaling and increased cell proliferation. Consequently, this molecular alteration is associated with a poor clinical prognosis in early-stage breast cancer in terms of shortened time to relapse, as well as shortened overall survival.[13,14] Initially, this finding was controversial, with many published studies failing to demonstrate an association between HER2/*neu* gene amplification and clinical outcome; but, in retrospect, it is clear that

* A modified version of this chapter appears in Advances in Breast Cancer Management, eds WJ Gradishar, WC Wood (Kluwer, 2000).

most of these contradictory studies were statistically underpowered (small sample sizes), had too short a duration of clinical follow-up, or were doomed to failure from the start because the reagents used to detect HER2/*neu* overexpression (usually antibodies) were insensitive.[16] It is now clear from larger published cohorts, with long clinical follow-up (some as much as 30 years) and suitable reagents, that HER2/*neu* overexpression is an independent prognostic factor predicting poor clinical outcome (increasing the relative risk of relapse by a factor of two to three for both node-positive and node-negative breast cancers.[17,18]

A significant body of laboratory and clinical data demonstrates that HER2/*neu* overexpression, as a result of its effects on mitogenic cell signaling pathways, plays an important role in the pathophysiology of malignancies containing the alteration. Cells with HER2/*neu* overexpression have increased cell proliferation, increased anchorage-independent cell growth (a marker of transformation), increased tumorigenicity, and increased rate of metastasis compared with

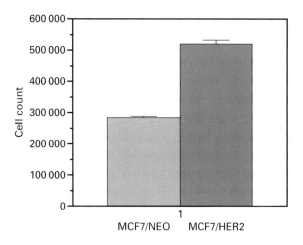

Figure 17.1
MCF7 breast carcinoma cells engineered to overexpress HER2/*neu* proliferate at nearly twice the rate of control (NEO) MCF7 cells: day 7 cell counts, seeding density 20 000/well; error bars indicate standard error.

control cells lacking HER2/*neu* overexpression (Figure 17.1). Since HER2/*neu* overexpression and co-ordinated increased kinase activity leads, at least in part, to the aggressive biological behavior of these tumors, it is an even more attractive target for therapeutic intervention by antibodies or other molecules that can oppose the effects of the HER2/*neu* kinase on cell signal transduction. The recombinant humanized monoclonal antibody Herceptin (trastuzumab) was approved by the US Food and Drug Administration (FDA) in September 1998 for the treatment of women with metastatic breast cancer.[19] The effects of Herceptin on downregulation of HER2/*neu* expression levels and/or its effects on HER2/*neu*-mediated signaling are likely to be critical to the clinical activity of this therapeutic antibody.

HER2/*neu* DETECTION IN CLINICAL TUMOR SPECIMENS

Clinicians are now faced with a challenge of accurate identification of patients with HER2/*neu* overexpression. Despite a number of marketing claims, detection of the HER2/*neu* alteration is not completely accurate using a number of the commercially available tests, including the FDA-approved HercepTest from DAKO. Many of these assays are suboptimal for detection of the HER2/*neu* alteration. A number of different approaches have been used to detect HER2/*neu* amplification at the DNA level (slot blot or Southern blot, fluorescence in situ hybridization (FISH), PCR-based techniques), at the transcript level (Northern analysis, RT-PCR), or at the protein level (Western blot, immunohistochemistry, ELISA). It is clear that all of the solid matrix blotting techniques suffer from potential dilutional artifacts resulting from admixture of normal stromal, inflammatory, and vascular cells in clinical tumor samples.[14,20] Techniques involving in situ detection are generally more sensitive in identifying gene amplification or protein over-expression. The most widely used technique for detection of HER2/*neu* overexpression at the protein level is immunohistochemistry. The problem with this technique is that multiple primary antibodies are currently in clinical use, each of which has differing sensitivity and speci-ficity, as well as different cutoff values to distin-guish overexpressing form non-overexpressing tumors.[16] It is therefore difficult to know whether a sample scored as HER2/*neu*-positive in one lab-oratory will be confirmed to be such by another laboratory. Another concern is that the degree of immunohistochemical staining for HER2/*neu* is subjective and qualitative. It is clear that forma-lin fixation of tumor samples and storage in paraffin results in epitope degradation, so that sensitivity is lost over time in archival clinical material.[14] To combat this problem, some assays resort to a technique called antigen retrieval, which consists of heating the tumor sample using a number of methods, including microwave radiation, water baths, ovens, etc., in order to 'retrieve' epitopes that have been lost during tissue fixation, embedding, and storage. This can create new problems in that normal tissues and non- HER2/*neu*-overexpressing malignancies, which all have physiologic levels of HER2/*neu* expression, can demonstrate enhancement of the signal from a small amount of HER2/*neu* protein, resulting in a false-positive interpretation of HER2/*neu* overexpression. Recent reports from the Mayo Clinic and from the University of North Carolina suggest a higher than expected false-positive rate using the FDA-approved HercepTest for detection of HER2/*neu* overexpression, and it is interesting to note that this assay also employs an antigen-retrieval step.[21,22] The ELISA assay to detect soluble HER2/*neu* protein in serum samples is not practical as a diagnostic assay for early-stage breast cancer, because soluble HER2/*neu* protein is only found in the serum of patients with both high disease burden and high-level HER2/*neu* overexpression, such as in cases of metastatic disease.[23] For patients with small primary tumors, this assay is almost always negative, even if the tumor overexpresses HER2/*neu* at the tissue level.

The most accurate technique currently avail-able for detection of HER2 gene alteration is DNA FISH.[18,20] In this assay, a fluorescent-labeled genomic DNA probe containing the HER2/*neu* gene and its flanking sequence is allowed to hybridize to tumor cell DNA within a standard paraffin-embedded tumor section mounted on a microscope slide. A second DNA probe, specific for chromosome 17 centromere and labeled with a different color than the HER2/*neu* probe, is used to distinguish true HER2/*neu* gene amplifi-cation from chromosome 17 ploidy. Using this technique, a quantitative copy number of HER2/*neu* genes per chromosome 17 centromere can be ascertained. One theoretical disadvantage of this assay is the inability to detect so-called 'single-copy overexpressors'. In such cases, the HER2/*neu* protein is overexpressed in the absence of HER2/*neu* amplification.[20] However, the frequency of single-copy HER2/*neu* overex-pression in breast cancers is estimated to be less than 5% of all overexpressing tumors. Moreover, these cases do not appear to have the poor prog-nosis of the amplified/overexpressors; therefore the advantages of FISH in terms of sensitivity and specificity far outweigh this disadvantage in terms of diagnostic accuracy.[20,24] The other potential problem with FISH methodology is its availability and cost. These problems will become inconsequential with the recent approval of FISH technology for HER2/*neu* analysis by the FDA. It is likely that cost will decrease with the increased economy of scale of HER2/*neu* testing using this technique.

Table 17.1   Association of HER2/*neu* overexpression with other clinicopathologic variables

- High S-phase fraction
- Aneuploidy
- Absence of ER/PgR expression[a]
- Presence of nodal metastasis
- High nuclear grade
- Short relapse-free interval
- Ductal (as opposed to lobular) histology

[a]ER, estrogen receptor; PgR, progesterone receptor.

It is critical to remember that HER2/*neu* overexpression correlates well with a number of other established prognostic factors and clinical parameters in breast cancer (Table 17.1). Therefore a clinician may be able to estimate the probability that a particular breast tumor will harbor HER2/*neu* overexpression based on these clinical parameters. If the results of a particular HER2/*neu* diagnostic assay are inconsistent with the clinical picture (particularly if an immunoassay was used for the HER2/*neu* analysis) then a different assay methodology should be used to retest the sample to confirm or refute the initial result. For example, a high-grade, lymph-node-positive, estrogen-receptor (ER)-negative tumor, with a high S-phase fraction and aneuploidy, is consistent with a HER2/*neu*-positive phenotype, especially if the patient relapses quickly. By contrast, a node-negative, diploid, ER-positive, well-differentiated breast carcinoma with low S phase is not likely to be HER2/*neu*-positive. Another important clinical observation is that HER2/*neu* overexpression is rarely seen in lobular carcinomas. Thus, despite the availability of sophisticated molecular diagnostic tools, good clinical judgment still applies.

DEVELOPMENT OF HERCEPTIN

Soon after the HER2/*neu* receptor subunit was shown to play a role in the pathogenesis of breast cancer, efforts were made to identify and characterize inhibitors of HER2/*neu* that would interrupt mitogenic signaling. To date, numerous agents have been identified that target HER2/*neu* such as tyrosine kinase inhibitors, inhibitors of various constituents of the Ras signaling pathway, neuregulin–toxin fusion proteins, single-chain antibodies, HER2/*neu* antisense molecules, small-molecule receptor antagonists, and monoclonal antibodies. Of these, one particular murine monoclonal antibody, 4D5, was found to have a significant and dose-dependent antiproliferative activity specifically against HER2/*neu*-overexpressing cancer cells, while having no effect on cells expressing physiologic levels of HER2/*neu*.[25] Murine monoclonal antibodies had been tested in clinical trials against numerous tumor targets in the past; however, most studies were negative. There were a number of reasons for this including the development of human anti-mouse antibodies (HAMA) that rapidly neutralized murine antibodies, rendering them useless as far as antitumor activity is concerned. New breakthroughs in biotechnology have allowed the possibility of overcoming this limiting clinical problem. Murine monoclonal antibodies may be now be 'humanized' by identifying the minimum set of amino acid residues in the complimentarity determining region (CDR) of the murine antibody required for antigen specificity and antigen-binding affinity, and substituting these regions into the CDRs of a consensus human IgG framework.[19] Maintaining both antigen specificity and binding affinity through this process is a painstaking exercise, but is essential in order to find a humanized variant with desired specifications. Ultimately, antibody humanization was achieved for 4D5, resulting in a recombinant humanized monoclonal antibody directed against HER2/*neu* (rhuMAb HER2/*neu*), now known as Herceptin (trastuzumab).[26] The specificity of 4D5 for HER2/*neu* was maintained, and the binding affinity ($K_d \approx 0.1$ nM) of the humanized variant was actually slightly improved over that of 4D5 ($K_d \approx 0.3$ nM).[26] In addition, Herceptin is based on an IgG1 consensus sequence, thus allowing for the possibility of antibody-mediated cellular cytotoxicity against tumor target cells by immune effector cells expressing Fc receptors.[27] Preclinical studies conducted in our laboratory at UCLA demonstrated that the antiproliferative effects of 4D5 and the dose-dependent antitumor efficacy against HER2/*neu* overexpressing xenografts in athymic mice were also maintained following antibody humanization.[28]

Based on the demonstration of preclinical efficacy, both the murine monoclonal and humanized versions were initially taken into humans in a series of single-dose and multidose phase I clinical trials conducted at UCLA in order to study tumor localization, toxicology, and pharmacokinetics of single-dose and multidose antibody administered intravenously to patients with HER2/*neu*-positive refractory metastatic breast cancer. The conclusions from these studies are summarized in Table 17.2. Herceptin has a favorable pharmacokinetic profile, achieving trough serum concentrations above the concentration needed for maximal antiproliferative effects in vitro, and also has a unique toxicological profile, with fevers during the first infusion and pain at sites of metastasis as the most commonly reported side-effects during phase I. For the most part, these symptoms were described as mild or moderate. Furthermore, there was no evidence of human anti-humanized antibodies against Herceptin. This was in contrast to a phase I trial conducted with murine 4D5 antibody, in which HAMA developed rapidly, as expected, in treated patients.

> ### Table 17.2   Conclusions from phase I clinical trials of Herceptin
>
> - Defined pharmacokinetics with a long serum half-life in high dose, achieving desired serum trough concentrations
> - Favorable toxicological profile (low-grade fevers)
> - No evidence of human anti-mouse antibodies (HAMA)
> - Demonstration of tumor localization with radio-iodinated 4D5

COMBINING HERCEPTIN WITH CYTOTOXIC CHEMOTHERAPY: RECEPTOR-ENHANCED CHEMOSENSITIVITY

By itself, Herceptin is not cytotoxic in vitro or in vivo, at least over short-term exposure. HER2/*neu*-positive cancer cells undergo cell cycle arrest with accumulation in the G_0/G_1 phase of the cell cycle on treatment with Herceptin, but there is no evidence of apoptosis or cytotoxicity (unless immune effector cells are introduced along with Herceptin), except occasionally after prolonged exposure.[27,29] One popular method of rendering antibodies cytotoxic envisioned by researchers in the anticancer antibody field was to covalently link cytotoxic drugs to therapeutic monoclonal antibodies. In one such effort, antibodies against epidermal growth factor receptor (EGFR, i.e. HER1) were coupled to cisplatin and tested against EGFR-expressing xenografts in vivo.[30] As controls for this experiment, the investigators also tested uncoupled, free anti-EGFR antibodies given concomitantly with free cisplatin. What resulted was surprising in that this combination had more antitumor activity than the covalently linked species and much more than either drug used alone. Because of the close homology between EGFR (HER1) and HER2/*neu*, we conducted a similar experiment in our laboratory and found the same result with the anti-HER2/*neu* antibody plus cisplatin.[29] Furthermore, we studied the nature of the interaction between anti-HER2/*neu* and cisplatin using a method to test for drug interactions, and we found the combination to be highly synergistic.[29] A mechanism of synergy in this case was a HER2/*neu* antibody-mediated attenuation of DNA repair activity, resulting in the accumulation of platinum–DNA adducts in the nucleus and concomitant enhanced cytotoxicity of cisplatin.[29] We have termed this effect receptor-enhanced chemosensitivity (REC) as it applies to both the HER1 and HER2/*neu* systems. We have now expanded our antibody/drug interaction studies to include combinations of Herceptin with antimetabolites, alkylating agents, taxanes, topoisomerase II inhibitors, vinca alkaloids, and anthracyclines. Of these, we have found the platinum analogs, docetaxel, vinorelbine, etoposide, thiotepa, and ionizing radiation to have synergistic cytotoxicity with Herceptin (Table 17.3).[31] One drug, 5-fluorouracil, is antagonistic with Herceptin. The mechanism of this antagonistic interaction remains unknown, but is the subject of ongoing investigation.

PHASE II HERCEPTIN CLINICAL TRIALS

Four phase II clinical trials of single-agent Herceptin or Herceptin in combination with cisplatin have been conducted. In a pilot phase II study of single-agent Herceptin for patients with HER2/*neu*-overexpressing breast cancer who failed prior chemotherapy for metastatic disease, an 11% response rate was observed.[32] In an expanded phase II study of Herceptin as a single agent for patients who had failed one or two prior chemotherapeutic regimens for metastatic

Table 17.3   Drug interactions with Herceptin

Drug	Interaction with Herceptin
Cisplatin/carboplatin	Synergistic
Docetaxel	Synergistic
Vinorelbine	Synergistic
Etoposide	Synergistic
Thiotepa	Synergistic
Ionizing radiation	Synergistic
Doxorubicin	Additive
Vinblastine	Additive
Paclitaxel	Additive
Methotrexate	Additive
5-Fluorouracil	Antagonistic

disease, a 14% response rate was noted.[33] More recently, results from single-agent Herceptin given as first-line therapy for HER2/*neu*-positive metastatic breast cancer were reported.[34] In this study, a higher response rate of about 25% was observed, suggesting that single-agent Herceptin may be more effective in patients less heavily pretreated with chemotherapy. In addition, this study randomized patients to two different dose levels of Herceptin. The first dose level was the standard 4 mg/kg loading dose followed by 2 mg/kg/week, and the second was double the standard dose (8 mg/kg load plus 4 mg/kg/week). No apparent difference in response rate was seen at the higher dose level, and the higher dose appeared to cause more frequent side-effects.[34] A significant contribution from all of these studies is a better understanding of the toxicology of Herceptin. For the most part, Herceptin is very well tolerated when administered as a single agent. Approximately 30–40% of patients experience fevers and/or chills during the initial

Table 17.4   Common side-effects of single-agent Herceptin (first infusion)

- Fever/chills
- Nausea/vomiting
- Pain at site of tumor
- Asthenia
- Diarrhea
- Headache

(4 mg/kg) loading dose.[26] These reactions, though sometimes dramatic because of the rigors, can usually be managed by administration of acetaminophen (paracetamol), diphenhydramine hydrochloride, or meperidine hydrochloride, and/or by slowing the rate of Herceptin infusion. Rarely, more serious reactions such as anaphylaxis have been observed. Other commonly reported side-effects of single-agent Herceptin are shown in Table 17.4

The first trial of the combination of Herceptin with chemotherapy in a clinical setting was performed at UCLA in 1992.[23] A unique feature of this phase II trial was that to gain entry into the study, all patients were required to have chemoresistant breast cancer as defined by objective evidence of disease progression *during* active chemotherapy treatment. The study population consisted of extensively pretreated advanced breast cancer patients with HER2/*neu* overexpression. Patients were treated with a loading dose of 250 mg intravenous Herceptin, followed by weekly doses of 100 mg intravenously for 9 weeks. Chemotherapy consisted of cisplatin (75 mg/m^2) on days 1, 29, and 57. Clinical response data in this study were confirmed by an independent, blinded, response evaluation committee. Objective partial clinical responses were seen in 24% of patients, and an additional 24% had either minor responses or disease stabiliza-

tion. This compares extremely favorably with both single-agent cisplatin (a reported response rate from five separate clinical trials of approximately 7%, 95% confidence limits 2–11%) and single-agent Herceptin (a response rate of about 12% in pretreated patients with metastatic disease).[23,32] In this study, the concomitant administration of cisplatin chemotherapy had no effect on Herceptin pharmacokinetics. This study was also the first comprehensive analysis of the relationship between Herceptin pharmacokinetics and serum levels of a soluble form of the HER2/*neu* protein. The extracellular domain of the HER2/*neu* protein can be cleaved from the surfaces of tumor cells, and can then be measured by a serum-based ELISA assay. There is a clear inverse relationship between serum-soluble HER2/*neu* protein and Herceptin trough concentration.[23] It has been suggested that soluble HER2/*neu* protein may be a marker of clinical response to Herceptin; however, our data demonstrate that a decrease in HER2/*neu* serum levels is not always associated with an objective clinical response. An increase in soluble HER2/*neu* protein was associated with disease progression in a majority of patients in the phase II program, suggesting that this may be a useful clinical marker to estimate probability of disease progression.[23] Pretreatment serum HER2/*neu* levels did not correlate with objective clinical response to Herceptin. Finally, a very important conclusion of this study was that Herceptin did not appear to increase the toxicity of cisplatin chemotherapy over that expected for cisplatin alone in this patient population. This is important, since renal epithelial cells are known to express HER2/*neu* protein at normal levels, and therefore were at risk of cisplatin-induced damage.

FIRST-LINE CHEMOTHERAPY PLUS HERCEPTIN FOR HER2/*neu*-OVEREXPRESSING METASTATIC BREAST CANCER

A large prospective randomized controlled trial of standard chemotherapy either alone or in combination with Herceptin has been completed.[35] The trial was conducted in 469 patients with HER2/*neu*-overexpressing metastatic breast cancer who had not previously been treated with chemotherapy for metastatic disease. Standard chemotherapy consisted of doxorubicin 60 mg/m^2 (or epirubicin 75 mg/m^2) plus cyclophosphamide 600 mg/m^2 intravenously every 21 days for anthracycline-naive patients (281 patients) or paclitaxel 175 mg/m^2 intravenously over 3 hours for those patients who had previously been treated with an anthracycline in the adjuvant setting (188 patients). A feature of the patient characteristics for this cohort was that the patients in the paclitaxel arm had worse prognostic features at diagnosis – as might be anticipated given their prior adjuvant treatment with an anthracycline. Patients on the paclitaxel arm were more likely to be premenopausal, have ER/PgR-negative tumors, more positive lymph nodes, and a higher incidence of prior radiation treatment, and about 20% had been treated with myeloablative chemotherapy followed by peripheral blood- or bone marrow derived hematopoietic stem cells. These patients also had a shorter time from diagnosis to relapse compared with patients treated on the doxorubicin/cyclophosphamide arm. Based on these pretreatment characteristics, one might expect that the response to treatment in the paclitaxel group would be lower than the response in the doxorubicin/cyclophosphamide-treated group in this study. However, even with this caveat, the response rate in the paclitaxel group was somewhat of a surprise in that the response rate for first-line single agent paclitaxel was only 15%, compared with 38% for the doxorubicin-containing arm. Patients randomized to receive Herceptin in combination with conventional chemotherapy had a higher overall response rate, a longer median response duration, a significantly longer time to disease progression, and an increased survival rate at two years.[35,36] With a median follow-up of 29 months, Herceptin combined with either chemotherapy regimen decreased the relative risk of death by 24% and increased the median survival from 20.3 months to 25.4 months.[36] This is particularly noteworthy given the fact that two-thirds of the women on the chemotherapy-alone arms subsequently received Herceptin, at the time of disease progression, on a companion study protocol following initial protocol treatment. It is also noteworthy that Herceptin, the first biologic agent to be approved by the FDA for breast cancer treatment, prolongs the survival of metastatic breast cancer patients.

Along with the clinical success of Herceptin came an unexpected toxicity: namely cardiac dysfunction, especially for those patients who received concomitant Herceptin and doxorubicin. The incidence of Herceptin-associated cardiotoxocity was also significantly increased in the paclitaxel/Herceptin-treated group.[35] The mechanism(s) of this unique toxicity is currently unknown. Expression of HER2/*neu* in adult myocardium was not previously well characterized, although it was presumed to be very low or absent on the basis of low-level HER2/*neu* transcript expression by PCR analysis, and undetectable levels of protein expression by immunohistochemistry. Two patients at UCLA who developed clinically symptomatic congestive heart failure had endomyocardial biopsy performed as part of their diagnostic evaluation. Both of these patients had pathological findings consistent with doxorubicin-associated myocardial cell damage by either ordinary light microscopy or electron microscopy (unpublished observation). Most of the patients with this syndrome had improvement in symptoms and/or an increase in left ventricular ejection fraction (LVEF) following treatment with ACE inhibitors, diuretics, or cardiac glycosides. Clearly, all patients receiving Herceptin should undergo baseline assessment of cardiac function and periodic monitoring of LV function, and if a significant decrease in LVEF is noted then the drug should probably be discontinued unless there is an eminent risk of dying from progressive cancer, which, in exceptional cases, may outweigh the risks of heart failure. The drug should be used cautiously or even avoided altogether in cases of known underlying serious cardiac illness – at least until the mechanism of cardiotoxicity is better defined, and/or until pretreatment risk factors for cardiotoxicity can be studied and understood more completely.

FUTURE CLINICAL DEVELOPMENT OF HERCEPTIN

At the time of this writing, there are a number of unknown questions regarding the potential clinical applications of Herceptin in cancer therapy. For example, the precise mechanism of action of Herceptin is still incompletely understood. Although inroads into this problem are being made, to date there is still no direct experimental evidence from clinical studies to confirm that Herceptin is a true immunotherapeutic. The optimum duration of Herceptin therapy is currently unknown. The clinical trials performed to date have been conducted with Herceptin treatment until the time of disease progression. Would a shorter duration of Herceptin be as efficacious? Or conversely, would continued Herceptin treatment beyond the time of progression in fact slow the rate of progression? Whether or

not Herceptin will have activity in other malignancies is not yet known, but many trials are either already underway or about to begin in ovarian cancer, non-small cell lung cancer, prostate cancer, colon cancer, gastric cancer, and many others. The preclinical studies would predict that Herceptin efficacy is likely to be restricted to amplified/overexpressing cancers. The initial clinical data seem to support this; however, the question is yet to be completely resolved. The integration of Herceptin with standard chemotherapy, hormonal therapy, and radiation therapy remains an active area of research. Clinical trials of a number of chemotherapy drug combinations with Herceptin are planned or underway.

The use of adjuvant Herceptin for HER2/*neu*-positive early-stage breast cancer is a very attractive treatment approach from both a theoretical and a practical point of view. As Herceptin is a therapeutic with a high molecular weight (approximately 150 kDa), penetration of the antibody into bulky tumor deposits is unfavourable owing to the high interstitial oncotic pressure and poor vascularization within metastatic solid tumors. Therefore, the efficacy of Herceptin would theoretically be maximal in a micrometastatic disease situation where intratumoral pharmacokinetic boundaries do not apply as much. Large-scale studies of adjuvant Herceptin for breast cancer are now beginning. These studies will require careful design in order to avoid the cardiotoxicity issues surrounding the use of Herceptin/Anthracycline administration. This is a difficult problem, given the fact that anthracyclines have now become a mainstay of adjuvant therapy and there is evidence that HER2/*neu*-positive patients may benefit most from anthracycline-based therapy.[37–39] Most of the adjuvant studies will use one year of adjuvant Herceptin, but the decision for this duration of Herceptin administration, though reasonable, is empiric. With the recognition of the cardiotoxicity potential, we have proposed a non-anthracycline adjuvant chemotherapy/Herceptin regimen consisting of a docetaxel/platinum combination, which will avoid anthracycline-associated cardiotoxicity issues in the adjuvant setting, where many women may be cured as a result of their initial surgery and radiation. More importantly, however, this approach will take advantage of the observed synergy between these agents. Whether or not Herceptin has activity in non-HER2/neu-overexpressing breast cancers is an issue that is being addressed in a number of ongoing clinical trials. Once again the scientific rationale for this approach is completely absent. The optimal dosing schedule and route of administration of Herceptin are continuing to be studied. Because Herceptin has a long serum half-life, it lends itself to less frequent administration, such as using twice the standard dose every other week. Also, formulations of Herceptin that may allow for subcutaneous administration of the drug are being pursued. Data from our laboratory at UCLA indicate that the efficacy of Herceptin is maintained when it is given subcutaneously in mouse models (unpublished observation). Very little is known about Herceptin resistance, but clearly such mechanisms must exist, since many breast cancer patients treated with the drug do not in fact have an objective clinical response. A better understanding of such mechanisms might allow for improved treatment approaches to HER2/neu-positive breast cancers.

Many clinical issues regarding HER2/neu amplification/overexpression remain unresolved. Its use as a prognostic factor, its use as a predictive marker for response to conventional breast cancer therapies, and its use as a target for future drug development provide a wealth of opportunities for future basic and clinical research. The fact that Herceptin prolongs the survival of patients with metastatic breast cancer is not only clinically significant for breast cancer therapy, but also the ultimate experimental proof from a scientific perspective that HER2/neu does play an important role in the pathophysiology of breast cancer – a fact that has long been disputed by investigators (a number of whom are now vocal proponents) who sharply criticized early laboratory investigations on HER2/neu biology, and who dismissed and/or rejected the concept of HER2/neu-targeted cancer therapeutics with monoclonal antibodies. The HER2/neu paradigm of targeted cancer therapy is now an important model for drug discovery and drug development in the biotechnology and pharmaceutical industries. Based on our experience with Herceptin, we believe that there will be other molecules that, like HER2/neu, will be targets for future novel cancer treatments. These new cancer therapeutic targets will require validation through careful scientific studies conducted in the laboratory, and through carefully designed clinical trials. Many physician/scientists in the field of oncology believe that the identification of new therapeutic targets will result in significant therapeutic benefits for future patients suffering not only from breast cancer but from many other human cancers.

REFERENCES

1. Shih C, Padhy L, Murray M et al, Transforming genes of carcinomas and neuroblastomas introduced into mouse fibroblasts. *Nature* 1981; **260**:261–4.
2. Coussens L, Yang-Feng TL, Liao YC et al, Tyrosine kinase receptor with extensive homology for EGF receptor shares chromosomal location with neu oncogene. *Science* 1985; **230**:1132–9.
3. King CR, Kraus MH, Aaronson SA, Amplification of a novel v-erb-B-2-related gene in human mammary carcinoma. *Science* 1985; **229**:974–6.

4. Carraway K, Cantley L, A neu acquaintance for erbB3 and erbB4: a role for receptor heterodimerization in growth signaling. *Cell* 1994; **78**:5–8.

5. Sliwkowski M, Schaefer G, Akita R et al, Coexpression of erbB2 and erbB3 proteins reconstitutes a high affinity receptor for heregulin. *J Biol Chem* 1994; **269**:15661–5.

6. Plowman G, Culouscou J-M, Whitney G et al, Ligand-specific activation of HER4/p180erB4, a fourth member of the epidermal growth factor receptor family. *Proc Natl Acad Sci USA* 1993; **90**:1746–50.

7. Reese DM, Slamon DJ, HER-2/neu signal transduction in human breast and ovarian cancer. *Stem Cells* 1997; **15**:1–8.

8. Wen D, Suggs SV, Karunagaran D et al, Structural and functional aspects of the multiplicity of neu differentiation factors. *Mol Cell Biol* 1994; **14**:1909–19.

9. Wen D, Peles E, Cupples R et al, Neu differentiation factor: a transmembrane glycoprotein containing and EGF domain and an immunoglobulin homology unit. *Cell* 1992; **69**:559–72.

10. Falls DL, Rosen KM, Corfas G et al, ARIA, a protein that stimulates acetylcholine receptor synthesis, is a member of the neu ligand family. *Cell* 1993; **72**:801.

11. Marchionni M, Goodearl A, Chen M et al, Glial growth factors are alternatively spliced erbB2 ligands expressed in the nervous system. *Nature* 1993; **362**:312.

12. Peles E, Ben-Levy R, Tzahor E et al, Cell-type specific interaction of neu differentiation factor (NDF/heregulin) with neu/HER-2 suggests complex ligand–receptor relationships. *EMBO J* 1993; **12**:961–71.

13. Slamon DJ, Clark GM, Wong SG et al, Human breast cancer: correlation of relapse and survival with amplification of the HER-2/neu oncogene. *Science* 1987; **235**:177–82.

14. Slamon DJ, Godolphin W, Jones LA et al, Studies of HER-2/neu proto-oncogene in human breast and ovarian cancer. *Science* 1989; **244**:707–12.

15. Seshadri R, Firgaira FA, Horsfall DJ et al, Clinical significance of HER-2/neu oncogene amplification in primary breast cancer. The South Australian Breast Cancer Study Group. *J Clin Oncol* 1993; **11**:1936–42.

16. Press MF, Hung G, Godolphin W et al, Sensitivity of HER-2/neu antibodies in archival tissue samples: potential source of error in immunohistochemical studies of oncogene expression. *Cancer Res* 1994; **54**:2771–7.

17. Toikkanen S, Helin H, Isola J, Joensuu H, Prognostic significance of HER-2 oncoprotein expression in breast cancer: a 30-year follow-up. *J Clin Oncol* 1992; **10**:1044–8.

18. Andrulis IL, Bull SB, Blackstein ME et al, for the Toronto Breast Cancer Study Group, neu/erbB-2 amplification identifies a poor-prognosis group of women with node-negative breast cancer. Toronto Breast Cancer Study Group. *J Clin Oncol* 1998; **16**:1340–9.

19. Carter P, Presta L, Gormon CM et al, Humanization of an anti-p185HER2 antibody for human cancer therapy. *Proc Natl Acad Sci USA* 1992; **89**:4285–9.

20. Pauletti G, Godolphin W, Press MF, Slamon DJ, Detection and quantitation of HER-2/neu gene amplification in human breast cancer archival material using fluorescence in situ hybridization. *Oncogene* 1996; **13**:63–72.

21. Roche PC, Ingle JN, Increased HER2 with U.S. FDA-approved antibody. *J Clin Oncol* 1999; **17**:434–5.

22. Maia D, Immunohistochemical assays for HER2 overexpression. *J Clin Oncol* 1999; **17**:434.

23. Pegram M, Lipton A, Hayes D et al, Phase II study of receptor-enhanced chemosensitivity using recombinant humanized anti-p185HER-2/neu monoclonal antibody plus cisplatin in patients with HER-2/neu overexpressing metastatic breast cancer refractory to chemotherapy treatment. *J Clin Oncol* 1998; **16**:2659–71.

24. Pegram MD, Pauletti G, Slamon DJ, HER-2/neu as a predictive marker of response

to breast cancer therapy. *Breast Cancer Res Treat* 1998; **52**:65–77.

25. Lewis GD, Figari I, Fendly B et al, Differential responses of human tumor cell lines to anti-p185[HER2] monoclonal antibodies. *Cancer Immunol Immunother* 1993; **37**:255–63.

26. Herceptin (trastuzumab) anti-HER2 monoclonal antibody. Product package insert. Genentech, Inc., South San Francisco, CA, September 1998.

27. Pegram MD, Baly D, Wirth C et al, Antibody dependent cell-mediated cytotoxicity in breast cancer patients in phase III clinical trials of a humanized anti-HER2 antibody. *Proc Am Assoc Cancer Res* 1997; **38**:602 (Abstract).

28. Pietras RJ, Pegram MD, Finn RS et al, Remission of human breast cancer xenografts on therapy with humanized monoclonal antibody to HER-2 receptor and DNA-reactive drugs. *Oncogene* 1998; **17**:2235–49.

29. Pietras RJ, Fendly BM, Chazin VR et al, Antibody to HER-2/neu receptor blocks DNA repair after cisplatin in human breast and ovarian cancer cells. *Oncogene* 1994; **9**:1829–38.

30. Aboud-Pirak E, Hurwitz E, Pirak ME et al, Efficacy of antibodies to epidermal growth factor receptor against KB carcinoma in vitro and in nude mice. *J Natl Cancer Inst* 1988; **80**:1605–11.

31. Pegram M, Hsu S, Lewis G et al, Inhibitory effects of combinations of HER-2/neu antibody and chemotherapeutic agents used for treatment of human breast cancers. *Oncogene* 1999; **18**:2241–51.

32. Baselga J, Tripathy D, Mendelsohn J et al, Phase II study of weekly intravenous recombinant humanized anti-p185HER2 monoclonal antibody in patients with HER2/neu-overexpressing metastatic breast cancer. *J Clin Oncol* 1996; **14**:737–44.

33. Cobleigh MA, Vogel CL, Tripathy D et al, Efficacy and safety of Herceptin (humanized anti-HER2 antibody) as a single agent in 222 women with HER2 overexpression who relapsed following chemotherapy for metastatic breast cancer. *Proc Am Soc Clin Oncol* 1998; **17**:376.

34. Vogel CL, Cobleigh MA, Tripathy D et al, Efficacy and safety of Herceptin (trastuzumab, humanized anti-HER2 antibody) as a single agent in first-line treatment of HER2 overexpressing metastatic breast cancer (HER2+/MBC). *Breast Cancer Res Treat* 1998; **50**:232a.

35. Slamon D, Leyland-Jones B, Shak S et al, Addition of Herceptin (humanized anti-HER-2 antibody) to first line chemotherapy for HER2 overexpressing metastatic breast cancer (HER2+MBC) markedly increases anticancer activity: a randomized, multinational controlled phase III trial. *Proc Am Soc Clin Oncol* 1998; **17**:377.

36. Norton L, Slamon D, Leyland-Jones B et al, Overall survival (OS) advantage to simultaneous chemotherapy (Crx) plus the humanized anti-HER2 monoclonal antibody Herceptin (H) in HER2-overexpressing (HER2+) metastatic breast cancer (MBC). *Proc Am Soc Clin Oncol* 1999; **18**:483.

37. Muss HB, Thor AD, Berry DA et al, c-erbB-2 expression and response to adjuvant therapy in women with node-positive early breast cancer. *N Engl J Med* 1994; **330**:1260–6.

38. Thor AD, Berry DA, Budman DR et al, erbB-2, p53, and efficacy of adjuvant therapy in lymph node-positive breast cancer. *J Natl Cancer Inst* 1998; **90**:1346–60.

39. Paik S, Bryant J, Parc C et al, erbB-2 and response to doxorubicin in patients with axillary lymph node-positive, hormone receptor-negative breast cancer. *J Natl Cancer Inst* 1998; **90**:1361–70.

18

Monitoring molecular outcomes of *E1A* gene therapy in breast and ovarian cancer

Naoto T Ueno, Gabriel N Hortobagyi, Mien-Chie Hung

ADENOVIRUS TYPE 5 *E1A* IS A TUMOR SUPPRESSOR GENE

Part of a 36-kilobase (kb) adenovirus genome, the *E1A* gene, encodes proline-rich nuclear-localized phosphoproteins that regulate the replication of adenovirus.[1] The primary function of *E1A* is to activate other adenoviral genes, to allow efficient replication of adenovirus.[1] Certain serotypes of E1A protein, such as adenovirus type 12, are strongly oncogenic and induce tumors at high frequency.[2] In contrast, adenovirus type 5 E1A protein and its close relative in terms of serotype, adenovirus type 2 E1A, are non-oncogenic.[3] As E1A proteins can transcriptionally transactivate proteins that can 'immortalize' transformed cells, *E1A* was considered an 'immortalization oncogene'.[4–6] The E1A proteins can stimulate transcription or repress the activity of certain viral and cellular transcriptional enhancers. In particular, we have found that *E1A* gene products inhibit HER2/*neu* overexpression in both rodent fibroblast and human cancer cells through transcriptional repression at the HER2/*neu* promoter.[7]

This finding prompted us to investigate whether *E1A* may function as a tumor suppressor in HER2/*neu*-overexpressing cancer cells by repressing HER2/*neu* overexpression. Initially, the *E1A* gene was introduced into genomic HER2/*neu*-transformed mouse fibroblasts. Indeed, *E1A* gene products suppressed the transformed phenotypes and inhibited the metastatic potential.[8,9] Interestingly, when HER2/*neu* was forcefully overexpressed in the former *E1A*-expressing HER2/*neu*-transformed mouse fibroblast, the tumorigenicity was restored, whereas metastatic tumor formation was still significantly inhibited by *E1A*.[10] We then examined whether *E1A* could reverse tumorigenicity in HER2/*neu*-overexpressing human ovarian cancer cells by transfecting the *E1A* gene into them. The *E1A*-expressing ovarian cancer cell lines expressed less HER2/*neu* protein, had fewer malignancies, and were less able to induce tumors in immunocompetent mice.[11]

Besides having tumor suppressive activity in HER2/*neu*-overexpressing tumors, *E1A* also appears to be associated with tumor-suppressive activities independent of HER2/*neu*, e.g. *E1A* repressed transcription of various proteases involved in tumor cell invasion and metastasis: type IV collagenase,[9,12] plasminogen activator,[13] stromelysin,[14,15] interstitial collagenase[12] and urokinase.[12] *E1A* also inhibited metastasis by elevating expression of the metastasis suppressor

$Nm23$ gene.[16–18] In another study, $E1A$ reduced anchorage-independent growth and tumorigenic growth of a variety of tumor cell lines, including human melanoma, fibrosarcoma,[19] A204 rhab-domyosarcoma, RD rhabdomyosarcoma, Saos-2 osteosarcoma, NCI-H23 non-small cell lung car-cinoma, MDA-MB-435s breast carcinoma, ras-transformed MDCK kidney epithelial cells[20] and murine melanoma.[21] $E1A$ has also been shown to induce apoptosis in different types of cells when $E1B$ is absent.[22–24] Further, $E1A$ increases the cytotoxic activity of tumor necrosis factor α (TNF-α) in $E1A$-transfected cells[25,26] and affects the susceptibility of target cells to TNF-α-independent cytolytic mechanisms by activated natural killer (NK) cells and macrophages.[27] $E1A$ also controls cell prolifera-tion by repressing the expression of growth factor-inducible gene.[15] In addition, it was recently found that $E1A$ could suppress at least one other tyrosine kinase besides HER2/neu, namely Axl, which is the prototype of a family of transmembrane receptors called UFO that include Sky and Eyk.[28]

Thus, previous findings clearly demonstrate that $E1A$ can function as a tumor suppressor gene by several different mechanisms: transcrip-tional repression of HER2/neu, inhibition of metastasis-related genes, activation of metastasis suppressor genes, induction of apoptosis, induc-tion of host immune responses, repression of growth factor-inducible genes and induction of differentiation (Table 18.1). The function of $E1A$ as a tumor suppressor may be dependent on the individual oncogenic backgrounds of cancer cells. Recently, it was reported that $E1A$ might induce the EWS–$FLI1$ rearrangement specific to Ewing's sarcoma;[29] however, we and other groups could not confirm this association between $E1A$ expression and oncogenicity of Ewing's sarcoma[30,31] (F Meric et al, unpublished observation). Indeed, when the $E1A$ was intro-

---

Table 18.1   Function of $E1A$ gene as tumor suppressor gene

Transcriptional repression of HER2/neu
Inhibition of metastasis-related genes
Activation of metastasis suppressor genes
Induction of apoptosis
Induction of host immune responses
Repression of growth factor-inducible genes
Induction of differentiation

---

duced into mouse fibroblasts, we did not detect any transforming phenotype.[9] Further, there is no epidemiologic evidence to suggest that aden-ovirus type 5 $E1A$ can cause tumors in human subjects. Therefore, for the time being, $E1A$ should not be considered an oncogene but a tumor suppressor gene.

PRECLINICAL ANIMAL DATA FOR $E1A$ GENE THERAPY IN HUMAN BREAST AND OVARIAN CANCER

Human gene delivery systems can largely be divided into viral and non-viral. Although viral delivery of DNA plasmids is efficient, there are disadvantages – retroviral vectors cannot trans-fect non-dividing cells and adenoviral vectors can be strongly immunogenic.[32] On the other hand, non-viral delivery systems may allow repetitive DNA transfection with minimum toxicity and immunogenicity; however, their transfection effi-ciency is limited when compared with that of viral vectors.[33] One of the best-known non-viral delivery systems is the cationic liposome. The first cationic liposome was developed for in vitro gene transfer in the late 1980s by Felgner et al.[34] The system is designed so that, even though the positive charge of the liposome interacts with the negative charge of the DNA, the overall charge remains positive even after the DNA–cationic liposome complex is formed. This, in turn, promotes the complex's interaction with the negatively charged cell membrane and transfection of the target cells.

The DC-Chol cationic liposome, which was developed by Leaf et al at the University of Pittsburgh, can facilitate gene delivery into mammalian cells both in vitro and in vivo, without major toxicities. It is also known for its biodegradable, non-mutagenic and non-immunogenic properties.[35–39] These properties were considered to be an advantage for allowing multiple repetitive injections of a therapeutic gene, and therefore led us to explore DC-Chol as the gene delivery system in a preclinical phase I trial of *E1A* gene therapy.

The potential of *E1A* as a therapeutic agent for human cancers was investigated in preclinical models of ovarian and breast cancer. First, a human breast cancer xenograft model was established by injecting human HER2/*neu*-overexpressing breast cells (MDA-MB-361) into the mammary fat pads of nude mice. After tumor formation was confirmed, *E1A* genes complexed with DC-Chol cationic liposomes (*E1A*/DC-Chol complex) were injected intratumorally.[40] As a result, the growth of HER2/*neu*-overexpressing breast cancer cells was inhibited. Similar results were observed in a human ovarian cancer xenograft model. In brief, human HER2/*neu*-overexpressing ovarian cancer cells (SKOV-3) were injected intraperitoneally into mice. Then, the *E1A*/DC-Chol complex was delivered into the peritoneal cavity of the tumor-bearing mice. Thus, the growth and dissemination of HER2/*neu*-overexpressing ovarian cancer cells were inhibited. About 70% of the mice survived at least 1 year, whereas all untreated controls developed severe tumor symptoms and died within 160 days.

PRECLINICAL STUDIES OF *E1A* GENE TOXICITY

Before moving into a phase I trial, we evaluated the toxicity (safety profile) of the *E1A*/DC-Chol complex by injecting it intraperitoneally into normal mice. In the short term, the cumulative dose, which was up to 40 times that proposed for use in the phase I trial, had no adverse effects on renal, hepatic or hematologic function in nude mice. No major pathologic changes were observed in any organs. Further, analysis was performed to demonstrate whether the *E1A* was still residing in normal cells after the *E1A*-treated mice had survived for a certain time. Nine months after treatment with the complex was discontinued, the mice were analyzed for the effect of treatment on major organs, including the genitals (uterus, fallopian tube and ovary), liver, lung, heart, kidney, spleen and brain. There was no macroscopic or microscopic effect. However, at 18 months after the last injection of *E1A*, *E1A* DNA was still detected in the lungs and kidneys but not in the liver, heart spleen, brain, uterus or ovary. Therefore, we concluded that the DC-Chol cationic liposome gene delivery system might allow repetitive injection of the *E1A*/DC-Chol complex into our patients without inducing any major toxicity; nevertheless, long-term follow-up is needed to determine the ultimate effect of *E1A*.[38,39] On the basis of our results, an Investigational New Drug (IND) application was filed with the US Food and Drug Administration (FDA) and approved. In 1996, a phase I trial of *E1A* gene therapy for breast and ovarian cancer was opened at the MD Anderson Cancer Center (Figure 18.1).

PHASE I TRIAL OF *E1A* GENE THERAPY IN HER2/*neu*-OVEREXPRESSING BREAST AND OVARIAN CANCER

This phase I clinical trial entitled 'Phase I study of *E1A* gene therapy for patients with metastatic

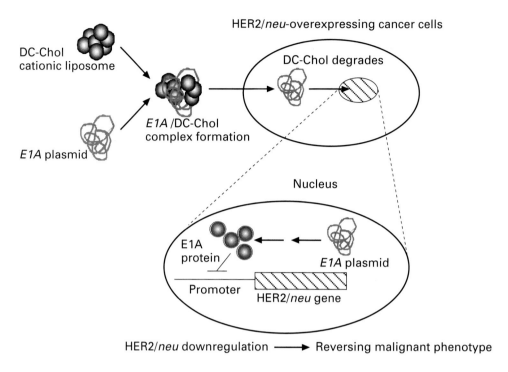

Figure 18.1
Phase I trial of *E1A* gene therapy for breast and ovarian cancer.

breast or ovarian cancer that overexpresses HER2/*neu*', was originally designed in 1995 and initiated at the MD Anderson Cancer Center in 1996.[41] At first, only patients with breast or ovarian tumors overexpressing HER2/*neu* were eligible; later, patients with tumors expressing low levels of HER2/*neu* became eligible. A tumor was considered positive for HER2/*neu* overexpression if more than 10% of tumor cells had an HER2/*neu* signal intensity stronger than 1+.[42] In the trial, each patient received a weekly injection of the *E1A*/DC-Chol cationic liposome complex through a Tenchkoff catheter placed in either the pleural cavity (in breast cancer patients) or the peritoneal cavity (in ovarian cancer patients). After three consecutive weekly injections, patients were given a week off (one cycle). The starting dose of the *E1A*/DC-Chol complex was

1.8 mg/m² (this dose was derived from the effective dose established in the preclinical animal studies).[37,40] The *E1A* dose was given at one of three doses: 1.8, 3.6 or 7.2 mg/m²/injection.

Several different outcomes can be monitored during a trial of cancer gene therapy: adverse event (toxicity), clinical outcome, molecular outcome and pharmacologic outcome (Table 18.2). The monitoring of outcome depends on the final objective of the study as well as on the technology available for monitoring the outcome (particularly in studies of molecular effect and pharmacology). The objective of our phase I trial was to determine the maximum tolerated dose (MTD) and maximum biological active dose (MBAD) of *E1A* plasmid (mg/m²) (Table 18.2). Our goal was to demonstrate the feasibility of delivering *E1A*/DC-Chol complexes into a

Table 18.2   Endpoints for gene therapy

	Endpoints	Methodology
Adverse event	MTD	NCI common toxicity criteria
Molecular effect	MBAD	See Table 18.3
Clinical effect	Tumor response rate	Restaging of disease by
	Overall survival	physical examination,
	Progression-free survival	radiographic and biochemical
		studies
Pharmacology	Drug level	Pharmacodynamic
		Pharmacokinetic

MTD, maximum tolerated dose; MBAD, maximum biological active dose.

patient's thoracic or peritoneal cavity, transducing *E1A* into tumor cells, and thus downregulating HER2/*neu* overexpression in the tumor. As no toxicity was detected during the preclinical toxicity study, the dose of *E1A* plasmid was escalated at 100% increments instead of by the Fibonacci method. Adverse event was monitored weekly and graded using the common toxicity criteria of the National Cancer Institute (NCI). As certain toxicities may not be easily distinguished from toxicities related to disease progression or toxicities not related to the regimen, all adverse events were recorded. These events were further graded on a scale of 1–5 to help determine whether there was a true cause-and-effect relationship between treatment and adverse event.

MONITORING *E1A* GENE EXPRESSION

Monitoring the expression level of a therapeutic gene in both targeted and non-targeted cells is very critical for cancer gene therapy. It can be done at three levels: at actual delivery of the plasmid DNA into the cells (transfection), at mRNA synthesis from DNA (transcription) and at protein synthesis from mRNA (translation). Each of these levels has different assays for monitoring this expression (Table 18.3). When designing a clinical trial, selecting the optimal assays is critical for several reasons. First, the assays can be expensive and time-consuming to perform. Second, the choice of assay is often affected by the type, source and volume of tumor tissue that can be collected from particular patients. In our phase I trial, we chose to use immunohistochemical staining, a useful method for determining the distribution of *E1A* gene expression in tissue, and reverse transcriptase polymerase chain reaction (RT-PCR), a highly sensitive method for detecting *E1A*. Western blotting was not feasible because of the large amounts of *E1A*-transfected tumor cells that would be needed.

In terms of collecting the tumor samples, we designed the study so that we could collect tumor tissue specimens in a serial time course. To achieve this goal, we initially limited the

Table 18.3   Monitoring gene expression

DNA	RNA	Proteins
Southern blotting	Northern blotting	Immunohistochemical staining
PCR	RT-PCR	Western blotting
FISH		

PCR, polymerase chain reaction; RT, reverse transcriptase; FISH, fluorescence in situ hybridization.

study to those patients who had either ascites or pleural effusions. This allowed us to collect intra-cavitary fluids, which are likely to contain tumor cells. By inserting a Tenchkoff catheter (chronic indwelling catheter), we could readily obtain the fluid on a weekly basis and, in this way, put our patients at less risk when accessing the tumor so frequently. Further, we also considered that this might allow us to determine the most optimal timing for analysis of maximum transfection and protein synthesis after injection the E1A/DC-Chol complex. Therefore, for this purpose, we collected specimens before the first injection of E1A/DC-Chol complex and then 3 days and 7 days later.

Before starting the study, we considered the following issues related to gene expression: efficiency, distribution and duration (Table 18.4). With regards to efficiency, the methodology for accurately determining the transfection efficiency of therapeutic genes in both tumor and non-tumor cells in human subjects has not yet been established. In preclinical models, one commonly describes DNA transfection efficiency or protein expression efficiency in terms of the percentage of positive gene or protein expression among the entire cell population transfected with the DNA. For intraperitoneal or intrapleural therapy, the transfection of E1A/DC-Chol complex into

human cells is probably limited to those cells that are physically exposed at the surface. Therefore, monitoring the gene expression efficiency in such trials cannot be determined easily. Indeed, similar findings have been reported for intratumoral gene therapy trials: when gene expression was examined, its gene expression was strongest next to the needle insertion site into the tumor.

As for the issue of distribution of therapeutic genes, even in a study using local injection, one needs to examine the gene distribution in all organ sites. We have attempted to do this in our current trial of E1A/DC-Chol by collecting normal organ tissue at the autopsy of study participants. This is particularly important because the cationic liposome is known for its capacity for systemic gene distribution when injected systemically.

With regard to the issue of duration, the stability of the gene expression can be an advantage or disadvantage for cancer gene therapy. Expression of genes delivered by cationic liposome is transient in cells, and the DNA plasmid will be degraded thereafter. However, we do not know how long the gene may be expressed in cells, nor do we know the efficiency of the integration of the transgene into the host chromosomes. This can be a critical safety concern in

Table 18.4   Issues involved in gene expression

Efficiency	Percentage of gene expression in the target tissue: low versus high
	Distribution of gene expression in a cell: central versus periphery
	How to determine the gene expression efficiency?
Distribution	*E1A* expression at the injection site (local) versus distant organ sites (systemic)
	E1A expression in tumor cells versus non-tumor cells
Duration	Transient expression: how long?
	Stable expression: does it integrate into host DNA?

Table 18.5   Monitoring physiological effect of gene expression

Biological endpoints	Assay	Phase I trial of *E1A* gene therapy
HER2/*neu*	ICH (quality)	Yes
	Imaging analysis (quantitative)	Yes
	Western blotting	No
Apoptosis	DNA fragmentation	No
	TUNEL assay	Yes
Proliferation index	FACS	Yes
	Ki67	No
Immunological approach	Cytokine level	Yes
	Lysis of autologous tumor cells transfected with *E1A*	No

ICH, immunohistochemical staining; FACS, fluorescence-activated cell sorting; TUNEL, terminal transferase UTP nick end labeling.

gene therapy. The integrated DNA can result in a chronic adverse event to normal host cells and can even be passed on to the next generation of cancer cells in fertility organs such as the ovaries.

MONITORING BIOLOGIC EFFECT OF *E1A* GENE (TABLE 18.5)

In our phase I trial, MBAD was defined as the dose of *E1A* plasmid (mg/m^2) that would have the expected biologic effect on the cancer cells (i.e. a more than 25% downregulation of HER2/*neu* expression) after *E1A*/DC-Chol complex-mediated gene delivery. HER2/*neu* downregulation by *E1A* was selected as the biologic end-point because it was the most established one at the time we designed the clinical trial.

In cancer gene therapy trials, the threshold for triggering the molecular effect of a therapeutic gene is generally not known. Yet we expect the MBAD we chose to become a pivotal dosage for our future phase II trial if the molecular effects (HER2/*neu* downregulation) triggered by the therapeutic gene (*E1A*) turn out to be the dominant mechanism of antitumor activity. For example, *E1A* may downregulate HER2/*neu* at dose A but, to induce rapid apoptosis, it may have to be given at one dose level higher or lower. Alternatively, low *E1A* gene expression may induce strong antitumor activity by triggering a bystander effect, which may be dependent on a therapeutic gene or a cancer genetic abnormality. Therefore, the MBAD dosage defined in our phase I trial may not actually turn out to be the effective dosage for a future phase II trial, depending on the biologic endpoints selected to monitor for MBAD. In planning gene therapy trials, one should always select the molecular endpoints that can be measured in the most objective manner, and be mindful that careful prospective clinical and molecular data analysis will be needed in defining the final dosage deployed in any pivotal phase II trial.

To assess HER2/*neu* downregulation, our plan was to use anti-HER2/*neu* antibody to stain immunohistochemically tumors collected from either ascites or pleural fluid of patients before and after *E1A* gene therapy. However, our main concern was whether HER2/*neu* downregulation could truly be quantified by simply reading for immunohistochemical staining when a heterogeneous collection of tumor cells might be present. Therefore, before starting the trial, we evaluated whether the SAMBA 4000 cell image analysis system could be used to obtain a quantitative mean optical density (MOD) and labeling index of HER2/*neu*. To assess the accuracy of the machine-read MOD, HER2/*neu*-overexpressing cancer cells (SK-OV-3 ip1) and low HER2/*neu*-expressing cells (MDA-MB-435) were mixed at different ratios and paraffinized into blocks for immunohistochemical staining with anti-HER2/*neu* antibody. Serial dilution of these tumor cells showed a decreased labeling index that reflected the ratio of cells with positive anti-HER2/*neu* antibody staining to all cells. The MOD remained at a level that reflected the machine reading of the intensity of anti-HER2/*neu* antibody signal strength. In addition, the MOD we obtained correlated with the standard four-grade system used by our team's pathologist when measuring the HER2/*neu* expression level in primary squamous cell carcinoma in a human mouth.[42] These results indicated that downregulation of HER2/*neu* could be objectively quantitated.

Further, we recognize that the possible therapeutic mechanisms suggested by preclinical experiments may not always match the real clinical anti-tumor mechanism. As described in the previous section, *E1A* can reverse the malignant phenotype by triggering the host immune system, inducing apoptosis and tumor lysis, and suppressing metastatic capability.[43] Therefore, even if anti-tumor activity can be detected in treated patients, it is possible that other activities associated with *E1A*/DC-Chol complexes will contribute to the anti-tumor activities in addition to downregulation of HER2/*neu*. Indeed, we collected multiple samples (tumor, intracavitary fluid and serum) in the phase I trial and later studied them for apoptosis and Ki67 expression (as a proliferation index), because *E1A* is known to induce apoptosis and suppress proliferation of certain cells. We also examined the cytokine levels such as TNF-α and interferon-γ in the cavitary fluid because *E1A* is known to sensitize cells to TNF-α. However, a retrospective analysis of the samples had its limitations, possibly as a result of not collecting the samples under optimal conditions or at appropriate times. Therefore, correlation generated from the study does not confirm the molecular mechanism of the *E1A*, although it has a greater tendency to generate new hypotheses to test in future trials.

PRELIMINARY OUTCOME OF PHASE I TRIAL OF *E1A* GENE THERAPY AND FINAL THOUGHTS

In our phase I trial of *E1A* gene therapy, the median number of injections of *E1A*/DC-Chol complex given was 6 (1–8); the most common adverse event was development of fever 2–3 days after each injection regardless of dose levels. A dose of $7.2 \, \text{mg/m}^2$ produced grade 3–4 nausea/vomiting or pain, which led to a reduction in the dose to $3.6 \, \text{mg/m}^2$. Three patients had catheter-related infections requiring discontinuation of the treatment. There were no drug-related fatalities. Several patients experienced stable disease with a transient decrease in their tumor marker levels (CA-125, carcinoembryonic antigen (CEA)). Immunohistochemical staining for HER2/*neu* expression in six patients showed downregulation of HER2/*neu* in all six. RT-PCR in one patient detected *E1A* expression in multiple organs (lungs, tumor, liver, kidneys), but not in the brain or ovaries. In addition, *E1A* expression, as detected by immunohistochemical staining, and induction of apoptosis were confirmed after *E1A*/DC-Chol complex treatment. Thus, we concluded that *E1A* delivery is feasible and that *E1A* expression can be detected in cancer cells.

CONCLUSION

In conclusion, the preliminary data from our phase I trial have actually given us more new hypotheses to test in both preclinical and clinical experiments. This generation of new hypotheses is important because it will keep the study of cancer gene therapy moving back and forth between the clinic and the laboratory. To improve the efficacy and safety of cancer gene therapy, the molecular effects that can trigger anti-tumor activity or side effects need to be investigated in a prospective manner. Simply performing a clinical trial will not help us in the future, especially as the field of cancer gene therapy is rapidly evolving in terms of both technology and gene delivery. Thus, flexibility in assessing samples during the trial will be very important for designing a clinical trial. The preliminary results of phase I trials of tumor suppression activities associated with *E1A* have already gone some way toward establishing this flexibility by laying a scientific background for the design of future phase II clinical trials of *E1A* as an anticancer agent.

REFERENCES

1. Berk AJ, Adenovirus promoters and E1A transactivation. *Annu Rev Genet* 1986; **20**:45–79.
2. Berk AJ, Functions of adenovirus E1A. *Cancer Surv* 1986; **5**:367–87.
3. Schrier PI, Bernards R, Vaessen RT, Houweling A, van der Eb AJ, Expression of class I major histocompatibility antigens switched off by highly oncogenic adenovirus 12 in transformed rat cells. *Nature* 1983; **305**:771–5.
4. Ruley HE, Adenovirus early region 1A enables viral and cellular transforming genes to transform primary cells in culture. *Nature* 1983; **304**:602–6.
5. Byrd PJ, Grand RJ, Gallimore PH, Differential transformation of primary human embryo retinal cells by adenovirus E1 regions and combinations of E1A + Ras. *Oncogene* 1988; **2**:477–84.
6. Montell C, Courtois G, Eng C, Berk A, Complete transformation by adenovirus 2 requires both E1A proteins. *Cell* 1984; **36**:951–61.
7. Yu D, Suen TC, Yan DH, Chang LS, Hung MC, Transcriptional repression of the neu protooncogene by the adenovirus 5 E1A gene products. *Proc Natl Acad Sci USA* 1990; **87**:4499–503.
8. Yu DH, Scorsone K, Hung MC, Adenovirus type 5 E1A gene products act as trans-

formation suppressors of the neu oncogene. *Mol Cell Biol* 1991; **11**:1745–50.

9. Yu D, Hamada J, Zhang H, Nicolson GL, Hung MC, Mechanisms of c-erbB2/neu oncogene-induced metastasis and repression of metastatic properties by adenovirus 5 E1A gene products. *Oncogene* 1992; 7:2263–70.

10. Yu D, Shi D, Scanlon M, Hung MC, Reexpression of neu-encoded oncoprotein counteracts the tumor-suppressing but not the metastasis-suppressing function of E1A. *Cancer Res* 1993; 53:5784–90.

11. Yu D, Wolf JK, Scanlon M, Price JE, Hung MC, Enhanced c-erbB-2/neu expression in human ovarian cancer cells correlates with more severe malignancy that can be suppressed by E1A. *Cancer Res* 1993; 53:891–8.

12. Frisch SM, Reich R, Collier IE, Genrich LT, Martin G, Goldberg GI, Adenovirus E1A represses protease gene expression and inhibits metastasis of human tumor cells. *Oncogene* 1990; 5:75–83.

13. Young KS, Weigel R, Hiebert S, Nevins JR, Adenovirus E1A-mediated negative control of genes activated during F9 differentiation. *Mol Cell Biol* 1989; 9:3109–13.

14. Timmers HT, van Dam H, Pronk GJ, Bos JL, Van der Eb AJ, Adenovirus E1A represses transcription of the cellular JE gene. *J Virol* 1989; 63:1470–3.

15. van Dam H, Offringa R, Smits AM, Bos JL, Jones NC, van d.E A, The repression of the growth factor-inducible genes JE, c-myc and stromelysin by adenovirus E1A is mediated by conserved region 1. *Oncogene* 1989; 4:1207–12.

16. Pozzatti R, McCormick M, Thompson MA, Khoury G, The *E1A* gene of adenovirus type 2 reduces the metastatic potential of ras-transformed rat embryo cells. *Mol Cell Biol* 1988; 8:2984–8.

17. Steeg PS, Bevilacqua G, Pozzatti R, Liotta LA, Sobel ME, Altered expression of NM23, a gene associated with low tumor metastatic potential, during adenovirus 2 E1A inhibition of

18. Rosengard AM, Krutzsch HC, Shearn A et al, Reduced Nm23/Awd protein in tumour metastasis and aberrant Drosophila development. *Nature* 1989; **342**:177–80.

19. Frisch SM, Antioncogenic effect of adenovirus E1A in human tumor cells. *Proc Natl Acad Sci USA* 1991; **88**:9077–81.

20. Frisch SM and Dolter KE, Adenovirus E1A-mediated tumor suppression by a c-erbB-2/neu-independent mechanism. *Cancer Res* 1995; **55**:5551–5.

21. Deng J, Xia W, Hung MC, Adenovirus 5 E1A-mediated tumor suppression associated with E1A-mediated apoptosis in vivo. *Oncogene* 1998; **17**:2167–75.

22. Rao L, Debbas M, Sabbatini P, Hockenbery D, Korsmeyer S, White E, The adenovirus E1A proteins induce apoptosis, which is inhibited by the E1B 19-kDa and Bcl-2 proteins. *Proc Natl Acad Sci USA* 1992; **89**:7742–6.

23. Lowe SW, Ruley HE, Stabilization of the p53 tumor suppressor is induced by adenovirus 5 E1A and accompanies apoptosis. *Genes Dev* 1993; 7:535–45.

24. Debbas M, White E, Wild-type p53 mediates apoptosis by E1A, which is inhibited by E1B. *Genes Dev* 1993; 7:546–54.

25. Chen MJ, Holskin B, Strickler J et al, Induction by E1A oncogene expression of cellular susceptibility to lysis by TNF. *Nature* 1987; 330:581–3.

26. Shao R, Hu MC, Zhou BP et al, E1A sensitizes cells to tumor necrosis factor-induced apoptosis through inhibition of IkappaB kinases and nuclear factor kappaB activities. *J Biol Chem* 1999; 274:21495–8.

27. Cook JL, May DL, Wilson BA et al, A. Role of tumor necrosis factor-alpha in E1A oncogene-induced susceptibility of neoplastic cells to lysis by natural killer cells and activated macrophages. *J Immunol* 1989; **142**:4527–34.

28. Lee WP, Liao Y, Robinson D et al, Axl-Gas6 interaction counteracts E1A-mediated cell

growth suppression and proapoptotic activity. *Mol Cell Biol* 1999; **19**:8075–82.

29. Sanchez-Prieto R, de Alava E, Palomino T et al, An association between viral genes and human oncogenic alterations: the adenovirus E1A induces the Ewing tumor fusion transcript EWS-FLI1. *Nature Med* 1999; **5**:1076–9.

30. Kovar H, E1A and the Ewing tumor translocation. *Nature Med* 1999; **5**:1331.

31. Melot T, Delattre O, E1A and the Ewing tumor translocation. *Nature Med* 1999; **5**:1331.

32. Friedmann T, Overcoming the obstacles to gene therapy. *Sci Am* 1997; **276**:96–101.

33. Felgner PL, Nonviral strategies for gene therapy. *Sci Am* 1997; **276**:102–6.

34. Felgner PL, Ringold GM, Cationic liposome-mediated transfection. *Nature* 1989; **337**:387–8.

35. Nabel EG, Gordon D, Yang ZY et al, Gene transfer in vivo with DNA-liposome complexes: lack of autoimmunity and gonadal localization. *Hum Gene Ther* 1992; **3**:649–56.

36. Nabel GJ, Nabel EG, Yang ZY et al, Direct gene transfer with DNA-liposome complexes in melanoma: expression, biologic activity, and lack of toxicity in humans. *Proc Natl Acad Sci USA* 1993; **90**:11307–11.

37. Yu D, Matin A, Xia W, Sorgi F, Huang L, Hung MC, Liposome-mediated in vivo E1A gene transfer suppressed dissemination of ovarian cancer cells that overexpress HER-2/*neu*. *Oncogene* 1995; **11**:1383–8.

38. Xing X, Liu V, Xia W et al, Safety studies of the intraperitoneal injection of E1A-liposome complex in mice. *Gene Ther* 1997; **4**:238–43.

39. Xing X, Zhang S, Chang JY et al, Safety study and characterization of E1A-liposome complex gene delivery in an ovarian cancer model. *Gene Ther* 1998; **5**:1538–44.

40. Chang JY, Xia W, Shao R et al, The tumor suppression activity of E1A in HER-2/*neu*-overexpressing breast cancer. *Oncogene* 1997; **14**:561–8.

41. Hortobagyi GN, Hung MC, Lopez-Berestein G, A Phase I multicenter study of E1A gene therapy for patients with metastatic breast cancer and epithelial ovarian cancer that overexpresses HER-2/*neu* or epithelial ovarian cancer. *Hum Gene Ther* 1998; **9**:1775–98.

42. Xia WY, Lau YK, Zhang HZ et al, Strong correlation between c-Erbb-2 overexpression and overall survival of patients with oral squamous cell carcinoma. *Clin Cancer Res* 1997; **3**:3–9.

43. Mymryk JS, Tumor suppressive properties of the adenovirus 5 *E1A* oncogene. *Oncogene* 1996; **13**:1581–9.

19

Angiogenesis, antiangiogenic therapy and breast cancer

Kathy D Miller, George W Sledge

What makes a collection of cells a cancer? This question has driven the research agenda of oncology since the field's inception. It is a question with more than one answer, but uncontrolled growth and distant spread are central to each answer. Angiogenesis, or new blood vessel formation, is now known to play an important role in both growth and metastasis. The recognition of the central importance of angiogenesis, and the understanding of how new blood vessels are formed, has led to novel therapies designed to interrupt the process. This chapter explores the mechanisms underlying angiogenesis, its specific role in breast cancer, and recent attempts both to measure and to interfere with new blood vessel formation. It also discusses the specific challenges posed by the development of anti-angiogenic agents.

ANGIOGENESIS – BACKGROUND

Growth of solid tumors in both primary and metastatic sites depends on angiogenesis to nourish the tumor. In pioneering work by Folkman,[1] cancer cells implanted in vascular sites in animals grew rapidly and formed large tumors. In contrast, cells implanted in avascular sites were unable to form tumor masses larger than 1–2 mm in size.[1] This work led Folkman to hypothesize that angiogenesis was obligatory for tumor growth.

Under physiologic conditions, angiogenesis involves initial *activation*, including sequential basement membrane degradation, cell migration, extracellular matrix invasion, endothelial cell proliferation and capillary lumen formation. The newly formed microvasculature matures through the process of *resolution*, which includes inhibition of proliferation, basement membrane reconstitution and junctional complex formation.[2] Both activation and resolution are tightly regulated processes, governed by specific stimulatory and inhibitory factors, many of which have been identified (Table 19.1).

In contrast to what is seen with physiologic angiogenesis, tumor microvessels frequently lack complete endothelial linings and basement membranes. They tend to be highly irregular and tortuous, with arteriovenous shunts and blind ends being common. Blood flow through tumors tends to be sluggish, and the tumor-associated vessels leakier than normal.[3]

Table 19.1   Positive and negative regulators of angiogenesis

Positive regulators
    VEGF
    bFGF
    TGF-β1[156]
    PDGF[157]
    Angiogenin[29,158]
    Thymidine phosphorylase[159,160]
    Angiopoietin-1[161,162]

Negative regulators
    Angiostatin
    Endostatin
    2-Methoxyestradiol
    Thrombospondin-1[163,164]
    Platelet factor IV[165]
    TIMPs
    IFN-α[2,88]
    Angiopoietin-2[166]
    Prostate-specific antigen[167,168]

VEGF, vascular endothelial growth factor; bFGF, basic fibroblast growth factor; TGF, transforming growth factor; PDGF, platelet-derived growth factor; TIMP, tissue inhibitor of metalloproteinase; IFN, interferon.

ROLE OF ANGIOGENESIS IN BREAST CANCER

Preclinical studies

Extensive laboratory data suggest that angiogenesis plays an essential role in breast cancer development, invasion and metastasis. Hyperplastic murine breast papillomas[4] and histologically normal lobules adjacent to cancerous breast tissue[5] support angiogenesis in preclinical models, suggesting that angiogenesis precedes transformation of mammary hyperplasia to malignancy. Transfection of tumor cells with an angiogenic stimulatory peptide, such as fibroblast growth factor-1 or -4,[6,7] vascular endothelial growth factor (VEGF)[8,9] or progelatinase-B (matrix metalloproteinase-9, MMP-9),[10] increases tumor growth, invasiveness, microvasculature and metastasis.[11] Conversely, transfection of tumor cells with inhibitors of angiogenesis, including thrombospondin-1[12] or tissue inhibitor of metalloproteinase-4 (TIMP-4),[13] decreases growth and metastasis.[14]

The MMP family of enzymes degrades the basement membrane and extracellular matrix and is associated with a family of endogenous inhibitors, TIMPs. Under normal physiologic conditions, the MMPs and TIMPs exist in an exquisite balance – a balance that is upset during active angiogenesis. Expression of MMPs increases with the progression from benign to *in situ*, invasive and metastatic breast cancer,[15] and is associated with increasing histologic tumor grade.[16] Microscopic metastases are growth restricted and remain dormant until they undergo an 'angiogenic switch', presumably a result of further mutation.[17,18] This angiogenic switch often results in increased expression of MMPs.[19]

Clinical evidence

Clinicopathologic correlations also confirm the central role of angiogenesis in breast cancer progression. Fibrocystic lesions with the highest vascular density are associated with a greater risk of breast cancer.[20] Two distinct vascular patterns have been described in association with ductal carcinoma in situ (DCIS): a diffuse increase in stromal vascularity between duct lesions and a dense rim of microvessels adjacent to the basement membrane of individual ducts.[21,22] Microvessel density is highest with histopathologically aggressive DCIS lesions[22] and associated with increased VEGF expression.[23] Multiple angiogenic factors are commonly expressed by invasive human breast cancers; at least six different proangiogenic factors were identified in each of 64 primary breast tumors studied by Relf and colleagues, with the 121-amino acid isoform of VEGF predominating.[24] Several studies have found an inverse correlation between VEGF expression and overall survival in both node-positive and node-negative patients.[25–28] Eppenberger et al confirmed the negative prognostic value of VEGF expression for both relapse and survival.[29]

Membrane-associated factors such as urokinase-type plasminogen activator (uPA) expression,[29] the ratio of uPA to plasminogen activator inhibitor-1 (PAI-1),[30] integrin $\alpha_v\beta_3$,[31] and collagenase IV[32] have also been associated with impaired survival or local relapse. In contrast, expression of many inhibitors of angiogenesis is lost or downregulated in tumors.[16,33]

Weidner and colleagues assessed tumor vasculature in primary breast tumors by specifically staining endothelial cells with antibodies directed against factor VIII-associated antigen, scanning to identify the area with the greatest microvessel density and meticulously counting microvessels in a single $200 \times$ field. In a preliminary study of 49 unselected patients, mean microvessel density (MVD) was 101 in patients who developed metastases compared with 45 in those who remained disease free ($p = 0.003$ in univariate analysis).[34] The prognostic significance of tumor MVD was then confirmed in a blinded study of 165 consecutive patients by the same investigators.[35] Tumor MVD was the only significant predictor of overall and relapse-free survival among the node-negative subset in this follow-up study.

Investigation in this area has flourished with other groups modifying the technique to use different endothelial antibodies[36,37] and counting strategies.[38] These studies have generally,[28,39,40] although not uniformly,[41,42] validated the poor prognosis and early relapse associated with increasing MVD. Differences in sample size, technique, methods and interobserver variability probably account for the discrepancies.[43–45] The extent of primary tumor vascularization has also been associated with tumor shedding at the time of surgery[46] and the probability of bone marrow micrometastases.[47]

ANGIOGENESIS: THE POTENTIAL AND PITFALLS OF A NEW THERAPEUTIC TARGET

Normal vasculature is quiescent in health adults with each endothelial cell dividing once every 10 years; active angiogenesis is required only for wound healing, endometrial proliferation, post-lactational mammary gland involution and pregnancy. In contrast, tissue remodeling and angiogenesis are crucial for the growth and metastasis of breast cancer and provide attractive therapeutic targets that may have limited (at least theoretically) toxicity. Redundancy in the angiogenic cascade offers both potential and problems. It may be possible to interrupt the process of angiogenesis at several different levels with the potential for synergy. Unfortunately, it may also be naïve to expect inhibition of only one angiogenic factor to alter the clinical course.

Antiangiogenic agents may be conceptually divided into two general categories. What might be called 'vasculotoxins' have a direct toxic effect on proliferating endothelium, inducing endothelial apoptosis and cell death. Assuming that a given number of endothelial cells are required to support a population of tumor cells, and that some more-or-less fixed ratio between the two exists, the vasculotoxins might be expected to have a multiplier effect in human tumors. As such they may produce clinical responses similar to traditional antineoplastics; standard drug development and clinical trials may be appropriate.

Conversely, we might term 'vasculostatins' agents that merely prevent further new blood vessel formation without directly damaging the existing microvasculature. Such vasculostatins may require prolonged administration to induce and maintain tumor dormancy. Classic phase II trials of the vasculostatins in patients with well-established tumors may result in few (if any) objective responses without refuting the theoretical basis for their use.[48] As such, delayed responses would be expected; prolonged stable disease might well be considered a 'win' for such agents.

Successful development of antiangiogenic therapy, particularly the vasculostatins, will require a new conceptual approach to clinical research. In this approach, physicians will need to think in terms of biologically active rather than maximal tolerated dose, chronic rather than intermittent therapy, and induction of tumor dormancy rather than tumor cell kill. Current testing of new clinical agents in the phase II setting regularly focuses on overall response rate; agents failing to pass some level of response are frequently discarded. This may represent a strategic error for agents that only prevent further tumor growth. It may be necessary for some agents to jump over the phase II setting into a randomized trial once appropriate safety concerns have been met.

Hahnfeldt and colleagues have recently explored a model of tumor growth under angiogenic signaling.[49] This model considers growth of the tumor vasculature to be explicitly time dependent (rather than dependent on tumor volume) and to be under the control of distinct positive and negative signals arising from the tumor. Overall, the model parallels gompertzian kinetics with tumor growth slowing as tumor size increases. Tumor growth eventually reaches a plateau as the action of stimulators of vascular growth are offset by the increasing production of vascular inhibitors by the primary tumor. Antiangiogenic therapies act to lower this plateau tumor size – hopefully to a level compatible with asymptomatic host survival. Importantly, the final tumor size is dependent only on the balance of positive and negative angiogenic factors and is *independent* of tumor size at the start of treatment. The model also predicts initial tumor *growth* with some inhibitors of angiogenesis (particularly angiostatin) before stabilization at the plateau size is achieved. This early growth could easily be interpreted (perhaps misinterpreted) as treatment failure unless surrogate markers of angiogenesis are used to guide therapy. If such a model is a correct approximation of clinical reality, then clinical trialists (and their patients) will need to learn to tolerate the prospect of initial disease progression. This will not be a comfortable prospect for many.

Surrogate end-points of angiogenesis

Correlative laboratory studies assessing biologically meaningful intermediate end-points of angiogenesis are a necessity. Unfortunately, the correlation between intermediate end-points, angiogenesis and biological activity remains unproven. Despite the wealth of laboratory data, direct clinical evidence linking antiangiogenic activity, changes in tumor MVD and objective tumor response is lacking. In addition to the need to establish the clinical relevance of antiangiogenic activity, the development of reliable surrogate markers of angiogenesis that could guide therapy without repeated tissue samples is urgently needed.

Although as yet no clear standard has emerged, the search for reliable surrogates of antiangiogenic activity has focused on two main areas: soluble factors and imaging of the tumor vasculature.

Soluble measures of angiogenesis

VEGF is a potent and specific stimulator of endothelial cell proliferation and angiogenesis.[50] VEGF expression, measured by immunohisto-chemistry or in tumor cytosolic extracts, correlates with MVD and is associated with early relapse in primary breast cancer.[25,27] VEGF can be measured in sera and is typically detected at higher levels in patients with cancer than in healthy volunteers.[51] Higher concentrations have been found in those patients with stage III compared with stage I and II breast cancer.[52] Serum concentrations of VEGF may primarily reflect platelet counts rather than tumor burden, so measurements in platelet-poor plasma have been recommended.[53,54] Although attempts to correlate single pre-treatment levels with response to therapy[55] and the ability of serial measurements to predict response[56] have been disappointing, neither of these preliminary studies directly assessed angiogenesis.

Fibroblast growth factor (FGF) is also commonly produced by breast cancers and can be measured in serum and urine. Similar to VEGF, FGF levels are increased in patients with breast cancer[57,58] and may predict survival.[59] The correlation of serial FGF measurements with changes in tumor microvasculature has not been reported.

Vascular cell adhesion molecule (VCAM-1) is transiently expressed on endothelial cells in response to stimulation by various cytokines, including VEGF.[60] Although the major physiologic role of VCAM-1 appears to be in the adhesion of leukocytes to endothelium, a role in the adhesion of malignant cells during the process of metastasis has been proposed.[61,62] Increased concentrations of serum soluble VCAM-1 are detected in patients with cancer, further supporting its role.[63] In a recently reported pilot study, serum VCAM-1 levels were more tightly correlated with breast cancer MVD than serum VEGF levels. Although initial levels in patients with known metastatic disease were not predictive of response, levels quickly rose in patients whose disease progressed but decreased or remained stable in responding patients.[56] Whether these changes in VCAM-1 levels were associated with changes in tumor MVD is not known.

The MMP family of enzymes degrade molecules of the basement membrane and extracellular matrix and are critical for the process of cellular movement and invasion.[64] The gelatinases (MMP-2 and MMP-9) have received particular attention as a result of their ability to degrade type IV collagen and the correlation of expression with tumor angiogenesis.[65] Overall expression of the gelatinases has been associated with grade and stage of breast cancer;[15,16] increased serum levels are found in patients with metastatic disease. Given the central role of these peptides in the angiogenic process, decreases in serum levels should theoretically correlate with changes in tumor MVD and may predict response to antiangiogenic therapy. This hypothesis has not yet been tested prospectively.

IMAGING TUMOR VASCULATURE

Assessment of tumor blood flow by color Doppler ultrasonography (CDUS) did not correlate with tumor microvessel density in one small study,[66] but nevertheless was an independent predictor of survival.[67] Other investigators, however, found a significant correlation between CDUS images and MVD; increased blood flow as detected by CDUS was predictive of lymph node metastasis in this pilot study.[68] The potential of this technique to monitor the effect of therapy was shown by investigators at the Royal Marsden Hospital. Thirty-four patients with large or centrally located breast tumors were followed with clinical examination, B-mode ultrasonography and CDUS. Changes in vascularity as measured by CDUS images were concordant with changes in tumor size at more than 75% of the time points assessed. Perhaps more striking, changes were apparent by CDUS at least 4 weeks before any change in tumor size was detected by physical examination or B-mode ultrasonography in 40% of patients.[69] The ability of serial imaging with CDUS to detect and quantify changes in tumor microvasculature with therapy is intriguing but as yet unproven.

Positron emission tomography (PET) uses small doses of radiopharmaceuticals to image the body based on metabolic activity or blood flow. Sequential PET imaging using radiolabeled 2-[^{18}F]fluoro-2-deoxyglucose (FDG) to quantify tumor metabolic activity predicted response to primary chemotherapy in three small pilot trials.[70–72] PET scans obtained with ^{15}O-labeled water and ^{11}O-labeled carbon monoxide have been used to image primary brain tumors and to quantitate regional cerebral blood flow.[73–75] PET studies have been used to study the local tumor microenvironment, including tumor vasculature in isolated human tumor xenografts.[76] A small pilot study in breast cancer patients using ^{15}O-labeled water found increased blood flow associated with the tumor compared with surrounding normal breast tissue but did not attempt any correlation with histology or MVD.[77] Yoon and colleagues evaluated 99m Tc-labeled sestamibi uptake and washout in 31 patients with untreated primary breast cancer. Both early and later tumor-to-normal breast ratios correlated well with tumor MVD.[78] Alterations in tumor-associated blood flow and blood volume, as measured by PET, with chemotherapy have not been correlated with changes in tumor histology.

Magnetic resonance imaging (MRI) has been used to evaluate tumor-associated vasculature by several groups, with mixed results. Esserman and colleagues used contrast-enhanced MRI with a triple acquisition, rapid gradient, echo technique (TARGET). In a pilot study of 32 patients, tumors with the most intense early signal enhancement and rapid contrast washout (high signal enhancement ratio) had the highest MVD.[79] A similar contrast-enhanced method with three time points correlated well with changes in tumor necrosis and increasing vascular permeability after treatment with tamoxifen[80] or a monoclonal antibody directed against VEGF.[81] Using a different dynamic image sequence, Stomper et al found an overall association between MRI gadolinium enhancement amplitude and vessel density, but the ability to predict vessel density did not reach a clinically useful level.[82] Other investigators found no significant correlation between dynamic echo-planar imaging and tumor MVD.[83]

ANTIANGIOGENIC ACTIVITY OF EXISTING AGENTS: OLD DOGS WITH NEW TRICKS?

Oncologists may have been unknowingly administering antiangiogenic therapy for years. Tamoxifen exerts a long-term suppressive effect on estrogen-sensitive breast cancer cell lines and has been used in the treatment of breast cancer for more than 20 years. Initially thought to be merely a competitive inhibitor of estradiol, estrogen-independent mechanisms of action have recently been proposed.[84] Tamoxifen inhibits VEGF- and FGF-stimulated embryonic angiogenesis in the chick chorioallantoic membrane (CAM) model. This effect was not reversed by excess estradiol, suggesting that the antiangiogenic mechanism is not dependent on estradiol concentration or estrogen receptor content.[85,86] Treatment with tamoxifen resulted in a more than 50% decrease in the endothelial density of viable tumor and an increase in the extent of necrosis in MCF-7 tumors growing in nude mice.[87] The inhibition of angiogenesis was detected before measurable effects on tumor volume.[88] Using differential display technology to assess gene expression in tumor and normal breast tissue from two patients, Silva and colleagues reported that brief treatment with tamoxifen resulted in downregulation of CD36, a glycoprotein receptor for matrix proteins thrombospondin-1 and collagen types I and IV.[89] Thrombospondin-1 is involved in hematogenous tumor dissemination, invasion and angiogenesis, so downregulation of CD36 represents a potential mechanism for the observed antiangiogenic effect.

The influence of sex steroids on angiogenesis is complex and may be tissue and steroid specific. Progestational agents increased secreted VEGF in the culture media of some but not all breast cancer cell lines.[90] The effect of sex steroids on FGF-stimulated angiogenesis in the rabbit corneal micropocket assay is also quite variable; significant inhibition is seen with dexamethasone and four analogs of medroxyprogesterone acetate (MPA), whereas 17β-estradiol and at least one other MPA analog had no effect.[91]

Several chemotherapeutic agents used routinely in breast cancer treatment have known antiangiogenic activity. The taxanes are antiangiogenic in in vitro and in vivo models. Paclitaxel inhibits endothelial proliferation, migration and tubule formation at levels significantly below those required for tumor cell kill.[92,93] The MVD of murine breast cancers was significantly decreased by treatment with paclitaxel at doses that did not affect the rate of tumor growth.[94] Docetaxel inhibits the proliferation of human endothelial cells and the ability of endothelial cells to form capillary tubules in a fibrin clot assay. Elevated levels of DNA nuclear matrix protein, a measure of apoptosis, were also seen with docetaxel treatment.[95]

Doxorubicin selectively inhibited collagenase I

(MMP-1) gene expression, but had not effect on MMP-2 or MMP-9, in the melanoma A2058 cell line. Doxorubicin treatment was associated with a decreased ability of the tumor cells to invade a collagen matrix independent of any antiproliferative effect.[96] In vivo angiogenesis by Caki-2 renal carcinoma xenografts was decreased by one-third after treatment with doxorubicin; no effect was seen with the Caki-1 cell line.[97] Pirarubicin and mitoxantrone both inhibited rat lung endothelial cells and diminished neovascularization in the CAM assay.[98]

ANGIOGENESIS INHIBITION ENTERS THE CLINIC: A VIEW OF THE FUTURE

The significant improvement in our understanding of angiogenesis has allowed for the development of agents targeting specific steps in the angiogenic cascade. Agents may be conceptually grouped into one of several categories: activation blockers, which either directly inhibit or otherwise interfere with the action of proangiogenic substances; endothelial toxins, which specifically target endothelial antigens; and resolution enhancers, which stimulate or mimic substances known to inhibit angiogenesis.

Activation blockers

Degradation of the basement membrane and surrounding stroma by the MMPs is crucial for direct tissue invasion and angiogenesis. Inhibition of the MMPs decreases angiogenesis in preclinical systems and mouse xenografts.[65,99−102] Several MMP inhibitors have been identified and are currently in preclinical and clinical trials. The tetracycline antibiotic doxycycline is a broad inhibitor of the MMPs; doxycycline treatment reduces invasion through a reconstituted basement membrane and arrests proliferation in breast cancer cell lines.[103] A phase I trial of doxycycline in patients with advanced cancer achieved steady-state trough levels above those needed for MMP inhibition in vitro, although no objective responses were seen.[104]

Batimastat is a synthetic inhibitor of MMPs that interacts with the critical zinc-binding site of the enzyme. Although batimastat does not alter the viability of MDA-MB-435 cells in culture, nude mice treated with batimastat after resection of MDA-MB-435 tumors grown in their mammary fat pads had significantly decreased local tumor regrowth and a lower incidence, number and total volume of lung metastasis compared with control mice.[105] Recent study has found synergistic antimetastatic activity with the combination of batimastat and doxycycline in this mouse xenograft model.[106]

Clinical development of batimastat has been eclipsed by marimastat, an orally available analog. Phase I trials achieved serum levels above those needed for enzyme inhibition but were limited by reversible tendonitis/bursitis.[107] Although not predicted to induce substantial clinical responses in patients with well-established bulky tumors, chronic therapy with an MMP inhibitor may delay or eliminate tumor regrowth after initial surgical excision or systemic chemotherapy. Two ongoing or recently completed trials investigate this potential. The Eastern Cooperative Oncology Group study ECOG-2196 randomizes patients with metastatic disease who are responding to treatment or stable after initial chemotherapy with either marimastat or placebo. The primary end-point is time to progression. A limited institution phase I pilot study was performed to provide the pharmacokinetic and safety data needed to justify a full-scale phase III adjuvant trial. Sixty-three patients with early stage breast cancer received marimastat at one of two dose levels either after doxorubicin-based chemotherapy or concomitantly with tamoxifen. Overall, marimastat was well tolerated but musculoskeletal toxicity

resulted in significant dose reductions and limited chronic administration to doses yielding plasma levels below the target range.[108] Two other orally available MMPs have entered clinical trials with ongoing phase III studies in a variety of tumor types.[109,110]

Angiogenesis requires stimulation of vascular endothelial cells through the release of angiogenic peptides including VEGF. An antibody directed against VEGF inhibited the growth of several human tumors in animal models,[111,112] stimulating interest in clinical development. A humanized recombinant version of anti-VEGF (rhuMAb-VEGF) has entered clinical trials in several tumor types; rhuMAb-VEGF was well tolerated and produced the expected decrease in free plasma VEGF levels in a multicenter phase I trial involving 25 patients. Three patients had tumor-related bleeding episodes, including an intracranial hemorrhage into an unrecognized cerebral metastasis in a patient with hepatocellular carcinoma. Although no objective responses were seen, 14 patients had stable disease at evaluation on day 72.[113] Preliminary results of an ongoing phase II trial of anti-VEGF in patients with refractory breast cancer have been reported. So far, 37 patients have been treated with clinical activity, including one confirmed complete response, observed. Therapy was generally well tolerated with mild hypertension in several patients; no bleeding episodes were noted.[114]

Inhibition of the VEGF receptor tyrosine kinase domain (Flk-1 and Flt-1) may also represent a fruitful therapeutic target. The critical role of Flk-1 in tumor angiogenesis was demonstrated using a dominant-negative Flk-1 transfectant. Eight of nine tumor cell lines with dominant negative Flk-1 showed growth inhibition and reduced MVD in athymic mice.[115] A synthetic inhibitor of the Flk-1 kinase has been developed (SU5416) that inhibits VEGF-dependent growth of endothelial cells without altering tumor growth in vitro. Systemic administration of SU5416 inhibited the growth of human tumors in mice without apparent toxicity.[116,117] SU5416 was well tolerated in a phase I clinical trial with the dose-limiting toxicity being projectile vomiting probably related to the diluent.[118,119] Proposals for combination phase I and disease-specific phase II trials are being coordinated by the NCI and are expected to have started in early 2000.

SU6668 inhibits the thymidine kinases associated with several receptors, including VEGF, FGF and platelet-derived growth factor.[120] SU6668 inhibited metastases (55.3%), microvessel formation (36.2%) and cell proliferation (27.3%), and increased tumor cell (4.3-fold) and endothelial cell (81.4-fold) apoptosis in Balb/c mice carrying CT-26 colon cancer xenografts.[121] Early clinical trials of SU6668 are ongoing.

PNU-145156E (formerly FCE26644), a sulfonated distamycine A derivative, is a noncytotoxic molecule whose anti-tumor activity is exerted through the formation of a reversible complex with growth/angiogenic factors.[122,123] In vitro PNU-145156E did not modify the cytotoxicity induced by several chemotherapeutic agents. However, in vivo, at the optimal dose of each compound, the anti-tumor activity was significantly increased in all combinations, with no associated increase in general toxicity. In healthy mice treated with cyclophosphamide or doxorubicin, the addition of PNU-145156E did not enhance the myelotoxic effect.[124] In phase I testing, PNU-145156E induced an unpredictable and short-lasting decrease in anti-thrombin III levels without effects on serum FGF or VEGF concentrations.[125]

Endothelial toxins

Disruption of endothelial cell chemotaxis and migration interferes with angiogenesis. The integrins, particularly $\alpha_v\beta_3$, provide critical attachment between the migrating endothelial cell and the extracellular matrix;[126] $\alpha_v\beta_3$ also localizes MMP-2 to the membrane of endothelial cells in the leading podosomes of new vessels, providing carefully targeted matrix destruction.[127] Moreover, immunohistochemical studies of clinical specimens from ocular pathologies suggest that both $\alpha_v\beta_3$ and $\alpha_v\beta_5$ are of importance for endothelial cell function in angiogenic neovascular disease.[128] Antibodies that block $\alpha_v\beta_3$ inhibit angiogenesis and tumor growth in vitro[129] and in vivo.[130] A humanized monoclonal antibody against $\alpha_v\beta_3$, vitaxin, was well tolerated and showed some activity in a phase I trial.[131] Phase II trials are ongoing.

Specific antibodies used to characterize the vitronectin receptors $\alpha_v\beta_3$ and $\alpha_v\beta_5$ in vitro were employed to study the function of these integrins in vivo.[132] The RGD (Arg-Gly-Asp) epitope is critical for the function of many β_1 integrins and is the same epitope that $\alpha_v\beta_3$ recognizes in its extracellular matrix ligands. This has led to the development of a family of RGD-containing peptides that can serve as potent and selective inhibitors of the vitronectin receptors. EMD121974 is the inner salt of a cyclized pentapeptide c-[Arg-Asp-DPhe-(NMeVal)] with significant antiangiogenic activity in a variety of preclinical in vitro and in vivo models. Phase I trials of EMD121974 have recently been initiated.

Resting endothelial cells are normally quiescent; proliferation increases dramatically in the leading podosomes of new capillaries. The protein endoglin is expressed much more strongly in growing tumor microvasculature than in the vasculature of surrounding normal tissues. Antibodies directed against endoglin decreased tumor growth in mice xenografts.[133,134] Anti-endoglin antibodies complexed to deglycosylated ricin A chain produced long-lasting complete remission of preformed tumors in immunocompromised mice.[135,136] The antiangiogenic activity of the antibiotic TNP-470 (AGM-1470) is also dependent on inhibition of endothelial cell proliferation.[137–139]

Resolution enhancers

Animal studies had suggested that some primary tumors may inhibit the growth of their metastases; resection of the primary tumor increases the growth rate of metastases in these tumors.[140–142] Investigation of these animal models has led to the identification of several naturally occurring inhibitors of angiogenesis. Angiostatin, a 38-kDa plasminogen fragment, inhibits growth of tumors and induces prolonged tumor dormancy in mice.[143,144] The exact mechanism of action is unclear, but mitosis arrest of endothelial cells has been demonstrated.[145] Treatment with angiostatin increases sensitivity to radiation;[146] potential interactions with cytotoxic agents are unknown. A phase I study began in April 2000.

Endostatin, a 20-kDa proteolytic fragment of collagen XVIII, has antiangiogenic activity similar to angiostatin.[147] Endostatin has a highly basic region with significant affinity for heparin, suggesting that binding to heparin sulfate proteoglycans involved in growth factor signaling may be responsible for its activity.[148] Treatment with endostatin produced regression of tumors in mice with prolonged dormancy; no apparent resistance developed during intermittent therapy (up to six cycles).[149] Endostatin has been synthesized and entered phase I trials as a single agent at three sites in the fall of 1999.

A naturally occurring metabolite of estradiol, 2-methoxyestradiol ($2ME_2$), has a dual mechanism of action: (1) as an antiproliferative drug acting directly on the tumor cell compartment and (2) as an antiangiogenic drug acting on tumor vasculature. In vitro, $2ME_2$ exhibits antiproliferative activity in tumor cells with IC_{50} (concentration that causes 50% inhibition)

values generally in the submicromolar to low micromolar range, independent of the estrogen responsiveness of the cell line. The inhibition of proliferation is believed to result primarily from the induction of apoptosis, possibly through the activation of *p53*. In addition, the rate, but not the degree, of tubulin (de)polymerization is inhibited by $2ME_2$ treatment in certain cell lines.[150] In vivo, $2ME_2$ is effective in xenograft and metastatic disease models. Oral administration of $2ME_2$ effectively reduces the rate of growth of tumor xenografts in mice in the absence of significant toxicity.[151,152] 2-Methoxyestradiol treatment also greatly reduces the number of lung metastases in murine models.[153]

The antiangiogenic activity of $2ME_2$ has been demonstrated in vivo in corneal micropocket[152] and CAM systems,[154] as well as by the observation of reduced tumor vasculature in $2ME_2$-treated mice. In vitro, $2ME_2$ inhibits tubule formation in bovine microvascular endothelial cells stimulated by basic FGF (bFGF)[151] and the proliferation of human umbilical vein endothelial cells.[155] 2-Methoxyestradiol should have entered phase I trials in early 2000.

CONCLUSION

As with any novel approach, angiogenesis inhibition will require testing in the setting of carefully conducted prospective trials. It is likely that this therapy will neither cure all cancers nor be without toxicity. Like all therapies, use of antiangiogenics will require a balance of risk and benefit. Yet there can be little question that the advent of antiangiogenic therapy will be widely welcomed by physicians and patients. In part this is the result of clever media advertising, almost unparalleled in the history of the disease. Below the layers of hype, however, lies a solid theoretical foundation, a large number of potential therapeutic targets and a growing number of testable agents. Unless we have totally misunderstood the biology of this disease, some form of angiogenesis inhibition should work. Dimming cancer's blood tide should go far to controlling the 'mere anarchy' of the disease. The next few years should see us measurably closer to that goal.

REFERENCES

1. Folkman J, What is the evidence that tumors are angiogenesis dependent? *J Natl Cancer Inst* 1990; **82**:4–6.

2. Pepper MS, Mandriota SJ, Vassalli JD et al, Angiogenesis-regulating cytokines: activities and interactions. *Curr Top Microbiol Immunol* 1996; **213**:31–67.

3. Brown JM, Giaccia AJ. The unique physiology of solid tumors: opportunities (and problems) for cancer therapy. *Cancer Res* 1998; **58**:1408–16.

4. Brem SS, Gullino PM, Medina D, Angiogenesis: a marker for neoplastic transformation of mammary papillary hyperplasia. *Science* 1997; **195**:880–2.

5. Jensen HM, Chen I, DeVault MR et al, Angiogenesis induced by 'normal' human breast tissue: a probable marker for precancer. *Science* 1982; **218**:293–5.

6. Kurebayashi J, McLeskey SW, Johnson MD et al, Quantitative demonstration of spontaneous metastasis by MCF-7 human breast cancer cells cotransfected with fibroblast growth factor 4 and LacZ. *Cancer Res* 1993; **53**:2178–87.

7. McLeskey SW, Zhang L, Kharbanda S et al, Fibroblast growth factor overexpressing breast carcinoma cells as models of angiogenesis and metastasis. *Breast Cancer Res Treat* 1996; **39**:103–17.

8. Zhang HT, Craft P, Scott PA et al, Enhancement of tumor growth and vascular density by transfection of vascular endothelial cell growth factor into MCF-7 human breast carcinoma cells. *J Natl Cancer Inst* 1995; **87**:213–19.

9. McLeskey SW, Tobias CA, Vezza PR et al, Tumor growth of FGF or VEGF transfected MCF-7 breast carcinoma cells correlates with density of specific microvessels independent of the transfected angiogenic factor. *Am J Pathol* 1998; **153**:1993–2006.

10. Nakajima M, Welch DR, Wynn DM et al, Serum and plasma M(r) 92,000 progelatinase levels correlate with spontaneous metastasis of rat 13762NF mammary adenocarcinoma. *Cancer Res* 1993; **53**:5802–7.

11. Giunciuglio D, Culty M, Fassina G et al, Invasive phenotype of MCF10A cells overexpressing c-Ha-ras and c-erbB-2 oncogenes. *Int J Cancer* 1995; **63**:815–22.

12. Weinstat-Saslow DL, Zabrenetzky VS, Van-Houtte K et al, Transfection of thrombospondin 1 complementary DNA into a human breast carcinoma cell line reduces primary tumor growth, metastatic potential, and angiogenesis. *Cancer Res* 1994; **54**:6504–11.

13. Wang M, Liu YE, Greene J et al, Inhibition of tumor growth and metastasis of human breast cancer cells transfected with tissue inhibitor of metalloproteinase 4. *Oncogene* 1997; **14**:2767–74.

14. Liotta LA, Steeg PS, Stetler-Stevenson WG, Cancer metastasis and angiogenesis: an imbalance of positive and negative regulation. *Cell* 1991; **64**:327–36.

15. Monteagudo C, Merino MJ, San-Juan J et al, Immunohistochemical distribution of type IV collagenase in normal, benign, and malignant breast tissue. *Am J Pathol* 1990; **136**:585–92.

16. Kossakowska AE, Huchcroft SA, Urbanski SJ et al, Comparative analysis of the expression patterns of metalloproteinases and their inhibitors in breast neoplasia, sporadic colorectal neoplasia, pulmonary carcinomas and malignant non-Hodgkin's lymphomas in humans. *Br J Cancer* 1996; **73**:1401–8.

17. Folkman J, Hanahan D, Switch to the angiogenic phenotype during tumorigenesis. *Princess Takamatsu Symp* 1991; **22**:339–47.

18. Holmgren L, O'Reilly MS, Folkman J, Dormancy of micrometastases: balanced proliferation and apoptosis in the presence of angiogenesis suppression [see comments]. *Nat Med* 1995; **1**:149–53.

19. Azzam HS, Arand G, Lippman ME et al, Association of MMP-2 activation potential with metastatic progression in human breast cancer cell lines independent of MMP-2 production. *J Natl Cancer Inst* 1993; **85**:1758–64.

20. Guinebretiere JM, Le Monique G, Gavoille A et al, Angiogenesis and risk of breast cancer in women with fibrocystic disease [letter; comment]. *J Natl Cancer Inst* 1994; **86**:635–6.

21. Engels K, Fox SB, Whitehouse RM et al, Distinct angiogenic patterns are associated with high-grade in situ ductal carcinomas of the breast. *J Pathol* 1997; **181**:207–12.

22. Guidi AJ, Fischer L, Harris JR et al, Microvessel density and distribution in ductal carcinoma in situ of the breast. *J Natl Cancer Inst* 1994; **86**:614–19.

23. Guidi AJ, Schnitt SJ, Fischer L et al, Vascular permeability factor (vascular endothelial growth factor) expression and angiogenesis in patients with ductal carcinoma in situ of the breast. *Cancer* 1997; **80**:1945–53.

24. Relf M, LeJeune S, Scott PA et al, Expression of the angiogenic factors vascular endothelial cell growth factor, acidic and basic fibroblast growth factor, tumor growth factor beta-1, platelet-derived endothelial cell growth factor, placenta growth factor, and pleiotrophin in human primary breast cancer and its relation to angiogenesis. *Cancer Res* 1997; **57**:963–9.

25. Gasparini G, Toi M, Gion M et al, Prognostic significance of vascular endothelial growth factor protein in node-negative breast carcinoma. *J Natl Cancer Inst* 1997; **89**:139–47.

26. Linderholm B, Tavelin B, Grankvist K et al, Vascular endothelial growth factor is of high prognostic value in node-negative breast carcinoma. *J Clin Oncol* 1998; **16**:3121–8.

27. Toi M, Kondo S, Suzuki H et al, Quantitative analysis of vascular endothelial growth factor in primary breast cancer. *Cancer* 1996; **77**:1101–6.

28. Toi M, Inada K, Suzuki H et al, Tumor angiogenesis in breast cancer: its importance as a prognostic indicator and the association with vascular endothelial growth factor expression. *Breast Cancer Res Treat* 1995; **36**:193–204.

29. Eppenberger U, Kueng W, Schlaeppi JM et al, Markers of tumor angiogenesis and proteolysis independently define high- and low-risk subsets of node-negative breast cancer patients. *J Clin Oncol* 1998; **16**:3129–36.

30. Thomssen C, Prechtl A, Polcher M et al, Interim analysis of a randomized trial of risk-adapted adjuvant chemotherapy in node-negative breast cancer patients guided by the prognostic factors uPA and PAI-1. *Breast Care Res Treat* 1999; **57**:25.

31. Gasparini G, Brooks PC, Biganzoli E et al, Vascular integrin alpha(v)beta3: a new prognostic indicator in breast cancer. *Clin Cancer Res* 1998; **4**:2625–34.

32. Daidone MG, Silvestrini R, D'Errico A et al, Laminin receptors, collagenase IV and prognosis in node-negative breast cancers. *Int J Cancer* 1991; **48**:529–32.

33. Zajchowski DA, Band V, Trask DK et al, Suppression of tumor-forming ability and related traits in MCF-7 human breast cancer cells by fusion with immortal mammary epithelial cells. *Proc Natl Acad Sci USA* 1990; **87**:2314–18.

34. Weidner N, Semple J, Welch W et al, Tumor angiogenesis and metastasis – correlation in invasive breast cancer. *N Engl J Med* 1991; **324**:1–8.

35. Weidner N, Folkman J, Pozza F et al, Tumor angiogenesis: a new significant and independent prognostic indicator in early stage breast carcinoma. *J Natl Cancer Inst* 1992; **84**:1875–87.

36. Horak E, Leek R, Klenk N, Angiogenesis, assessed by platelet/endothelial cell adhesion molecule antibodies, as indicator of node metastasis and survival in breast cancer. *Lancet* 1992; **340**:1120–4.

37. Martin L, Green B, Renshaw C et al, Examining the technique of angiogenesis assessment in invasive breast cancer. *Br J Cancer* 1997; **76**:40–3.

38. Simpson J, Ahn C, Battifora H et al, Endothelial area as a prognostic indicator for invasive breast carcinoma. *Cancer* 1996; **77**:2077–85.

39. Bevilacqua P, Barbareschi M, Verderio P et al, Prognostic value of intratumoral microvessel density, a measure of tumor angiogenesis, in node-negative breast carcinoma – results of a multiparametric study. *Breast Cancer Res Treat* 1995; **36**:205–17.

40. Bosari S, Lee A, DeLellis R et al, Microvessel quantitation and prognosis in invasive breast carcinoma. *Hum Pathol* 1992; **23**:755–61.

41. Hall N, Fish D, Hunt N et al, Is the relationship between angiogenesis and metastasis in breast cancer real? *Surg Oncol* 1992; **1**:223–9.

42. Van Hoef M, Knox W, Dhesi S et al, Assessment of tumor vascularity as a prognostic factor in lymph node negative invasive breast cancer. *Eur J Cancer* 1993; **29A**:1141–5.

43. Vermeulen PB, Libura M, Libura J et al, Influence of investigator experience and microscopic field size on microvessel density in node-negative breast carcinoma. *Breast Cancer Res Treat* 1997; **42**:165–72.

44. Vermeulen PB, Gasparini G, Fox SB et al, Quantification of angiogenesis in solid human tumours: an international consensus on the methodology and criteria of evaluation. *Eur J Cancer* 1996; **32A**:2474–84.

45. Weidner N, Current pathologic methods for measuring intratumoral microvessel density within breast carcinoma and other solid tumors. *Breast Cancer Treat Res* 1995; **36**: 169–80.

46. McCulloch P, Choy A, Martin L, Association between tumour angiogenesis and tumour cell shedding into effluent venous blood during breast cancer surgery [see comments]. *Lancet* 1995; **346**:1334–5.

47. Fox S, Leek R, Bliss J et al, Association of tumor angiogenesis with bone marrow micrometastases in breast cancer patients. *J Natl Cancer Inst* 1997; **89**:1044–9.

48. Sledge G, Gordon M, Therapeutic implications of angiogenesis inhibition. *Semin Oncol* 1998; **25**:59–65.

49. Hahnfeldt P, Panigrahy D, Folkman J et al, Tumor development under angiogenic signaling: A dynamic theory of tumor growth, treatment response, and postvascular dormancy. *Cancer Res* 1999; **59**:4770–5.

50. Ferrara N, Davis-Smyth T, The biology of vascular endothelial growth factor. *Endocrinol Rev* 1997; **18**:4–25.

51. Dirix L, Vermeulen P, Pawinski A et al, Elevated levels of the angiogenic cytokines basic fibroblast growth factor and vascular endothelial growth factor in the sera of cancer patients. *Br J Cancer* 1997; **76**:238–43.

52. Yamamoto Y, Toi M, Kondo S et al, Concentrations of vascular endothelial growth factor in the sera of normal controls and cancer patients. *Clin Cancer Res* 1996; **2**:821–6.

53. Verheul H, Hoekman K, Luykx-de Bakker S et al, Platelet: Transporter of vascular endothelial growth factor. *Clin Cancer Res* 1997; **3**: 2187–90.

54. Wynendaele W, Derua R, Hoylaerts M et al, Vascular endothelial growth factor measured in platelet poor plasma allows optimal separation between cancer patients and volunteers: A key to study an angiogenic marker in vivo? *Ann Oncol* 1999; **10**:965–71.

55. Zon R, Neuberg D, Wood W et al, Correlation of plasma VEGF with clinical outcome in patients with metastatic breast cancer. *Proc Am Soc Clin Oncol* 1998; **17**:185.

56. Byrne G, Blann A, Venizelos J et al, Serum soluble VCAM: A surrogate marker of angiogenesis. *Breast Cancer Treat Res* 1998; **50**:330.

57. Dirix LY, Vermeulen PB, Pawinski A et al,

Elevated levels of the angiogenic cytokines basic fibroblast growth factor and vascular endothelial growth factor in sera of cancer patients. *Br J Cancer* 1997; **76**:238–43.

58. Nguyen M, Watanabe H, Budson A et al, Elevated levels of an angiogenic peptide, basic fibroblast growth factor, in the urine of patients with a wide spectrum of cancers. *J Natl Cancer Inst* 1994; **86**:356–61.

59. Folkman J, Tumour angiogenesis: Diagnostic and therapeutic implications. *Am Assoc Cancer Res* 1993; **34**:571–2.

60. Osborn L, Hession C, Tizard R et al, Direct expression cloning of vascular cell adhesion molecule 1, a cytokine-induced endothelial protein that binds to lymphocytes. *Cell* 1989; **59**:1203–11.

61. Rice GE, Bevilacqua MP, An inducible endothelial cell surface glycoprotein mediates melanoma adhesion. *Science* 1989; **246**:1303–6.

62. Zetter BR, Adhesion molecules in tumor metastasis [see comments]. *Semin Cancer Biol* 1993; **4**:219–29.

63. Banks RE, Gearing AJ, Hemingway IK et al, Circulating intercellular adhesion molecule-1 (ICAM-1), E-selectin and vascular cell adhesion molecule-1 (VCAM-1) in human malignancies. *Br J Cancer* 1993; **68**:122–4.

64. Matrisian LM, Metalloproteinases and their inhibitors in matrix remodeling. *Trends Genet* 1990; **6**:121–5.

65. Kurizaki T, Toi M, Tominaga T, Relationship between matrix metalloproteinase expression and tumor angiogenesis in human breast carcinoma. *Oncol Rep* 1998; **5**:673–7.

66. Peters-Engl C, Medl M, Mirau M et al, Color-coded and spectral Doppler flow in breast carcinomas – relationship with the tumor microvasculature. *Breast Cancer Res Treat* 1998; **47**:83–9.

67. Peters-Engl C, Frank W, Medl M, Tumor flow in malignant breast tumors measured by doppler ultrasound: An independent predictor of survival. *Breast Cancer Treat Res* 1998; **50**:228.

68. Bhlomer J, Gohlke A, Hufnagel P et al, Correlation between morphologic parameters of vascularization, color doppler image features and lymph node metastasis in breast cancer. *Breast Cancer Res Treat* 1998; **50**:331.

69. Kedar RP, Cosgrove DO, Smith IE et al, Breast carcinoma: measurement of tumor response to primary medical therapy with color Doppler flow imaging. *Radiology* 1994; **190**:825–30.

70. Jansson T, Westlin JE, Ahlstrom H et al, Positron emission tomography studies in patients with locally advanced and/or metastatic breast cancer: a method for early therapy evaluation? *J Clin Oncol* 1995; **13**:1470–7.

71. Bassa P, Kim EE, Inoue T et al, Evaluation of preoperative chemotherapy using PET with fluorine-18-fluorodeoxyglucose in breast cancer. *J Nucl Med* 1996; **37**:931–8.

72. Wahl RL, Zasadny K, Helvie M et al, Metabolic monitoring of breast cancer chemohormonotherapy using positron emission tomography: initial evaluation. *J Clin Oncol* 1993; **11**:2101–11.

73. Jarden JO, Pathophysiological aspects of malignant brain tumors studied with positron emission tomography. *Acta Neurol Scand Suppl* 1994; **156**:1–35.

74. Lammertsma AA, Wise RJ, Jones T, In vivo measurements of regional cerebral blood flow and blood volume in patients with brain tumours using positron emission tomography. *Acta Neurochir* 1983; **69**:5–13.

75. Jones SC, Greenberg JH, Reivich M, Error analysis for the determination of cerebral blood flow with the continuous inhalation of ^{15}O-labeled carbon dioxide and positron emission tomography. *J Comput Assist Tomogr* 1982; **6**:116–24.

76. Kallinowski F, Schlenger KH, Runkel S et al, Blood flow, metabolism, cellular microenvironment, and growth rate of human tumor xenografts. *Cancer Res* 1989; **49**:3759–64.

77. Wilson CB, Lammertsma AA, McKenzie CG et al, Measurements of blood flow and exchanging water space in breast tumors using

positron emission tomography: a rapid and noninvasive dynamic method. *Cancer Res* 1992; **52**:1592–7.

78. Yoon J-H, Bom H-S, Song H-C et al, Double-phase Tc-99m sestamibi scintimammography to assess angiogenesis with P-glycoprotein expression in patients with untreated breast cancer. *Clin Nucl Med* 1999; **24**:314–18.

79. Esserman L, Hylton N, George T et al, Contrast-enhanced magnetic resonance imaging to assess tumor histopathology and angiogenesis in breast carcinoma. *Breast Journal* 1999; **5**:13–21.

80. Furman-Haran E, Grobgeld D, Margalit R et al, Response of MCF7 human breast cancer to tamoxifen: evaluation by the three-time point, contrast-enhanced magnetic resonance imaging method. *Clin Cancer Res* 1998; **4**:2299–304.

81. Pham C, Roberts T, van Bruggen N et al, Magnetic resonance imaging detects suppression of tumor vascular permeability after administration of antibody to vascular endothelial growth factor. *Cancer Invest* 1998; **16**:225–30.

82. Stomper P, Winston J, Klippenstein D et al, Angiogenesis and dynamic MR imaging gadolinium enhancement of malignant and benign breast lesions. *Breast Cancer Res Treat* 1997; **45**:39–46.

83. Hulka C, Edmister W, Smith B et al, Dynamic echo-planar imaging of the breast: experience in diagnosing breast carcinoma and correlation with tumor angiogenesis. *Radiology* 1997; **205**:837–42.

84. Wiseman H, Tamoxifen: new membrane-mediated mechanisms of action and therapeutic advances. *Trends Pharmacol Sci* 1994; **15**:83–9.

85. Gagliardi A, Collins DC, Inhibition of angiogenesis by antiestrogens. *Cancer Res* 1993; **53**:533–5.

86. Gagliardi AR, Hennig B, Collins DC, Anti-estrogens inhibit endothelial cell growth stimulated by angiogenic growth factors. *Anticancer Res* 1996; **16**:1101–6.

87. Haran EF, Maretzek AF, Goldberg I et al, Tamoxifen enhances cell death in implanted MCF7 breast cancer by inhibiting endothelium growth. *Cancer Res* 1994; **54**:5511–14.

88. Lindner DJ, Borden EC, Effects of tamoxifen and interferon-beta or the combination on tumor-induced angiogenesis. *Int J Cancer* 1997; **71**:456–61.

89. Silva ID, Salicioni AM, Russo IH et al, Tamoxifen down-regulates CD36 messenger RNA levels in normal and neoplastic human breast tissues. *Cancer Res* 1997; **57**:378–81.

90. Hyder SM, Murthy L, Stancel GM, Progestin regulation of vascular endothelial growth factor in human breast cancer cells. *Cancer Res* 1998; **58**:392–5.

91. Yamamoto T, Terada N, Nishizawa Y et al, Angiostatic activities of medroxyprogesterone acetate and its analogues. *Int J Cancer* 1994; **56**:393–9.

92. Klauber N, Parangi S, Flynn E et al, Inhibition of angiogenesis and breast cancer in mice by the microtubule inhibitors 2-methoxyestradiol and taxol. *Cancer Res* 1997; **57**:81–6.

93. Belotti D, Vergani V, Drudis T et al, The microtubule-affecting drug paclitaxel has antiangiogenic activity. *Clin Cancer Res* 1996; **2**:1843–9.

94. Lau D, Young L, Xue L et al, Paclitaxel: an angiogenesis antagonist in a metastatic breast cancer model. *Proc Am Soc Clin Oncol* 1998; **17**:107.

95. Sweeney C, Sledge GJ, Chemotherapy agents as antiangiogenic therapy. *Cancer Conference Highlights* 1999; **3**:2–4.

96. Benbow U, Maitra R, Hamilton J et al, Selective modulation of collagenase 1 gene expression by the chemotherapeutic agent doxorubicin. *Clin Cancer Res* 1999; **5**:203–8.

97. Schirner M, Hoffmann J, Menrad A et al, Antiangiogenic chemotherapeutic agents: characterization in comparison to their tumor growth inhibition in human renal cell carcinoma models. *Clin Cancer Res* 1998; **4**:1331–6.

98. Ligo M, Shimamura M, Sagawa K et al,

Characteristics of the inhibitory effect of mitoxantrone and pirarubicin on lung metastases of colon carcinoma 26. *Jpn J Cancer Res* 1995; **86**:867–72.

99. Fisher C, Gilbertson-Beadling S, Powers EA et al, Interstitial collagenase is required for angiogenesis in vitro. *Dev Biol* 1994; **162**:499–510.

100. Low JA, Johnson MD, Bone EA et al, The matrix metalloproteinase inhibitor batimastat (BB-94) retards human breast cancer solid tumor growth but not ascites formation in nude mice. *Clin Cancer Res* 1996; **2**:1207–14.

101. Taraboletti G, Garofalo A, Belotti D et al, Inhibition of angiogenesis and murine hemangioma growth by batimastat, a synthetic inhibitor of matrix metalloproteinases. *J Natl Cancer Inst* 1995; **87**:293–8.

102. Tamargo RJ, Bok RA, Brem H, Angiogenesis inhibition by minocycline. *Cancer Res* 1991; **51**:672–5.

103. Fife RS, Sledge GW Jr, Effects of doxycycline on in vitro growth, migration, and gelatinase activity of breast carcinoma cells. *J Lab Clin Med* 1995; **125**:407–11.

104. Gordon M, Battiato L, Jones D et al, A phase I trial of doxocycline in patients with cancer. *Proc Am Soc Clin Oncol* 1997; **16**: 226a.

105. Sledge GW Jr, Qulali M, Goulet R et al, Effect of matrix metalloproteinase inhibitor batimastat on breast cancer regrowth and metastasis in athymic mice. *J Natl Cancer Inst* 1995; **87**:1546–50.

106. Sledge G, Qulali M, Bone E et al, Combination matrix metalloproteinase inhibition in an athymic mouse xenograft model of human breast cancer metastasis. *Proc Am Assoc Cancer Res* 1996; **37**:A639.

107. Wojtowicz-Praga S, Torri J, Johnson M et al, Phase I trial of Marimastat, a novel matrix metalloproteinase inhibitor, administered orally to patients with advanced lung cancer. *J Clin Oncol* 1998; **16**:2150–6.

108. Miller K, Gradishar W, Schuchter L et al, A randomized phase II pilot trial of adjuvant marimastat in patients with early stage breast cancer. *Proc Am Soc Clin Oncol* 2000; in press.

109. D'Olimpio J, Hande K, Collier M et al, Phase I study of the matrix metalloprotease inhibitor AG3340 in combination with paclitaxel and carboplatin for the treatment of patients with advanced solid tumors. *Proc Am Soc Clin Oncol* 1999; **18**:160a.

110. Tolcher A, Rowinsky E, Rizzo J et al, A phase I and pharmacokinetic study of the oral matrix metalloproteinase inhibitor Bayer 12-9566 in combination with paclitaxel and carboplatin. *Proc Am Soc Clin Oncol* 1999; **18**:160a.

111. Warren RS, Yuan H, Matli MR et al, Regulation by vascular endothelial growth factor of human colon cancer tumorigenesis in a mouse model of experimental liver metastasis. *J Clin Invest* 1995; **95**:1789–97.

112. Kim KJ, Li B, Winer J et al, Inhibition of vascular endothelial growth factor-induced angiogenesis suppresses tumour growth in vivo. *Nature* 1993; **362**:841–4.

113. Gordon M, Talpaz M, Margolin K et al, Phase I trial of recombinant humanized monoclonal anti-vascular endothelial growth factor (anti-VEGF Mab) in patients with metastatic cancer. *Proc Am Soc Clin Oncol* 1998; **17**:210a.

114. Sledge G, Miller K, Novotny W et al, A phase II trial of single-agent rhuMAb VEGF (recombinant humanized monoclonal antibody to vascular endothelial cell growth factor) in patients with relapsed metastatic breast cancer. *Proc Am Soc Clin Oncol* 2000; in press.

115. Millauer B, Longhi MP, Plate KH et al, Dominant-negative inhibition of Flk-1 suppresses the growth of many tumor types in vivo. *Cancer Res* 1996; **56**:1615–20.

116. Fong TA, Shawver LK, Sun L et al, SU5416 is a potent and selective inhibitor of the vascular endothelial growth factor receptor (Flk-1/KDR) that inhibits tyrosine kinase catalysis, tumor vascularization, and growth of multiple tumor types. *Cancer Res* 1999; **59**:99–106.

117. Shaheen R, Davis D, Liu W et al, Antiangiogenic therapy targeting the tyrosine kinase

receptor for vascular endothelial growth factor receptor inhibits the growth of liver metastasis and induces tumor and endothelial cell apoptosis. *Cancer Res* 1999; **59**:5412–16.

118. Rosen L, Kabbinavar F, Rosen P et al, Phase I trial of SU5416, a novel angiogenesis inhibitor in patients with advanced malignancies. *Proc Am Soc Clin Oncol* 1998; **17**:218a.

119. Rosen L, Mulay M, Mayers A et al, Phase I dose-escalating trial of SU5416, a novel angiogenesis inhibitor in patients with advanced malignancies. *Proc Am Soc Clin Oncol* 1999; **18**:161a.

120. Klohs WD, Hamby JM, Antiangiogenic agents [In Process Citation]. *Curr Opin Biotechnol* 1999; **10**:544–9.

121. Shaheen RM, Davis DW, Liu W et al, Antiangiogenic therapy targeting the tyrosine kinase receptor for vascular endothelial growth factor receptor inhibits the growth of colon cancer liver metastasis and induces tumor and endothelial cell apoptosis. *Cancer Res* 1999; **59**:5412–16.

122. Ciomei M, Pastori W, Mariani M et al, New sulfonated distamycin A derivatives with bFGF complexing activity. *Biochem Pharmacol* 1994; **47**:295–302.

123. Zamai M, Caiolfa VR, Pines D et al, Nature of interaction between basic fibroblast growth factor and the antiangiogenic drug 7,7-(carbonyl-bis[imino-N-methyl-4,2-pyrrolecarbonylimino[N-methyl-4,2-pyrrole]-carbonylimino]) bis-(1,3-naphthalene disulfonate). *Biophys J* 1998; **75**:672–82.

124. Sola F, Capolongo L, Moneta D et al, The antitumor efficacy of cytotoxic drugs is potentiated by treatment with PNU 145156E, a growth-factor-complexing molecule. *Cancer Chemother Pharmacol* 1999; **43**:241–6.

125. deVries E, Groen H, Wynendaele W et al, PNU-145156E – a novel angiogenesis inhibitor in patients with solid tumors: an update of a phase I and pharmacokinetic study. *Proc Am Soc Clin Oncol* 1999; **18**:161a.

126. Brooks PC, Clark RA, Cheresh DA, Require-ment of vascular integrin alpha v beta 3 for angiogenesis. *Science* 1994; **264**:569–71.

127. Brooks PC, Silletti S, von Schalscha TL et al, Disruption of angiogenesis by PEX, a non-catalytic metalloproteinase fragment with integrin binding activity. *Cell* 1998; **92**:391–400.

128. Friedlander M, Theesfeld C, Sugita M et al, Involvement of integrins avb3 and avb5 in ocular neovascular disease. *Proc Natl Acad Sci USA* 1996; **93**:9764–9.

129. Brooks PC, Montgomery AM, Rosenfeld M et al, Integrin alpha v beta 3 antagonists promote tumor regression by inducing apoptosis of angiogenic blood vessels. *Cell* 1994; **79**: 1157–64.

130. Brooks PC, Stromblad S, Klemke R et al, Anti-integrin alpha v beta 3 blocks human breast cancer growth and angiogenesis in human skin [see comments]. *J Clin Invest* 1995; **96**:1815–22.

131. Gutheil J, Campbell T, Pierce J et al, Phase I study of vitaxin, an anti-angiogenic humanized monoclonal antibody to vascular integrin $\alpha v\beta 3$. *Proc Am Soc Clin Oncol* 1998; **17**:215a.

132. Cheresh D, Spiro R, Biosynthetic and functional properties of an Arg-Gly-Asp directed receptor involved in human melanoma cell attachment to vitronectin. *J Biol Chem* 1987; **262**:17703–11.

133. Thorpe PE, Burrows FJ, Antibody-directed targeting of the vasculature of solid tumors [see comments]. *Breast Cancer Res Treat* 1995; **36**:237–51.

134. Burrows FJ, Derbyshire EJ, Tazzari PL et al, Up-regulation of endoglin on vascular endothelial cells in human solid tumors: implications for diagnosis and therapy. *Clin Cancer Res* 1995; **1**:1623–34.

135. Seon B, Matsuno F, Haruto Y et al, Long-lasting complete inhibition of human solid tumors in SCID mice by targeting endothelial cells of tumor vasculature with antihuman endoglin immunotoxin. *Clin Cancer Res* 1997; **3**:1031–44.

136. Matsuno F, Haruto Y, Kondo M et al, Induc-

tion of lasting complete regression of pre-formed distinct solid tumors by targeting the tumor vasculature using two new anti-endoglin monoclonal antibodies. *Clin Cancer Res* 1999; **5**:371–82.

137. McLeskey SW, Zhang L, Trock BJ et al, Effects of AGM-1470 and pentosan polysulphate on tumorigenicity and metastasis of FGF-transfected MCF-7 cells. *Br J Cancer* 1996; **73**: 1053–62.

138. Sasaki A, Alcalde RE, Nishiyama A et al, Angiogenesis inhibitor TNP-470 inhibits human breast cancer osteolytic bone metastasis in nude mice through the reduction of bone reception. *Cancer Res* 1998; **58**:462–7.

139. Singh Y, Shikata N, Kiyozuka Y et al, Inhibition of tumor growth and metastasis by angiogenesis inhibitor TNP-470 on breast cancer cell lines in vitro and in vivo. *Breast Cancer Res Treat* 1997; **45**:15–27.

140. Fisher B, Saffer E, Rudock C et al, Presence of a growth stimulating factor in serum following primary tumor removal in mice. *Cancer Res* 1989; **49**:1996–2001.

141. Fisher B, Gunduz N, Saffer EA, Influence of the interval between primary tumor removal and chemotherapy on kinetics and growth of metastases. *Cancer Res* 1983; **43**:1488–92.

142. Simpson-Herren L, Sanford AH, Holmquist JP, Effects of surgery on the cell kinetics of residual tumor. *Cancer Treat Rep* 1976; **60**: 1749–60.

143. O'Reilly MS, Holmgren L, Shing Y et al, Angiostatin: a novel angiogenesis inhibitor that mediates the suppression of metastases by a Lewis lung carcinoma [see comments]. *Cell* 1994; **79**:315–28.

144. O'Reilly MS, Holmgren L, Chen C et al, Angiostatin induces and sustains dormancy of human primary tumors in mice. *Nat Med* 1996; **2**:689–92.

145. Griscelli F, Li H, Bennaceur-Griscelli A et al, Angiostatin gene transfer: inhibition of tumor growth in vivo by blockage of endothelial cell proliferation associated with a mitosis arrest.

Proc Natl Acad Sci USA 1998; **95**:6367–72.

146. Gorski DH, Mauceri HJ, Salloum RM et al, Potentiation of the antitumour effect of ionizing radiation by brief concomitant exposures to angiostatin. *Cancer Res* 1998; **58**:5686–9.

147. O'Reilly MS, Boehm T, Shing Y et al, Endostatin: an endogenous inhibitor of angiogenesis and tumor growth. *Cell* 1997; **88**:277–85.

148. Hohenester E, Sasaki T, Olsen BR et al, Crystal structure of the angiogenesis inhibitor endostatin at 1.5 A resolution. *EMBO J* 1998; **17**: 1656–64.

149. Boehm T, Folkman J, Browder T et al, Antiangiogenic therapy of experimental cancer does not induce acquired drug resistance [see comments]. *Nature* 1997; **390**:404–7.

150. Attalla H, Makela TP, Adlercreutz H et al, 2-Methoxyestradiol arrests cells in mitosis without depolymerizing tubulin. *Biochem Biophys Res Commun* 1996; **228**:467–73.

151. Fotsis T, Zhang Y, Pepper MS et al, The endogenous oestrogen metabolite 2-methoxyoestradiol inhibits angiogenesis and suppresses tumour growth. *Nature* 1994; **368**: 237–9.

152. Klauber N, Parangi S, Flynn F et al, Inhibition of angiogenesis and breast cancer in mice by the microtubule inhibitors 2-methoxyestradiol and Taxol. *Cancer Res* 1997; **57**:81–6.

153. Schumacher G, Kataoka M, Roth J et al, Potent antitumor activity of 2-methoxyestradiol in human pancreatic cancer cell lines. *Clin Cancer Res* 1999; **5**:493–9.

154. Yue TL, Wang X, Louden CS et al, 2-Methoxyestradiol, an endogenous estrogen metabolite, induces apoptosis in endothelial cells and inhibits angiogenesis: possible role for stress-activated protein kinase signaling pathway and Fas expression. *Mol Pharmacol* 1997; **51**:951–62.

155. Reiser F, Way D, Bernas M et al, Inhibition of normal and experimental angiotumor endothelial cell proliferation and cell cycle progression by 2-methoxyestradiol. *Proc Soc Exp Biol Med* 1998; **219**:211–16.

156. Walker RA, Dearing SJ, Transforming growth factor beta 1 in ductal carcinoma in situ and invasive carcinomas of the breast. *Eur J Cancer* 1992; **28**:641–4.

157. de Jong JS, van Diest PJ, van der Valk P et al, Expression of growth factors, growth-inhibiting factors, and their receptors in invasive breast cancer. II: Correlations with proliferation and angiogenesis. *J Pathol* 1998; **184**:53–7.

158. Piccoli R, Olson KA, Vallee BL et al, Chimeric anti-angiogenin antibody cAb 26-2F inhibits the formation of human breast cancer xenografts in athymic mice. *Proc Natl Acad Sci USA* 1998; **95**:4579–83.

159. Fox SB, Engels K, Comley M et al, Relationship of elevated tumour thymidine phosphorylase in node-positive breast carcinomas to the effects of adjuvant CMF. *Ann Oncol* 1997; **8**:271–5.

160. Engels K, Fox SB, Whitehouse RM et al, Up-regulation of thymidine phosphorylase expression is associated with a discrete pattern of angiogenesis in ductal carcinomas in situ of the breast. *J Pathol* 1997; **182**:414–20.

161. Koblizek TI, Weiss C, Yancopoulos GD et al, Angiopoietin-1 induces sprouting angiogenesis in vitro. *Curr Biol* 1998; **8**:529–32.

162. Suri C, Jones PF, Patan S et al, Requisite role of angiopoietin-1, a ligand for the TIE2 receptor, during embryonic angiogenesis [see comments]. *Cell* 1996; **87**:1171–80.

163. Guo NH, Krutzsch HC, Inman JK et al, Antiproliferative and antitumor activities of D-reverse peptides derived from the second type-1 repeat of thrombospondin-1. *J Pept Res* 1997; **50**:210–21.

164. Wang TN, Qian XH, Granick MS et al, Inhibition of breast cancer progression by an antibody to a thrombospondin-1 receptor. *Surgery* 1996; **120**:449–54.

165. Soncin F, Shapiro R, Fett JW, A cell-surface proteoglycan mediates human adenocarcinoma HT-29 cell adhesion to human angiogenin. *J Biol Chem* 1994; **269**:8999–9005.

166. Maisonpierre PC, Suri C, Jones PF et al, Angiopoietin-2, a natural antagonist for Tie2 that disrupts in vivo angiogenesis [see comments]. *Science* 1997; **277**:55–60.

167. Fortier AH, Nelson BJ, Grella DK et al, Antiangiogenic activity of prostate-specific antigen. *J Natl Cancer Inst* 1999; **91**:1635–40.

168. Heidtmann HH, Nettelbeck DM, Mingels A et al, Generation of angiostatin-like fragments from plasminogen by prostate-specific antigen. *Br J Cancer* 1999; **81**:1269–73.

SECTION 5: Special Issues in Surgical Treatment

Section Editor: EP Mamounas

20

Historical perspective and present and future challenges

Eleftherios P Mamounas

EVOLUTION IN BREAST CANCER UNDERSTANDING AND MANAGEMENT

During the last quarter of the twentieth century, the surgical management of breast cancer has undergone significant evolution as a result of the profound changes that have occurred in the biological understanding and clinical presentation of the disease. The postulation of an alternative hypothesis of tumor disemination challenged the previously accepted halsteadian principles that had governed the surgical management of the disease up to that time.[1] This hypothesis was supported by results from randomized clinical trials demonstrating that the extent of surgical resection did not significantly impact on patient outcome.[2-5] Based on results from several such trials, the radical procedures, developed at the turn of the century, were abandoned and replaced by those conserving the breast. The alternative hypothesis was further supported by results from clinical trials indicating that the administration of systemic therapy improves the disease-free and overall survival of patients with early stage breast cancer.[6-8] As a result, systemic therapy – either as adjuvant chemotherapy, adjuvant hormonal therapy or a combination of both – is currently recommended for most such patients.

Challenges of the alternative hypothesis have recently been mounted.[9,10] The 'oligometastases' hypothesis was formulated as a result of clinical data indicating excellent prognosis in patients with small breast cancers treated with locoregional therapy only. This hypothesis was further supported by more recent clinical data indicating an improvement in outcome with more extensive locoregional therapy (postmastectomy locoregional radiotherapy) in patients who have received adequate systemic chemotherapy.[11,12] According to the 'oligometastases' hypothesis, breast cancer is – in some cases – still a locoregional disease at the time of diagnosis. In those cases, persistent disease locally or regionally after treatment may give rise to distant metastases, and therefore locoregional therapy is important.

The weakness of the hypothesis is that there is no proposed method of determining which patients have just locoregional disease and which already have systemic micrometastases. Furthermore, with the development of new, sensitive, immunohistochemical techniques that detect tumor cells in bone marrow and peripheral blood, there is mounting evidence confirming that most patients with invasive breast cancer have tumor cells present systemically at the time of diagnosis.[13-15] Thus, as we enter the next century, the systemic hypothesis still remains the one in accordance with most of the clinical and experimental data regarding breast cancer behavior. Technologic advancements in the molecular level are now beginning to provide us with a better understanding of the biologic profile and – as a result – clinical behavior of the breast cancer cell. In the future, this detailed 'molecular mapping' will ultimately determine in which patients the micrometastatic tumor cells will eventually grow to form overt metastases and in which they will be destroyed by the host and/or appropriate systemic therapy. As a result, a new series of hypotheses will be formulated that will govern breast cancer understanding and management into the next millennium.

NEW SURGICAL QUESTIONS AND CHALLENGES

The development and widespread use of mammography during the last quarter of the century have had a dramatic impact on the clinical presentation and, consequently, on management of breast cancer. As more breast cancers are found at an earlier stage, the percentage of patients who present with axillary nodal involvement is constantly decreasing. Thus, more axillary dissections are currently performed in patients with negative nodes, making it imperative to develop new methods that allow less invasive staging and avoid the morbidity of an axillary dissection. The demonstration of validity of the sentinel node concept in breast cancer[16-20] has created a great deal of enthusiasm for establishing sentinel node biopsy as the preferred method of axillary staging. However, along with the enthusiasm come significant new questions and challenges that will need to be addressed as this method gains popularity. These will be reviewed in detail in Chapter 21.

With the establishment of breast-conserving surgery as the surgical treatment of choice for most stage I and II breast cancer patients, and with the demonstration of benefit from systemic chemotherapy administration, the question arose of whether, by administering systemic chemotherapy before surgical removal, one might be able – by decreasing primary tumor size – to allow patients, who would otherwise require a mastectomy, to undergo breast-conserving surgery. More importantly, biologic hypotheses regarding the relationship of the primary tumor and micrometastatic disease had been formulated and required testing in the clinical setting.[21-24] As a result of the biologic and clinical rationale for evaluating preoperative chemotherapy, nonrandomized and randomized trials were conducted in the 1980s which eventually established the worth of this approach.[25-34] Although a disease-free survival or overall survival was not demonstrated by administering chemotherapy in the preoperative (neoadjuvant) setting when compared with the standard adjuvant approach,[33,34] neoadjuvant chemotherapy may offer some advantages from both a clinical and a biologic standpoint.[35] The decrease in primary tumor size with preoperative chemotherapy has resulted in the performance of more breast-conserving procedures.[26,31-33] More importantly, a correlation between primary tumor response and long-term outcome has been demonstrated in several prospective studies,[26,32,33] making tumor response an important intermediate end-point for use in clinical trials evaluating new agents or new regimens. As a result of the expansive use of preoperative chemotherapy, a number of surgical issues and questions have surfaced that relate to the surgical management of both primary breast tumors and axillary lymph nodes. These will also be reviewed in detail in Chapter 22.

In this section, rather than revisiting in detail the historical evolution of breast cancer surgery during the twentieth century, we concentrate on new surgical questions that have surfaced during the past few years, and the challenges that they will pose in the years to come.

REFERENCES

1. Fisher B, Laboratory and clinical research in breast cancer – a personal adventure: the David A. Karnofsky Memorial Lecture. *Cancer Res* 1980; **40**:3863–74.

2. Fisher B, Redmond C, Fisher E et al, Ten-year results of a randomized clinical trial comparing radical mastectomy and total mastectomy with or without radiation. *N Engl J Med* 1985; **312**:674–81.

3. Fisher B, Redmond C, Poisson R et al, Eight-year results of a randomized clinical trial comparing total mastectomy and lumpectomy with or without irradiation in the treatment of breast cancer. *N Engl J Med* 1989; **320**:822–8.

4. Fisher B, Anderson S, Redmond C et al, Reanalysis and results after 12 years of follow-up in a randomized clinical trial comparing total mastectomy with lumpectomy with or without irradiation in the treatment of breast cancer. *N Engl J Med* 1995; **333**:1456–61.

5. Early Breast Cancer Trialists' Collaborative Group, Effects of radiotherapy and surgery in early breast cancer: An overview of the randomized trials. *N Engl J Med* 1995; **333**: 1444–55.

6. Early Breast Cancer Trialists' Collaborative Group, Systemic treatment of early breast cancer by hormonal, cytotoxic, or immune therapy: 33 randomised trials involving 31,000 recurrences and 24,000 deaths among 75,000 women. *Lancet* 1992; **339**:1–15.

7. Early Breast Cancer Trialists' Collaborative Group, Systemic treatment of early breast cancer by hormonal, cytotoxic, or immune therapy: 33 randomised trials involving 31,000 recurrences and 24,000 deaths among 75,000 women. *Lancet* 1992; **339**:71–85.

8. Early Breast Cancer Trialists' Collaborative Group, Tamoxifen for early breast cancer: an overview of the randomized trials. *Lancet* 1998; **351**:1451–67.

9. Hellman S, Natural history of small breast cancers. *J Clin Oncol* 1994; **12**:2229–34.

10. Hellman S, Stopping metastases at their source. *N Engl J Med* 1997; **337**:996–7.

11. Overgaard M, Hansen PS, Overgaard J et al, Postoperative radiotherapy in high-risk premenopausal women with breast cancer who receive adjuvant chemotherapy. *N Engl J Med* 1997; **337**:949–95.

12. Ragaz J, Jackson S, Le N et al, Adjuvant radiotherapy and chemotherapy in node-positive premenopausal women with breast cancer. *N Engl J Med* 1997; **337**:956–62.

13. Krag DN, Ashikaga T, Moss TJ et al, Breast cancer cells in the blood: A pilot study. *Breast J* 1999; **5**:354–8.

14. Naume B, Borgen E, Beiske K et al, Immuno-magnetic techniques for the enrichment and detection of isolated breast carcinoma cells in the bone marrow and peripheral blood. *J Hematother* 1997; **6**:103–14.

15. Diel IJ, Kaufmann M, Costa SD et al, Micrometastatic breast cancer cells in bone marrow at primary surgery: prognostic value in comparison with nodal status. *J Natl Cancer Inst* 1996; **88**:1652–8.

16. Krag D, Weaver D, Ashikaga T et al, The sentinel node in breast cancer: A multicenter validation study. *N Engl J Med* 1998; **339**:941–6.

17. Veronesi U, Paganelli G, Galimberti V et al, Sentinel node biopsy to avoid axillary dissection in breast cancer with clinically negative nodes. *Lancet* 1997; **349**:1864–7.

18. Giuliano AE, Kirgan DM, Guenther JM et al, Lymphatic mapping and sentinel lymphadenectomy for breast cancer. *Ann Surg* 1994; **220**:391–8.

19. Giuliano AE, Jones RC, Brennan M et al, Sentinel lymphadenectomy in breast cancer. *J Clin Oncol* 1997; **15**:2345–50.

20. Albertini JJ, Lyman GH, Cox C et al, Lymphatic mapping and sentinel node biopsy in

the patient with breast cancer. *JAMA* 1996; 276:1818–22.

21. Skipper HE, Kinetics of mammary tumor cell growth and implications for therapy. *Cancer* 1971; 28:1479–99.

22. Goldie JH, Coldman AJ, A mathematical model for relating the drug sensitivity of tumors to their spontaneous mutation rate. *Cancer Treat Rep* 1979; 63:1727–33.

23. Gunduz N, Fisher B, Saffer EA, Effect of surgical removal on the growth and kinetics of residual tumor. *Cancer Res* 1979; 39:3861–5.

24. Fisher B, Gunduz N, Saffer EA, Influence of the interval between primary tumor removal and chemotherapy on kinetics and growth of metastases. *Cancer Res* 1983; 43:1488–92.

25. Jacquillat C, Weil M, Baillet F et al, Results of neoadjuvant chemotherapy and radiation therapy in breast conserving treatment of 250 patients with all stages of infiltrative breast cancer. *Cancer* 1990; 66:119–29.

26. Bonadonna G, Veronesi U, Brambilla C et al, Primary chemotherapy to avoid mastectomy in tumors with diameters of three centimeters or more. *J Natl Cancer Inst* 1990; 82:1539–45.

27. Tubiana-Hulin M, Malek M, Briffod M et al, Preoperative chemotherapy of operable breast cancer, (stage IIIA). Prognostic factors of distant recurrence. *Eur J Cancer* 1993; 29A(suppl 6):S76.

28. Belembaogo E, Feillel V, Chollet P et al, Neoadjuvant chemotherapy in 126 operable breast cancers. *Eur J Cancer* 1992; 28A: 896–900.

29. Smith IE, Jones AL, O'Brien MER et al, Primary medical (neo-adjuvant) chemotherapy for operable breast cancer. *Eur J Cancer* 1993; 29A:1796–9.

30. Mauriac L, Durand M, Avril A, Dilhuydy J-M, Effects on primary chemotherapy in conservative treatment of breast cancer patients with operable tumors larger than 3 cm. *Ann Oncol* 1991; 2:347–54.

31. Scholl SM, Fourquet A, Asselain B et al, Neoadjuvant versus adjuvant chemotherapy in premenopausal patients with tumours considered too large for breast conserving surgery: preliminary results of a randomized trial. *Eur J Cancer* 1994; 30(suppl 6):645–52.

32. Powles TJ, Hickish TF, Makris A et al, Randomized trial of chemoendocrine therapy started before or after surgery for treatment of primary breast cancer. *J Clin Oncol* 1995; 13:547–52.

33. Fisher B, Brown A, Mamounas E et al, Effect of preoperative chemotherapy of local-regional disease in women with operable breast cancer: findings from National Surgical Adjuvant Breast and Bowel Project B-18. *J Clin Oncol* 1997; 15:2483–93.

34. Fisher B, Bryant J, Wolmark N et al, Effect of preoperative chemotherapy on the outcome of women with operable breast cancer. *J Clin Oncol* 1998; 16:2672–85.

35. Fisher B, Mamounas EP, Preoperative chemotherapy: a model for studying the biology and therapy of primary breast cancer. *J Clin Oncol* 1995; 13:537–40.

21

Should surgeons abandon routine axillary dissection for sentinel node biopsy in early breast cancer?

Frederick L Moffat, David N Krag

Regional lymph node status is the most significant pathologic determinant of prognosis in early carcinoma of the breast. Patients with axillary node metastases are at much higher risk of distant metastasis and breast cancer mortality than pathologic node-negative (pN-negative) patients, especially those with small primary tumors.[1] Postoperative adjuvant systemic therapy significantly reduces the risk of development of systemic disease and death in pathologic node-positive (pN-positive) patients. Although pN-negative patients also benefit from adjuvant systemic therapy, the regimens used often differ from those employed for pN-positive disease. The number of positive nodes is considered by many medical oncologists in the selection of systemic adjuvant therapy in individual patients. Detailed information on the tumor status of the regional lymphatics can therefore be very important in clinical decision-making in early breast cancer, and is frequently a prerequisite for entry into trials sponsored by the National Cancer Institute (NCI) and other clinical trials.

There is a great deal of enthusiasm among general and oncologic surgeons for sentinel lymph-node biopsy (SLNB), a term that encompasses several technical variations on a new, minimally invasive, surgical procedure for nodal staging of cancer. SLNB was brought to the attention of the surgical community at large by Morton et al,[2] who demonstrated that the first node(s) to receive lymph flow (and therefore metastasizing malignant cells) from a primary melanoma can be identified by peritumoral intradermal injection of vital blue dye. Blue-stained lymphatic vessels were visualized through an incision made in the skin overlying the lymph node basin(s) at risk, and dissected to one or more blue-stained sentinel lymph nodes (SLNs). SLNB was performed in 223 patients and completion lymphadenectomy was immediately performed in all cases for comparison of the histopathology of the SLN(s) to that of the lymph-node basin at risk. In all but two SLNBs, the status of the SLNs reflected that of the regional nodal basin. As there were 40 pN-positive nodal basins among these 223 patients, the false-negative (FN) rate for the SLNBs in this series was no higher than 5%.

Since that landmark paper, a wealth of published data has affirmed the validity of the sentinel lymph-node hypothesis in melanoma patients. Interestingly, in only two other reports[3,4] was confirmatory lymphadenectomy performed with SLNB. Nevertheless, a consensus has been reached that, in the hands of experienced surgeons, SLNB in patients with clinical node-negative (cN-negative) melanoma is superior to either of the conventional options, these being observation alone or elective lymphadenectomy of at-risk nodal basins. This conclusion is currently valid only for melanoma, a disease in which occult nodal metastases almost invariably progress if left undisturbed and these metastases are highly prejudicial to cure and survival. Melanoma metastases to regional nodes are 'instigators' as well as 'indicators' or markers of risk of disseminated disease and cancer mortality.

Alex et al[5] and Krag et al[6] described a method of SLNB in which a radiolabeled colloid, technetium-99m sulfur colloid (^{99m}TcSC), was used as the SLN marking agent and SLNB was performed using a γ detection probe (GDP) to guide dissection directly to the SLN(s) by the shortest route from the overlying skin. A cutaneous 'hot spot' denoting an underlying SLN was identified using the GDP, and SLNB was performed through an incision made at that point.

Krag et al[6] and Alex and Krag[7] were the first to describe SLNB in breast cancer using this technique. Of 70 consecutive patients in whom SLNB and immediate axillary node dissection (AND) were performed, 21 proved to be pN positive. In none of these was SLNB falsely negative. This and a number of other pilot studies, in which blue dye, radiolabeled colloids or both were used as node-labeling agents, demonstrated that SLNs could be localized in 65–95% of patients with cN-negative breast cancer.

EVIDENCE OF EFFICACY OF SLNB IN BREAST CANCER

To date only one NCI-sponsored, prospective, multicenter study of SLNB with confirmatory AND in breast cancer patients has been published.[8] Numerous single institution studies of SLNB in breast cancer patients using a variety of SLNB methodologies are now in print (Table 21.1). There are also many reports on methodological variables such as type of radiolabeled colloid, volume of radiolabeled colloid injectate, route of radiocolloid or blue dye injection (peritumoral/intraparenchymal, subdermal, intradermal) and time dependence of the various methods.[30]

Faced with a rapidly expanding literature on SLNB in breast cancer, in which the results and conclusions are significantly more variable than those in melanoma, surgeons understandably have mixed opinions about whether SLNB is sufficiently well developed and studied to permit its safe substitution for routine AND in clinical practice.

The University of Vermont Multicenter Validation Study

Krag et al[8] recently reported the results of this NCI-sponsored prospective multicenter trial of SLNB in cN-negative unifocal invasive breast cancer, the only study of its kind on SLNB in breast cancer that is currently in print. Eleven surgeons in academic and community practice participated in this trial. All patients underwent SLNB using 1 mCi unfiltered ^{99m}TcSC in 4 ml physiological saline injected peritumorally, and confirmatory AND was performed in all patients. Preoperative lymphoscintigraphy (LS) was not mandatory and blue dye was not used.

Of the 443 patients accrued, at least one cutaneous hot spot was localized in 413 patients (93.2%), and 114 patients proved to be pN-positive. SLNs were found outside the axilla (primarily in the internal mammary chain) in 8% of cases, and in 3% of all patients from whom one or more SLNs were removed the positive SLNs were exclusively non-axillary in location. The accuracy of the histologic status of SLNs compared with the status of the axillary nodes was 97%, and the negative predictive value of SLNB

Table 21.1 Single institution experience with SLNB in breast cancer

	No. of patients	No. of pN-positives	SLN Localized (%)	NPV (%)	FN rate (%)
Blue dye only					
Giuliano et al[9]	174	62	66	94	11.9
Giuliano et al[10]	114	25	64	96	8.0
Giuliano et al[11]	107	42	93	100	0
Guenther et al[12]	145	31	71	96	9.7
Flett et al[13]	68	21	82	94	14.3
Radiolabeled colloid/GDP only					
Alex and Krag[7]	70	21	71	100	0
Veronesi[a] et al[14]	163	85	98	95	4.7
Roumen et al[15]	68	23	69	97	4.3
Borgstein et al[16]	104	45	94	98	2.2
Crossin et al[17]	50	8	84	97	12.5
Miner et al[18]	42	7	98	97	14.3
Snider et al[19]	80	14	88	93	7.0
Rubio et al[20]	55	17	96	95	11.8
Moffat et al[21]	70	20	89	96	10.0
Offodile et al[22]	41	18	98	100	0
Veronesi[a] et al[23]	376	168	99	94	6.7
Both methods					
Albertini et al[24]	62	18	92	100	0
Reintgen et al[25]	174	38	92	99	2.6
Barnwell et al[26]	42	15	90	100	0
Nwariaku et al[27]	119	27	81	99	3.7
O'Hea et al[28]	60	20	93	93	15.0
Hill et al[29]	104	47	92	92	10.6

[a] Subdermal injection of radiolabeled colloid (all other series were intraparenchymal/peritumoral).
SLN, sentinel lymph node; SLNB, sentinel lymph-node biopsy; pN, pathologic node; NPV, negative predictive value; FN, false-negative.

was similarly favorable at 96%. However, among the 114 pN-positive patients, the SLNs were negative for tumor in 13, an FN rate of 11.4%. There was marked variation in the FN rates of individual surgeons, ranging from 0% to 28.6%. Although this variance did not reach statistical significance, it is nevertheless clinically important. Limitations in the methodology accounted for much of the discrepancy in FN rates between surgeons (see over).

Factors predictive of failure to find a cutaneous hot spot were age over 50 years (reduced radiolabeled colloid labeling caused by atrophy and fatty replacement of nodal parenchyma), prior excisional rather than incisional or core biopsy of the primary cancer (greater disruption of local lymphatics) and medial situation of the primary cancer. All 13 patients with FN SLNBs had laterally situated cancers ($p = 0.004$). These false negatives occurred because of proximity to the axilla of the radioactive diffusion zone in the breast, resulting from the intraparenchymal peritumoral injection of ^{99m}TcSC.

The radiolabeled colloid diffusion zone in the breast significantly interferes with GDP localization of all SLNs,[21,31] and is almost certainly an important factor in between-surgeon variation in FN rates. This diffusion zone, the size of which can vary markedly between patients, is a significant factor in the surgical learning curve and FN rates. Nevertheless, SLN localization rates in this study and in single institution series in which radiolabeled colloid/GDP methods are used often exceed 90%.

The National Surgical Adjuvant Breast and Bowel Project (NSABP) is sponsoring the B-32 protocol, a prospective randomized trial of SLNB plus AND versus SLNB alone, based on results of the Vermont study. Isosulfan blue dye will be used in addition to radiolabeled colloid, the blue dye being injected around the primary tumor intraoperatively because SLN labeling with this marker is very time dependent, unlike unfiltered ^{99m}TcSC. The use of blue dye will add a second lymph-node-marking agent which is not sensitive to the high radiation background produced by radiolabeled colloid injection at the primary tumor site.

Single institution series in which confirmatory AND was performed

The surgical learning curve is much longer when vital blue dye is used alone compared with radiolabeled colloid methods with or without blue dye. Moreover, the dissection required to find blue-labeled nodes is much more extensive without the aid of a GDP, because the dissection must trace blue-stained lymph vessels back toward the injection zone as well as to SLNs, to ensure that any SLNs situated between the SLNB incision and the primary tumor are identified. The extent of dissection may occasionally approach that of AND.

In addition, localization rates tend to be lower when vital blue dye is used alone, ranging from 64% to 93%. By comparison, the localization rates for radiolabeled colloid/GDP methods range from 71% to 99% and, for both methods used in combination, 81–100% (see Table 21.1).

Until recently, most single institution series have cited negative predictive value (NPV) when discussing the diagnostic efficacy of SLNB. The reported NPV for SLNB ranges from 94% to 100% when blue dye is used alone, from 93% to 100% for radiolabeled colloid alone, and from 93% to 100% when both radiolabeled colloid and blue dye are used (see Table 21.1).

On the face of it, these are highly impressive numbers, but a closer look reveals the deficiency in this approach. NPV is defined as the number of true negatives divided by the sum of true negatives and false negatives. Given that 20–30% of the current breast cancer patient population is pN positive, if every SLNB were false negative in every patient the NPV could still be as high as 80%! A far more useful statistic is the FN rate, calculated as the number of false negatives divided by the sum of false negatives and true positives.

The SLNB FN rates vary considerably irrespective of the method used, and no method has an advantage over any other with respect to this very important statistic. For radiolabeled colloid/GDP methods used alone, blue dye alone and both nodal markers used in combination, FN rates were in the ranges 0–14.3%, 0–14.3% and 0–15%, respectively (see Table 22.1). This between-series variation mirrors the between-surgeon variability observed in the Vermont trial and, as with the Vermont trial, bespeaks a number of technical challenges with current methods of SLNB rather than significant differences in expertise between surgeons.

Single institution studies in which AND was not routinely performed

There are a few recent series reporting SLNB in breast cancer without confirmatory AND in most of the patients reported on.[25,29,32,33] These are from large academic institutions that have invested considerable time and resources into developing SLNB for use in breast cancer. For the most part, these series consist of large numbers of patients operated upon consecutively by several surgeons in the institution. At varying times in the course of accruing the studied patients, a number of variables such as type of radiolabeled colloid, route of radiolabeled colloid administration, type of GDP, etc. have been changed.

A number of guidelines and principles have been gleaned from these experiences, which may be of value to surgeons as they begin to learn how to do SLNB and acquire experience with this procedure.

The very low FN rates reported in some of these series, although calculated from only a subset of the patients studied, are a credit to the participating surgeons and institutions. It is unclear whether surgeons with less background, commitment or institutional resources will have the same uniformly high rates of success. The results of these series fall well short of convincing evidence that SLNB should now replace AND in the management of breast cancer.

ONGOING METHODOLOGICAL DEVELOPMENTS IN SLNB FOR BREAST CANCER

SLNB is technically more challenging in breast cancer than in melanoma, as noted above. The amount of dissection required when blue dye is used alone can be excessive, and the radioactive diffusion zone that results from intraparenchymal peritumoral injection of radiolabeled colloid interferes significantly with GDP localization of some or all SLNs in individual patients.

A rapidly increasing number of communications in the peer-reviewed literature are focused on technical issues and modifications of existing methods.[30] For example, Krag et al[31,34] and Linehan et al[35] demonstrated SLN localization rates with unfiltered compared with filtered ^{99m}TcSC. Krag et al[31,34] have shown that the size of the radioactive diffusion zone does not vary significantly for volumes of radiolabeled colloid injectate about 4 ml, but larger volumes do improve SLN localization rates.

Alternative routes of radiocolloid administration are being investigated. Borgstein et al[36] tested the hypothesis that the skin and parenchyma of the breast drain by the same lymphatic pathways to one or more common SLNs. In 30 consecutive patients, intradermally injected blue dye and peritumorally injected ^{99m}Tc-labeled colloidal albumin labeled the same lymph node(s). Other pilot studies have yielded similar results and excellent SLN localization rates. Intradermal, subdermal and periareolar routes of injection avoid the problem of inadvertent injection of radiolabeled colloid into the underlying pectoralis muscle or into breast biopsy cavities. With their expertise in radiolabeled colloid injection and lymphoscintigraphy in melanoma, nuclear medicine physicians are more comfortable with these routes of administration. Moreover, the size of the diffusion zone at the injection site is much smaller, which may facilitate superior SLN localization and reduced FN rates.

However, there is concern that the subdermal, intradermal or subareolar routes of radiolabeled colloid injection may significantly underestimate the incidence of non-axillary sentinel lymphatic drainage. Sentinel drainage of melanomas of the breast skin and anterior chest wall to the internal mammary and mediastinal nodes is rare. It has yet to be proved that these routes of injection are superior or even equivalent to peritumoral injection for SLNB in breast cancer.

PROSPECTIVE RANDOMIZED COOPERATIVE GROUP TRIALS IN PROGRESS

Two prospective randomized cooperative group trials have just recently been opened for accrual in North America. The NSABP B-32 protocol randomly assigns patients with unifocal cN-negative breast cancer to SLNB plus AND or SLNB alone. The SLNs from patients randomized to SLNB alone are examined by touch preparation (prep) technique intraoperatively. If the SLNs are found to be involved by tumor on touch preps or on subsequent paraffin section histology, AND is performed. Patients are followed for morbidity (serial volumetric assessments for arm lymphedema), goniometry for range of motion in the ipsilateral shoulder, and locoregional, distant and disease-free survival.

Surgeons participating in the NSABP B-32 trial are carefully trained and monitored through their early experience. An experienced surgeon–mentor is sent out to train surgeons in their own institutions. The surgeon–mentor also meets with institutional personnel and professionals from the operating room, nuclear medicine, radiology and pathology. The surgeon–mentor subsequently monitors and reviews with the trainee a series of training cases to verify that the surgeon is ready to accrue randomized patients to the study. Once approved, the surgeon–trainee continues to be monitored by the mentor for at least the first 20 randomized cases.

The American College of Surgeons' Oncology Group has chosen a different experimental design. All registered patients undergo SLNB. Those with negative SLNs by histology will have no further surgery, but their SLNs will undergo analysis by immunohistochemistry; these patients will be followed on a register. Patients with pN-positive SLNs will be randomized to observation or AND.

Other prospective cooperative trials of SLNB in breast cancer are planned or under way elsewhere, such as the Medical Research Council ALMANAC trial in the UK and a randomized trial in Italy.

CONCLUSION

There are several decades of data and experience with AND in cooperative trial groups. These demonstrate that the results obtained by breast surgeons in different practice settings in North America and Europe are excellent and highly reproducible. Regional control after lymphadenectomy approaches 100%. The same cannot be said of SLNB. There are no long-term data on outcomes from sentinel node resection only in breast cancer patients. Only a minority of the surgeons who currently manage breast cancer have had any experience with SLNB, and the results to date are much more variable than consistent. This is especially true for FN rates, the most significant (albeit hard to measure) parameter of clinical efficacy.

Clearly, much remains to be done before SLNB can be considered a comparable or superior alternative for staging of the regional lymphatics in breast cancer. Surgeons who have not yet begun to learn this technique now have the opportunity to get trained under well-supervised conditions, by participating in one of the cooperative group trials that have recently been opened. In the NSABP B-32 trial they receive hands-on training in their own operating rooms and their experience is carefully monitored by their surgeon–mentors. These trials offer the best hope that expertise in this new procedure can be disseminated to surgeons in a controlled manner, assuring a high, uniform standard of performance which will eventuate in SLNB replacing AND as the standard of care for regional nodal staging in breast cancer.

REFERENCES

1. Dees EC, Shulman LN, Souba WW et al, Does information from axillary dissection change treatment in clinically node-negative patients with breast cancer? An algorithm for assessment of impact of axillary dissection. *Ann Surg* 1997; **226**:279–87.

2. Morton DL, Wen D-R, Wong JH et al, Technical details of intraoperative lymphatic mapping for early stage melanoma. *Arch Surg* 1992; **27**:392–9.

3. Reintgen DS, Cruse CW, Wells K et al, The orderly progression of melanoma nodal metastases. *Ann Surg* 1994; **220**:759–67.

4. Thompson JF, McCarthy WH, Bosch CMJ et al, Sentinel lymph node status as an indicator of the presence of metastatic melanoma in regional lymph nodes. *Melanoma Res* 1995; **5**:255-60.

5. Alex JC, Weaver DL, Fairbank JT, Rankin BS, Krag DN, Gamma probe guided lymph node localization in malignant melanoma. *Surg Oncol* 1993; **2**:303–8.

6. Krag DN, Weaver DL, Alex JC, Fairbank JT, Surgical resection and radiolocalization of the sentinel node in breast cancer using a gamma probe. *Surg Oncol* 1993; **2**:335–40.

7. Alex JC, Krag DN, The gamma probe-guided resection of radiolabeled primary lymph nodes. *Surg Oncol Clin North Am* 1996; **5**:33–41.

8. Krag DN, Weaver DL, Ashkaga T et al, The sentinel node in breast cancer. A multicenter validation study. *N Engl J Med* 1998; **339**:941–6.

9. Giuliano AE, Kirgan DM, Guenther JM et al, Lymphatic mapping and sentinel lymphadenectomy for breast cancer. *Ann Surg* 1994; **220**:391–401.

10. Giuliano AE, Barth AM, Spivack B et al, Incidence and predictors of axillary metastasis in T1 carcinoma of the breast. *J Am Coll Surg* 1996; **193**:185–9.

11. Giuliano AE, Jones RC, Brennan M et al, Sentinel lymphadenectomy in breast cancer. *J Clin Oncol* 1997; **15**:2345–50.

12. Guenther JM, Krishnamoorthy M, Tan LR, Sentinel lymphadenectomy for breast cancer in a community managed care setting. *Cancer J Sci Am* 1997; **3**:336–40.

13. Flett MM, Going JJ, Stanton PD et al, Sentinel node localization in patients with breast cancer. *Br J Surg* 1998; **85**:991–3.

14. Beronesi U, Paganelli G, Galimberti V et al, Sentinel node biopsy to avoid axillary dissection in breast cancer with clinically negative nodes. *Lancet* 1997; **349**: 1864–7.

15. Roumen RMH, Valkenburg JGM, Geuskens LM, Lymphoscintigraphy and feasibility of sentinel node biopsy in 83 patients with primary breast cancer. *Eur J Surg Oncol* 1997; **23**:495–502.

16. Borgstein PJ, Pijpers R, Comans EF et al, Sentinel lymph node biopsy in breast cancer: guidelines and pitfalls of lymphoscintigraphy and gamma probe detection. *J Am Coll Surg* 1998; **186**:275–83.

17. Crossin JA, Johnson AC, Stewart PB et al, Gamma probe guided resection of the sentinel lymph node in breast cancer. *Am Surg* 1998; **64**:666–8.

18. Miner TJ, Shriver CD, Jaques DP et al, Ultrasonographically guided injection improves

localization of the radiolabeled sentinel lymph node in breast cancer. *Ann Surg Oncol* 1998; 5:315–21.

19. Snider HS, Dowlatshahi K, Fan M et al, Sentinel node biopsy in the staging of breast cancer. *Am J Surg* 1998; 176:305–10.

20. Rubio IT, Korourian S, Cowan C et al, Sentinel lymph node biopsy for staging breast cancer. *Am J Surg* 1998; 176:305–10.

21. Moffat FL, Gulec SA, Sittler SY et al, Unfiltered sulphur colloid and sentinel node biopsy for breast cancer: technical and kinetic considerations. *Ann Surg Oncol* 1999; 6:746–55.

22. Offodile R, Hoh C, Barsky SH et al, Minimally invasive breast carcinoma staging using lymphatic mapping with radiolabeled dextran. *Cancer* 1998; 82:1704–8.

23. Veronesi U, Paganelli G, Viale G et al, Sentinel lymph node biopsy and axillary dissection in breast cancer: results in a large series. *J Natl Cancer Inst* 1999; 91;368–73.

24. Albertini JJ, Lyman GH, Cox C et al, Lymphatic mapping and sentinel node biopsy in patients with breast cancer. *JAMA* 1996; 276:1818–22.

25. Reintgen DS, Joseph E, Lyman GH et al, The role of selective lymphadenectomy in breast cancer. *Cancer Control (MCC)* 1997; 4:211–19.

26. Barnwell JM, Arredondo MA, Kollmorgen D et al, Sentinel node biopsy in breast cancer. *Ann Surg Oncol* 1998; 5:126–30.

27. Nwariaku FE, Euhus DM, Beitsch PD et al, Sentinel lymph node biopsy, an alternative to elective axillary dissection for breast cancer. *Am J Surg* 1998; 176:529–31.

28. O'Hea BJ, Hill ADK, El-Shirbiny AM et al, Sentinel lymph node biopsy in breast cancer: initial experience at Memorial Sloan–Kettering Cancer Center. *J Am Coll Surg* 1998; 186:423–7.

29. Hill ADK, Tran KN, Akhurts T et al, Lessons learned from 500 cases of lymphatic mapping for breast cancer. *Ann Surg* 1999; 229:528–31.

30. Keshtegar MRS, Ell PJ, Sentinel lymph node detection and imaging. *Eur J Nucl Med* 1999; 26:57–67.

31. Krag DN, Ashikaga T, Harlow SP et al, Development of sentinel node targeting technique in breast cancer patients. *Breast J* 1998; 4:67–74.

32. Cox CE, Pendas S, Cox JM et al, Guidelines for sentinel node biopsy and lymphatic mapping in patients with breast cancer. *Ann Surg* 1998; 227:645–53.

33. Cox CE, Haddad F, Bass S et al, Lymphatic mapping in the treatment of breast cancer. *Oncology* 1998; 12:1283–98.

34. Krag DN, Minimal access surgery for staging regional lymph nodes: the sentinel node concept. *Curr Probl Surg* 1998; 35:951–1018.

35. Linehan DC, Hill ADK, Tran KN et al, Sentinel lymph node biopsy in breast cancer: unfiltered isotope is superior to filtered. *J Am Coll Surg* 1999; 188:377–81.

36. Borgstein PJ, Meijer S, Pijpers R, Intradermal blue dye to identify sentinel lymph node in breast cancer. *Lancet* 1997; 349:1668–9.

22

Surgical considerations in breast cancer patients treated with preoperative chemotherapy

Harry D Bear

Since Haagensen outlined criteria of inoperability for breast cancer, primary surgery, even radical mastectomy, has been considered inappropriate for certain patients, particularly those now staged as IIIB.[1] For these women with locally advanced breast cancers (LABC), surgery did not alter the clinical outcome, which in nearly all cases was to succumb to systemic metastases. This issue aside, surgery was frequently unsuccessful even at controlling local disease. From the time of Haagensen through the 1970s, radical radiotherapy was used as the primary form of treatment, to which hormonal therapy was often added. Both local control and survival were quite poor with this approach.[2,3] When effective chemotherapy became available in the 1970s, this became the primary or first treatment modality offered to these patients. The addition of chemotherapy for LABC has arguably increased survival for these patients, although it has not been shown convincingly that it is really the sequence of treatments rather than the addition of effective systemic treatment at any time that is responsible for this improvement. While the question of sequencing treatments may be relevant in women with operable LABC, in those with categorically inoperable disease (e.g inflammatory breast cancer or cancer fixed to the chest wall), primary chemotherapy clearly has the potential to make these tumors operable.[4–7]

As primary chemotherapy (also called neoadjuvant, induction, preoperative, or up-front chemotherapy) has improved, the responses of primary tumors have become more impressive and patient survival for LABC has increased. The local treatment philosophy has evolved from considering surgical intervention as futile towards more aggressive local treatment for patients who now have a reasonable chance at long-term survival. More recently, the dramatic shrinkage in local and regional disease induced by chemotherapy (particularly anthracycline-containing regimens) has even led to consideration of breast conservation in these patients. Moreover, the concept of primary chemotherapy has now 'crept' down the stages to operable breast cancers, based on theoretical considerations related to the possibility of improved survival. One of the greatest potential advantages to preoperative treatment regimens is the ability to predict patient outcomes from the response of the local and regional disease. If, as seems likely from studies reported in the past few years, the local response predicts systemic response and patient outcome, then comparisons of different systemic treatment regimens can yield meaning-

Table 22.1   Rationale for preoperative chemotherapy

Biologic rationale	Refs
Removal of primary tumor may accelerate growth of micrometastases:	
Serum growth factors	8, 9
Removal of source of angiostatins	10, 11
Increased likelihood of chemoresistant clones with increased tumor burden	12
Test of Skipper hypothesis, that primary and metastatic clones may respond differently to chemotherapy	13

Clinical rationale	Refs
Make unresectable tumors operable	4–7
Make breast conservation feasible for large tumors	14–19
Allows objective assessment of response	14
More rapid assessment of new drugs and regimens	
Correlation of pathologic and molecular markers with response to treatment	

ful results much more rapidly than if we had to wait for survival results to mature. Furthermore, correlating breast tumor responses with biologic and molecular markers should provide important clues to predict tumor sensitivity or resistance to a particular treatment. The biologic and clinical rationale favoring primary or 'neoadjuvant' chemotherapy is summarized in Table 22.1. Even more recently, the use of primary chemotherapy has been proposed for less advanced cancers for the purpose of making breast conservation treatment feasible in women with large primary tumors. For both locally advanced and early-stage breast cancer, elimination of any surgical treatment of the primary tumor and/or lymph nodes after primary chemotherapy has also been described.

The surgical issues that will be addressed here relate to several key questions about patients with breast cancer who, for whatever reason, are treated with primary chemotherapy. These questions include the following:

- Should women with LABC, either inflammatory or non-inflammatory, undergo mastectomy even if they respond well to chemotherapy, or can breast conservation be attempted?
- In women with operable breast cancer, is it appropriate to use primary chemotherapy for

the purpose of making breast conservation feasible?

- If a clinical complete response (i.e. disappearance of palpable tumor) occurs with chemotherapy, is any surgical excision or 'lumpectomy' necessary?
- If lumpectomy is to be done, how does one ensure that the site of the original tumor is actually resected after a clinical complete response (CR)?
- Is surgical/pathologic staging of the axillary nodes after chemotherapy useful for prognostic information and/or regional disease control?
- Can the new technique of sentinel node mapping be used instead of full axillary node dissection in the postchemotherapy setting?

Each of these issues will be considered, and the evidence for or against different surgical approaches will be reviewed. While there are relevant data available from prospective randomized trials comparing primary chemotherapy with standard postoperative adjuvant therapy, few, if any, trials have evaluated the choice of local therapy after chemotherapy in a prospective fashion. It is important to note, moreover, that in many reports, the choice of local therapy was dependent on the response to systemic treatment and not a result of random allocation. When this is the case, it is difficult to derive reliable conclusions about surgical treatment. When the evidence is inconclusive, appropriate options will be offered, based on what evidence does exist.

IS MASTECTOMY NECESSARY AFTER PRIMARY CHEMOTHERAPY FOR LABC?

As one reviews the history of the development of primary chemotherapy for LABC, it is important to remember that the starting assumption during the 1950s, 60s and 70s was that surgery was con-

traindicated for most of these patients. Until effective systemic agents became available, the primary modality used in this setting was radiotherapy.[2,3] This was only moderately effective at controlling local disease, but since most of these patients succumbed fairly rapidly to systemic disease, long-term local/regional control was not a major issue. The experience with surgery alone for operable LABC at our institution led to a trial of preoperative radiotherapy followed by surgery. Although local control was modestly improved, the five-year disease-free survival rate was still only 17%.[20] Similar results were reported by others, as well.[21]

When effective systemic therapy became available and was used for patients with LABC, the commonly used approach to local therapy remained radiotherapy. With more prolonged survival, however, the inability of standard doses of radiation to control the local disease became evident.[22–24] This led to the use of higher doses of radiation and the re-introduction of surgery, including mastectomy, to the mix of treatments. While higher doses of radiation may be more effective than standard doses, the morbidity tends to be higher, with a higher frequency of poor cosmetic outcomes.[24,25] A number of series have evaluated the choice of local treatment options in the context of LABC treated with 'up-front' chemotherapy. We shall consider inflammatory and non-inflammatory LABC separately, although some series include both types of patients.

NON-INFLAMMATORY LOCALLY ADVANCED BREAST CANCER

As noted earlier, a number of theoretical advantages have been attributed to primary chemotherapy for breast cancer. Once it had been shown that chemotherapy might improve survival in patients with LABC and could convert previously inoperable patients into surgical candidates, the possibility that breast conservation might be utilized with good long-term local control began to be considered. Interpretation of the literature in this area is hampered by the fact that some series mix widely varying groups of patients together, including some that are not really inoperable. In a sense, the breast-conserving approach for LABC grew out of a somewhat paradoxical convergence of the hopelessness of mastectomy for LABC, the rise of breast-conserving treatment (BCT) for early breast cancer, and the dramatic tumor regressions seen with primary chemotherapy. In 1986, Héry et al[26] reported on 25 patients with LABC treated with primary chemotherapy followed by breast and nodal irradiation. Unfortunately, almost a quarter of these women later required mastectomy for local recurrences. A number of randomized trials have examined the issue of local treatment options for LABC after primary chemotherapy, but these have mostly been comparisons of surgery alone versus radiation alone (without mastectomy or even gross tumor excision). At the National Cancer Institute of Milan, mastectomy was compared with radiotherapy after three cycles of doxorubicin plus vincristine, with more chemotherapy after local treatment.[22] Although survival and other endpoints were not different between the treatment groups, both groups experienced a local-regional recurrence rate of approximately 30%. A US trial conducted by the CALGB also evaluated mastectomy alone versus radiation alone after primary chemotherapy.[26] Again, as expected, local treatment did not significantly affect survival or distant metastases, but it should be noted that the evaluable patients were already a selected subset (91 out of 113) who became 'operable' after chemotherapy. And, although local control rates were similar in the two groups, local relapse rates were 19% and 27% for surgery and radiotherapy, respectively. Although not com-

pared directly with BCT or with mastectomy, the highest local control rates have generally been obtained with the combination of mastectomy plus radiation after chemotherapy.[23,25,27] In 1992, however, the MD Anderson group reported on a retrospective analysis of mastectomy specimens from women who had undergone induction chemotherapy for locally advanced breast cancer, and concluded that 23% of the evaluable patients could theoretically have undergone BCT.[28] More recently, they have reported on a high success rate for treatment of non-inflammatory LABC with breast conservation following induction chemotherapy, as long as strict selection criteria were used.[17,29] Others have also reported on the selective use of BCT after chemotherapy for women presenting with LABC.[16]

Pierce et al[25] at the US National Cancer Institute (NCI) reported a prospective series of patients with LABC treated with primary chemotherapy and then selected for BCT if they had a clinical CR and multiple needle biopsies showed no tumor. These 31 patients (out of an initial group of 107) were treated with radiation only, and 16% developed a local-regional failure. This was higher than the local failure rate (4%) following mastectomy plus radiotherapy, and led the authors to conclude that mastectomy was the preferred treatment for these patients, regardless of local response to chemotherapy. This recurrence rate, while it may not be ideal, is still lower than the rates seen when radiation alone has been used less selectively. Moreover, the accuracy of needle biopsies in this report may be questioned, particularly in the light of pathologic CR rates with chemotherapy in most series in the range of 10% or less. Thus, they probably underestimated the frequency and extent of residual disease in the breast. Local control might have been improved, in this and other series in which radiation was used alone, by the inclusion of local tumor resection (i.e. 'lumpectomy'), without necessarily resorting to mastectomy. A more recent update of the NCI experience indicated that patients with non-inflammatory LABC, negative biopsies after chemotherapy, and treated with radiation alone had only a 4.5% rate of breast recurrence.[30] In part, the forces that drive decisions about local therapy and understanding results in patients treated with primary chemotherapy relate to the prognostic relevance of response to chemotherapy (discussed in detail below). Because a poor response to chemotherapy indicates a higher likelihood of distant failure and death, local control is less likely to be a problem in these patients. Thus, if mastectomy is used only for patients who respond poorly to chemotherapy, then one might get the impression that mastectomy is associated with a poor outcome. Conversely, if patients with LABC who respond poorly to chemotherapy are treated with radiation only, then one might erroneously conclude that mastectomy actually improves outcome.

Thus, for LABC patients with a poor response to primary chemotherapy, the choice of local treatment depends on technical operability. If a patient's tumor is inoperable after chemotherapy, then radiotherapy should be used, and mastectomy added if the tumor becomes operable after radiation. An alternative that now should be considered after a trial of doxorubicin-based chemotherapy would be to try a taxane next, and then reassess for operability.[31–38] For patients who become operable after chemotherapy but who fail to meet the criteria for BCT (tumor smaller than 5 cm, absence of 'grave signs', and no multicentric disease), mastectomy should be performed, and probably followed by radiation to the chest wall, particularly if they have positive nodes or a tumor greater than 7 cm in diameter. For those who do meet the BCT criteria, segmental mastectomy can be performed, and if negative margins can be achieved, the breast should then

be irradiated. Until we have a good way to determine that a patient has had a complete pathologic CR, the use of radiation alone should probably not be considered standard treatment for most patients who present with a large mass. However, we have used this approach very selectively in a few patients with aggressive twice-daily radiotherapy to the breast, if there is no evidence of residual tumor and multiple needle biopsies are negative. Our current treatment algorithm for non-inflammatory LABC is shown in Figure 22.1. A final note on the timing of surgery after chemotherapy: as long as one waits until the patient's leukocyte count has recovered to normal following the last dose of chemotherapy, the risk of complications should not exceed the expected rate for patients undergoing primary surgery.[30,39] This generally takes four to six weeks.

INFLAMMATORY BREAST CANCER

The treatment and prognosis for inflammatory breast cancer has also changed dramatically over the past two decades, based mainly on the effectiveness of systemic chemotherapy. This group of patients historically has had the worst prognosis of all women with non-metastatic breast cancer, with five-year survival rates of 10% or less. With aggressive systemic therapy, the expected five-year survival for these women now approaches 50%.[40] Local control was, relatively speaking, a less important problem when most of these women succumbed early to distant disease, but control of disease in the breast now has become a significant issue. It is generally agreed that these women should be treated with aggressive systemic chemotherapy and regional radiotherapy, but the role of mastectomy in these women has been controversial. A 1996 report from MD Anderson[40] indicated that the results for patients with inflammatory breast cancer were similar

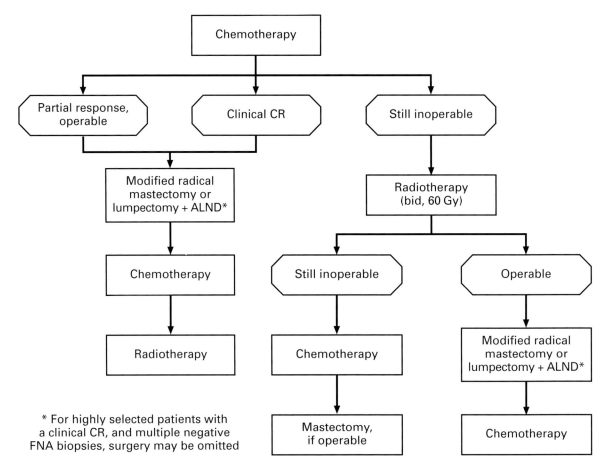

Figure 22.1
Algorithm illustrating strategy for management of non-inflammatory locally advanced inoperable breast cancer.
CR, complete response; ALND, axillary lymph node dissection.

with mastectomy plus radiotherapy compared with radiotherapy alone, and the overall locoregional control rate was 82%. A more recent report from the same institution,[41] however, suggests that local control and survival may actually be improved by the addition of mastectomy. The choice of local therapy in these 172 patients with inflammatory breast cancer was made according to criteria that evolved during the course of the experience reported. All patients were treated with primary doxorubicin-based chemotherapy.

Patients who underwent mastectomy plus radiotherapy had a lower incidence of local recurrence (16.3%) than those treated with radiation alone (35.7%), but this advantage was confined to the patients with a partial response to chemotherapy. These authors also indicated an improvement in disease-free survival with mastectomy for those patients who had either a complete or partial response to induction chemotherapy. Although they claim no systematic bias in favor of mastectomy, patients were not randomly allocated to locoregional treatment. Similar conclusions have been reached by others, and it has also been suggested that negative surgical margins may be important in inflammatory breast cancer.[42,43] Although the significance of negative margins was taken as evidence that an aggressive surgical approach is justified, this correlation more likely reflects the response to chemotherapy rather than the adequacy of surgery. In some series, the decision to proceed to mastectomy was based on the response to systemic treatment, and those patients with the best responses to chemotherapy tend to be chosen for mastectomy, with non-responders being relegated to radiation alone. Obviously, this biases the results against those treated without mastectomy.[43–47] In contrast, in the subset of patients with inflammatory breast cancer treated at the NCI and who received radiation alone after an apparent pathologic CR to chemotherapy, the local recurrence rate was 38.9%, which was much worse than for other LABC patients treated with breast conservation.[30]

We have prospectively evaluated the use of accelerated superfractionated radiation alone after chemotherapy in women with inflammatory breast cancer, and found that most of a subset of patients who had a CR to chemotherapy plus aggressive radiotherapy were able to avoid mastectomy in the long term.[48] The overall breast preservation rate was 74%. Among the 15 patients with a CR after induction chemotherapy, 87% remained locally controlled without mastectomy. It should be noted, however, that breast conservation was carefully chosen for those patients with no evidence of disease after chemotherapy plus radiotherapy, as determined by physical examination, mammography and multiple fine-needle aspiration biopsies. The latter technique, because of its ability to sample multiple areas of the breast tissue, may actually be more accurate than surgical or core needle biopsy.

Thus, we have shown that breast conservation is feasible and safe in some of these patients, particularly if they have a good response to induction chemotherapy, but this is the same group that the MD Anderson data suggest benefits most from mastectomy. In the absence of good level I evidence on either side, the decision to perform or omit mastectomy for patients with inflammatory breast cancer must be individualized and based partly on philosophy. To some physicians and patients, the importance of breast conservation seems less in these patients who have such a serious threat to survival. On the other hand, as survival has improved, breast conservation has become a reasonable secondary objective, as long as it does not compromise survival. A suggested algorithm for inflammatory breast cancer, which we use as a guide to treatment decisions, is shown in Figure 22.2. Note that for women with a large mass and inflammatory changes, the local treatment follows the guidelines for other LABC patients, as shown in Figure 22.1. If a large mass, in addition to the inflammatory component, is present at diagnosis, then a lumpectomy or mastectomy should be performed, as dictated by the residual mass after chemotherapy.

CAN PRIMARY CHEMOTHERAPY BE USED TO 'SHRINK' OPERABLE BREAST CANCERS TO MAKE BREAST CONSERVATION FEASIBLE?

A number of non-randomized series have described the use of preoperative chemotherapy in patients with operable breast cancers. As with LABC, many of these publications include a 'mixed bag' of patients, ranging from stage II to stage IIIB. Recently, the National Cancer Institute of Milan reported on a series of 536 patients with tumors greater than 2.5 cm in diameter. Using a variety of different chemotherapy

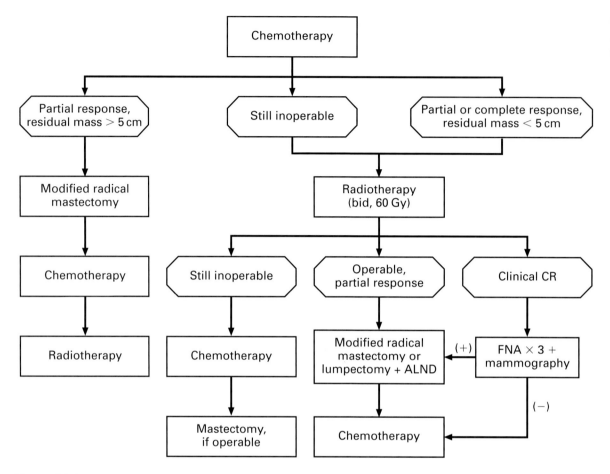

Figure 22.2
Algorithm illustrating strategy for management of inflammatory breast cancer. CR, complete response; FNA, fine-needle aspiration biopsy; ALND, axillary lymph node dissection.

regimens, 85% of these patients could be treated with breast conservation (lumpectomy plus radiation).[15] Although the rate of breast conservation in this report was high, many of these patients would likely have been considered suitable for BCT in the USA without prior chemotherapy. Despite a high rate of overall objective responses (76%), only 16% of the Milan patients had clinical CRs, and only 3% had pathologic CRs (no cancer in the breast resection specimen). Calais et al[49] reported a series of 158 patients with

tumors larger than 3 cm who were treated with primary chemotherapy in a prospectively designed protocol. Subsequent therapy was altered according to response. Patients with a clinical CR underwent radiation followed by more cycles of the same chemotherapy as given initially. Those with a partial response and tumor smaller than 3 cm after chemotherapy underwent lumpectomy plus radiation and more of the same chemotherapy. Non-responders underwent mastectomy plus radiation and then chemotherapy with different agents. Approximately 60% of the patients had objective responses, and 20% had clinical CRs. BCT was possible in 49% of the patients, and only 6 of these experienced local recurrences. Not surprisingly, the five-year survival rate was higher for responders (89.7%) than for non-responders (57.3%). While this study could have been interpreted as showing that mastectomy did not offer any survival advantage, the selection criteria for local treatment, rather than the local treatment itself, accounts for this difference. Like the Milan series, this trial included some patients who could have had a lumpectomy primarily, but it did help to establish the feasibility of this approach to BCT for larger operable breast cancers.

A number of randomized trials have been carried out comparing primary chemotherapy with the more standard approach of adjuvant chemotherapy administered after local treatment. While these studies were not designed to address local therapy issues per se, they do offer important insights into the biology of local control after primary chemotherapy. Mauriac et al[18] randomized 272 women with breast cancers larger than 3 cm to modified radical mastectomy followed by chemotherapy versus chemotherapy followed by local treatment. In the latter group, 62.6% had BCT, and 44 patients had radiation only as local treatment (see below). Although the preoperative chemotherapy group experienced a higher survival rate, it is important to note that chemotherapy was only given to patients in the primary mastectomy group if they were node-positive or estrogen receptor-negative. Thus, while all of the primary chemotherapy patients received chemotherapy, only 104 of the 138 primary mastectomy patients received chemotherapy. This alone, rather than the sequence of treatments, could account for the survival difference. The local recurrence rate, on the other hand, was higher in the primary chemotherapy group,

which is not unexpected, but does not necessarily mean that breast conservation is inappropriate for this group of patients. Scholl et al[19] randomized 414 patients (T2 or T3, N0 or N1) to four cycles of cyclophosphamide, doxorubicin, and 5-fluorouracil (CAF) followed by radiation versus radiation followed by four cycles of CAF. Interestingly, surgery was only used in patients who had a persistent mass after completing radiotherapy, regardless of sequence. Breast conservation was possible in 82% of the primary chemotherapy group and in 77% of the primary radiation group. Survival was also slightly better in the primary chemotherapy group (86% versus 78%), but the neoadjuvant chemotherapy patients received treatment at higher dose intensity. In terms of local treatment, this series again shows that BCT is feasible in women with larger tumors, but could be achieved with primary radiation or with primary chemotherapy. Whether it is appropriate to omit surgery altogether in selected patients, as described in the Scholl report, will be addressed below. In the UK, Powles et al[50] also carried out a randomized trial comparing neoadjuvant chemotherapy plus postoperative chemotherapy with 'standard' chemotherapy given for the same number of cycles after surgery. Using the preoperative chemotherapy approach decreased the need for mastectomy from 28% to 13%, but since there were only 200 patients in the trial, it is underpowered to reach any firm conclusions. Interestingly, however, the overall response rate of 85% was similar to that of other series, as was the low rate of pathologic CRs (only 10%).

The largest randomized trial to date comparing primary chemotherapy with standard postoperative chemotherapy was National Surgical Adjuvant Breast and Bowel Project (NSABP) Protocol B-18.[14,51] Among 683 evaluable patients randomized to preoperative chemotherapy, the overall response rate to primary chemotherapy was 79%. Although 36% of patients had clinical CRs, only 13% had pathologic CRs, including 4% who had residual in situ disease, but no invasive cancer. Preoperative chemotherapy with four cycles of doxorubicin and cyclophosphamide (AC) was associated with a statistically significant increase in the rate of BCT compared with primary surgical treatment (68% versus 60%), and survival at five years was virtually identical in the two treatment groups. Although this trial did not indicate any significant advantage for primary chemotherapy in terms of survival, it does provide a sound basis and level I evidence for the conclusion that primary or preoperative chemotherapy is just as effective as standard postoperative adjuvant chemotherapy. Thus, it can be considered safe to use chemotherapy 'up-front' to shrink tumors in order to offer BCT to women with large operable tumors, without compromising survival. However, it should be noted that the rate of ipsilateral breast tumor recurrence (IBTR) was higher (15%) in the subset of patients who were converted to lumpectomy candidates by administering preoperative chemotherapy, even though negative margins were required for BCT in all patients.[14] This result raises questions about what actually happens when a tumor 'shrinks' during chemotherapy and about the meaning of margins in this setting. We really do not know whether a particular patient's tumor actually shrinks, contracting toward the center, while other tumors really just become more indistinct, with residual rests of tumor being left at the original tumor's perimeter (see the schematic in Figure 22.3). If the latter occurs, is the amount of residual disease similar to what is left behind by a margin-negative lumpectomy done primarily? If so, then radiation should be able to control the residual cancer in most of these patients, just as it does in the 40% or more of patients who have some cancer left in the breast after lumpec-

tomy.[52,53] Conversely, if there is more disease remaining in the breast, similar to what remains after a standard lumpectomy with positive margins, then we would expect the rate of local recurrence to be higher, as in fact it was in women converted to BCT. This might have been improved upon by the use of radiation boosts to the tumor bed (not allowed by the protocol) or by administration of tamoxifen to premenopausal women, whose risk for local recurrence was higher than for older women.

An issue that has seldom been addressed in the literature is whether the cosmetic result of BCT is improved by using preoperative chemotherapy to shrink the tumor and reduce the amount of tissue to be removed at lumpectomy. While this seems plausible, the possibility that higher than usual doses of radiation may be needed to reduce the IBTR rate to acceptable levels after removal of a tumor that has been reduced in size by chemotherapy could negate much of this advantage. Future trials of preoperative chemotherapy should include careful assessment of the cosmetic outcome, as well as the local and systemic recurrence rates.

IN WOMEN WHO ARE CANDIDATES FOR BREAST CONSERVATION AFTER PRIMARY CHEMOTHERAPY, IS A LUMPECTOMY NECESSARY?

Based on the results of NSABP Trial B-06, we know that segmental mastectomy or lumpectomy, even with negative margins, leaves microscopic foci of cancer in the breast in at least 40% of patients.[52,53] The addition of radiotherapy can reduce the incidence of IBTR from this theoretical 40% level to 10% or less. With positive margins, the IBTR rate has been shown to be higher than with negative margins.[54] Thus, the purpose of lumpectomy can be viewed as reducing the tumor burden in the breast to a level

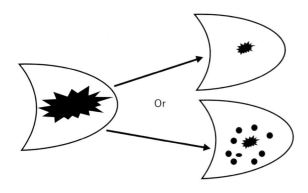

Figure 22.3
Schematic showing alternative hypotheses about what happens during primary chemotherapy for a large breast cancer. In some cases, the tumor mass contracts inwards, leaving the surrounding tissue tumor-free. In other patients, the tumor may seem to disappear, but significant residual 'rests' of tumor are left at the periphery of the original tumor mass.

that can be controlled with radiation. Can chemotherapy accomplish the same goal, particularly in patients with an apparent CR to primary chemotherapy?

Some data relevant to this question can be extrapolated from the pathologic data in trials of preoperative chemotherapy. In virtually all of the trials reporting on the use of neoadjuvant chemotherapy followed by surgical excision of the primary lesion, only a small minority of patients had no residual invasive cancer in the breast. Bonadonna et al,[15] as noted above, reported that with five different regimens, and despite a clinical CR rate of 16%, only 3% of patients had no microscopic cancer in the breast. In NSABP Trial B-18, using four cycles of doxorubicin plus cyclophosphamide preoperatively, the clinical complete response rate was 36%, but only 13% of patients had no invasive cancer in the breast, including 4% who still had ductal carcinoma in situ.[14,51] Likewise, Powles et al,[50] in a small randomized trial of preoperative plus postoperative versus postoperative chemotherapy,

observed pathologic CRs in only 10% of the patients receiving four cycles of preoperative chemotherapy. The theoretical issue that this raises is whether the residual cancer remaining in at least two-thirds of patients with a clinical CR from chemotherapy is analogous to the microscopic disease present after a lumpectomy with negative margins or is more like that remaining after an 'inadequate' lumpectomy with positive margins.

A number of trials, particularly from European centers, have documented experience with the use of radiation alone, without surgery, for local treatment of operable breast cancer treated initially with chemotherapy. However, while some of these trials were randomized prospective studies of neoadjuvant chemotherapy, few if any specifically address local treatment of operable breast cancer after chemotherapy. For example, Calais et al[49] used a selective approach to the local treatment of tumors larger than 3 cm at diagnosis and treated initially with mitoxantrone or epirubicin plus vindesine plus cyclophosphamide plus 5-fluorouracil for three cycles. Of 158 patients, 32 clinical complete responders were treated with radiotherapy alone, using 45 Gy to the whole breast and a 35 Gy brachytherapy boost to the tumor area. Only 2 of these 32 patients had a local recurrence at a median follow-up of 38 months for the entire study. As described above, Scholl et al[19] performed a randomized trial of primary chemotherapy versus chemotherapy given after local treatment. Surgery was only performed if there was a residual mass after radiation treatment to the breast. The breast conservation rate was the same in both groups, and approximately half of each group was treated with radiotherapy only. While concluding that combined chemotherapy plus radiotherapy can increase breast preservation in patients with T2 or larger tumors, the actuarial breast preservation rates in this trial were just over 60% at five years, even though approximately 80% of patients were initially treated with breast preservation. Despite a radiation-boosting strategy bringing the total dose up to 75–80 Gy for patients with a CR and no surgery, the authors later noted that these patients in particular had high local recurrence rates, leading them to conclude that routine surgical excision should be considered, regardless of the response to primary chemotherapy.[55] Baillet et al,[56] in Paris, having found that high-dose radiotherapy (45 Gy external beam plus 30–35 Gy interstitial) led to unsatisfactory cosmetic results, decided to decrease the boost selectively in patients with a good response to primary chemotherapy. In 135 patients with tumors larger than 5 cm, 26 had failure in the breast, and the cosmetic result was considered excellent in 66% of those alive at five years. Using a selective approach to local therapy, another French group used radiotherapy alone in 41 patients who had a clinical CR or near CR.[57] With a median follow-up of only 30 months, they reported that only 3 of these 41 had experienced a local recurrence. Interestingly, however, among the 64 patients who had residual tumor amenable to lumpectomy, there had been no local recurrences. Although this difference is small, it is actually the reverse of what one would expect, given the prognostic significance of response to chemotherapy. In the Bourdeaux randomized trial of neoadjuvant versus adjuvant chemotherapy described previously, 44 patients who had a clinical CR after primary chemotherapy were selectively treated with radiation only, and no breast surgery.[18] Of these 44 patients, 4 experienced a breast recurrence at a median follow-up for the entire trial of 34 months. This accounted for two-thirds of all the breast recurrences in the breast conservation patients, despite the apparent CR to chemotherapy. One of the most striking series relevant to the pos-

sible omission of surgery for breast cancer also comes from France. Jacquillat et al[58] reported on a prospective protocol in which 250 women with stage I–IIIB breast cancer were treated with neoadjuvant chemotherapy, followed by radiation alone to the breast, regardless of the response to chemotherapy. Two different radiation regimens were used, both biologically equivalent to 45 Gy to the whole breast, and an interstitial boost of 20–30 Gy was added, with the boost dose being based on initial tumor size and residual disease. All patients achieved a clinical CR at the end of treatment, and no patient underwent initial mastectomy. With a median follow-up of over five years, the total breast recurrence rate was less than 10%, and the actuarial rate of breast preservation was 94%. The authors also indicate that, despite the aggressive radiotherapy regimen used, 88% of the patients had an excellent or good cosmetic result. Such good cosmesis, however, has not been uniformly observed with the high doses of radiation often used in patients who do not undergo lumpectomy, but careful evaluation of cosmesis is often missing. It remains an open question whether lumpectomy with moderate doses of radiation or omitting surgery and using more aggressive radiation produces better cosmetic outcomes.

It is important to remember that, regardless of the apparent clinical response, the pathologic CR rate is generally around 10%. Whether or not lumpectomy after chemotherapy provides better cosmesis or improved local control, it may provide potentially important prognostic information relative to patient survival. A number of groups have shown that pathologic CR is an excellent predictor of overall outcome. Bonadonna et al,[15] for example, found that the small subset of patients with a histologic CR had a better eight-year relapse-free survival rate (86%) than those with a good partial response but with residual microscopic disease (56%).

Likewise, the MD Anderson series found that patients with a histologic CR in the breast to induction chemotherapy had a higher likelihood of negative nodes, and those with no tumor in the breast or lymph nodes had a significantly higher overall survival rate at five years (89%) compared with those with a lesser response (64%).[29] In NSABP B-18, clinical complete response was a significant predictor of disease-free, relapse-free, and distant disease-free survival (DFS, RFS, and DDFS), but not overall survival.[14] Pathologic CR was the most potent response parameter and the only one that came close to significance in predicting overall survival ($p = 0.06$). The differences in DFS, RFS, and DDFS remained significant after adjusting for clinical tumor size, clinical nodal status, and age. However, in a Cox regression model, breast tumor response was a less powerful prognostic factor than tumor size or pathologic nodal status. As observed in the MD Anderson series, pathologic breast tumor response and pathologic nodal status after chemotherapy were strongly related. Until recently, the importance of prognostication based on response to chemotherapy was largely theoretical, since there was little that could be added to doxorubicin-based chemotherapy that would be likely to alter the outcome. With the demonstration of the efficacy of the taxanes against anthracycline-resistant breast cancer, there is now the potential for adding a systemic treatment that may improve outcomes in these poor-prognosis patients.[31–38] This question is currently being addressed in NSABP Protocol B-27, which may determine whether the addition of a taxane after doxorubicin plus cyclophosphamide will improve survival in those patients who have less than a complete response to the initial chemotherapy.

Among the trials described above, only Jacquillat et al[58] omitted surgical tumor excision in all patients after chemotherapy without regard to tumor response. Even in the selected subset of patients with a CR, outcomes have not been uniformly favorable with the omission of surgery. This, along with the knowledge that very few patients receiving primary chemotherapy will be pathologically tumor-free and the importance of that pathologic information for predicting prognosis, make it seem most prudent, at present, to proceed with lumpectomy, regardless of the clinical response to chemotherapy. However, this issue could be specifically addressed in future trials. If we could identify patients likely to have a pathologic CR, then it might be appropriate to omit lumpectomy in those patients. Another question that would then need to be addressed is the most reliable way to measure/predict the response of the tumor to chemotherapy. Biologic and molecular markers that may predict response are currently being examined in ancillary trials to B-27. Candidates for measuring the response in a way that correlates with pathologic response include mammography, sonography, magnetic resonance imaging, and PET scanning of the breast, which are being actively investigated.[59–62]

ASSUMING THAT LUMPECTOMY IS INDICATED AFTER CHEMOTHERAPY, HOW IS THE LOCATION AND EXTENT OF RESIDUAL TUMOR DETERMINED?

Having made the case for breast conservation and for lumpectomy after primary chemotherapy when the response to chemotherapy allows, it is important that the site of residual tumor be located. After a CR, however, this may be difficult. A number of methods have been used successfully to overcome this problem. In many patients, the tumor site can be marked with small skin tattoos, similar to those used by radiation oncologists to mark treatment fields. Either a single spot over the center of the tumor or four spots marking the peripheral 'corners' of the lesion can be used. The latter also helps to ensure that any measurements taken during the course of treatment will be comparable from week to week. Another method that has been used successfully has been to use mammographically or ultrasound guided placement of a small clip in the tumor before beginning treatment or before it disappears. Then, wire localization 'targeted' on this clip can be used to guide tumor excision. In some patients, especially those with microcalcifications at the tumor site initially, a residual mammographic abnormality may remain after chemotherapy, even if no palpable tumor is present. This can be used for targeting of a needle as a guide to excision, without the need for a clip. Whatever the method used, if excision of the primary tumor site is desirable, it is important to be sure that the appropriate tissue is removed.

WHAT IS THE ROLE OF AXILLARY LYMPH NODE DISSECTION AFTER CHEMOTHERAPY?

Axillary lymph node dissection (ALND) has been performed as a standard part of breast cancer treatment because pathologic node status is a strong predictor of prognosis and the need for systemic therapy, because clinical assessment of the axillary nodes is inaccurate, and because ALND provides good regional control without high-dose radiation to the axilla. It has been argued by some that the need for ALND and its attendant morbidity has decreased markedly.[63–67] In part, this has resulted from the increasing use of adjuvant chemotherapy in node-negative as well as node-positive patients. However, recent data now suggest that node-positive patients may benefit from the addition of a taxane after standard doxorubicin-based chemotherapy.[68] Thus, for patients with a significant likelihood of nodal metastases, pathologic staging may have become

important again, at least for the moment. It has also been argued that the use of preoperative chemotherapy may obviate the need for axillary node staging, since chemotherapy is being given as primary treatment, based on clinical staging, and in many regimens, additional chemotherapy and/or radiation are given to all patients who present with locally advanced breast cancer. Several reports on preoperative chemotherapy, however, have demonstrated that axillary node pathology profoundly impacts prognosis for such patients.[14,15,69,70] In the report by Bonadonna et al,[15] for example, the eight-year relapse-free survival rate varied from 75% in node-negative patients down to 35% in patients with more than three positive nodes. A similar effect of nodal status was seen in NSABP B-18.[14] A close association of nodal status with pathologic tumor response in the breast was also observed in this study; 87% of patients with a pathologic CR in the breast had negative nodes. In fact, the MD Anderson group has argued that this association may make it possible to omit ALND in certain patients, although only 63% of their patients with a pathologic CR in the breast had negative nodes.[71] This group has also suggested that axillary assessment with physical examination and ultrasound may identify those patients with 0 to three nodes involved, who may not need ALND if the axilla is to be irradiated.[72] They have also suggested that a good partial response in the breast (more than 50% reduction in tumor size) correlates with a low rate of axillary node involvement and few positive nodes (86% node-negative for clinical N0 patients and 65% for clinical N1 patients).[73] However, the number of patients in this latter study was small, and, for some reason, 6 patients who had a pathologic CR in the breast (and who might have been expected to have the lowest rate of nodal involvement after chemotherapy) were excluded. Danforth et al[30] similarly noted that only 2.4% of patients with a pathologic CR in the breast and clinically negative regional nodes had an axillary recurrence with the use of axillary radiation. If the pathologic response in the breast is a predictor of axillary nodal status, or if the breast pathology is used by itself to predict prognosis and to decide on the need for further treatment after primary chemotherapy, then ALND will add little important information. Furthermore, it seems clear that microscopic disease in lymph nodes can be controlled with radiation, which can be added to breast radiation with little increase in morbidity.[74-77] However, since few patients have pathologic CRs with current regimens, and up to a third of patients without tumor in the breast may still have cancer in the lymph nodes, depending entirely on breast pathology at this time would seem inappropriate for most patients treated with primary chemotherapy. Furthermore, the presence of tumor in both the breast and the axillary nodes may predict a worse prognosis than either alone.[29] Although it seems clear that axillary nodal status after chemotherapy has prognostic significance, it is not clear what to do about it. Possibilities range from more of the same chemotherapy used preoperatively, to chemotherapy with non-cross-resistant drugs (e.g. taxanes), or even to high-dose chemotherapy with stem cell transplantation. It is hoped that the results of the ongoing NSABP B-27 trial will help to answer this question.

ASSUMING THAT AXILLARY NODE STATUS IS USEFUL INFORMATION AFTER CHEMOTHERAPY, CAN SENTINEL NODE MAPPING AND BIOPSY BE USED IN PLACE OF FULL ALND IN THIS SETTING?

In recent years, procedures for mapping the so-called 'sentinel lymph nodes' (SLN) have been described, and the pathologic status of the sentinel node has been shown to be a highly accurate predictor of axillary node status.[78-83] The sentinel nodes, identified by radionuclide tracers and/or by colored dyes, are felt to be the first nodes in the pathway of lymphatic spread. False-negative rates vary from a few percent up to 11% in different series. For patients in whom primary chemotherapy is indicated, the idea of using SLN mapping as an alternative to ALND has some appeal, especially if decisions about subsequent additional therapy are going to be made on the basis of residual nodal metastases. However, there are currently few data to support the use of SLN mapping in this setting. The accuracy of SLN status as an indicator of nodal pathology after chemotherapy hinges on two fundamental assumptions: first, that nodal spread occurs sequentially, starting with the sentinel node; and, second, that regression of nodal disease occurs in reverse order during systemic treatment. While data from multiple studies seem to support the first assumption, the second has not been established. As yet, there are only anecdotal reports of small numbers of patients undergoing SLN mapping and ALND after primary chemotherapy. At least one of these, albeit involving only 14 patients, indicates that SLN biopsy has a high (21%) false-negative rate after chemotherapy.[84] This is certainly an area that deserves more prospective study. An alternate strategy to avoid the morbidity of ALND in patients receiving neoadjuvant chemotherapy would be to perform SLN mapping and biopsy prior to chemotherapy. If the SLN is pathologically negative, then there would be no need for ALND after chemotherapy. For those patients with a positive SLN at presentation, lumpectomy or mastectomy plus ALND should be performed after chemotherapy, if surgery is indicated.

Table 22.2   Summary of surgical issues after primary chemotherapy for breast cancer

Question	Recommendation	Level of evidence	Comments
Mastectomy for LABC (non-inflammatory)?	BCT may be used selectively. Most patients should have surgical	I for BCT II for excision	
Mastectomy for inflammatory breast cancer?	BCT may be used selectively	III	If a large mass is present, it should be resected by lumpectomy or mastectomy, as needed
Can primary chemotherapy be used to facilitate BCT for large tumors?	Yes	I	Uncertainty about postchemotherapy margins and extent of residual disease may lead to higher IBTR rates than 'standard' BCT for small cancers
Is lumpectomy necessary after chemotherapy, even after a clinical CR?	Yes. (Might selectively eliminate lumpectomy for apparent CR patients, especially if pathologic CR could be predicted accurately.)	II	Prognostic information may be useful. Pathologic CR is uncommon. There is a need for high-dose radiation if no surgery is performed
How does one find residual tumor after CR?	Tattoo, clip, or needle localization of residual calcifications	IV	
Role of ALND after primary chemotherapy?	Should be used in most patients, especially in patients who do not have a CR in the breast. Might be omitted for few patients with a pathologic CR in the breast	III	Provides good regional control. It is unclear how information will affect subsequent treatment at present
SLN mapping after chemotherapy?	Unknown	IV	

SUMMARY

Conclusions about each of the issues and questions discussed here and the grade of evidence for each are listed in Table 22.2. For LABC, a number of large series of patients provide fairly convincing evidence (level I) that BCT can be used selectively after neoadjuvant chemotherapy. For most patients, surgical excision of the residual tumor or tumor site should be performed, to optimize local control and to provide important prognostic information (level II). The question of whether mastectomy is necessary for patients with inflammatory cancer remains controversial, with data on both sides (level III). There is good evidence (level I) provided by a number of prospective trials of primary chemotherapy (especially NSABP Protocol B-18) that it is safe and appropriate to use primary chemotherapy to reduce the size of breast tumors in order to make BCT feasible. As with LABC, the available data (level II) suggest that the tumor site should be excised, even after an apparent clinical CR, rather than using radiotherapy alone. Some results do indicate that surgery might be omitted in selected patients, but cosmetic outcomes, IBTR rates, and the utility of prognostic information have not been analyzed in a prospective fashion. If the primary tumor site is to be excised, a number of techniques can be used to localize it accurately, but no real systematic study on this issue has been published. Data are inconsistent (level III) on the role of ALND after chemotherapy, but for now, we continue to recommend it for most patients receiving primary chemotherapy. As with ALND as part of primary surgery, the role of ALND will ultimately depend on how the pathologic nodal status affects subsequent treatment. The potential role of SLN mapping after chemotherapy has appeal, but little hard data are available to justify its use in this setting (level IV).

REFERENCES

1. Haagensen CD, Stout AP, Carcinoma of the breast. II. Criteria of operability. *Ann Surg* 1943; **118**:859–68.
2. Rubens RD, Armitage P, Winter PJ et al, Prognosis in inoperable stage III carcinoma of the breast. *Eur J Cancer* 1977; **13**:805–11.
3. Zucali R, Uslenghi C, Kenda R, Bonadonna G, Natural history and survival of inoperable breast cancer treated with radiotherapy followed by radical mastectomy. *Cancer* 1976; **37**:1442–31.
4. Hortobagyi GN, Blumenschein GR, Spanos W et al, Multimodal treatment of locoregionally advanced breast cancer. *Cancer* 1983; **51**:763–8.
5. Gardin G, Rosso R, Campora E et al, Locally advanced non-metastatic breast cancer: analysis of prognostic factors in 125 patients homogeneously treated with a combined modality approach. *Eur J Cancer* 1995; **31A**:1428–33.
6. Hortobagyi GN, Multidisciplinary management of advanced primary and metastatic breast cancer. *Cancer* 1994; **74**:416–23.
7. Perez EA, Foo ML, Fulmer JT, Management of locally advanced breast cancer. *Oncology* 1997; **11**(Suppl 9):9–17.
8. Fisher B, Gunduz N, Saffer EA, Influence of the interval between primary tumor removal and chemotherapy on kinetics and growth of metastases. *Cancer Res* 1983; **43**:1488–92.
9. Gunduz N, Fisher B, Saffer EA, Effect of surgical removal on growth and kinetics of residual tumor. *Cancer Res* 1979; **39**:3861–5.
10. O'Reilly MS, Holmgren L, Shing Y et al, Angiostatin: a circulating endothelial cell inhibitor that suppresses angiogenesis and tumor growth. *Cold Spring Harbor Symp Quant Biol* 1994; **59**:471–82.
11. O'Reilly MS, Holmgren L, Chen C, Folkman J, Angiostatin induces and sustains dormancy of human primary tumors in mice. *Nature Med* 1996; **2**:689–92.
12. Goldie JH, Coldman AJ, A mathematical

model for relating the drug sensitivity of tumors to their spontaneous mutation rate. *Cancer Treat Rep* 1979; **63**:1727–33.

13. Skipper HE, Kinetics of mammary tumor cell growth and implications for therapy. *Cancer* 1971; **28**:1479–99.

14. Fisher B, Bryant J, Wolmark N et al, Effect of preoperative chemotherapy on the outcome of women with operable breast cancer. *J Clin Oncol* 1998; **16**:2672–85.

15. Bonadonna G, Valagussa P, Brambilla C et al, Primary chemotherapy in operable breast cancer: eight-year experience at the Milan Cancer Institute. *J Clin Oncol* 1998; **16**:93–100.

16. Schwartz GF, Birchansky CA, Komarnicky LT et al, Induction chemotherapy followed by breast conservation for locally advanced carcinoma of the breast. *Cancer* 1994; **73**:362–9.

17. Hortobagyi GN, Buzdar AU, Strom EA et al, Primary chemotherapy for early and advanced breast cancer. *Cancer Lett* 1995; **90**:103–9.

18. Mauriac L, Durand M, Avril A, Dilhydy JM, Effects of primary chemotherapy in conservative treatment of breast cancer patients with operable tumors larger than 3 cm. Results of a randomized trial in a single centre. *Ann Oncol* 1991; **2**:347–54.

19. Scholl SM, Fourquet A, Asselain B et al, Neoadjuvant versus adjuvant chemotherapy in premenopausal patients with tumors considered too large for breast conserving surgery: preliminary results of a randomised trial: S6. *Eur J Cancer* 1994; **30A**:645–52.

20. Terz JJ, Romero CA, Kay S et al, Preoperative radiotherapy for stage III carcinoma of the breast. *Surg Gynecol Obstet* 1978; **147**:497–502.

21. Townsend CM Jr, Abston S, Fish JC, Surgical adjuvant treatment of locally advanced breast cancer. *Ann Surg* 1985; **201**:604–10.

22. DeLena M, Varini M, Zucali R, Rovini D, Multimodal treatment for locally advanced breast cancer: results of chemotherapy–radiotherapy versus chemotherapy-surgery. *Cancer Clin Trials* 1981; **4**:229–36.

23. Perez CA, Graham ML, Taylor ME et al, Management of locally advanced carcinoma of the breast: I. Noninflammatory. *Cancer* 1994; **74**:453–65.

24. Héry M, Namer M, Moro M et al, Conservative treatment (chemotherapy/radiotherapy) of locally advanced breast cancer. *Cancer* 1986; **57**:1744–9.

25. Pierce LJ, Lippman M, Ben-Baruch N et al, The effect of systemic therapy on local-regional control in locally advanced breast cancer. *Int J Radiat Oncol Biol Phys* 1992; **23**:949–60.

26. Perloff M, Lesnick GJ, Korzun A et al, Combination chemotherapy with mastectomy or radiotherapy for stage III breast carcinoma: a Cancer and Leukemia Group B study. *J Clin Oncol* 1988; **6**:261–9.

27. Hortobagyi GN, Ames FC, Buzdar AU et al, Management of stage III breast cancer with primary chemotherapy, surgery, and radiation therapy. *Cancer* 1988; **62**:2507–16.

28. Singletary SE, McNeese MD, Horotbagyi GN, Feasibility of breast-conservation surgery after induction chemotherapy for locally advanced breast carcinoma. *Cancer* 1992; **69**:2849–52.

29. Kuerer HM, Newman LA, Smith TL et al, Clinical course of breast cancer patients with complete pathologic primary tumor and axillary lymph node response to doxorubicin-based neoadjuvant chemotherapy. *J Clin Oncol* 1999; **17**:460–9.

30. Danforth DN, Zujewski J, O'Shaughnessy J et al, Selection of local therapy after neoadjuvant chemotherapy in patients with stage IIIA,B breast cancer. *Ann Surg Oncol* 1998; **5**:150–8.

31. Seidman AD, Reichman BS, Crown JPA et al, Paclitaxel as second and subsequent therapy for metastatic breast cancer: activity independent of prior anthracycline response. *J Clin Oncol* 1995; **13**:1152–9.

32. Ravdin PM, Burris HA III, Cook G et al, Phase II trial of docetaxel in advanced anthracycline-resistant or anthracenedione-resistant breast cancer. *J Clin Oncol* 1995; **13**:2879–85.

33. Valero V, Holmes FA, Walters RS et al, Phase

II trial of docetaxel: a new, highly effective antineoplastic agent in the management of patients with anthracycline-resistant metastatic breast cancer. *J Clin Oncol* 1995; **13**:2886–94.

34. Holmes FA, Walters RS, Theriault RL et al, Phase II trial of Taxol, an active drug in the treatment of metastatic breast cancer. *J Natl Cancer Inst* 1991; **83**:1797–805.

35. Gianni L, Munzone E, Capri G et al, Paclitaxel in metastatic breast cancer: a trial of two doses by a 3-hour infusion in patients with disease recurrence after prior therapy with anthracyclines. *J Natl Cancer Inst* 1995; **87**:1169–75.

36. Fountzilas G, Athanassiades A, Giannakakis T et al, A phase II study of paclitaxel in advanced breast cancer resistant to anthracyclines. *Eur J Cancer* 1996; **32A**:47–51.

37. Archer CD, Lowdell C, Sinnett HD et al, Docetaxel: response in patients who have received at least two prior chemotherapy regimes for metastatic breast cancer. *Eur J Cancer* 1998; **34A**:816–19.

38. Gradishar WJ, Docetaxel as neoadjuvant chemotherapy in patients with stage III breast cancer. Phase II study: preliminary results. *Oncology* **11**(Suppl 8):15–18.

39. Broadwater JR, Edwards MJ, Kuglen C et al, Mastectomy following preoperative chemotherapy: strict operative criteria control operative morbidity. *Ann Surg* 1991; **213**:126–9.

40. Valero V, Buzdar AU, Hortobagyi GN, Inflammatory breast cancer: clinical features and the role of multimodality therapy. *Breast* 1996; **2**:345–52.

41. Fleming RYD, Asmar L, Buzdar AU et al, Effectiveness of mastectomy by response to induction chemotherapy for control in inflammatory breast carcinoma. *Ann Surg Oncol* 1997; **4**:452–61.

42. Curcio LD, Rupp E, Williams WL et al, Beyond palliative mastectomy in inflammatory breast cancer – a reassessment of margin status. *Ann Surg Oncol* 1999; **6**:249–54.

43. Sener SF, Imperato JP, Khandekar JD et al, Achieving local control for inflammatory carcinoma of the breast. *Surg Gynecol Obstet* 1992; **175**:141–4.

44. Singletary SE, Editorial. Current options for inflammatory breast cancer. *Ann Surg Oncol* 1999; **6**:228–9.

45. Hagelberg RS, Joly PS, Anderson RP, Role of surgery in the treatment of inflammatory breast carcinoma. *Am J Surg* 1984; **148**:124–31.

46. Schafer P, Alberto P, Forni M et al, Surgery as part of a combined modality approach for inflammatory breast carcinoma. *Cancer* 1987; **59**:1063–7.

47. Brun B, Otmezguine Y, Feuilhade F et al, Treatment of inflammatory breast cancer with combination chemotherapy and mastectomy versus breast conservation. *Cancer* 1988; **61**: 1096–103.

48. Arthur DW, Schmidt-Ullrich RK, Riedman RB et al, Accelerated superfractionated radiotherapy for inflammatory breast carcinoma: complete response predicts outcome and allows for breast conservation. *Int J Radiat Oncol Biol Phys* 1999; **44**:289–96.

49. Calais G, Berger C, Descamps P et al, Conservative treatment feasibility with induction chemotherapy, surgery, and radiotherapy for patients with breast carcinoma larger than 3 cm. *Cancer* 1994; **74**:1283–8.

50. Powles TJ, Hickish TF, Makris A et al, Randomized trial of chemoendocrine therapy started before or after surgery for treatment of primary breast cancer. *J Clin Oncol* 1995; **13**:547–52.

51. Fisher B, Brown A, Mamounas E et al, Effect of preoperative chemotherapy on local-regional disease in women with operable breast cancer: findings from National Surgical Adjuvant Breast and Bowel Project B-18. *J Clin Oncol* 1997; **15**:2483–93.

52. Fisher B, Redmond C, Poisson R et al, Eight-year results of a randomized clinical trial comparing total mastectomy and lumpectomy with or without irradiation in the treatment of breast cancer. *N Engl J Med* 1989; **320**:822–8.

53. Fisher B, Anderson S, Redmond CK et al, Reanalysis and results after 12 years of follow-up in a randomized clinical trial comparing total mastectomy with or without irradiation in the treatment of breast cancer. *N Engl J Med* 1995; **333**:1456–61.

54. Gage I, Schnitt SJ, Nixon AJ et al, Pathologic margin involvement and the risk of recurrence in patients treated with breast-conserving therapy. *Cancer* 1996; **78**:1921–8.

55. Scholl SM, Pierga JY, Asselain B et al, Breast tumour response to primary chemotherapy predicts local and distant control as well as survival. *Eur J Cancer* 1995; **31A**:1969–75.

56. Baillet F, Rozec C, Ucla L, Chauveinc L et al, Treatment of locally advanced breast cancer without mastectomy: 5- and 10-year results of 135 tumors larger than 5 centimeters treated by external beam therapy, brachytherapy, and neoadjuvant chemotherapy. *Ann NY Acad Sci* 1993; **698**:264–70.

57. Bélembaogo E, Feillel V, Chollet P et al, Neoadjuvant chemotherapy in 126 operable breast cancers. *Eur J Cancer* **28A**:896–900.

58. Jacquillat C, Weil M, Baillet F et al, Results of neoadjuvant chemotherapy and radiation therapy in the breast-conserving treatment of 250 patients with all stages of infiltrative breast cancer. *Cancer* 1990; **66**:119–29.

59. Abraham DC, Jones RC, Jones SE et al, Evaluation of neoadjuvant chemotherapeutic response of locally advanced breast cancer by magnetic resonance imaging. *Cancer* 1996; **78**:91–100.

60. Vinnicombe SJ, MacVicar AD, Guy RL et al, Primary breast cancer: mammographic changes after neoadjuvant chemotherapy, with pathologic correlation. *Radiology* 1996; **198**:333–40.

61. Herrada J, Iyer RB, Atkinson EN et al, Relative value of physical examination, mammography, and breast sonography in evaluating the size of the primary tumor and regional lymph node metastases in women receiving neoadjuvant chemotherapy for locally advanced breast carcinoma. *Clin Cancer Res* 1997; **3**:1565–9.

62. Bassa P, Kim EE, Inoue T et al, Evaluation of preoperative chemotherapy using PET with fluorine-18-fluorodeoxyglucose in breast cancer. *J Nucl Med* 1996; **37**:931–8.

63. Cady B, Stone MD, Schuler JG et al, The new era in breast cancer – invasion, size, and nodal involvement dramatically decreasing as a result of mammographic screening. *Arch Surg* 1996; **131**:301–7.

64. Cady B, Is axillary lymph node dissection in routine management of breast cancer? No. *Breast J* 1997; **3**:246–60.

65. Silverstein MJ, Gierson ED, Waisman JR et al, Axillary lymph node dissection for T1a breast carcinoma: is it indicated? *Cancer* 1994; **73**:664–7.

66. Morrow M, Axillary dissection: when and how radical? *Semin Surg Oncol* 1996; **12**:321–7.

67. Dent DM, Axillary lymphadenectomy for breast cancer – paradigm shifts and pragmatic surgeons. *Arch Surg* 1996; **131**:1125–78.

68. Henderson IC, Berry D, Demetri G et al, Improved disease-free (DFS) and overall survival (OS) from the addition of sequential paclitaxel (T) but not from the escalation of doxorubicin (A) dose level in the adjuvant chemotherapy of patients (PTS) with node-positive breast cancer (BC). *Proc Am Soc Clin Oncol* 1998; **17**:101a.

69. McCready DR, Hortobagyi GN, Kau SW et al, The prognostic significance of lymph node metastases after preoperative chemotherapy for locally advanced breast cancer. *Arch Surg* 1989; **124**:21–5.

70. Machiavelli MR, Romero AO, Pérez JE et al, Prognostic significance of pathological response of primary tumor and metastatic axillary lymph nodes after neoadjuvant chemotherapy for locally advanced breast carcinoma. *Cancer J Sci Am* 1998; **4**:125–31.

71. Kuerer HM, Newman LA, Buzdar AU et al, Pathologic tumor response in the breast following neoadjuvant chemotherapy predicts axillary lymph node status. *Cancer J Sci Am* 1998; **4**:230–6.

72. Kuerer HM, Newman LA, Fornage BD et al, Role of axillary lymph node dissection after tumor downstaging with induction chemotherapy for locally advanced breast cancer. *Ann Surg Oncol* 1998; **5**:673–80.

73. Lenert JT, Vlastos G, Mirza NQ et al, Primary tumor response to induction chemotherapy as a predictor of histologic status of axillary nodes in operable breast cancer patients. *Ann Surg Oncol* 1999; **6**:762–7.

74. Fisher B, Redmond C, Fisher ER et al, Ten-year results of a randomized clinical trial comparing radical mastectomy and total mastectomy with or without radiation. *N Engl J Med* 1985; **312**:674–81.

75. Baeza MR, Sole J, Leon A et al, Conservative treatment of early breast cancer. *Int J Radiat Oncol Biol Phys* 1988; **14**:669–76.

76. Delouche G, Bachelot F, Premont M, Kurtz JM, Conservation treatment of early breast cancer: long term results and complications. *Int J Radiat Oncol Biol Phys* 1987; **13**:29–34.

77. Cabanes PA, Salmon RJ, Vilcoq JR et al, Value of axillary dissection in addition to lumpectomy and radiotherapy in early breast cancer. *Lancet* 1992; **339**:1245–8.

78. Giuliano AE, Jones RC, Brennan M, Statman R, Sentinel lymphadenectomy in breast cancer. *J Clin Oncol* 1997; **15**:2345–50.

79. Veronesi U, Paganelli G, Galimberti V et al, Sentinel-node biopsy to avoid axillary dissection in breast cancer with clinically negative lymph-nodes. *Lancet* 1997; **349**:1864–7.

80. Turner RR, Ollila DW, Krasne DL, Giuliano AE, Histopathologic validation of the sentinel lymph node hypothesis for breast carcinoma. *Ann Surg* 1997; **226**:271–8.

81. Veronesi U, Paganelli G, Viale G et al, Sentinel lymph node biopsy and axillary dissection in breast cancer: results in a large series. *J Natl Cancer Inst* 1999; **91**:368–73.

82. Gulec SA, Moffat FL, Carroll RG et al, Sentinel lymph node localization in early breast cancer. *J Nucl Med* 1998; **39**:1388–93.

83. Krag D, Weaver D, Ashikaga T et al, The sentinel node in breast cancer – a multicenter validation study. *N Engl J Med* 1998; **339**:941–6.

84. Anderson BO, Jewell K, Eary JF et al, Neoadjuvant chemotherapy contraindicates sentinel node mapping in breast cancer. *Proc Am Soc Clin Oncol* 1999; **18**:71a.

SECTION 6: Radiation Therapy

Section Editor: BG Haffty

23

Radiation therapy in the management of breast cancer

Bruce G Haffty

BREAST-CONSERVING THERAPY

Breast-conserving therapy with lumpectomy followed by radiation therapy (RT) to the intact breast is an acceptable and preferable standard of care in the management of early stage invasive breast cancer.[1-4] There have been several prospective randomized trials that have clearly established breast-conserving surgery with lumpectomy followed by radiation to the intact breast as an alternative to mastectomy. All of the modern randomized trials have demonstrated that those patients treated conservatively (pathologic node negative as well as pathologic node positive) have disease-free, distant metastasis-free and overall survival rates that are equivalent to those of their counterparts treated by mastectomy. Relapses occurring in the conservatively treated breast can be effectively salvaged by mastectomy, without any overall compromise in survival rates.

Although most patients with operable breast cancer are candidates for conservative surgery followed by RT to the intact breast, there are a number of relative contraindications and a number of factors that may predict an adverse outcome after breast conservation therapy.[5-10] Factors that have been identified as potential

contraindications to breast-conservation therapy based on increased risk of complications include, but are not limited to, pregnancy, history of prior irradiation, presence of collagen vascular disease, and technical and anatomic factors that may result in poor cosmetic outcome or increased complications.[5-10]

Prognostic factors for ipsilateral breast tumor recurrence

There have been a number of studies evaluating prognostic factors that may result in an increased risk of local recurrence. Gross multicentric or multifocal disease, detected either clinically or mammographically, is generally considered to be a contraindication to breast conservation. Although selected patients with two or more lesions may be considered candidates for breast conservation, patients with gross multicentric disease have been shown to have a high risk of local recurrence.[10,11] The high incidence of breast recurrence may be secondary to the presence of significant residual tumor burden in the breast after conservative surgery. Another factor, which must be considered in evaluating patients with gross multicentric disease, is the cosmetic result, which may be significantly compromised by the surgical removal of two or more lesions from the same breast. Despite the relative contraindication of multicentric disease, there have been retrospective studies from several institutions of selected patients with two synchronous ipsilateral breast masses who underwent wide local excision of all gross disease and subsequently underwent RT. Although the local recurrence rate was slightly higher in this group of patients, selected patients with synchronous ipsilateral breast tumors may be considered for this approach, provided that they understand the potential of an increased risk of local recurrence.[11]

Extensive intraductal component (EIC) is a pathologic entity defined as having an invasive ductal carcinoma with an intraductal component comprising 25% or more of the primary invasive tumor, with intraductal carcinoma in the surrounding normal breast tissue.[12] A lesion composed of predominantly ductal carcinoma in situ with focal areas of invasion is also categorized as an EIC-positive tumor. Initial reports indicated that extensive intraductal component was found to be a powerful predictor of local failure. It is important to note, however, that patients in these studies were treated at a time when microscopic assessment of the margins of resection was not routinely performed. In a recent update, the inter-relationship of microscopic margins of resection, the presence of extensive intraductal component and ipsilateral breast tumor recurrence (IBTR) after breast-conserving therapy was evaluated. In that analysis, the 5-year rate of IBTR for all patients with negative margins was 2% and for all patients with focally positive margins 9%. The authors recommended that breast-conservation therapy be considered in patients with negative margins or focally involved margins whether or not EIC is present.[7] In patients with greater than focally involved margins, the IBTR rate was high. It is apparent that patients with extensive intraductal component with diffusely involved margins, which cannot be cleared on re-excision, are not optimal candidates for breast-conserving therapy. Whether or not EIC is present, the currently available literature suggests that achievement of a negative surgical margin is likely to result in a lower and acceptable local relapse rate.[7,8]

There have been a number of other clinical and/or pathologic factors that have been associated with high local recurrence rates. Although there have been some consistencies, there have been a number of conflicting reports regarding clinical and/or pathologic factors that may be predictive of IBTR. Factors typically predictive of a high rate of systemic metastasis, such as number of axillary lymph nodes involved, primary tumor size, lymph vascular invasion, DNA ploidy and high S-phase fraction, have not been consistently shown to be predictive of IBTR.[5,10]

One prognostic factor for local recurrence, which has been reported in several studies, has been the association of young age with high local recurrence rates.[5,10,13–16] Although a highly significant correlation with young age and local recurrence has been reported, there is no evidence that young patients electing breast-conserving therapy have a compromised survival and we continue to offer young patients lumpectomy followed by RT as an acceptable standard of care. To date, there is no evidence that patients with strong family history and/or hereditary forms of breast cancer have a high rate of local recurrence, although data regarding the risk of local recurrence in patients with BRCA1 and BRCA2 positivity are limited.[13–16]

In summary, it is apparent that the vast majority of patients with operable breast cancer, provided adequate excision of the tumor can be obtained with an acceptable cosmetic result, are acceptable candidates for breast-conservation therapy.

Radiation therapy after breast-conservation surgery should be employed using careful treatment planning techniques that minimize treatment of the underlying heart and lung. To achieve the optimal cosmetic result, an effort should be made to obtain homogeneous dose distribution throughout the breast. Doses of 180–200 cGy/day in the intact breast to a total dose of 4500–5000 cGy are considered standard. Administration of a boost using an electron beam or interstitial implant to bring the tumor bed to a total dose of 6000–6600 cGy is frequently employed. Although the necessity of a boost is controversial, and has been the subject of debate, most of the radiation oncologists in the USA continue to use a boost. In a recently published randomized clinical trial, delivery of a boost of 10 Gy to the tumor bed after 50 Gy to the whole breast resulted in a statistically significant reduction in local recurrence, although the local recurrence rate in patients treated with or without the boost was quite acceptable.[17]

In patients undergoing breast-conserving therapy who have had an axillary lymph-node dissection, the role of regional nodal irradiation is controversial.[18–20] In general, patients with pathologically negative axillary nodes would be treated to the breast only, eliminating RT to the internal mammary or supraclavicular fossa. In patients with node-positive disease, RT to the supraclavicular fossa and/or internal mammary chain may be considered, although the benefits are uncertain. Extrapolation from the results of recent randomized trials, indicating a survival benefit to regional nodal irradiation in the postmastectomy setting, indicates that regional nodal irradiation in node-positive, conservatively treated patients may be beneficial.[21–23]

SUBSETS OF PATIENTS IN WHOM RADIATION THERAPY MAY BE AVOIDED

Currently, for patients with invasive breast cancer, RT after lumpectomy remains the standard of care. A number of prospective randomized trials have addressed the issue of lumpectomy alone versus lumpectomy with radiation, and have consistently shown RT to reduce the risk of IBTR significantly.[1–4] Although there has been no clearly established survival benefit from RT to the intact breast after lumpectomy, local recurrence rates in patients treated with lumpectomy alone have been shown to be as high as 40–50%, despite the use of adjuvant systemic therapy. A recently reported, prospective, single-arm trial attempted to employ lumpectomy alone in a highly selected group of patients with small tumors, negative margins and negative lymph nodes. Even in this select group of patients, local recurrence rate approached 25% with relatively limited follow-up.[24] Currently, there is an Intergroup trial evaluating lumpectomy alone versus lumpectomy and RT in a select group of patients aged over 70 years with tumors less than 2.0 cm, positive estrogen receptors and negative pathologic margins. For patients with invasive carcinoma, the use of lumpectomy alone should currently be limited to prospective trials.

Sequencing of chemoradiation

Most patients undergoing lumpectomy followed by RT to the intact breast for invasive breast carcinoma will be receiving some form of systemic therapy, in the form of either cytotoxic chemotherapy or adjuvant hormonal treatment. For those patients undergoing cytotoxic chemotherapy, the optimal sequencing of radiowith chemotherapy remains an active area of investigation and an ongoing debate.[25] There have been conflicting reports in the literature regarding the issue of whether a delay in RT compromises local control. Although initial reports indicated a high local recurrence rate in those patients in whom a course of definitive RT was delayed more than 16 weeks, a number of other series have failed to confirm these findings.[25–28] Furthermore, a randomized clinical trial addressing the issue of the sequencing of chemotherapy and RT from the Joint Center for Radiation Therapy (JCRT) indicated that, although delaying RT resulted in a slightly higher local recurrence rate, a delay in chemotherapy compromised distant metastasis.[29] The vast majority of patients in this trial, however, were node positive. Currently, in most node-positive patients in whom systemic cytotoxic chemotherapy is being considered, initiation of chemotherapy before radiation appears reasonable. Concurrent chemo-radiotherapy has, however, also been employed and, although some have reported an increased risk of acute reactions and complications with this approach, others have not. Clearly, concomitant chemo-radiotherapy may be considered in selected patients, provided that radiation is not administered with concomitant doxorubicin-based chemotherapy.

For patients with node-negative disease, the issue of the timing of chemotherapy with RT is more controversial. Currently, decisions regarding the timing of chemotherapy with RT is highly individualized, depending on risk factors for systemic and/or local disease, along with the patients' own preferences.

POSTMASTECTOMY RADIATION

A number of prospective and retrospective series in patients treated with mastectomy have demonstrated that patients with primary tumors larger than 5 cm in size and/or involvement of four or more lymph nodes have a high risk of locoregional failure after mastectomy.[21–23,30–32] Even in patients who have undergone high-dose chemotherapy with or without stem cell rescue, locoregional failure is a significant problem in this group of patients without the use of postmastectomy radiation. Most current, ongoing, clinical trials evaluating dose-intensive chemotherapy, with or without bone marrow stem cell transplantation, routinely include postmastectomy RT to the chest wall and/or regional lymph nodes to minimize locoregional recurrence in patients with locally advanced cancer and multiple positive nodes.

The use of postmastectomy RT in patients with earlier stages of disease is more controversial.[21–23,30–32] Three recently conducted randomized clinical trials, however, demonstrated a disease-free survival and overall survival advantage with postmastectomy radiation in node-positive patients.[21–23] In two of these trials, premenopausal patients were treated with mastectomy and cytotoxic chemotherapy and were randomized to receive or not receive postmastectomy radiation to the chest wall and regional lymph nodes. In the third trial, postmenopausal women were treated with tamoxifen and randomized to postmastectomy radiation or observation. Long-term follow-up of these trials has shown an improvement in distant metastasis and overall survival, not only in patients with four or more nodes, but also in patients with one to three nodes.

Thus, these trials have resurrected the issue of postmastectomy RT in patients with earlier stages of disease and limited nodal involvement. Although there are a number of controversies regarding the extent of axillary lymph node dissection in these patients, subset analysis, as well as RT techniques employed, these trials have highlighted the issue of considering postmastectomy radiation in patients with earlier stages of disease. Currently, there are plans for a randomized American Intergroup trial, addressing the issue of postmastectomy radiation in patients with one to three positive nodes. It is hoped that this trial will address the question of which subsets of patients with one to three nodes, using modern, currently accepted radiation techniques and chemotherapy programs, derive the greatest benefit from postmastectomy radiation.

In those patients in whom postmastectomy RT is employed, careful treatment techniques and field arrangements that minimize overlap between adjacent fields and minimize the dose to underlying cardiac and pulmonary structures are required. Whether to include the internal mammary (IM) chain, supraclavicular fossa and/or axilla remains controversial and an unsettled issue. Although the randomized trials reported above employed techniques treating IM and axillary nodes, the risk:benefit of the extent of nodal irradiation is unclear. A current ongoing trial in Europe randomizing patients to tangential fields alone compared with tangential fields with IM and supraclavicular radiation is ongoing, although the results of that trial will not be available for several years.

LOCAL REGIONAL RECURRENCE OF DISEASE

Local regional recurrence of disease remains a major clinical problem for patients carrying the diagnosis of breast cancer. Depending on the patient's initial presentation and subsequent management, local regional recurrence rates as high as 50% have been reported. Obviously, appropriate use of surgery, systemic therapy and radiation should be employed, as outlined earlier, in an effort to minimize the chance of local regional recurrence. Despite adequate and appropriate local regional and systemic therapy, however, between 5% and 20% of patients will experience local regional recurrence of disease. With over 150 000 new cases of breast cancer per year, local regional recurrence obviously remains a major problem facing the clinical oncologist. Local regional recurrences can be divided into the following categories: tumors in the ipsilateral breast after conservative surgery; postmastectomy

chest wall recurrences; and regional nodal recurrences after conservative surgery or mastectomy.

Local relapse after lumpectomy with or without radiation

For those patients who develop a local failure after breast-conserving surgery for invasive breast cancer or ductal carcinoma in situ (DCIS), tumor usually develops in the region of the initial primary tumor. Although the prognosis after IBTR is more favorable than other local regional relapses, early IBTRs after lumpectomy and RT have been associated with a relatively high rate of systemic metastasis.[33] For those patients who have undergone lumpectomy alone without radiation, re-excision at the time of local recurrence followed by RT may be an option, although there are limited data on this approach.

For patients experiencing an IBTR after lumpectomy with RT, mastectomy is the most commonly employed standard treatment modality. Although there have been some studies reporting acceptable results with repeat wide local excision, or repeat wide local excision with additional radiation, selection criteria for this approach are unclear and long-term follow-up regarding this management option is lacking. Studies from the University of Pennsylvania, evaluating salvage mastectomy specimens of patients who sustained an IBTR, failed to identify a subgroup of patients in whom local excision of the tumor bed would provide adequate local treatment.[34] There is a subgroup of patients, however, who are unwilling to consider salvage mastectomy. Based on available data, these patients may be managed by wide local excision with or without the addition of limited field re-irradiation, provided that these patients are willing to accept some uncertainty regarding this treatment approach.

After definitive surgical treatment with salvage mastectomy for those patients experiencing an

IBTR, reconstruction with autologous tissue using a TRAM (transverse rectus abdominis myocutaneous) flap may be considered. Acceptable long-term results in previously irradiated patients have been reported using these surgical techniques. Reconstruction with saline or silicon implants after radiation have been associated with a high rate of complications and should generally be avoided.[35]

There are limited data regarding the role of systemic therapy after salvage mastectomy for IBTR. Although patients with early IBTRs have a relatively high rate of subsequent systemic metastasis, the benefit of adjuvant systemic therapy in this setting is unclear. Given the high rate of metastasis in more aggressive IBTRs, however, some patients and/or their oncologists may consider the use of adjuvant systemic therapy in those patients with aggressive early local recurrences. In those patients not previously on hormonal therapy with estrogen receptor (ER)-positive recurrences, adjuvant tamoxifen may also be considered.[36] For patients with late local recurrences, which may represent new primary tumors and may be distinctly removed from the original tumor bed, evaluation of the tumor for prognostic factors such as tumor size, ER status, DNA ploidy, S-phase fraction and other prognostic factors may aid the clinician in making a decision about the use of adjuvant systemic therapy. As a result of the lack of available data on adjuvant systemic therapy in the setting of an IBTR, the approach to these patients is, by necessity, highly individualized.

Chest wall recurrences after mastectomy

Patients who develop a postmastectomy chest wall recurrence have a relatively high rate of subsequent systemic metastasis. Many of these patients will experience long disease-free intervals and, for those patients with isolated chest wall recurrences, long-term 5- to 10-year disease-free survivals of more than 50% have been reported.[36] It is therefore important to attempt to obtain adequate local regional control in these patients who may experience a relatively long survival after chest wall recurrence. In patients suspected of having chest wall recurrence, biopsy is clearly indicated. When feasible, excision of the mass should be attempted followed by comprehensive RT to involve the chest wall and/or regional lymph nodes. Radiation treatment techniques are generally similar to those employed with standard postmastectomy radiation therapy and consist of a photon and/or electron beam directed at the chest wall and adjacent lymph nodes. Treatment planning should strive for homogeneous dose distributions throughout the target area, while minimizing the dose to the underlying cardiac and pulmonary structures. Conventional fractionation of 180–200 cGy/day to the area of local regional recurrence and immediately adjacent areas at risk to a total dose of 4500–5000 cGy, with a boost to the area of recurrence or gross residual disease to a dose of 6000–6500 cGy, results in acceptable long-term local regional control.

In patients who experienced a chest wall recurrence and had previously undergone RT, additional limited-field RT may be considered. Re-irradiation to the chest wall with limited fields has been associated with acceptable long-term complications. Several reports regarding the use of hyperthermia with concomitant RT in this setting have also shown acceptable local control and complication rates.[37,38]

Clearly, patients with chest wall recurrences after mastectomy have a relatively high rate of systemic metastasis. There are limited data, however, about the use of adjuvant systemic therapy in this setting. A recently reported randomized trial demonstrated disease-free survival benefit with the use of adjuvant tamoxifen after RT at the time of postmastectomy chest wall recurrence in patients with ER-positive tumors.[36]

Patients with ER-negative tumors and aggressive local regional recurrences may be considered for cytotoxic chemotherapy given their relatively poor prognosis and high rate of distant metastasis, although the prospective randomized trials addressing the use of adjuvant systemic therapy in this setting are non-existent.

Treatment of regional nodal recurrences

Regional nodal relapses after mastectomy or conservative surgery with RT carry a relatively poor prognosis. Although patients initially treated with a simple mastectomy experiencing an axillary recurrence had a favorable prognosis, most patients sustaining recurrences in the IM chain, supraclavicular fossa or axilla after dissection and/or RT have a high rate of systemic metastasis. Nevertheless, adequate local regional control in these patients at the time of regional relapse is an important goal. After biopsy and/or surgical resection, when feasible, RT can provide adequate long-term local regional control. Depending on the location of the regional relapse, RT to the nodal relapse and adjacent areas at risk can be accomplished using treatment techniques as previously described. Conventional doses of 180–200 cGy/fraction to total doses of 4500–5000 cGy, with a cone down to the area of residual disease to doses of between 5000 and 6000 cGy, should result in adequate long-term local regional control. These patients have an extremely high risk of systemic metastasis but, as with postmastectomy chest wall recurrences and IBTRs, there are limited data about the role of adjuvant systemic therapy in this setting. Again, owing to the lack of available data, adjuvant systemic therapy can be employed on an individualized basis. For those patients who have not previously been on hormonal therapy and are receptor positive, it would be reasonable to consider tamoxifen in addition to any other systemic therapy.

Clearly, the role of systemic therapy at the time of local regional relapse has not been well defined. Given the significant numbers of patients who experience local regional relapse, along with the relatively high rate of subsequent systemic disease in these patients, consideration of systemic therapy is reasonable. This area is clearly in need of well-designed multi-institutional trials to address the issue of adjuvant systemic therapy at the time of local relapse.

MANAGEMENT OF DUCTAL CARCINOMA IN SITU

For patients with DCIS, lumpectomy alone versus lumpectomy with RT continues to be an active area of investigation and debate. The National Surgical Adjuvant Breast and Bowel Project (NSABP) B-17 trial, which randomized patients with DCIS to lumpectomy versus lumpectomy and RT, clearly showed a benefit to RT in reducing the risk of local recurrence.[39] The benefit of RT was noted in all subsets of patients, including those with low-grade non-comedo-type DCIS. Similar results from a randomized trial in Europe have recently been reported.[40] As in the NSABP trial, all subgroups of patients benefited from RT with respect to a reduction in the local relapse rate. The radiation technique is similar to that described above for invasive cancer, with 4500–5000 cGy to the whole breast, generally followed by a boost to the tumor bed.

There have been a number of retrospective series with limited follow-up reporting acceptable local recurrence rates in selected patients with DCIS treated by lumpectomy alone (without radiation). A recently published study employed careful treatment techniques with detailed attention to surgical margins. Based on their experience, the authors do not advocate radiation therapy in patients with DCIS that was excised with margins of 10 mm or more.[41] Currently, the authors continue to offer RT to most patients with DCIS, although results of ongoing trials and longer follow-up of patients treated with lumpectomy alone with careful attention to surgical margins are likely to identify a subset of patients with DCIS who may be treated with excision alone.

Radiation therapy in lobular carcinoma in situ

Many patients with invasive breast cancer or with DCIS will have an associated histologic component of lobular carcinoma in situ (LCIS). Although data addressing this entity are limited, the available retrospective literature indicates that there is no adverse impact of a component of LCIS with respect to local or systemic relapse.[42] In general, the underlying DCIS or invasive breast cancer is treated appropriately and the LCIS component does not impact on the management decision or outcome.

For patients with pure LCIS, there is no role for radiation after biopsy or lumpectomy. These patients may be surgically managed or observed. Although these patients have a high probability of subsequently developing a frankly invasive malignancy of DCIS, and clearly may benefit from chemoprophylaxis, there is no established role for radiation therapy for the patient with the histologic diagnosis of pure LCIS.

REFERENCES

1. Haffty BG, Ward BA, Is breast-conserving surgery with radiation superior to mastectomy in selected patients? *Cancer J Sci Am* 1997; 3:2–3.
2. Fisher B, Redmond C, Poisson R et al, Eight-year results of a randomized clinical trial comparing total mastectomy and lumpectomy with or without irradiation in the treatment of breast cancer. *N Engl J Med* 1989; 320:822–8.
3. Veronesi U, Sacozzi R, Del Vecchio M et al, Comparising radical mastectomy with quadrantectomy, axillary dissection and radiotherapy in patients with small cancers of the breast. *N Engl J Med* 1981; 305:6–11.
4. Fowble B, Solin LJ, Schultz DJ, Conservative surgery and radiation for early stage breast cancer. In: Fowble B, Goodman RL, Glick JH et al, eds. *Breast Cancer Treatment. A Comprehensive Guide to Management.* St Louis, MO: Mosby, 1991: 3–88.
5. Haffty BG, Fischer D, Rose M et al, Prognostic factors for local recurrence in the conservatively treated breast cancer patient: A cautious interpretation of the data. *J Clin Oncol* 1991; 9:997–1003.
6. Harris J, Recht A, Almaric R et al, Time course and prognosis of local recurrence following primary radiation therapy for early breast cancer. *J Clin Oncol* 1984; 2:37–41.
7. Gage I, Schnitt SJ, Nixon AJ et al, Pathologic margin involvement and the risk of recurrence in patients treated with breast-conserving therapy. *Cancer* 1996; 78:1921–8.
8. Smitt MC, Nowels JW, Zdeblich MJ et al, The importance of the lumpectomy surgical margin status in long term results of breast conservation. *Cancer* 1995; 76:259–67.
9. Fleck R, McNeese MD, Ellerbroek NA et al, Consequences of breast irradiation in patients with pre-existing collagen vascular disease. *Int J Radiat Oncol Biol Phys* 1989; 17:829–33.
10. DiPaola RS, Orel SG, Fowble BL. Ipsilateral breast tumor recurrence following conservative surgery and radiation therapy. *Oncology* 1994; 8:59–68.
11. Wilson LD, Beinfield M, McKhann CF, Haffty BG, Conservative surgery and radiation in the treatment of synchronous ipsilateral breast cancers. *Cancer* 1993; 72:137–42.
12. Schnitt SJ, Connolly JL, Harris JR et al, Pathologic predictors of early local recurrence in stage I and II breast cancer treated by primary radiation therapy. *Cancer* 1984; 53:1049.
13. Turner BC, Harold E, Matloff E et al, BRCA1/BRCA2 germline mutations in locally recurrent breast cancer patients following lumpectomy and radiation therapy: implications for breast conserving management in

patients with BRCA1/BRCA2 mutations. *J Clin Oncol* 1999; 17:2001–9.

14. Fowble BL, Schultz DJ, Overmoyer B et al, The influence of young age on outcome in early stage breast cancer. *Int J Radiat Oncol Biol Phys* 1994; 30:23–33.

15. Chabner E, Nixon AJ, Garber J et al, Family history suggestive of an inherited susceptibility to breast cancer and treatment outcome in young women after breast-conserving therapy. *Int J Radiat Oncol Biol Phys* 1997; 39:137.

16. Peterson M, Fowble B, Solin LJ et al, Family history status as a prognostic factor for breast cancer patients treated with conservative surgery and irradiation. *Breast J* 1995; 1: 202–9.

17. Romestaing P, Lehingue Y, Carrie C et al, Role of 10-Gy boost in the conservative treatment of early breast cancer: results of a randomized clinical trial in Lyon, France. *J Clin Oncol* 1997; 15:963–8.

18. Haffty BG, Ward B, Pathare P et al, Reappraisal of the role of axillary lymph node dissection in the conservative treatment of breast cancer. *J Clin Oncol* 1997; 15:691–700.

19. Recht A, Pierce SM, Abner A et al, Regional nodal failure after conservative surgery and radiotherapy for early-stage breast carcinoma. *J Clin Oncol* 1991; 9:988–96.

20. Haffty BG, Fischer D, Fischer JJ, Regional nodal irradiation in the conservative treatment of breast cancer. *Int J Radiat Oncol Biol Phys* 1990; 19:859–65.

21. Overgaard M, Hansen PS, Overgaard J et al, Postoperative radiotherapy in high-risk premenopausal women with breast cancer who receive adjuvant chemotherapy. *N Engl J Med* 1997; 337:949–55.

22. Ragaz J, Jackson SM, Le N et al, Adjuvant radiotherapy and chemotherapy in node-positive premenopausal women with breast cancer. *N Engl J Med* 1997; 337:956–62.

23. Overgaard M, Jensen MB, Overgaard J et al, Postoperative radiotherapy in high risk postmenopausal breast cancer patients given adju-

vant tamoxifen: Danish breast cancer cooperative group DBCG 82c randomised trial. *Lancet* 1999; 353:1641–8.

24. Schnitt SJ, Hayman J, Gelman R et al, A prospective study of conservative surgery alone in the treatment of selected patients with Stage I breast cancer. *Cancer* 1996; 77: 1094–100.

25. Haffty BG, Who's on first? Sequencing chemotherapy and radiation therapy in conservatively managed node-negative breast cancer. *Cancer J Sci Am* 1999; 5:147–9.

26. Wallgren A, Bernier J, Gelbar RD et al, Timing of radiotherapy and chemotherapy following breast conserving surgery for patients with node positive breast cancer. International Breast Study Group. *Int J Radiat Oncol Biol Phys* 1996; 35:649–59.

27. McCormick B, Norton L, Yao TJ et al, The impact of the sequence of radiation and chemotherapy on local control after breast conserving surgery. *Cancer J Sci Am* 1996; 2:39–45.

28. Bucholz TA, Hunt KK, Amosson CM et al, Sequencing of chemotherapy and radiation in lymph node negative breast cancer. *Cancer J Sci Am* 1999; 5:159–64.

29. Recht A, Come SE, Henderson C et al, The sequencing of chemotherapy and radiation therapy after conservative surgery for early-stage breast cancer. *N Engl J Med* 1996; 334:1356–99.

30. Fowble B, Gray R, Gilchrist K et al, Identification of a subgroup of patients with breast cancer and histologically positive nodes receiving adjuvant chemotherapy who may benefit from postoperative radiotherapy. *J Clin Oncol* 1988; 6:1107–17.

31. Olson JE, Neuberg D, Pandya K et al, The role of radiotherapy in the management of operable locally advanced breast carcinoma: results of a randomized trial by the Eastern Cooperative Oncology Group. *Cancer* 1997; 79:1138–49.

32. Early Breast Cancer Trialists Collaborative

Group, Effects of radiotherapy and surgery in early breast cancer: an overview of the randomized trials. *N Engl J Med* 1995; **333**: 1444–55.

33. Haffty BG, Reiss M, Beinfield M et al, Ipsilateral breast tumor recurrence as a predictor of distant disease: Implications for systemic therapy at the time of local relapse. *J Clin Oncol* 1996; **13**:52–7.

34. Fowble B, Solin LJ, Schultz DJ, Weiss MC, Breast recurrence and survival related to primary tumor location in patients undergoing conservative surgery and radiation for early stage breast cancer. *Int J Radiat Oncol Biol Phys* 1992; **23**:933–9.

35. Forman DL, Chiu J, Restifo RJ et al, Breast reconstruction in previously irradiated patients using tissue expanders and implants: a potentially unfavorable result. *Ann Plast Surg* 1998; **40**:360–3.

36. Borner M, Bacchi M, Goldhirsch A et al, First isolated loco-regional recurrence following mastectomy for breast cancer: Results of a phase III multicenter study comparing systemic treatment with observation after excision and radiation. *J Clin Oncol* 1994; **12**: 2071–7.

37. Van der Zee J, van der Holt B, Rietveld PJ et al, Reirradiation combined with hyperthermia in recurrent breast cancer results in a worthwhile local palliation. *Br J Cancer* 1999; **79**:483–90.

38. Lee HK, Antell AG, Perez CA et al, Superficial hyperthermia and irradiation for recurrent breast carcinoma of the chest wall: prognostic factors in 196 tumors. *Int J Radiat Oncol Biol Phys* 1998; **40**:365–75.

39. Fisher B, Costintino J, Redmond C et al, Lumpectomy compared with lumpectomy and radiation therapy for the treatment of intraductal breast cancer. *N Engl J Med* 1993; **328**:1581–6.

40. Recht A, Rutgers EJ, Fentiman IS et al, The fourth EORTC DCIS Consensus meeting. *Eur J Cancer* 1998; **34**:1664–9.

41. Silverstein MJ, Lagios MD, Groshen S et al, The influence of margin width on local control of ductal carcinoma in situ of the breast. *N Engl J Med* 1999; **340**:1455–61.

42. Moran M, Haffty BG, Lobular carcinoma in situ as a component of breast cancer: The long term outcome treated with breast conservation therapy. *Int J Radiat Oncol Biol Phys* 1998; **40**:353–8.

24

Survival gains of locoregional radiation in early breast cancer

Joseph Ragaz, Stewart M Jackson

This chapter reviews the outcome of postmastectomy locoregional radiation therapy (RT) in stage I–II breast cancer patients, as seen in the radiation trials published in the 1990s. The outcome is defined as recurrence (locoregional or systemic) or deaths by breast cancer or other causes (breast cancer mortality, overall survival). Locoregional radiation therapy is defined as adjuvant postmastectomy radiation treatment encompassing the chest wall and nodal regions. Evidence will be categorized, whenever possible, into three categories (levels I, II or III), according to the strength of data supporting the conclusions.

BACKGROUND

Adjuvant therapy – old RT trials

The avoidance of locoregional and systemic recurrence in breast cancer is the most important therapeutic achievement of adjuvant treatment modalities, because their reduction will ultimately increase breast cancer survival. Since the mid-1980s, systemic adjuvant therapeutic modalities including chemotherapy and tamoxifen have consistently shown a significant reduction of breast cancer-associated mortality,[1,2] as a result of their impact on systemically disseminated micrometastases.

On the other hand, radiation therapy has been considered a treatment modality primarily aimed at reducing local events. The Oxford overview meta-analysis of all randomized radiation trials initiated before 1995 confirmed level I evidence, in virtually all trials, of a significant reduction of locoregional events.[3] However, the meta-analysis showed that, despite a substantial reduction of locoregional recurrences, the overall survival was not improved significantly.[3] Of importance were observations of a reduction of systemic recurrences by RT, and a small magnitude of breast cancer mortality improvement, counterbalanced, however, in the overall survival analysis by increased cardiac deaths in irradiated patients.[4]

Adjuvant RT trials – new trials

More recently, several large randomized trials of postoperative wide-field RT have shown not only a significant reduction of locoregional recurrences due to RT (Table 24.1), but also a substantial reduction of systemic events[5–8] and of breast cancer mortality.[6–8] This may be the result of several reasons. Introduction of megavoltage equipment and improved RT planning in the late 1970s and 1980s resulted in improved breast cancer cell kill and lower cardiotoxicity, compared with the techniques used in the 1950s and

Table 24.1   Locoregional recurrences: all patients

| Study | Follow-up (years) | Recurrences (%) | | |
		CT	CT + RT	Absolute percentage
Arriagada et al[5]	15	26	6	20
Overgaard et al[7]	10	33	13	20
Ragaz et al[6]	15	23	13	10
Overgaard et al[8]	10	35	8	27
Marks et al[12a]	3	25	6	19

[a]Patients with more than 10 positive nodes treated with high-dose chemotherapy (CT) + autologous bone marrow transplantation. CT, chemotherapy; RT, radiation therapy.

1960s. Also, adjuvant chemotherapy has been used increasingly since the late 1970s, and several mechanisms have been offered to explain a positive CT–RT interaction.[9] Specifically, with combined adjuvant CT and RT, the increased cell kill of systemic clones by CT would assist the RT effect. This aspect of the CT–RT interaction would emphasize that, while reducing locoregional disease, RT given alone fails to affect the pre-existing systemic micrometastases that may be eliminated by CT. Therefore, the untreated pre-existing *systemic* micrometastases would contribute towards breast cancer death, regardless of local control by RT. Also, CT can act as an effective radiosensitizer, improving the cell kill of RT in clones exposed to CT – a very important additional aspect favoring the combined chemoradiation approaches in the therapy of solid tumors in general.

Oxford overview and the new RT trials

The combination of the above arguments could offer a very plausible explanation into why the recent randomized RT trials reported in the 1990s emerged with positive RT effects, involving not only a reduction of locoregional recurrences, but also of systemic events and overall mortality. On the other hand, the overview meta-analysis incorporating a prevalent majority of 'old trials' failed to do so. Of importance regarding this discrepancy is the large heterogeneity of studies reviewed by the Oxford meta-analysis, which included a mix of studies with older and newer RT technologies and planning, when compared with the more uniform use of RT equipment and planning techniques in the newer trials. Also, the newer trials included larger numbers of randomized patients per trials (i.e. >300), who were followed up for a minimum of 10 years, compared with many smaller trials in the meta-analysis followed up for shorter time periods. These points may be of great importance because the significance for overall survival will be directly proportional to number of events (i.e. deaths) – a product of length of follow-up and number of patients. In summary, therefore, although meta-analyses, in general, contribute greatly in interpreting small outcome differences that may not emerge as significant in small trials, the obligatory condition for successful conduct of meta-analysis is a homogeneity and comparability of trials included. Therefore, the evidence from the recent large randomized individual trials may offer an important insight into the impact of RT in the management of early breast cancer, and may offer more reliable evidence of its impact than the meta-analysis.

The main objective of this review is to document whether or not the modern era radiation trials or locoregional RT given for stage I–II breast cancer as published in the 1990s have shown RT to impact on locoregional and systemic metastases, and on breast cancer and overall survival. Also, attempts will be made to quantitate these benefits in various patient subsets, in order to recommend to community oncologists in which situations to use RT routinely. A question of whether the benefits of RT (mostly documented in trials using 'moderate' dose chemotherapy regimens such as cyclophosphamide, methotrexate, 5-fluorouracil (5-FU) combinations (CMF) would also apply to the modern era of chemotherapy, including anthracyclines and taxanes, is also addressed.

REVIEW OF THE NEW RT TRIALS

Trial I: the Swedish trial – impact of radiation in the absence of chemotherapy

One of the first 'modern' era radiation trials using five-field radiation after mastectomy, which showed RT benefit with long follow-up, is the Swedish Stockholm trial as updated by Arriagada et al.[5] This trial was launched in 1971 using a megavoltage radiation technique, with 960 breast cancer patients treated with modified radical mastectomy. Patients were randomized to three groups: group I – preoperative RT; group II – postoperative RT; and group III – surgical controls. Approximately 45% of all patients were

premenopausal and 60% of all cases were node negative. The radiotherapy schedule in both radiation arms included a total of 45 Gy over 5 weeks, using a five-field technique, which encompassed the chest wall, the axilla, supraclavicular area and internal mammary nodes. As the interim analysis showed no difference between the pre- and postoperative radiation arms, the two RT groups were merged, with the final analysis restricted to: group I – radiation vs group II – controls. Analysis was reported at 15-year follow-up.[5]

Taking all patients (i.e. node-negative and node-positive, pre- and postmenopausal), locoregional recurrences were seen in 26% of controls versus 6% in the RT arm (relative risk, RR = 0.2, $p < 0.0001$), combined locoregional and distant metastases in 68% versus 55% (RR = 0.69, $p < 0.0001$) and deaths (from any cause) in 49% vs 44% (RR = 0.85, $p = 0.1$). Of importance is the analysis of distant metastases according to the nodal status. Although not altered significantly in the node-negative patients, the rate of distant metastases was significantly reduced by RT in the node-positive cohorts (72 versus 54%, RR = 0.66, $p = 0.01$). In addition, although in the node-negative patients the overall survival was only minimally affected by RT (RR = 0.92), the 20% mortality reduction reflecting the avoidance of systemic events by RT in the node-positive group is quite substantial, and in line with the mortality reduction shown in the next generation trials from British Columbia and Denmark, using adjuvant CT in conjunction with RT, although perhaps of lower magnitude than in those CT–RT trials. Thus, the large Swedish Stockholm trial is one of the first radiation studies using megavoltage technique, just before the era of adjuvant chemotherapy, which showed a significant RT benefit in improving systemic recurrences and breast cancer mortality in node-positive cases.

Conclusion

This trial provides level I evidence for reduction of locoregional recurrences in node-negative and node-positive patients, level I evidence for a reduction of systemic metastases in node-positive patients and level II evidence for reduction of breast cancer mortality in node-positive cases.

Trial II: the British Columbia trial – impact of radiation in association with chemotherapy schedules of medium dose intensity

The British Columbia study was a two-arm randomized trial, conducted between 1979 and 1986. Inclusion criteria included premenopausal node-positive breast cancer patients, treated with mastectomy and adjuvant chemotherapy, who were randomized to CT alone versus CT + RT. RT was applied between the third and fourth chemotherapy cycles (the 'sandwich' technique). All cases had a modified radical mastectomy with level I/level II axillary dissection and a median of 11 lymph nodes were removed; all patients received megavoltage radiation with a cobalt source, with a planned dose of 3750 cGy/16 fractions over $3\frac{1}{2}$ weeks, encompassing all regional nodal areas including internal mammary fields. CT included cyclophosphamide 600 mg/m^2, methotrexate 40 mg/m^2 and 5-FU 600 mg/m^2 given every 3 weeks × 8. Long-term follow-up (over 15 years) was needed before the significance in favor of RT emerged.[6,10]

Results at 15 years of follow-up[6] showed a significant reduction of locoregional and systemic recurrences by RT (RR = 0.44, p = 0.003; RR = 0.66, p = 0.006, respectively), with a substantial and significant 29% improvement of breast cancer mortality (RR = 0.71, p = 0.05). The recent update of this trial[10] showed not only a persistence of this benefit, but also more significance in improving overall survival, with a

30% reduction of overall mortality in patients randomized to RT (RR = 0.7, p = 0.02). Subsets with one to three positive axillary nodes benefited with a similar magnitude as the cases with more than four nodes (RR 0.65 versus 0.74, respectively).

Conclusion

This trial confirms, in node-positive premenopausal patients treated with modified radical mastectomy and a medium-dose adjuvant chemotherapy (a modified CMF regimen), a significant reduction in locoregional and systemic recurrences, with a resulting reduction in breast cancer and overall mortality. The benefits of RT were of similar magnitude among cases with one to three as those with more than four positive nodes. Evidence was level I for all outcomes.

Trial III: the Danish premenopausal study – RT impact in chemotherapy schedules of medium–high-dose intensity

The Danish Breast Cancer Cooperative Group (DBCG) radiation trials took place between the years 1982 and 1989. Included were pre- and postmenopausal menopausal patients, with premenopausal patients receiving CMF chemotherapy reported separately (DBCG 82b trial[7]), and postmenopausal cases, treated with tamoxifen (82c trial[8]). The premenopausal study randomized 1708 breast cancer patients, who had undergone mastectomy and adjuvant chemotherapy, into CT + RT versus CT alone. CT was a modified Bonadonna regimen, with cyclophosphamide 600 mg/m^2, methotrexate 40 mg/m^2 and 5-FU 600 mg/m^2 given every 4 weeks. Of all patients, 135 had node-negative disease, but a high-risk primary tumor (tumor size >5 cm, or invasion of skin/pectoral fascia); the remaining cases were node positive, with 1061 having one to three positive axillary nodes (N1–3), and 409 having

Table 24.2   Locoregional recurrences: analysis according to the nodal subsets

Study	Follow-up (years)	Recurrences (%)		
		CT	CT + RT	Absolute percentage
Overgaard et al[7] (premenopause)	10			
All patients		32	9	23
Node negative		17	3	14
N1–3		30	7	23
N4+		42	14	28
Arriagada et al[5]	15			
All patients		26	6	20
Node-negative		18	2	16
Node-positive		37	10	27
Ragaz et al[6]	15			
All patients		23	13	10
N1–3		15	9	6
N4+		32	17	15
Overgaard et al[8] (postmenopause)	10			
All patients		35	8	27
Node negative		23	6	17
N1–3		31	6	25
N4+		46	11	35

CT, chemotherapy; RT, radiation therapy.

more than four nodes (N4+) involved. At mastectomy, a median of seven lymph nodes were removed, with 255, 1042 and 409 patients having had two to three, four to nine and more than nine nodes removed, respectively.

Results at 10 years showed, in patients from the RT arm, a significant reduction of locoregional recurrences and a significant improvement of overall survival. Tables 24.2–24.6 show that the locoregional + systemic recurrences, as well as overall survival rates, were all improved in the radiation arm. The RR reductions seen were of similar magnitude in all patients, as in various subsets including node-negative, N1–3 and N4+ cohorts, as well as cases with zero to three, three to nine or more than ten lymph nodes removed (Tables 24.3 and 24.5). These observations provide evidence for the survival improvement of RT for the node-positive cohorts, and also that the relative odds reduction of events caused by RT is constant across most subsets treated.

Conclusion

The Danish trial 82b involving a very large number of cases showed, as in the British Columbia study, that, in premenopausal cases

Table 24.3   Analysis of locoregional recurrences in subsets according to number of nodes removed

Study	Follow-up (years)	Recurrences (%)		
		CT	CT + RT	Absolute percentage
Overgaard et al[7] (premenopause)	10			
All patients		32	9	23
No. of nodes removed:				
0–3		40	10	30
4–9		32	8	24
9+		27	9	18
Overgaard et al[8] (postmenopause)	10			
All patients		35	8	27
No. of nodes removed:				
<8		36	7	29
>8		34	8	26

CT, chemotherapy; RT, radiation therapy.

Table 24.4   Impact of RT: any recurrences (locoregional + systemic)

Study	Follow-up (years)	Recurrences (%)		
		No RT	RT	Absolute percentage
Arriagada et al[5]	15	49	35	14
Overgaard et al[7]	10	58	43	15
Ragaz et al[6]	15	63	48	15
Overgaard et al[8]	10	60	47	13
Marks et al[12a]	3	19	9	10

[a]Patients with more than 10 positive nodes treated with high-dose chemotherapy + autologous bone marrow transplantation. RT, radiation therapy.

with high-risk stage I–II breast cancer treated with mastectomy + medium-dose intensity CT, RT resulted in a significant reduction of recurrences (locoregional as well as systemic), and a reduction of overall mortality. Improvement was seen in subsets with high-risk node-negative disease, as well as in subsets with N1–3 as for N4+ cases.

Table 24.5 Impact of RT: analysis of recurrences (locoregional + systemic) according to the nodal subsets

Study	Follow-up (years)	Recurrences (%)		
		No RT	RT	Absolute percentage
Arriagada et al[5]	15			
All patients		49	35	14
Node-negative		34	26	12
Node-positive		71	53	15
Overgaard et al[7] (premenopause)	10			
All patients		58	43	15
Node negative		34	22	12
N1–3		53	37	15
N4+		76	60	16
Ragaz et al[6]	15			
All patients		63	48	17
N1–3		48	36	12
N4+		83	62	21
Overgaard et al[8] (postmenopause)	10			
All patients		60	47	13
Node-negative		53	34	19
N1–3		52	40	12
N4+		78	63	13

RT, radiation therapy.

There is level I evidence for RT improvements of all outcomes in premenopausal breast cancer subsets as randomized.

Trial IV: the Danish postmenopausal study – RT impact in the presence of tamoxifen

The Danish postmenopausal trial, as in the premenopausal study, started in 1982. Until 1990, over 1370 postmenopausal women with stage I–II breast cancer were randomized into groups with or without locoregional RT. All patients took tamoxifen 30 mg/day for 1 year, as part of their systemic adjuvant therapy. Similar to the premenopausal cases, node-positive as well as node-negative cases were eligible; node-positive cases were grouped into those with fewer than eight axillary nodes removed vs those with more than eight axillary nodes removed.[8]

At 10-year follow-up, irradiated patients had significantly fewer recurrences (47%) compared with 60% in cases without RT. Overall survival was also improved significantly (45 versus 36%, $p = 0.03$). Although all subsets had a substantial reduction of recurrences and improvement in

Table 24.6   Analysis of recurrences (locoregional + systemic) in subsets according to number of nodes removed

Study	Follow-up (years)	Recurrences (%)		
		No RT	RT	Absolute percentage
Overgaard et al[7] (premenopause)	10			
All patients		58	43	15
Nodes removed:				
N0–3		57	44	13
N3–9		58	41	17
N9+		57	44	13
Overgaard et al[8] (postmenopause)	10			
All patients		60	47	13
Nodes removed:				
<8		59	45	14
>8		61	49	12

RT, radiation therapy.

Table 24.7   Impact of RT: frequency of deaths – all patients

Study	Follow-up (years)	Deaths (%)		
		No RT	RT	Absolute percentage
Arriagada et al[5]	15	49	44	5
Overgaard et al[7a] (premenopause)	10	55	46	9
Ragaz et al[6a]	15	54	46	8
Overgaard et al[8a] (postmenopause)	10	64	55	9

[a]Estimates from percentage of overall survival.

overall survival (see Tables 24.1–24.6), when compared with the premenopausal patients, in whom the survival benefit was seen already after the second year, the beneficial survival impact emerged substantially later in time, after 5 years, probably reflecting the slower rate of developing breast cancer events in the older patients.

Conclusion

This trial shows a significant reduction of locoregional and distant recurrences in post-menopausal patients treated with 1 year of tamoxifen, and an improvement of overall survival by RT. The evidence is level I for cases eligible for the study.

Trial V: RT impact in chemotherapy schedules of high-dose intensity – the pilot study of the CALGB trial with or without radiation

The Cancer Leukemia Group B (CALGB) study of high-dose intensity chemotherapy with bone marrow support provides some data regarding the RT effect in patients treated with high-dose chemotherapy. This pilot study led to the first of the large-scale, randomized, adjuvant, high-dose chemotherapy trials requiring bone marrow/stem cell transplantation in the adjuvant setting. Initiated by Peters et al[11] from the CALGB group in the late 1980s, for patients with stage II disease at high risk with more than 10 positive axillary nodes involved, it later extended to become an Inter-group trial involving several US collaborative groups as well as the Canadian National Cancer Institute (NCI).[11] Marks et al[12] reported on the first 43 patients from this trial assessing the role of RT.

All patients were treated in a pilot study of the CALGB high-dose chemotherapy program using the Duke University phase I–II high-dose chemotherapy plus bone marrow transplantation schedule. All cases had, induction chemotherapy after a modified radical mastectomy, with four cycles of cyclophosphamide 600 mg/m^2, doxorubicin 60 mg/m^2, 5-FU 600 mg/m^2 (the CAF regimen). This was followed in cases randomized to the high-dose chemotherapy arm by cyclophosphamide 5625 mg/m^2, cisplatin 165 mg/m^2, carmustine 600 mg/m^2 (the high-dose CDB regimen), with cytokines and stem cell transplantation. Patients in the second arm were treated with the same CT but lower doses (the lower-dose CDB regimen), not requiring bone marrow/stem cell transplantation, but only cytokines. In the high-dose arm, the first nine patients had no RT. Of those, three (33%) developed locoregional recurrence within the first 12 months and three developed distant metastases. As a result, all the subsequent 34 cases in the described study had five-field radiation added at the end of the chemotherapy. At the 3-year follow-up, these cases were updated and reported. Patients were well balanced for prognostic factors, with a median of 13 positive nodes in both groups. Summary results are shown in Tables 24.1 and 24.4 and indicate that, despite the high-dose chemotherapy, locoregional recurrences were seen in 27% versus 3% in unirradiated versus irradiated cases, and systemic recurrences were seen in 27% versus 9%, respectively. Thus, despite the intensive chemotherapy schedule used, locoregional micrometastases were not eliminated, local and systemic recurrences not avoided, and RT was confirmed as a required adjuvant treatment modality.

Conclusion

In this study, there was a significant reduction of locoregional and distant recurrences by RT, despite the high-dose chemotherapy using anthracyclines and high-dose alkylators requiring stem cell transplantation. There is level III evidence regarding the impact of RT on recurrences; there were no data on survival.

COMMENTS

Radiation impact on locoregional recurrences
Incidence of locoregional events
(see Tables 24.1 and 24.2)

In summary, data from the old literature, like those from the new trials, provide consensus for RT reducing locoregional recurrences significantly. The difference is the incidence of locoregional events and the magnitude of the RT benefit among trials. As seen in Table 24.1, although the incidence of locoregional events in cases *without RT* differs widely among trials, with ranges of 10–46% according to subsets, all studies show a similar proportional rate of locoregional event reduction. The main reason for the wide absolute local recurrence heterogeneity is manyfold: the inclusion of different subsets among different trials; different follow-up duration in various studies; and different methodologies for reporting local events. Specifically, some trials report a locoregional recurrence only if it occurs before the systemic event, some include a local event if it occurs either before or after systemic events, and some restrict a local event to a true 'isolated local recurrence', counting local relapses as events only if occurring more than 3–6 months before the systemic event.

Of great interest is the possibility that the impact of RT is restricted only to cases with inadequate axillary surgery. The Scandinavian and the British Columbia trials offer insight into this issue because the median number of removed axillary lymph nodes in the Danish trial was seven, compared with the median of 11 from the British Columbia trial, or compared with what is expected from a level I/II axillary node dissection. Table 24.2 indicates that the Swedish and the British Columbia trials, with 'adequate' surgery, show significant benefits regarding the reduction of local events, but so do the Danish trials with less adequate surgery. Furthermore, Table 24.3 shows that, within the Danish trial 82b, cases with less than three, three to nine or more than nine nodes removed all derive a substantial RT benefit, and that patients with more than nine nodes removed had still very high (27%) locoregional recurrences if not irradiated, despite the apparently adequate number of axillary nodes removed; and recurrence was reduced significantly (to 9%) by RT.

These data provide evidence for a rather constant relative risk reduction by RT in most subsets, whether node positive or node negative, among N1–3 or N4+ cases or among cohorts with fewer than three nodes removed, three to nine or more than nine nodes removed.

Radiation impact on systemic recurrences/breast cancer mortality

As seen in Tables 24.4–24.7, the reviewed trials show a substantial improvement of either systemic recurrences (including the Swedish, British Columbia, Danish and the CALGB trials) or breast cancer mortality/overall survival (the British Columbia and Danish trials).

The unresolved issue is more detailed interaction of local and systemic events, especially the impact of avoiding the locoregional recurrence by RT and the systemic dissemination. The British Columbia trial provides evidence that most cases with a locoregional event will eventually develop, in long-term follow-up (15 years), a systemic recurrence (i.e. >80%), and will suffer a breast cancer death.[13] Therefore, the salvage RT or CT at the time of locoregional recurrence after mastectomy does not have the same curative potential as the same treatments delivered in the adjuvant setting. What is less clear, but important, is the origin of systemic recurrences and, specifically, whether systemic events originate from the locoregional recurrences or from the *locoregional microscopic source* (i.e. lymph nodes/chest wall) disseminating before the diagnosis of locoregional recurrence. In the latter case, both the locoregional and the systemic recurrences would have a common source (i.e. the locoregional microscopic micrometastases). Data for avoiding systemic recurrences by RT in the absence of locoregional failures (i.e. as seen in most trials with adequate follow-up showing the number of systemic events to be substantially higher than locoregional recurrences) are also compatible with the hypothesis that both the locoregional and the systemic events originate from the locoregional microscopic micrometastases. Thus, although some systemic recurrences could originate from clones disseminating from the site of the locoregional recurrence, the prevalent majority of systemic disease originates from the subclinical locoregional metastases. Thus, they could be the subject of curative treatments with combined chemoradiation treatment approaches. Accordingly, both locoregional and systemic recurrences probably originate from the same source, which, although microscopic, may be sufficiently extensive to be resistant to chemotherapy and therefore demands RT; and therefore locoregional recurrences are a marker rather than the source of systemic events.

SUMMARY

The above review allows several conceptual conclusions to be made about the impact of RT in breast cancer patients with high-risk stage I–II disease.

Impact of RT in patients treated without systemic CT[5]

- Level I evidence for a reduction of locoregional events in node-negative and node-positive cases.
- Level I evidence for reduction of systemic events in node-positive cases.
- Level II evidence for reduction of breast cancer mortality in node-positive cases.

Impact of RT in patients treated with medium-intensity adjuvant CT[6,7]

- Level I evidence in premenopausal patients for a reduction of locoregional and systemic events.
- Level I evidence for reduced breast cancer mortality.

- Level I evidence for improved overall survival.

Impact of RT in postmenopausal patients treated with adjuvant tamoxifen[8]

- Level I evidence in postmenopausal breast cancer patients treated with tamoxifen (30 mg for 1 year) for reduction of locoregional and systemic recurrences.
- Level I evidence for reduced breast cancer mortality and for improved overall survival in cases as randomized.

Impact of RT in high-risk patients (N10+) treated with anthracycline-containing adjuvant CT followed by high-dose intensity alkylating CT requiring stem cell transplantation[12]

- Level III evidence for reduction of locoregional recurrences.
- Level III evidence for reduction of systemic recurrences.

EVIDENCE-BASED RECOMMENDATIONS AND CONCLUDING REMARKS

- This review provides evidence for the benefit of modern era radiation in subsets of high-risk patients with early breast cancer using megavoltage RT equipment, encompassing chest wall and all regional nodes.
- The benefit is defined as a significant reduction of both locoregional and systemic recurrences, reduced breast cancer mortality and improved overall survival.
- Although the level I evidence for breast cancer mortality/overall survival is restricted to trials using RT in conjunction with systemic treatments, it is very likely that there are substantial survival gains also in RT treatments using modern RT equipment alone, without systemic treatment. It is, however, possible that in these situations, the survival benefits may

be less evident than in studies using chemotherapy in conjunction.

- As the RT benefit, in cases with more than ten positive nodes treated with anthracycline adjuvant CT followed by high-dose CT requiring stem cells, is derived from non-randomized trials, it is defined as level III evidence. However, because of high absolute recurrent rates without RT in these very high-risk stage II cases, and because absolute and relative reductions of recurrences by RT in those situations are of similar magnitude to those seen in stage I–II cases treated with medium CT dose, the RT gains in these situations are considered to be substantial and clinically relevant.

- These observations provide some clinical evidence for the hypothesis that even the most dose-intense chemotherapy will not be likely to offer curative results for 'bulk' diseases. In those situations, RT may be required in conjunction, similar to treatment approaches with other solid tumors.

- Although some investigators consider it reasonable to re-test the RT impact with the modern era chemotherapy regimens (i.e. anthracycline/taxanes), others feel that many lives may be lost in the process if high-risk stage II breast cancer cases in the control arm are treated without RT. This is particularly because it is evident that *no currently available* chemotherapy regimen given alone without RT can adequately control locally advanced microscopic disease.

- The issue of great importance is the toxicity of RT in conjunction with anthracycline/taxane regimens (e.g. cardiotoxicity). The magnitude of this problem may have to be determined in clinical trials, and the testing of routine implementation of cardioprotective agents such as dexrazoxane (Zinecard), shown from randomized trials[14] to reduce the anthracycline-associated cardiotoxicity (level I evidence), may have to be considered.

- Data in this overview provide evidence for RT benefit in most subsets with high risk for recurrence, including node-negative cohorts, as well as in subsets with N1–3 vs N4+ disease. Although the test for interaction failed to test any difference of this benefit among the N1–3 compared with N4+ cohorts,[6] the more subtle differences among different cohorts may have to be determined. Preliminary evidence indicates more RT benefit in N1–3 patients with high-risk features (such as extensive nodal spread/extracapsular spread), which is compelling enough to consider stratification for these factors and implementation of early stopping rules in any new generation randomized RT trials.[10] In the situations in which clinicians do not participate in randomized trials, it would be reasonable to consider routine use of adjuvant locoregional RT combined with optimum adjuvant CT for any high-risk cohorts.

CONCLUSION

For the present community practice guidelines, it would be appropriate to use locoregional RT for any situations where the risk of locoregional or systemic recurrences is high, no RT where risk is low and participation in randomized trials if the risk is intermediate.

REFERENCES

1. Early Breast Cancer Trialists' Collaborative Group, Polychemotherapy for early breast cancer: an overview of the randomized trials. *Lancet* 1998; **352**:930–42.
2. Early Breast Cancer Trialists' Collaborative Group, Tamoxifen for early breast cancer: an overview of the randomized trials. *Lancet* 1998; **351**:1451–67.

3. Early Breast Cancer Trialists' Collaborative Group, Effective radiotherapy and surgery in early breast cancer: an overview of the randomized trials. *N Engl J Med* 1995; **333**: 144–55.

4. Cuzick J, Stewart H, Rutqvist LE, Cause specific mortality in long term survivors of breast cancer who participated in trials of radiotherapy. *J Clin Oncol* 1994; **12**:447–53.

5. Arriagada R, Rutqvist LE, Mattson A et al, Adequate locoregional treatment for early breast cancer may prevent secondary dissemination. *J Clin Oncol* 1995; **13**:2869–78.

6. Ragaz J, Jackson SM, Le N et al, Adjuvant radiotherapy and chemotherapy in node positive premenopausal women with breast cancer. *N Engl J Med* 1997; **337**:956–62.

7. Overgaard M, Hanxen PS, Carsten R et al, Postoperative radiotherapy in high risk premenopausal women with breast cancer who receive adjuvant chemotherapy. *N Engl J Med* 1997; **337**:949–55.

8. Overgaard M, Jensen MB, Overgaard J et al, Postoperative radiotherapy in high-risk postmenopausal breast-cancer patients given adjuvant tamoxifen: Danish Breast Cancer Cooperative Group DBCG 82c randomised trial. *Lancet* 1999; **353**:1641–8.

9. Ragaz J, Survival impact of wide field radiation in high risk cases with early breast cancer: controversy or settled issue? *Clin Breast Cancer* 2000 (in press).

10. Ragaz J, Jackson SM, Le N et al, Postmastectomy radiation outcome in node positive breast cancer patients among N1–3 versus N4+ subsets: impact of extracapsular spread. Update of the British Columbia randomized trial. *Proc Am Soc Clin Oncol* 1999; **18**:73a.

11. Peters WP, Ross M, Vredenburgh JJ et al, High-dose chemotherapy and autologous bone marrow support as consolidation after standard dose adjuvant therapy for high-risk primary breast cancer. *J Clin Oncol* 1993; **11**:1132.

12. Marks LB, Halperin EC, Prosnitz LR et al, Post-mastectomy radiotherapy following high-dose adjuvant chemotherapy and bone marrow transplantation for breast cancer patients with more than 10 positive axillary lymph nodes. *Int J Radiat Oncol Biol Phys* 1992; **23**:1021–6.

13. Chia S, Ragaz J, Jackson S et al, Locoregional disease in breast cancer: Marker or a source of systemic disease? Recurrence pattern analysis of the British Columbia randomized trial. *Proc Am Soc Clin Oncol* 1998; **17**:168.

14. Swain SM, Whaley FS, Gerber MC et al, Delayed administration of dexrazoxane provides cardioprotection for patients with advanced breast cancer treated with doxorubicin-containing therapy. *J Clin Oncol* 1997; **15**:1318–32.

SECTION 7: Supportive Therapy

Section Editors: AHG Paterson, M-A Lindsay

25

The place of bisphosphonates in the management of breast cancer

Alexander HG Paterson

Bone pain, fractures and hypercalcemia are important causes of morbidity in patients with metastatic breast cancer despite recent advances in hormone and cytotoxic therapy. These skeletal complications arise because of progressive focal or generalized osteolysis. Osteolysis occurs because of osteoclast activation, either directly by tumor products or by products secreted by nearby host cells in response to tumor cell products.[1] As the osteoclast plays a central role in focal or generalized osteolysis, inhibitors of osteoclast function may lead to palliation and, in some cases, to prevention of osteolytic destruction and its complications.[2] It is also possible that the growth and development of bone metastases may be inhibited in a proportion of patients, and the bone loss associated with premature menopause induced by adjuvant chemotherapy may be prevented.

THE CLINICAL PROBLEM

Skeletal pain, fracture and hypercalcemia are well recognized by oncologists as major causes of morbidity in patients with breast cancer. Verte-bral fractures not only cause pain and disability, but may also lead to spinal cord compression. In women, the problems of bone metastases are compounded by the propensity to osteoporosis. Women have a lower total bone mass than men and the fracture threshold is reached at an earlier age in women than in men. In addition, in pre-menopausal women with breast cancer, the increasing use of adjuvant cytotoxic chemotherapy leads to earlier menopause with subsequent earlier accelerated loss of bone.

NORMAL AND ABNORMAL BONE REMODELING

Bone remodeling is a dynamic process occurring in response to poorly understood physical and chemical forces along lines of stress.[3] Remodeling may result from initial stimulation by osteoblastic cells, which are derived from bone marrow stromal cells.[4] Osteoclasts are recruited to an area of damaged or worn bone, which is then broken down, forming a bone resorption bay, by the action of lytic substances secreted by the osteoclast. Osteoblasts then move into the bone resorption bay (Howship's lacuna), and new bone precursor substances, largely consisting of type I collagen, are laid down in layers, which, over time, become mineralized. The formation of new bone after orderly resorption in the resorption cavities is termed 'coupling'. Bone remodeling normally occurs, therefore, as the result of a balance between bone destruction and new bone formation.

When malignant cells infiltrate bone spaces, the balance of new bone formation and bone destruction is perturbed, and bone remodeling and turnover become abnormal. Under these circumstances, three mechanisms contribute to abnormalities of bone remodeling.[5] The first occurs when a wave of bone resorption is initiated, usually focally, but sometimes generally, leading to increased bone turnover; loss of bone occurs because the resorption phase precedes the formation phase. A second mechanism comes into play when the normal connection between bone resorption and formation is disrupted and new bone is formed at sites other than where resorption has recently taken place. A third mechanism ('uncoupling') occurs when the amount of new bone formed in the resorption bays does not match quantitatively the amount of bone resorbed.

Carcinoma cells can secrete a variety of substances, such as parathyroid hormone-related peptide (PTHrP), prostaglandin E and transforming growth factors, which might stimulate tumor growth by autocrine or paracrine mechanisms, but which also have stimulatory effects on osteoclast function. Most of these effects occur locally, but these substances can also be secreted into the circulation, and have a generalized effect on bone metabolism.[6] In prostate cancer, where osteoblastic metastases predominate, the excessive, deranged and uncoupled new bone formation can lead to the 'bone hunger syndrome', a situation in which Ca^{2+} entrapment in bone leads to lower than normal plasma Ca^{2+} levels, with subsequent elevation of parathyroid hormone (PTH). This secondary hyperparathyroidism can lead to further generalized bone loss. In breast cancer, PTHrP release also leads to increased proximal tubular reabsorption of Ca^{2+} within the kidney, and this is an important mechanism for the appearance of hypercalcemia in breast and other cancers.[8]

'SEED AND SOIL' THEORIES

The concept of a malignant-cell–matrix interaction is an old one, and hypotheses have been developed to explain the appearance of metastases at specific sites. These have been termed 'seed and soil' theories. Experiments designed to investigate the relationship between malignant cells and their surrounding tissues at sites of metastases suggest that chemical interactions form the basis of the association.[9]

The association of breast cancer with the development of bone metastases was first expressed in print by Paget in 1889 when he wrote:[10]

The evidence seems to be irresistible that in cancer of the breast, the bones suffer in a special way, which cannot be explained by any theory of embolism alone.

The notion that there might be a local reason for the development of metastases at specific sites beyond a chance colonization after embolism was further developed by Batson,[11] who described the connection between the vertebral venous plexus and the bone marrow spaces, hypothesizing a retrograde spread that would allow metastases from a primary prostate cancer to lodge preferentially in the lower vetebrae. Once within the marrow space, metastases have a blood supply for further growth. Mundy has taken the seed and soil idea one step further by adding the concept of a 'vicious cycle', with products from tumor-induced breakdown of bone leading to stimulation and further growth of malignant cells.[12]

BONE METASTASES

Incidence and morbidity

The association of osteolytic, osteosclerotic and mixed lytic/sclerotic bone metastases with breast cancer is well known to clinicians. In the experience of a major clinical trials group, the National Surgical Adjuvant Breast and Bowel Project (NSABP) in the USA, bone metastases account for the highest proportion of first sites of relapse in breast cancer patients who have recurrence of their disease after adjuvant therapy with hormones and/or chemotherapy. Approximately one-third of patients who develop distant metastases do so in bone either as the sole site of recurrence or simultaneously with other sites of disease. As the disease progresses, most patients will develop bone metastases; their median survival from diagnosis of bone metastases is between 18 and 20 months.[13,14] Recently, we have shown that patients presenting with breast cancer have a four to five times higher rate of vertebral fracture than an age-matched group of well women.[15] This is most probably related to chemotherapy-induced premature menopause with accelerated bone loss.

Bone pain

When malignant cells invade the intertrabecular spaces, the malignant cells may form a mass to a size where secreted substances have an impact on local physiology. It is too simplistic to explain bone pain on purely mechanistic grounds, by suggesting that a bone metastasis causes pain because trabecular fractures occur and bone collapses, leading to compression and distortion of the periosteum – a site known to be innervated by pain fibers. It is difficult to understand how bone pain can occur in the absence of fracture, but this does happen commonly. Bone marrow spaces are innervated by nociceptive C-fibers that are sensitive to changes in pressure, and it is probable that the malignant cells secrete pain-provoking factors such as substance P, bradykinins, prostaglandins and other cytokines, which lead to stimulation of C-type fibers within bone. Prostaglandins may also play a role by sensitizing free nerve endings to vasoactive amines and kinins released.[16] The precise interaction between the tumor and bone microenvironment is unknown. The subject of bone pain caused by metastases has been well reviewed.[17]

BONE METASTASES: GENERAL PRINCIPLES OF MANAGEMENT

Although this review focuses on the place of bisphosphonates in the treatment of bone metastases in breast cancer (mainly because this area has provided some of the most exciting research in recent years), other modalities continue to provide the mainstay of therapy.

Bone pain management includes a thorough history and physical examination, full discussion with the patient about a plan of action, and attempts to modify the pathologic process. These attempts include external-beam radiotherapy (still the most effective remedy for alleviation of localized bone pain) and palliative chemotherapy. A good response to chemotherapy includes subjective relief of symptoms. Hormone therapy in breast cancer can provide a high-quality remission in patients with bone metastases. Radionuclide therapy with strontium-89 can be effective in alleviating the bone pain of breast cancer. Patients may require sequential therapy with bisphosphonates and strontium-89. Trials of both modalities used together are overdue.

Elevation of the pain threshold with the use of

non-pharmacologic methods, as well as analgesics, interruption of pain pathways by local or regional anaesthesia or neurolysis, and modification of lifestyles, is helpful, but invariably opiate and other adjuvant analgesic management will be required.

Prophylactic surgery and radiation therapy for patients with cortical erosion caused by metastasis in the femur and humerus will prevent the distress of a pathologic fracture.

BISPHOSPHONATES

Many bisphosphonates have been assessed in the management of malignant hypercalcemia. These include etidronate, pamidronate, clodronate, risedronate, mildronate, neridronate, alendronate, ibandronate and zoledronate. Etidronate, pamidronate and clodronate have been the most extensively tested bisphosphonates, and are widely available for the treatment of hypercalcemia and Paget's disease of bone. We have previously demonstrated the action of etidronate in the treatment of hypercalcemia.[18] Pamidronate, clodronate and etidronate lead to an effective lowering of serum calcium, which is attributable to decreased bone resorption, but etidronate appears to impair the mineralization of bone and must be given intermittently to allow normal bone formation to occur.[19] Pamidronate, an aminobisphosphonate, may not be ideal for oral use because of dose-related gastrointestinal toxicity. There is some evidence that long-term pamidronate administered orally may also induce osteomalacia.[20] Clodronate is effective when given intravenously for hypercalcemia and bone pain, and can be used orally. Its long-term administration is not associated with a defect in the mineralization of bone.[21]

The geminal bisphosphonates are analogs of pyrophosphate characterized by a stable P–C–P bond. They bind with high affinity to hydroxyapatite crystals in bone, and are potent inhibitors of normal and pathologic bone resorption.[22] Several mechanisms of action seem to operate, the dominant mechanism differing in different compounds, but all appear to have a final common effect of inhibition of osteoclast function. The osteoblast might be the initial target cell for bisphosphonates, exerting an effect on the osteoclast by modulation of stimulating and inhibiting factors that control osteoclast function.[23] Transforming growth factor β (TGF-β) is known to induce osteoclast apoptosis, and its production by bone surface osteoblasts as a result of bisphosphonate stimulation may explain this phenomenon.

These agents appear to promote apoptosis in murine osteoclasts both in vivo and in vitro, the more potent bisphosphonates exhibiting the greatest apoptotic action.[24] In the absence of apoptosis, inhibition of osteoclast function appears to be mediated by osteoblasts, which produce a factor that inhibits osteoclastic function.[25] This action does not interfere with the ability of cells of the monocyte–macrophage lineage to produce colonies.[26] Bisphosphonates can also inhibit the proliferation and promote the cell death of macrophages.[27,28] Again, the process is one of apoptosis rather than necrosis and may, in part, explain the pain-relieving properties of bisphosphonates. More recently, Shipman et al[29] have described the induction of apoptosis by bisphosphonates in human myeloma cell lines.

CLINICAL TRIALS OF BISPHOSPHONATES IN BREAST CANCER

Hypercalcemia

As a result of secretion of factors from infiltrating malignant ductal cells acting focally and humorally, osteoclast activity is markedly increased, with a reduction in osteoblast activity, leading to 'uncoupling' of bone resorption and formation.[30] PTHrP appears to play a central role in malignant hypercalcemia.[31]

We have recently reviewed the evidence for the treatment of hypercalcemia and have offered some broad guidelines.[32] Saline rehydration will usually effect a median reduction of 0.25 mmol/l but its effect is transient.[33] Rehydration is useful for treating mild degrees of hypercalcemia, but should usually be accompanied by bisphosphonate therapy. Symptomatic hypercalcemia, especially with levels of Ca^{2+} greater than 3.0 mmol/l, requires vigorous rehydration (physiological saline 150–200 ml/h with KCl 20–40 mmol/l added, and the administration of clodronate 1500 mg in 500 ml physiological saline over 2–3 hours or pamidronate 60–90 mg in 500 ml physiological saline over 2–3 hours). Pamidronate may give a longer duration of maintenance of normocalcemia[34] action than clodronate (28 days median versus 14 days), but in many countries is significantly more expensive. Newer bisphosphonates, such as ibandronate and zoledronate, are currently being studied.

Skeletal complications

Early clinical investigations of bisphosphonates were carried out in uncontrolled trials of patients with advanced disease or small, non-placebo-controlled, open studies.[35] Although it has been shown that these investigators were correct in their conclusions, it is difficult to determine the extent to which patient selection and the placebo effect influenced the positive results of the investigations.

One of the first randomized controlled studies to be published was an open trial of the aminobisphosphonate, pamidronate, given orally for 2 years at 300 mg daily in patients with bone metastases from breast cancer.[36] The investigators demonstrated a reduction in the skeletal complications of hypercalcemia and vertebral fractures. Radiation treatment for bone pain was also reduced, but there was difficulty in patient compliance due to gastrointestinal side effects.

In a double-blind, randomized, placebo-controlled trial of oral clodronate 1600 mg given daily for 2 years, we confirmed this beneficial effect on skeletal morbidity in patients with bone metastases from breast cancer.[37] The number of patients who had episodes of hypercalcemia and the total number of episodes were reduced; the number of major vertebral fractures and the vertebral deformity rate were also reduced; finally, the number of radiotherapy treatments was lower in the clodronate-treated patients. No survival benefit was evident. McCloskey et al[38] reviewed the pre-entry and follow-up vertebral fracture prevalence in 163 of the 173 patients in this trial, and found that 46% of the patients had evidence of vertebral fracture at trial entry. The patients deriving the greatest benefit from the oral clodronate were those who had already sustained vertebral fractures and were therefore at greatest risk for sustaining further fractures.

Pamidronate, which can occasionally induce sclerosis in osteolytic lesions when used as the only therapy,[39] has been investigated in several trials. Tumor response in bone and duration of response were assessed in a double-blind, randomized trial, which showed similar response rates in bone but an increased duration of response for patients receiving pamidronate given intravenously every 3 weeks.[40] Measurement of response in bone can be a difficult process and, unless differences in the arms of a trial are large, small but significant differences can be missed. Hortobagyi et al[41] have reported a randomized trial of 380 patients with recurrent breast cancer in bone and demonstrated a convincing reduction in the skeletal complications of vertebral fracture, pain and hypercalcemia with intravenous pamidronate 90 mg given monthly for 2 years. No survival benefit was apparent.

As a result of these well-controlled trials, we

currently recommend the use of either oral clodronate 1600 mg daily (preferably taken at least 30 minutes before breakfast or at least 2 hours away from food) or intravenous pamidronate 90 mg every 4 weeks in patients with radiologically established bone metastases from breast cancer.

Bone pain

The idea that bisphosphonates might decrease bone pain in some patients with bone metastases arose from clinical observations of patients receiving bisphosphonates for hypercalcemia. Patients not only experienced normalization of serum Ca^{2+} and relief of the symptoms of hypercalcemia, but also reported relief of pain.

Ernst et al[42] demonstrated, in a double-blind crossover trial of intravenous clodronate in patients with bone pain caused by a variety of malignancies, that clodronate had useful analgesic properties. This was confirmed in a larger, randomized, double-blind, controlled trial of intravenous clodronate in patients with metastatic bone pain.[43] No dose–response relationship was seen. Improvement in pain and mobility scores had been described in a previously reported trial of oral pamidronate, although these patients had not been selected specifically because of bone pain but because they had osteolytic metastases.[44] Pain relief has also been described with intravenous pamidronate in a placebo-controlled trial in patients with bone metastases from breast cancer.[41] The mechanism of pain relief is unknown, but may be related to the previously described mechanisms of action on osteoclast and macrophage apoptosis or an inhibition of pain-provoking cellular factors.

TRIALS OF ADJUVANT BISPHOSPHONATES

Patients with recurrent disease but no bone metastases

Some intriguing pioneer data were generated in a small, randomized, placebo-controlled, clinical trial of continuous oral clodronate in patients who had recurrent breast cancer, but with no evidence of bone metastases on bone scanning and conventional radiology.[45] Although overall survival in the two arms was similar, there was an expected significant reduction in skeletal complications. When the incidence of new bone metastases was assessed, a significant reduction in the number of new bone metastases in the clodronate-treated group was found. However, the number of patients developing bone metastases, although lower in the clodronate-treated group, was not significantly different from that in the control group. This study is one of the first of its kind to suggest that the intervention of a bisphosphonate, which primarily acts on osteoclasts, can have an impact on the behavior of bone metastases.

One other trial has assessed oral pamidronate in a similar group of patients with advanced or recurrent disease but no bone metastases. The trial was randomized but not placebo-controlled, and was also relatively small, with an accrual of 124 patients. A large number of patients withdrew from the trial because of the gastrointestinal side effects of oral pamidronate, and compliance was a problem. Results showed no effect on rate of development of skeletal metastases, quality of life or survival.[46]

PATIENTS WITH OPERABLE BREAST CANCER

As Goldhirsch has pointed out in reviewing the trials of the International Breast Cancer Study

Group, the main effect of the adjuvant therapy used in the Group's trials has been to reduce local, regional and distant soft tissue recurrences. First recurrences in bone and viscera have been minimally affected.[47]

At menopause, bone resorption accelerates in women, and they reach the fracture threshold at an earlier mean age than men, largely because of their lower peak bone mass. Combination chemotherapy is now used in premenopausal women with all stages of breast cancer. Many women with multiple positive lymph nodes receive high-dose chemotherapy with stem cell rescue. One of the effects of these treatments, particularly when high-dose chemotherapy is used, or when the protocol contains alkylating agents, is to cause ovarian ablation leading to premature menopause. The skeletal effects of oophorectomy in rats are predictable, and consist of an early acceleration of bone turnover with loss of bone substance, especially cancellous bone. This accelerated bone turnover can be reduced by estrogen or the bisphosphonate, risedronate. The effect of estrogen is lost 90 days after cessation of estrogen therapy. In contrast, the bisphosphonate is still effective 180 days after withdrawal.[48] The bone loss after premature menopause in patients can be substantial, reaching as much as 7% in the first year in some women, but can be prevented by clodronate[49] and risedronate.[50]

The results of adjuvant chemotherapy and hormone therapy show that there is room for improvement in dealing with bone metastasis as a site of disease recurrence. Tamoxifen does appear to reduce the incidence of new bone metastases as well as metastases at other sites.[5] This reduction in the incidence of bone metastasis as the site of first recurrence is not seen with chemotherapy. Tamoxifen is also known to have a beneficial effect on reducing bone resorption in postmenopausal women.[52] Early attempts to reduce the incidence of bone metastases in patients with operable breast cancer using prostaglandin inhibitors, such as aspirin and indomethacin, were unsuccessful. This was despite in vitro data from the Walker carcinoma and in vivo data in the osteolytic rabbit VX2 tumor, which suggested that osteolysis and bone metastases could be inhibited by early treatment with prostaglandin inhibitors.[53] These agents, although useful for the relief of pain, have little effect on the skeletal complications of established bone metastases. Bisphosphonates, which have an established record in reducing the skeletal complications of bone metastases, are a more promising group of compounds for prevention trials.

If clodronate and pamidronate can reduce the skeletal complications of patients with breast cancer, myeloma and possibly other malignancies, do they achieve this by means of a protective 'anti-osteolytic' mechanism, as implied by their known mechanisms of action, or is it possible that their final pathway mode of action, the inhibition of osteoclast function, has a feedback effect leading to inhibition of the growth of bone metastases? Can we, by affecting the 'soil' of the microenvironment in which deposits of tumor cells grow, influence the behavior of the 'seeds', the tumor micrometastases themselves? Production of PTHrP by breast carcinoma cells in bone is enhanced by growth factors such as activated TGF-β, produced as a result of both normal bone remodeling and accelerated osteolysis; this sets up a vicious cycle. It is also known that breast cancer cells secrete low-molecular-weight factors that specifically affect human osteoblast cell lines, inhibiting their proliferation and increasing their cAMP response to PTH.

Is it possible that we are merely interfering with the mechanisms of diagnosis, for example by inhibiting the uptake of radiolabeled technetium pertechnetate in the bone reaction surrounding a metastasis, thereby reducing the tumor : background ratio of radionuclide uptake? This is unlikely, given the extensive experience of bone scanning in patients with bone metastases who have received oral or intravenous bisphosphonates. There have been no reports of inhibition of uptake of bone-seeking radionuclides by bisphosphonates. Pecherstorfer et al[54] have demonstrated that there was no effect on bone scintigraphy in 11 patients with breast cancer scanned after receiving daily intravenous clodronate for 3 weeks. Similarly, there was no inhibition of uptake documented on scans taken after bisphosphonate treatment compared with baseline scans after intravenous pamidronate had been administered as little as 24 hours previously.[55]

A body of animal experimental data suggests that bisphosphonates have an inhibitory effect on the development of bone metastases. Pretreatment with bisphosphonates protects against the development of bone metastases in rats. When the Walker 256B carcinosarcoma is implanted intraosseously into Wistar–Lewis rats, pre-treatment with clodronate inhibits the development of bone metastases compared with controls.[56] Shorter intervals between the bisphosphonate therapy and the inoculation of tumor cells gave the best results, suggesting that, in the human setting, early therapy might give better results. This protective effect diminished with time after inoculation. Low-dose, continuous therapy also provided protection against metastatic growth.

Cell adhesion molecules are likely to be involved in the growth and invasion of breast cancer cells in bone.[57] van der Pluijm et al[58] have demonstrated that the more potent bisphosphonates can inhibit the adhesion of breast cancer cells to neonatal murine bone matrices (cortical bone slices and trabecular bone cryostat sections), although no effect was seen with etidronate or clodronate in this system. This anti-adhesion effect has been confirmed by Boissier et al,[59] who examined both prostate and breast cancer cells. No direct cytotoxicity on tumor cells was seen.

These animal studies suggest that it is possible to use bisphosphonates not only as a treatment for skeletal complications of cancer in humans, but also as a protectant against the development of metastases in bone.

Trials have shown that bisphosphonates can prevent the accelerated bone loss after the menopause and that this might prevent the development of osteoporosis. Saarto et al[60] demonstrated that 2 years of clodronate therapy reduced bone loss compared with controls in all groups of patients, including those receiving chemotherapy, although the effect was greatest in those women receiving tamoxifen, some of whom gained bone density.

The ideal setting for testing whether bisphosphonates can have a beneficial effect on the rate of development of bone metastases is in the setting of the adjuvant therapy of operable breast cancer. The diagnosis of new bone metastases and differentiation from vertebral osteopenic fractures is manageable in patients who are relatively fit, and the development of metastasis can be correlated with measurements of bone density and other parameters. One interesting trial of adjuvant bisphosphonates has been reported.[61] In this study, 142 patients with primary breast cancer and no evidence of distant metastases were randomized to receive oral clodronate 1600 mg daily, and a further 142 were randomized into a non-placebo control group. These patients all had bone marrow involvement, with tumor cells detectable using the technique described by this group.[62] After a median follow-up of 3 years, 21 patients in the clodronate group had developed distant metastases, compared with 42 patients in the control group. There were 10 patients relapsing in the bone, with an average of 3.1 metastases per patient in the clodronate group, compared with 19 patients relapsing in the bone, with an average of 6.3 metastases per patient in the control group. The relapse-free interval for bone was 23 months for the clodronate group, compared with 16 months for the control patients. Not only was there a reduction in new bone metastases, there was also a significant reduction in new visceral metastases and a survival advantage in the clodronate-treated group.

In an interim analysis of a larger, randomized, placebo-controlled trial, we have been unable to confirm the effect of oral clodronate on the incidence of visceral metastases or on survival; there does appear to be an effect, however, on the incidence of bone metastases.[63] These conflicting data require further assessment in larger, placebo-controlled, randomized trials. At this point, we are unable to recommend the use of bisphosphonates specifically as antitumor agents for the prevention of bone metastases in patients with operable breast cancer.

CONCLUSIONS

The following suggestions are submitted for consideration by physicians treating patients with breast cancer:

- Hypercalcemia: intravenous pamidronate or clodronate with rehydration as described in the text.
- Presence of bone metastases (symptomatic or asymptomatic): oral clodronate 1600 mg daily or intravenous pamidronate 90 mg every 4 weeks.
- Bone pain: intravenous pamidronate 90 mg every 4 weeks, intravenous clodronate 1500 mg every 2 weeks.
- Post-chemotherapy bone loss: oral clodronate 1600 mg daily if, on bone densitometry, the T-score is >2.5 (the T-score is a comparison of bone density in standard deviations with the normal peak bone mass), the annual rate of bone loss is >10% or fragility fractures are documented.
- Operable breast cancer: further controlled trials are required.

REFERENCES

1. Mundy GR, Ibbotson KJ, DeSouza SM et al, The hypercalcemia of cancer. Clinical implication and pathogenic mechanisms. *N Engl J Med* 1984; **310**:1718.
2. Taubt T, Elomaa I, Blomqvist C et al, Histomorphometric evidence for osteoclast medicated bone resorption in metastatic breast cancer. *Bone* 1994; **15**:161–6.
3. Kaplan FS, Osteoporosis: Pathophysiology and prevention. *Clin Symp* 1987; **39**:1–32.
4. Mundy GR, Bone resorption and turnover in health and disease. *Bone* 1987; **8**(Suppl 1): S9–16.
5. Kanis JA, McCloskey EV, Bone turnover and biochemical markers in malignancy. *Cancer* 1997; **80**(Suppl 8):1538–45.
6. Mundy GR, Hypercalcemia of malignancy revisited. *J Clin Invest* 1988; **82**:1–6.
7. Berruti A, Sperone P, Fasolis G et al, Pamidronate administration improves the secondary hyperparathyroidism due to 'bone hunger sydrome' in a patient with osteoblastic metastases from prostate cancer. *Prostate* 1997; **1**:252–5.
8. Kanis JA, Percival RC, Yates AJP, Urwin GH, Handy NAT, Effects of diphosphonates in hypercalcemia due to neoplasia. *Lancet* 1986; i:615–16.
9. Kamenor B, Kieran MW, Barrington-Leigh I, Longenecker BM, Homing receptors as functional markers for classification, prognosis, and therapy of leukemia and lymphomas. *Proc Soc Exp Biol Med* 1984; **177**:211–19.
10. Paget S, The distribution of secondary growths in cancer of the breast. *Lancet* 1889; i:571–3
11. Batson OV, The function of the vertebral veins

and their role in the spread of metastases. *Ann Surg* 1940; **112**:138.

12. Munday GR, Mechanisms of bone metastasis. *Cancer* 1997; **80**(Suppl 8):1546–56.

13. Smith R, Jiping W, Bryant J et al, Primary Breast Cancer (PBC) as a risk factor for bone recurrence (BR): NSABP experience. *Proc Am Soc Clin Oncol* 1999; **18**:Abst 457.

14. Paterson AHG, Natural history of skeletal complications of breast cancer, prostate cancer and myeloma. *Bone* 1987; **8**(Suppl 1):S17–S22.

15. Kanis JA, McCloskey EV, Powles T et al, A high incidence of vertebral fractures in women with breast cancer. *Br J Cancer* 1999; **79**:1179–81.

16. Ferreira SH, Prostaglandins: peripheral and central analgesia. *Adv Pain Res Ther* 1983; **5**:627–34.

17. Ernst DS, Role of bisphosphonates and other bone resorption inhibitors in metastatic bone pain. *Topics Palliat Care* 1997; **3**:117–37.

18. Ryzon B, Martodam RR, Troxell M et al, Intravenous etidronate in the management of malignant hypercalcemia. *Arch Intern Med* 1985; **145**:449–52.

19. Kanis JA, Urwin GH, Gray RES et al, Effects of intravenous etidronate disodium on skeletal and calcium metabolism. *Am J Med* 1984; **82**(Suppl 2A):55.

20. Adamson BB, Gallacher SJ, Byars J et al, Mineralization defects with pamidronate therapy for Paget's disease. *Lancet* 1993; **342**:1459–60.

21. Taube T, Elomaa I, Blomqvist C et al, Comparative effects of clodronate and calcitonin in metastatic breast cancer. *Eur J Clin Oncol* 1993; **29**:1677–81.

22. Fleisch H, *Bisphosphonates in Bone Disease – From the Laboratory to the Patient*, 3rd edn. New York: Parthenon Publishing Group, 1997.

23. Sahni M, Guenther HL, Fleisch H et al, Bisphosphonates act on rat bone resorption through the mediation of osteoblasts. *J Clin Invest* 1993; **91**:2004–11.

24. Hughes DE, Wright KR, Uy HL et al, Bisphosphonates promote apoptosis in murine osteoclasts in vitro and in vivo. *J Bone Miner Res* 1995; **10**:1478–87.

25. Siwek B, Lacroix M, DePllak C et al, Secretory products of breast cancer cells specifically affect human osteoblastic cells: partial characterization of active factors. *J Bone Miner Res* 1997; **12**:552–60.

26. Nishikawa M, Akatsu T, Katayama Y et al, Bisphosphonates act on osteoblastic cells and inhibit osteoclast formation in mouse marrow cultures. *Bone* 1996; **18**:9–14.

27. Selander KS, Monkkonen J, Karhukorpi EK et al, Characteristics of clodronate-induced apoptosis in osteoclasts and macrophages. *Mol Pharmacol* 1996; **50**:1127–38.

28. Rogers MJ, Chilton KM, Coxon FP et al, Bisphosphonates induce apoptosis in mouse macrophage-like cells in vitro by a nitric oxide independent mechanism. *J Bone Miner Res* 1996; **11**:1482–91.

29. Shipman CM, Rogers MJ, Apperley JF et al, Bisphosphonates induce apoptosis in human myeloma cell lines: a novel anti-tumour activity. *Br J Haematol* 1997; **98**:665–72.

30. Body JJ, Delmas PD, Urinary pyridinium cross-links as markers of bone resorption in tumor-associate hypercalcemia. *J Clin Endocrinol Metab* 1992; **74**:471–5.

31. Grill V, Ho P, Body JJ et al, Parathyroid hormone-related protein: elevated levels in both humoral hypercalcemia of malignancy and hypercalcemia complicating metastatic breast cancer. *J Clin Endocrinol Metab* 1991; **73**:1309–15.

32. Body JJ, Bartl R, Burckhardt P et al, Current use of bisphosphonates in oncology. International Bone and Cancer Study Group. *J Clin Oncol* 1998; **16**:3890–9.

33. Singer FR, Ritch PS, Lad TE et al, for the Hypercalcemia Study Group, Treatment of hypercalcemia of malignancy with intravenous etidronate. A controlled, multicenter study. *Arch Intern Med* 1991; **151**:471–6.

34. Purohit OP, Radstone CR, Anthony C et al, A randomized double-blind comparison of intra-

venous pamidronate and clodronate in the hypercalcemia of malignancy. *Br J Cancer* 1995; **72**:1289–93.

35. Elomaa I, Blomqvist C, Porrka L et al, Treatment of skeletal disease in breast cancer: a controlled clinical trial. *Bone* 1987; **8**(Suppl 1):S53–6.

36. van-Holten-Verzanvoort AT, Bijvoet OL, Cleton FJ et al, Reduced morbidity from skeletal metastases in breast cancer patients during long-term bisphosphonates (APD) treatment. *Lancet* 1987; **ii**:983–5.

37. Paterson AHG, Powles TJ, Kanis JA et al, Double-blind controlled trial of oral clodronate in patients with bone metastases from breast cancer. *J Clin Oncol* 1993; **11**:59–65.

38. McCloskey EV, Spector TD, Eyres KS et al, The assessment of vertebral deformity: a method for use in population studies and clinical trials. *Osteoporosis Int* 1993; **3**:138–47.

39. Coleman RE, Woll PJ, Miles M et al, Treatment of bone metastases from breast cancer with (3-amino-1-hydroxy-propylidene)-1,1-bisphosphonate (APD). *Br J Cancer* 1988; **58**:621–5.

40. Conte PF, Latreille J, Mauriac L et al, Delay in progression of bone metastases in breast cancer patients treated with intravenous pamidronate: results from a multinational randomized controlled trial. *J Clin Oncol* 1996; **14**:2552–9.

41. Hortobagyi GN, Theriault RL, Porter L et al, Efficacy of pamidronate in reducing skeletal complications in patients with breast cancer and lytic bone metastases. *N Engl J Med* 1996; **335**:1785–91.

42. Ernst DS, MacDonald N, Paterson AHG et al, A double-blind cross-over trial of intravenous clodronate in metastatic bone pain. *J Pain Sympt Manage* 1992; **7**:4–11.

43. Ernst DS, Brasher P, Hagen N et al, A randomized, controlled trial of intravenous clodronate in metastatic bone disease and pain. *J Pain Sympt Manage* 1997; **13**:319–26.

44. van-Holten-Verzanvoort AT, Zwinderman AH, Aaranson NK et al, The effect of supportive pamidronate treatment on aspects of quality of life of patients with advanced breast cancer. *Eur J Cancer* 1991; **27**:544–9.

45. Kanis JA, Powles T, Paterson AH et al, Clodronate and skeletal metastases. *Bone* 1996; **19**:663–7.

46. van-Holten-Verzanvoort AT, Hermans J, Beex LV et al, Does supportive pamidronate treatment prevent or delay the first manifestations of bone metastases in breast cancer patients? *Eur J Cancer* 1996; **32A**:450–4.

47. Goldhirsch A, Gelber RD, Price KN et al, Effect of systemic adjuvant treatment on first sites of breast cancer relapse. *Lancet* 1994; **343**:377–81.

48. Wronski TJ, Dann LM, Qi H, Yen SF, Skeletal effects of withdrawal of estrogen and diphosphonate treatment in ovariectomised rats. *Calcif Tissue Int* 1993; **53**:210–16.

49. Powles TJ, McCloskey E, Paterson AHG et al, Oral clodronate will reduce the loss of bone mineral density in women with primary breast cancer. *Proc Am Soc Clin Oncol* 1997; **16**:460.

50. Delmas PD, Balena R, Confraveux E, The bisphosphonate residronate prevents bone loss in women with artificial menopause due to chemotherapy of breast cancer: a double-blind, placebo-controlled study. *J Clin Oncol* 1997; **15**:955–62.

51. Fisher B, Constantino J, Redmond C et al, A randomized clinical trial evaluating tamoxifen in the treatment of patients with node-negative breast cancer who have estrogen receptor-positive tumours. *N Engl J Med* 1989; **320**:479–84.

52. Turken S, Siris E, Seldin D et al, Effects of tamoxifen on spinal bone density in women with breast cancer. *J Natl Cancer Inst* 1989; **81**:1086–8.

53. Powles TJ, Muindi J, Coombes C, Mechanisms for development of bone metastases and effects of anti-inflammatory drugs. In: Powles TJ, ed. *Prostaglandins and Cancer: First International Conference.* New York: Alan R Liss, 1982:541–3.

54. Pecherstorfer M, Schilling T, Janisch S et al, Effect of clodronate treatment on bone scintigraphy in metastatic breast cancer. *J Nucl Med* 1993; **34**:1039–44.

55. Macro M, Bouvard G, LeGangneux E et al, Intravenous aminohydroxy-propylidine bisphosphonate does not modify 99mTc-hydroxy-methylene bisphosphonate bone scintigraphy. A prospective study. *Rev Rheum Engl Ed* 1995; **62**:99–104.

56. Krempien B, Morphological findings in bone metastasis, tumorosteopathy and anti-osteolytic therapy. In: Diel IJ, Kaufmann M, Bastert G, eds. *Metastatic Bone Disease. Fundamental and Clinical Aspects.* Berlin: Springer, 1994.

57. Yoneda T, Sasaki A, Mundy G, Osteolytic bone metastasis in breast cancer. *Breast Cancer Res Treat* 1994; **32**:72–84.

58. van der Pluijm G, Vloedgraven H, van Beek E et al, Bisphosphonates inhibit the adhesion of breast cancer cells to bone matrices in vitro. *J Clin Invest* 1996; **98**:698–705.

59. Boussier S, Magnetto S, Frappart L et al, Bisphosphonates inhibit prostate and breast cancer cell adhesion to unmineralized and mineralized bone extracellular matrices. *Cancer Res* 1997; **57**:3890–4.

60. Saarto T, Blomqvist C, Valimaki M et al, Chemical castration induced by adjuvant cyclophosphamide, methotrexate and fluorouracil chemotherapy causes rapid bone loss that is reduced by clodronate: a randomized study in premenopausal breast cancer patients. *J Clin Oncol* 1997; **15**:1341–7.

61. Diel IJ, Solomayer EF, Costa SD et al, Reduction in new metastases in breast cancer with adjuvant clodronate treatment. *N Engl J Med* 1998; **339**:357–63.

62. Diel IJ, Kaufmann M, Costa SD et al, Micrometastatic breast cancer cells in bone marrow at primary surgery: Prognostic value in comparison with nodal status. *J Natl Cancer Inst* 1996; **88**:1652–8.

63. Powles TJ, Paterson AHG, Navantaus A et al, Adjuvant clodronate reduces the incidence of bone metastases in patients with operable primary breast cancer. *Proc Am Soc Clin Oncol* 1998; **17**:468.

26

Erythropoietin in the management of cancer patients

Alexander HG Paterson, Mary-Ann Lindsay

FATIGUE IN CANCER PATIENTS

Fatigue is a frequent symptom in cancer patients. Estimates of its prevalence range from 30 to 70% and are dependent on the background malignancy and the stage of the disease.[1] Fatigue has a multifactorial causation and may be related to the disease process itself, treatment of the disease or treatment of symptoms of the disease.

In the trajectory of the cancer disease process, fatigue is therefore seen as a symptom of the anemia of chronic malignant disease or as a direct symptom related to the effects of the tumor itself or as a symptom within the various syndromes of secretion of ectopic hormones. An example of the last is seen in the paraneoplastic syndromes such as cancer-related myopathies. Anemias in cancer patients can result from not only the anemia of chronic disease, but also deficiency states such as iron deficiency anemia caused by blood loss directly from the tumor as in carcinomas of the cecum. Iron, vitamin B_{12} and folate deficiencies may also occur from poor nutrition secondary to the anorexia associated with advanced malignant disease. Hemolytic anemias such as microangiopathic hemolysis occurring secondary to malignancies are also seen.

Treatment-related anemias are seen with cyto-toxic drugs. Mitomycin C, for example, causes anemia particularly after three or four cycles of the drug; however, all cytotoxic drugs when used to the point of marrow suppression will cause a reduction in erythropoiesis. Anemias in cancer patients should be investigated as in any other patient with testing for serum iron, vitamin B_{12} and folate, and examination of the blood smear.

Fatigue is also seen in the management of cancer-related symptoms, for example, when patients are on opiates, antidepressants and anxiolytics. In most patients, the fatigue is therefore a mix of causative factors – a result of the multi-system effects of the disease and a side effect of treatment.

Recently, erythropoietin has been examined as a treatment for patients with chronic anemia of malignant disease. Erythropoietin is an established treatment in managing patients with chronic renal disease and has been investigated thoroughly in patients on dialysis.[2] In this setting, the hormone has been shown to improve quality of life significantly with a substantial elevation of hemoglobin levels and reduced requirements for transfusion. The use of erythropoietin in renal dialysis patients has revolutionized the quality of life and diminished frequency of the symptom of fatigue in these patients; many will have an extraordinary increase in the sense of well-being after commencing erythropoietin.

Randomized controlled trials in patients receiving chemotherapy for the treatment of cancer, and controlled trials of erythropoietin in cancer patients with the anemia of chronic disease have recently been instituted.

CLINICAL TRIALS IN PATIENTS WITH MALIGNANT DISEASE

Initially, anecdotal evidence suggesting that erythropoietin might be helpful in the management of cancer patients with the anemia of chronic disease or anemias associated with chemotherapy suggested that there might be a benefit in terms of quality of life. However, the extent of the benefit, the overall effectiveness as well as the cost implications of such treatment were not clear. It should be remembered that, in contrast to patients with chronic renal disease, an alternative does exist for cancer patients – blood transfusions; these are not appropriate in patients with chronic renal disease. There continues to be some public concern regarding the safety of blood transfusions and indications for transfusions are being strictly monitored. Red cell transfusions are associated with febrile illnesses, urticarial reactions and sometimes fluid overload: occasionally serious incompatibility reactions occur. In cancer patients, depending on the stage and prognosis of the malignancy, there may be less concern about the small risks of hepatitis C, HIV and cytomegalovirus. Nevertheless, these risks should be borne in mind.

Trials using blood transfusions as an outcome

A number of randomized controlled trials have been performed to assess the value of erythropoietin in patients treated with chemotherapy. These trials differ in quality, dose of erythropoietin, hematologic status, types of malignancy and types of chemotherapy. Abels et al[3] showed, in a variety of patients with malignant disease who had hemoglobin concentrations of less than 105 g/l that an erythropoietin regimen given for 12 weeks reduced the number of patients requiring transfusion; these patients received platinum chemotherapy and the trial was placebo controlled. In 1993, Welch et al[4] published a study in patients with advanced ovarian carcinoma who were receiving chemotherapy and who had normal initial hemoglobin levels. In this open label trial, 30 patients received platinum-based chemotherapy with or without erythropoietin. A significant difference in the mean hemoglobin concentration maximum at cycles two to four was noted ($p < 0.001$). These investigators found that only 3 patients of 15 required transfusion in the erythropoietin arm, compared with 7 patients of 15 on the chemotherapy-alone arm. Delmastro et al[5] randomly allocated 43 patients with early breast cancer to receive either erythropoietin given at 150 IU/kg subcutaneously three times weekly with six cycles of non-platinum-based chemotherapy or just the chemotherapy alone (control). Results showed reduced transfusion requirements in patients receiving the erythropoietin with non-platinum-based chemotherapy, and lower hemoglobin levels in patients in the control group. Cascinu et al[6] showed a very significant reduction in blood transfusion requirements with erythropoietin 100 IU/kg given subcutaneously three times weekly in patients with a variety of malignancies receiving cis-platinum chemotherapy. Thatcher et al randomized 130 non-anemic patients with small cell lung cancer receiving four to six cycles of platinum-based chemotherapy to receive either erythropoietin 150 IU/kg subcutaneously three times weekly ($n = 42$), 300 IU/kg subcutaneously three times weekly ($n = 44$) or no erythropoietin ($n = 44$).[7] Fewer patients in the two arms receiving erythropoietin experienced anemia defined as hemoglobin of less than 10 g/dl, compared with the non-erythropoietin arm throughout treatment with chemotherapy ($p < 0.05$).

Transfusions were significantly less in the patients receiving the erythropoietin 300 IU/kg ($p < 0.001$) and 150 IU/kg ($p < 0.05$) versus the non-erythropoietin arm. In Littlewood et al, 375 cancer patients receiving six cycles of non-platinum-containing chemotherapy were randomized 2 : 1 in a multinational, double-blind, placebo-controlled study to evaluate the effect erythropoietin on hemoglobin levels and transfusion requirements. By the end of week 4 until the end of the study, defined as 4 weeks post-chemotherapy, 24.7% of patients in the erythropoietin group versus 39.5% of patients in the placebo group received transfusions ($p = 0.0057$). From baseline to the end of study, the mean change in hemoglobin in the erythropoietin group was 2.2 g/dl versus 0.5 g/dl in the placebo group ($p < 0.001$).[8]

Trials using quality of life as an outcome

Reducing transfusion requirements may be useful in terms of the patient's concern of safety of blood supply. It cannot be said that use of erythropoietin is economically effective if transfusion requirements were the only parameter to be measured because blood transfusions can be given efficiently and relatively cheaply at frequent intervals in the day care units of most hospitals and cancer centers. However, a blood transfusion by its nature gives a rapid rise of hemoglobin followed by a decline in hemoglobin levels, with recurrence of symptoms over a period of weeks. If erythropoietin can both elevate and maintain hemoglobin levels over time, one might expect quality of life to improve. This has been assessed in a number of studies. Assessment of quality of life is performed using a variety of instruments: disease-specific questionnaires and/or global questionnaires can be used. Thatcher,[7] using a simple three-item questionnaire regarding energy level, daily activity and quality of life, showed a significant improvement from baseline in overall quality of life in a group of patients receiving erythropoietin 150 IU/kg ($p < 0.05$). Littlewood et al[8] used the Linear Analog Self-Assessment (LASA) score, as well as a fatigue and general health score. They showed that patients treated with erythropoietin had higher scores on LASA scales (energy $p < 0.001$; activities $p < 0.01$; overall quality of life $p = 0.01$), as well as an improved fatigue score ($p < 0.01$) and general quality of life ($p < 0.05$). In Abel's study,[3] there was an improvement in energy level, daily activities and overall quality of life, but the effects were relatively small. In a retrospective analysis of this study, it seemed that the patients with most improvement were those who experienced an increase in hemoglobin levels.

More recently, Gabrilove et al,[9] in an open-label single-arm study, showed that a once-weekly dose of erythropoietin did lead to higher hemoglobin levels, with a decrease in the need for transfusions and an improvement in quality of life in anemic patients. In this study, 40 000 IU erythropoietin given subcutaneously once weekly with an increase in dose to 60 000 IU, if required, was used. Hemoglobin levels increased significantly from a mean of 9.4 g/dl at baseline to 11.6 g/dl at the final observation ($p < 0.001$). Transfusion requirements were reduced ($p < 0.001$) and quality-of-life parameters improved.

Another study by Quirt et al[10] was performed in patients with the anemia of malignant disease who were not receiving concomitant chemotherapy. In this larger study, 183 patients were treated with erythropoietin 150 IU/kg subcutaneously three times a week. Response was defined as an increase of 20 g/l or more hemoglobin without transfusion and was seen in 48% of patients (88 patients). The quality-of-life improvement was seen only in the patients experiencing a hemoglobin response. Erythropoietin also reduced transfusion rates (p values not available at time of abstract publication).

ADVERSE EFFECTS

Adverse effects related to erythropoietin administration are generally mild and rarely reported. Occasionally, pain at the injection site can be seen,[11–14] and flu-like symptoms with general constitutional malaise[14] and skin rash occur.[11,12,15] There has been one report of erythropoietin injections being related to an increase in blood pressure.[16] In general, the medication is well tolerated and may even engender some placebo effects in patients who are looking for an improvement in their symptoms.

INDICATIONS FOR ERYTHROPOIETIN USE

The indications for erythropoietin are still open for clinical investigation, and further research is required. Patients who have a documented anemia and an expectancy of life greater than 4 months should be considered for treatment. Patients who develop anemia with chemotherapy might also be considered for treatment, although blood transfusions when required may be a more effective and economic way to manage the situation when the chemotherapy is being given for a limited time period.

PHARMACOECONOMIC STUDIES

In Canada the current cost of a month's therapy with erythropoietin given at 150 IU/kg subcutaneously three times a week to an individual with an average adult body weight is approximately $US1200. Blood transfusion costs are variable across the country but are in the region of $US133 to $US200 per unit when given in a typical day care center.

Ortega et al[17] used an economic analysis approach whereby the concept of 'willingness to pay' was used; 100 patients were chosen at random and interviewed. Those receiving chemotherapy on average were willing to pay between $US550 and $US630. These amounts were subtracted from the cost of erythropoietin in assessing the overall costs. Using this technique, around $US3000 was the increased treatment cost per course of chemotherapy. Ortega et al concluded that intermittent transfusion is a more cost-effective treatment.

A study by Meadowcroft et al[18] retrospectively reviewed patients with breast cancer receiving chemotherapy. This group also showed that the cost of managing anemia in breast cancer patients was lower using blood transfusions.

GUIDELINE RECOMMENDATIONS

The Canadian Cancer and Anemia Guideline Development Group[19] have recommended that patients whose anemia is directly or indirectly related to malignancy, in particular: (1) where symptomatic anemia affects functional capacity or quality of life; or (2) where there are low baseline Hb levels ($\leq$100 g/l) at the start of cancer chemotherapy; or (3) baseline Hb levels ($\leq$120 g/l) where symptomatic anemia is anticipated; or (4) where there is a drop in Hb of 10–20 g/l at each cycle of chemotherapy where at least 3 cycles remain to be administered, use of erythropoietin is an alternative if blood transfusion is not an acceptable option. The review of evidence suggests that patients receiving platinum-based chemotherapy obtain the greatest benefit. The Group has recommended a starting dose of erythropoietin at 150 IU/kg subcutaneously three times per week. Patients should be evaluated for serum iron and iron-binding capacity before treatment and iron supplementation should be administered if necessary using ferrous gluconate 200 mg three times daily taken by mouth with food. Other causes of anemia should be excluded.

After 4 weeks of treatment, if the hemoglobin increase is 10 g/l or more, or the reticulocyte count increase is 40 000 cells/μl or more above baseline, the above dosage can be continued until the target hemoglobin level is achieved. In patients who do not achieve this response, the dose of erythropoietin can be increased to 300 IU/kg for the following 4 weeks. Using this higher dosage, if a hemoglobin increase of less than 10 g/l is achieved, or a reticulocyte site count of less than 40 000 cells/μl is measured, treatment should be stopped. Hemoglobin elevations more than 20 g/l per month is reason to reduce the erythropoietin dose by approximately 25%. Levels of hemoglobin exceeding 140 g/l should lead to discontinuation of therapy until the hemoglobin falls below 120 g/l, at which time erythropoietin can be restarted.

Some groups have suggested that erythropoietin levels can be used as a guide to therapy. However, in most instances this is not practicable.

CONCLUSIONS

After its success in improving the quality of life in patients with chronic renal disease, erythropoietin has been investigated in patients with the chronic anemia of malignancy and anemias associated with chemotherapy. There is now good evidence that erythropoietin can be used to increase hemoglobin levels in cancer patients and it can lead to a significant improvement in quality of life in responding patients. It is not clear whether this increased quality of life can be achieved using frequent intermittent blood transfusions. Evidence suggests that erythropoietin is more likely to improve quality of life than intermittent visits to the day care unit for blood transfusions.

Cost is a major concern, so that appropriate initial selection of patients and maintenance based on response should be made according to guidelines, such as those discussed above. One can record a useful clinical response by documenting alleviation of the symptoms of fatigue, lack of concentration, irritability and general malaise as criteria of effectiveness. Further research is required to assess whether chemotherapy responses might be improved in patients receiving erythropoietin with subsequent maintenance of ideal hemoglobin levels. Further modification of the guideline requirements for the use of erythropoietin will be required. Concern about availability of blood transfusion products in certain countries or regions may make the use of erythropoietin more attractive in the future.

REFERENCES

1. Del Mastro L, Venturini M, Strategies for the use of epoetin alfa in breast cancer patients. *Oncologist* 1998;3:314–18.
2. Eschback JW, Adamson JW, Cooperative Multicenter r-HuEPO Trial Group, Correction of the anaemia of hemodialysis (HD) patients with recombinant human erythropoietin (r-HuEPO); results of a multicenter study. *Kidney Int* 1968;33:189.
3. Abels RI, Larholt KM, Krantz KD, Bryant ED, Recombinant human erythropoietin for the treatment of anaemia of cancer. *Proceedings of the Beijing Symposium.* Dayton, OH: AlphaMed Press, 1991:121–41.
4. Welch RS, James RD, Wilkinson, PM, Belli F, Cowan RA, Recombinant human erythropoietin and platinum based chemotherapy in metastatic ovarian carcinoma. *Proc Am Soc Clin Oncol* 1993;**12**:A804.

5. Del Mastro L, Venturini M, Garrone O et al, Erythropoietin in the prevention of chemotherapy induced anaemia: results from a randomized trial in early breast cancer patients. *Proc Am Soc Clin Oncol* 1995;**14**:A697.

6. Cascinu S, Fedeli A, Del Ferro E, Fedeli SL, Catalano G, Recombinant human erythropoietin treatment in cisplatin-associated anaemia: a randomized, double-blind trial with placebo. *J Clin Oncol* 1994;**12**:1058–62.

7. Thatcher N, Controlled study of the efficacy and safety or r-Hu erythropoietin in the prevention of anemia in patients with small cell lung cancer receiving chemotherapy. *Proc Int Soc Hematol* 1994;**188**:A15.

8. Littlewood TJ, Bajetta E, Cella D, European Epoetin Alfa Study Group, Efficacy and quality of life outcomes of epoetin alfa in a double-blind, placebo-controlled multicenter study of cancer patients receiving non-platinum containing chemotherapy. *Proc Am Soc Clin Oncol* 1999;**18**:A2217.

9. Gabrilove JL, Einhorn LH, Livingstron RB, Winer E, Cleeland CS, Once-weekly dosing of epoetin alfa is similar to three-times-weekly dosing in increasing haemoglobin and quality of life. *Proc Am Soc Clin Oncol* 1999;**18**:A2216.

10. Quirt I, Kovacs M, Burdette-Radoux S, Dolan S, McKenzie M, Tang SC, Epoetin alfa reduces transfusion requirements, increases haemoglobin (Hb) and improves quality of life (QofL) in cancer patients with anaemia who are not receiving concomitant chemotherapy. *Proc Am Soc Clin Oncol* 1999;**18**:A2295.

11. Del Mastro L, Venturini M, Lionetto R et al, Randomized phase III trial evaluating the role of erythropoietin in the prevention of chemotherapy-induced anaemia. *J Clin Oncol* 1997;**15**:2715–21.

12. Csaki D, Ferencz T, Schyler D, Borsi JD, Recombinant human erythropoietin in the prevention of chemotherapy-induced anaemia in children with malignant solid tumors. *Eur J Cancer* 1998;**34**:364–7.

13. Thatcher N, De Campos ES, Bell DR et al, Epoietin alpha prevents anaemia and reduces transfusion requirements in patients undergoing primarily platinum-based chemotherapy for small cell lung cancer. *Br J Cancer* 1999;**80**:396–402.

14. tenBokkel Huinink WW, de Swart CAM, van Toorn DS et al, Controlled multicentre study of the influence of subcutaneous recombinant human erythropoietin on anaemia and transfusion dependency in patients with ovarian carcinoma treated with platinum-based chemotherapy. *Med Oncol* 1998;**15**:174–82.

15. de Campos E, Radford J, Steward W et al, Clinical and in vitro effects of recombinant human erythropoietin in patients receiving intensive chemotherapy for small-cell lung cancer. *J Clin Oncol* 1995;**13**:1623–31.

16. Varan A, Buyukpamukcu M, Kutluk T, Akyuz C, Recombinant human erythropoietin treatment for chemotherapy-related anaemia in children. *Pediatrics* 1999;**103**:E16.

17. Ortega A, Dranitsaris G, Puodziunas ALV, What are cancer patients willing to pay for prophylactic epoietin alfa? *Cancer* 1998;**83**:2588–96.

18. Meadowcroft AM, Gilbert CJ, Maravich-May D, Hayward SL, Cost of managing anaemia with and without prophylactic epoetin alfa therapy in breast cancer patients receiving combination chemotherapy. *Am J Health-Syst Pharm* 1998;**55**:1898–902.

19. Canadian Cancer and Anemia Guideline Development Group: In preparation by Integrated Healthcare Communications, Toronto, Ontario, funded through an unrestricted educational grant from Janssen-Ortho Inc, 2000.

27

Chemotherapy-induced nausea and vomiting

Sheryl Koski, Peter Venner

Nausea and vomiting are a frequent side effect of cytotoxic chemotherapy used for the treatment of malignancy. Untreated, 70–80% of patients will experience nausea and vomiting. Even in treated patients it is estimated that 40–50% will experience this side effect, which can have a significant impact on a patient's quality of life and compliance with treatment.[1] The incidence and severity of chemotherapy-induced emesis are dependent on several factors, including the emetogenicity of the chemotherapeutic agent and the risk factors of the patient.

EMETOGENICITY OF CYTOTOXIC CHEMOTHERAPY

Highly emetogenic chemotherapeutic agents are those that cause severe emesis in more than 90% of patients. Cisplatin is considered the most highly emetogenic agent, but other agents in this category include dacarbazine, nitrogen mustard and high doses of cyclophosphamide (> 1500 mg/m²). Moderately emetogenic agents cause emesis in 30–90% of patients, e.g. doxorubicin and lower doses of cyclophosphamide. Mildly emetogenic agents induce emesis in a minority of patients, 10–30%, but they may still warrant antiemetic prophylaxis. Examples

include mitoxantrone and etoposide. Minimally emetogenic agents seldom require the use of prophylactic antiemetic therapy (e.g. the vinca alkaloids).[1,2] There is some disagreement on the classification of combination chemotherapy regimens. The general consensus is that the emetogenicity of a combination should be the same as that of the most highly emetogenic drug within the regimen.[3] Table 27.1 gives the emetogenic classification of common chemotherapeutic agents and regimens.

RISK FACTORS AND PATHOPHYSIOLOGY

Acute emesis
Definition
Acute emesis is defined as nausea and vomiting occurring during the first 24 hours after chemotherapy. With most agents it starts within 1–2 hours of receiving chemotherapy; however, with some agents there can be a late onset of acute emesis – starting 9–18 hours after receiving chemotherapy (e.g. carboplatin, high-dose cyclophosphamide).[1]

Risk factors
Characteristics that have been associated with a

Table 27.1   Classification of emetogenicity[1,3]

Highly emetogenic	Moderately emetogenic	Mildly emetogenic	Minimally emetogenic
Cisplatin > 50 mg/m^2	Cisplatin 20–50 mg/m^2	Mitoxantrone	5-Fluorouracil
Cyclophosphamide	Carboplatin	Etoposide	Bleomycin
> 1500 mg/m^2	Doxorubicin	Irinotecan	Vinca alkaloids
Dacarbazine	Epirubicin	Docetaxel	Methotrexate
Nitrogen mustard	Idarubicin	Paclitaxel	Hydroxyurea
	Cyclophosphamide	Gemcitabine	Chlorambucil
	Ifosfamide		Fludarabine
	Cytarabine		Cladribine
	CMF (i.v. or p.o.)		
	FEC/FAC		

CMF, cyclophosphamide, methotrexate, 5-fluorouracil (5-FU); FEC, 5-FU, epirubicin, cyclophosphamide; FAC, 5-FU, doxorubicin, cyclophosphamide.

higher risk of acute emesis, include: (1) emesis with prior chemotherapy cycles, (2) younger age, (3) female sex and (4) low chronic ethanol intake.[2,3]

Pathophysiology

The precise pathophysiology of chemotherapy-induced nausea and vomiting is not completely understood. The mechanisms for acute emesis have received the greatest amount of study. Pathways involved in the emetic response include the central nervous system (CNS), gastrointestinal tract and vestibular system. Traditionally, it is believed that there are two key areas within the CNS that are involved in the emetic response. These are: (1) the vomiting centre, which is located in the lateral reticular formation of the medulla, and (2) the chemoreceptor trigger zone (CTZ), which is located in the area postrema (AP). The CTZ is located outside the blood–brain barrier and senses humoral stimuli within the blood and cerebrospinal fluid. Signals are then transmitted to the vomiting center which coordinates the motor mechanisms of emesis. Other sources of stimulation to the vomiting center include the vestibular system, the pharynx, the gastrointestinal tract and higher cortical centres. The vestibular system has a primary role in motion sickness, whereas the higher cortical centres may play a role in anticipatory emesis.[4] It is the CTZ, the gastrointestinal tract and higher cortical centers that are involved in the emetic response after cytotoxic chemotherapy.[2] More recently, studies suggest that it is the nucleus tractus solitarius (NTS) that is important in the emetic response. The NTS is located below the AP and coordinates the function of visceral and somatic afferents within the brain stem. Its neurons terminate within the AP and it may in fact be the NTS, rather than the CTZ, that is important in the emetic pathway.[5]

There are a number of neurotransmitters involved in the emetic response. Those that play a role in the pathophysiology of chemotherapy-induced emesis include: (1) dopamine, (2) serotonin and (3) substance P. Receptors for these neurotransmitters are found in the CTZ, the vomiting centre and the gastrointestinal tract. Early studies focused on the role of the dopamine receptor in chemotherapy-induced emesis and resulted in the development of the dopamine antagonists (e.g. metoclopramide, domperidone). The use of high-dose metoclopramide was the standard therapy for patients receiving cisplatin-based chemotherapy. However, in the 1970s it was discovered that the use of metoclopramide at high doses resulted in the inhibition of serotonin receptors, not dopamine receptors. This discovery led to the development of the serotonin (5-hydroxytryptamine, 5HT) receptor antagonists, which inhibit the $5HT_3$ receptor.[4,6]

Cytotoxic chemotherapy results in the release of serotonin from the enterochromaffin cells of the gastrointestinal tract which then stimulates the $5HT_3$ receptors. This stimulus is relayed back to the vomiting center in the CNS via abdominal vagal afferents. The $5HT_3$ receptor has also been identified within the AP. Therefore, $5HT_3$-receptor antagonists may act through these central receptors to mediate the development of chemotherapy-induced nausea and vomiting.[2,6] The mechanism by which cytotoxic chemotherapy results in the release of serotonin from the enterochromaffin cells is not known, but it may occur via free radical generation.[5]

Studies in cancer patients receiving high-dose cisplatin have shown that there is an increase in the plasma level and urinary excretion of 5-hydroxyindolacetic acid (5HIAA), a metabolite of serotonin, which parallels the onset of emesis. These levels then return to baseline between 9 and 16 hours after the infusion of cisplatin. This rise in 5HIAA is not affected by the use of $5HT_3$-receptor antagonists. This suggests that these agents do not prevent the release of serotonin but instead inhibit its action at the level of the $5HT_3$ receptor.[2,7,8] A similar rise in plasma and urinary 5HIAA is seen after the administration of dacarbazine, cyclophosphamide and low-dose cisplatin. The magnitude of the rise in 5HIAA is similar for high-dose cisplatin and dacarbazine. In the cyclophosphamide and low-dose cisplatin patients, the increase in 5HIAA is smaller and more delayed in onset. Therefore, the emetogenicity of a chemotherapy regimen may be related to its ability to release serotonin.[7]

More recently, inhibitors of the natural killer, NK-1 receptor have shown promise for the treatment of both acute and delayed emesis after cisplatin-based chemotherapy.[9] This suggests that substance P, the natural ligand for the NK-1 receptor, also has a role in the pathophysiology of the emetic response.

Delayed emesis
Definition
Delayed emesis is defined as nausea and vomiting occurring more than 24 hours after chemotherapy. This is most commonly seen in patients receiving cisplatin-based chemotherapy regimens.

Risk factors
The single most important risk factor for the development of delayed emesis is poor control of acute emesis.[3]

Pathophysiology
The pathophysiology of delayed emesis is very poorly understood. The studies, which followed the plasma and urinary levels of 5HIAA after the infusion of cisplatin, found that the levels of 5HIAA returned to baseline between 9 and 16 hours after cisplatin administration. Therefore, it is unlikely that serotonin plays a significant role in the etiology of delayed nausea and vomiting.[8] This is supported by the finding that the $5HT_3$-

receptor antagonists are less effective for the treatment of delayed emesis. It is possible that alterations in gut motility may contribute to the development of delayed emesis.[5] More recently, studies have shown that the use of an NK-1-receptor antagonist can decrease the incidence of delayed emesis. Therefore, substance P, the ligand for the NK-1 receptor, may play a role in the pathophysiology of delayed emesis.[9,10]

Anticipatory emesis
Definition
Anticipatory nausea and vomiting (ANV) generally begins 24 hours before the onset of chemotherapy. This is reported in approximately 30% of patients by the fourth cycle of chemotherapy.[11]

Risk factors
Patients who experience ANV seem to be more psychologically distressed by chemotherapy than those who do not develop it. The development of post-treatment nausea and vomiting is also a risk factor because ANV is seldom seen in patients who have not experienced post-treatment nausea and vomiting.[1,11]

Pathophysiology
The pathophysiology of ANV is not well understood, but it is believed to be a conditioned response. Its frequency increases with the number of chemotherapy cycles received and is related to the frequency and severity of post-treatment nausea and vomiting.

TREATMENT OF CHEMOTHERAPY-INDUCED NAUSEA AND VOMITING

Acute emesis
The introduction of the $5HT_3$-receptor antagonists in the 1980s has revolutionized the treatment of acute emesis as a result of highly and moderately emetogenic chemotherapy regimens.

Before their introduction, the standard therapy was the use of dopamine antagonists. Multiple studies and overviews have confirmed the superiority of the $5HT_3$-receptor antagonists for emetic control.[12,13] However, the prescribing practices for these agents have been quite variable. In 1999, the authors performed an overview of the literature to determine the equivalency of $5HT_3$-receptor antagonists currently available in Canada (ondansetron, granisetron and dolasetron) in order to develop guidelines for dosing and route of administration. The guidelines developed from this systematic review form the basis for the following treatment recommendations.

Highly emetogenic chemotherapy
Studies of highly emetogenic chemotherapy have been done almost exclusively with cisplatin-based chemotherapy regimens. A dose of cisplatin $\geqslant 50$ mg/m^2, in single or fractionated doses, is the gold standard for highly emetogenic chemotherapy. However, these recommendations can probably be generalized to other highly emetogenic chemotherapy regimens (e.g. dacarbazine).

The lowest effective doses for the $5HT_3$-receptor antagonists in the prophylaxis of acute emesis after highly emetogenic chemotherapy are: (1) ondansetron 8 mg i.v., (2) granisetron 10 µg/kg i.v. (about 1 mg i.v.), (3) dolasetron 1.8 mg/kg i.v., (4) ondansetron 24 mg p.o. and (5) granisetron 2 mg p.o.[14–28] The use of multiple-dose schedules or continuous infusion did not confer any additional benefit.[14–16,21,29,30] The three $5HT_3$-receptor antagonists have equivalent efficacy.[17,20,23,24,31–34]

The oral dosing of the $5HT_3$-receptor antagonists has not been well studied in highly emetogenic chemotherapy regimens. There have been no comparative studies with oral dolasetron and therefore it has not been recommended for use.

Although the above recommendations for oral dosing are based on current evidence, further study is warranted.

There has been extensive study of the role of adjunctive corticosteroids. Multiple studies have confirmed that the addition of a corticosteroid to a $5HT_3$-receptor antagonist results in superior control of acute emesis.[35–43] There have been no comparative studies of the different corticosteroids; however, dexamethasone is the agent most commonly used. There is only one study assessing the dose–response for dexamethasone.[44] In this study, patients received ondansetron 8 mg i.v. and then were randomized to dexamethasone 4, 8, 12 or 20 mg i.v. There was a linear trend for increasing protection from vomiting with increasing doses of dexamethasone. Dexamethasone 12 mg i.v. was statistically superior to dexamethasone 4 mg and 8 mg i.v.; however, the benefit of dexamethasone 20 mg i.v. vs 12 mg i.v. was restricted to the subgroup of patients receiving lower doses of cisplatin ($50–90$ mg/m^2 vs > 90 mg/m^2).

The recommended antiemetic regimen for the prophylaxis of acute emesis after highly emetogenic chemotherapy is a combination of a $5HT_3$-receptor antagonist and dexamethasone (see Table 27.2 for dosing guidelines). This should result in complete control of acute emesis in approximately 75% of patients.[3]

Moderately emetogenic chemotherapy

Clinical trials assessing the role of the $5HT_3$-receptor antagonists for the prophylaxis of nausea and vomiting after moderately emetogenic chemotherapy using a variety of chemotherapy regimens have been performed. Agents in this category have been discussed earlier in this chapter.

The lowest effective doses for the three $5HT_3$-receptor antagonists in the prophylaxis of acute emesis after moderately emetogenic chemotherapy are: (1) ondansetron 8 mg i.v., (2) granisetron 10 µg/kg i.v. (about 1 mg i.v.), (3) ondansetron 8 mg p.o. twice daily, (4) granisetron 2 mg p.o. four times daily, (5) granisetron 1 mg p.o. twice daily and (6) dolasetron 100 mg p.o. four times daily.[45–53] When the different $5HT_3$-receptor antagonists were compared, ondansetron and granisetron have equivalent efficacy.[47,49,54,55] There are only two studies comparing ondansetron and dolasetron, and the doses used in these studies differ from the recommended dosing; therefore, it is difficult to draw any conclusions about equivalency.[56,57] There have been no studies comparing granisetron and dolasetron in moderately emetogenic chemotherapy regimens.

As with the highly emetogenic chemotherapy regimens, the addition of a corticosteroid to a $5HT_3$-receptor antagonist results in improved control of acute emesis after moderately emetogenic chemotherapy.[57–60] Dexamethasone was used in all four studies in doses of 8–12 mg i.v. There have been no studies to compare the appropriate dosing of the corticosteroids in the setting of moderately emetogenic chemotherapy.

The recommended antiemetic regimen for the prophylaxis of acute emesis after moderately emetogenic chemotherapy is a $5HT_3$-receptor antagonist in combination with dexamethasone (see Table 27.2 for dosing guidelines). This should result in complete control of acute emesis in approximately 85–90% of patients.[3]

Mild and minimally emetogenic chemotherapy

There have been few comparative trials using chemotherapy agents in this class. An expert panel convened by the American Society of Clinical Oncology (ASCO) recommends that patients receiving mildly emetogenic chemotherapy should receive a single dose of corticosteroid, such as dexamethasone 4–8 mg p.o., before chemotherapy. This should result in the control

Table 27.2 Dosing guidelines for antiemetic prophylaxis

Chemotherapy regimen	Acute phase	Delayed phase
Highly emetogenic	Dexamethasone 12–20 mg i.v. *plus one of:* Ondansetron 8 mg i.v. Granisetron 1 mg i.v. Dolasetron 1.8 mg/kg i.v. Ondansetron 24 mg p.o. Granisetron 2 mg p.o.	1st line: Dexamethasone 8 mg p.o. twice daily, days 2–4 Metoclopramide 20 mg p.o. four times daily, days 2–4 (optional) 2nd line:[*] Dexamethasone 8 mg p.o. twice daily, days 2–4 *plus one of:* Ondansetron 8 mg p.o. twice daily Granisetron 1 mg p.o. twice daily Dolasetron 100 mg p.o. four times daily
Moderately emetogenic	Dexamethasone 8–12 mg i.v. *plus one of:* Ondansetron 8 mg i.v. Granisetron 1 mg i.v. Ondansetron 8 mg p.o. twice daily Granisetron 2 mg p.o. Granisetron 1 mg p.o.	1st line: Dexamethasone 8 mg p.o. twice daily, days 2–4 2nd line:[*] Dexamethasone 8 mg p.o. twice daily, days 2–4 *plus one of:* Ondansetron 8 mg p.o. twice daily Granisetron 1 mg p.o. twice daily
Mildly emetogenic	Dexamethasone 4–8 mg p.o.	No routine prophylaxis
Minimally emetogenic	No routine prophylaxis	No routine prophylaxis

[*] Failed 1st line or inadequate control of acute emesis.

of acute emesis in approximately 90% of patients. No routine antiemetic prophylaxis is recommended for patients receiving minimally emetogenic chemotherapy.[3]

Delayed emesis

The control of delayed emesis has long been a difficult treatment dilemma. Part of this difficulty is that the pathophysiology of delayed emesis is poorly understood. The only significant risk factor for the development of delayed emesis is the development of acute emesis. Therefore, the best method to treat or prevent delayed emesis is to provide adequate prophylaxis for acute emesis.

Studies on the treatment of delayed emesis have been poorly designed. For the most part, they are designed comparing different antiemetic regimens during both the acute and the delayed phases. As improved control of acute emesis will result in improved control of delayed emesis, it is difficult to determine whether the regimen administered during the delayed phase resulted in an improvement in the symptoms. A few well-designed studies have helped to direct recommendations for the treatment of delayed emesis. The use of the $5HT_3$-receptor antagonists has proved disappointing. Dexamethasone thus far appears to be the most effective drug for the treatment of delayed emesis.

Highly emetogenic chemotherapy

Studies have shown the superiority of dexamethasone, dopamine receptor antagonists, $5HT_3$-receptor antagonists and combinations of these agents in the control of delayed emesis versus placebo.[61–66]

There have been three well-designed trials addressing the optimal regimen for the treatment of delayed emesis after cisplatin-based chemotherapy. In all three trials, patients received the same antiemetic regimen for the prophylaxis of acute emesis, a $5HT_3$-receptor antagonist and dexamethasone, and were then randomized to one of two different regimens during the delayed phase. In two of these studies, the effectiveness of dexamethasone alone was compared with a combination of granisetron and dexamethasone.[67,68] In both studies the two regimens were equivalent. However, in one of the studies, the subgroup of patients who did not achieve complete control of acute emesis had better control of delayed emesis with the combi-

nation of granisetron and dexamethasone.[68] In this subgroup, control of delayed symptoms was unacceptably low in both arms (22.5% granisetron and dexamethasone versus 10% dexamethasone alone). In the third study, a combination of metoclopramide and dexamethasone was compared with a combination of ondansetron and dexamethasone during the delayed phase.[69] The two regimens were of equal efficacy, although there was a slight advantage for the combination of metoclopramide and dexamethasone in the control of delayed nausea. Again, the subgroup of patients who did not achieve complete control of acute emesis had better control of delayed symptoms with the combination of dexamethasone and a $5HT_3$-receptor antagonist. Only one study has compared the use of dexamethasone alone with a combination of dexamethasone and metoclopramide in the delayed phase.[70] In this study, the combination of metoclopramide and dexamethasone resulted in better control of delayed symptoms. However, this was before the routine use of $5HT_3$-receptor antagonists for the prophylaxis of acute emesis, so patients in this study were treated with high-dose metoclopramide before chemotherapy. Whether improved control of acute emesis with $5HT_3$-receptor antagonists would alter this result is unknown. There have not been any studies examining the dose or scheduling of corticosteroids or dopamine antagonists for the treatment of delayed emesis.

The recommended antiemetic regimen for the prevention of delayed emesis after highly emetogenic chemotherapy is dexamethasone alone or in combination with metoclopramide. If the above regimen fails, or if there is poor control of acute emesis, a combination of dexamethasone and a $5HT_3$-receptor antagonist should be used (see Table 27.2 for dosing guidelines). This should result in control of delayed emesis in 50–70% of patients.[3]

Moderately emetogenic chemotherapy

Dexamethasone, $5HT_3$-receptor antagonists and a combination of these two agents have been shown to be superior to placebo for the control of delayed emesis after moderately emetogenic chemotherapy.[71,72]

A single well-designed trial has compared these two regimens. Patients receiving moderately emetogenic chemotherapy were given a combination of a $5HT_3$-receptor antagonist and dexamethasone before chemotherapy for the prophylaxis of acute emesis. The patients were then randomized to receive dexamethasone alone or a combination of a $5HT_3$-receptor antagonist (ondansetron or dolasetron) and dexamethasone during the delayed phase. In this trial, the complete control rate (no emesis, no worse than mild nausea and no use of rescue therapy) was equivalent in the two arms. The combination of a $5HT_3$-receptor antagonist and dexamethasone resulted in the statistically superior control of delayed nausea. However, the difference between the two arms using a visual analog score was 6/100 mm vs 9/100 mm; therefore, this difference is not likely to be clinically relevant.[73]

The recommended antiemetic regimen for the prophylaxis of delayed emesis after moderately emetogenic chemotherapy is dexamethasone as a single agent. If this fails, or if there is poor control of acute emesis, a combination of dexamethasone and a $5HT_3$-receptor antagonist should be used (see Table 27.2 for dosing guidelines). The added efficacy of this regimen when used as salvage therapy is not known, but it would seem prudent to add the 5-HT_3 receptor antagonist at this time.

Mildly and minimally emetogenic chemotherapy

There has been very little study of the incidence or prevention of delayed emesis after mildly and minimally emetogenic chemotherapy. The expert consensus panel convened by ASCO does not recommend routine use of antiemetics for the prevention of delayed emesis in patients receiving these chemotherapy regimens.[3]

Anticipatory emesis

As discussed earlier, the etiology of ANV appears to be a conditioned response. It generally occurs in individuals who have had poor control of acute or delayed emesis with previous cycles of chemotherapy and its incidence increases with an increasing number of chemotherapy cycles received. The best approach for the treatment of ANV is prevention by administering optimal prophylaxis for acute and delayed emesis as described above. Once ANV develops, it is generally unresponsive to antiemetic therapy. Low doses of the anxiolytic, alprazolam, and behavioral therapy may be effective.[3,11,74]

CONCLUSION

Nausea and vomiting secondary to cytotoxic chemotherapy occur in a significant number of patients and are some of the most feared side effects. The pathophysiology is poorly understood but significant headway has been made. The advent of the $5HT_3$-receptor antagonists has resulted in a dramatic improvement in control of chemotherapy-induced acute emesis. However, delayed and anticipatory emesis still present treatment challenges. This chapter has presented guidelines for the optimal management of chemotherapy-induced emesis based on current evidence. There is still room for improvement and research into this area should continue.

REFERENCES

1. Osoba D, Warr D, Fitch M, Guidelines for the optimal management of chemotherapy-induced nausea and vomiting: a consensus. *Can J Oncol* 1995; **5**:381–99.

2. Gregory RE, Ettinger DS, 5-HT3 receptor antagonists for the prevention of chemotherapy-induced nausea and vomiting. A comparison of their pharmacology and clinical efficacy. *Drugs* 1998; **55**:173–89.

3. Gralla RJ, Osoba D, Kris MG et al, Recommendations for the use of antiemetics: evidence-based, clinical practice guidelines. *J Clin Oncol* 1999; **17**:2971–94.

4. Grunberg SM, Hesketh PJ, Control of chemotherapy-induced emesis. *N Engl J Med* 1993; **329**:1790–6.

5. Andrews PLR, Naylor RJ, Joss RA, Neuropharmacology of emesis and its relevance to anti-emetic therapy. *Support Care Cancer* 1998; **6**:197–203.

6. Andrews PL, Bhandari P, The 5-hydroxytryptamine receptor antagonists as antiemetics: preclinical evaluation and mechanism of action. *Eur J Cancer* 1993; **29A**:S11–16.

7. Cubeddu LX. Mechanisms by which cancer chemotherapeutic drugs induce emesis. *Semin Oncol* 1992; **19**:2–13.

8. Wilder-Smith OH, Borgeat A, Chappuis P et al, Urinary serotonin metabolite excretion during cisplatin chemotherapy. *Cancer* 1993; **72**:2239–41.

9. Navari RM, Reinhardt RR, Gralla RJ et al, Reduction of cisplatin-induces emesis by a selective neurokinin-1-receptor antagonist. *N Engl J Med* 1999; **340**:190–5.

10. Kris MG, Roila F, De Mulder PHM, Marty M, Delayed emesis following anticancer chemotherapy. *Support Care Cancer* 1998; **6**:228–32.

11. Morrow GR, Roscoe JA, Kirshner JJ et al, Anticipatory nausea and vomiting in the era of 5-HT3 antiemetics. *Support Care Cancer* 1998; **6**:244–7.

12. Jantunen IT, Kataja V, Muhonen TT, An overview of randomised studies comparing 5-HT3 receptor antagonists to conventional anti-emetics in the prophylaxis of acute chemotherapy-induced vomiting. *Eur J Cancer* 1997; **33**:66–74.

13. Fauser AA, Fellhauer M, Hoffmann M et al, Guidelines for anti-emetic therapy: acute emesis. *Eur J Cancer* 1999; **35**:361–70.

14. Seynaeve C, Schuller J, Buser K et al, Comparison of the anti-emetic efficacy of different doses of ondansetron, given as either a continuous infusion or a single intravenous dose, in acute cisplatin-induced emesis. A multicentre, double-blind, randomised, parallel group study. Ondansetron Study Group. *Br J Cancer* 1992; **66**:192–7.

15. Beck TM, Hesketh PJ, Madajewicz S et al, Stratified, randomized, double-blind comparison of intravenous ondansetron administered as a multiple-dose regimen versus two single-dose regimens in the prevention of cisplatin-induced nausea and vomiting. *J Clin Oncol* 1992; **10**:1969–75.

16. Hainsworth JD, Hesketh PJ, Single-dose ondansetron for the prevention of cisplatin-induced emesis: efficacy results. *Semin Oncol* 1992; **19**:14–19.

17. Ruff P, Paska W, Goedhals L et al, Ondansetron compared with granisetron in the prophylaxis of cisplatin-induced acute emesis: a multicentre double-blind, randomised, parallel-group study. The Ondansetron and Granisetron Emesis Study Group [published erratum appears in *Oncology* 1994 May–Jun; **51**:243]. *Oncology* 1994; **51**:113–18.

18. Riviere A, Dose finding study of granisetron in patients receiving high-dose cisplatin chemotherapy. The Granisetron Study Group. *Br J Cancer* 1994; **69**:967–71.

19. Navari RM, Kaplan HG, Gralla RJ et al, Efficacy and safety of granisetron, a selective 5-hydroxytryptamine-3 receptor antagonist, in the prevention of nausea and vomiting induced by high-dose cisplatin. *J Clin Oncol* 1994; **12**:2204–10.

20. Navari R, Gandara D, Hesketh P et al, Comparative clinical trial of granisetron and ondansetron in the prophylaxis of cisplatin-induced emesis. The Granisetron Study Group. *J Clin Oncol* 1995; **13**:1242–8.

21. Harman GS, Omura GA, Ryan K et al, A randomized double-blind comparison of single-dose and divided multiple-dose dolasetron for cisplatin-induced emesis. *Cancer Chemother Pharmacol* 1996; **38**:323–8.

22. Yeilding A, Bertoli L, Eisenberg P et al, Antiemetic efficacy of two different single intravenous doses of dolasetron in patients receiving high-dose cisplatin-containing chemotherapy. *Am J Clin Oncol* 1996; **19**:619–23.

23. Hesketh P, Navari R, Grote T et al, Double-blind, randomized comparison of the antiemetic efficacy of intravenous dolasetron mesylate and intravenous ondansetron in the prevention of acute cisplatin-induced emesis in patients with cancer. Dolasetron Comparative Chemotherapy-induced Emesis Prevention Group. *J Clin Oncol* 1996; **14**:2242–9.

24. Audhuy B, Cappelaere P, Martin M et al, A double-blind, randomised comparison of the anti-emetic efficacy of two intravenous doses of dolasetron mesilate and granisetron in patients receiving high dose cisplatin chemotherapy. *Eur J Cancer* 1996; **32A**:807–13.

25. Perez EA, Navari RM, Kaplan HG et al, Efficacy and safety of different doses of granisetron for the prophylaxis of cisplatin-induced emesis [see comments]. *Support Care Cancer* 1997; **5**:31–7.

26. Fumoleau P, Giovannini M, Rolland F et al, Ondansetron suppository: an effective treatment for the prevention of emetic disorders induced by cisplatin-based chemotherapy. French Ondansetron Study Group. *Oral Oncol* 1997; **33**:354–8.

27. Krzakowski M, Graham E, Goedhals L et al, A multicenter, double-blind comparison of i.v. and oral administration of ondansetron plus dexamethasone for acute cisplatin-induced emesis. Ondansetron Acute Emesis Study Group [In Process Citation]. *Anticancer Drugs* 1998; **9**:593–8.

28. Needles B, Miranda E, Rodriguez FM et al, A multicenter, double-blind, randomized comparison or oral ondansetron 8 mg b.i.d., 24 mg q.d., and 32 mg q.d. in the prevention of nausea and vomiting associated with highly emetogenic chemotherapy. S3AA3012 Study Group. *Support Care Cancer* 1999; **7**:347–53.

29. Tsavaris N, Fountzilas GNM, A randomized comparative study of antiemetic prophylaxis with ondansetron in a single 32 mg loading dose versus 8 mg every 6 h in patients undergoing cisplatin-based chemotherapy. *Oncology* 1998; **55**:513–16.

30. Birch R, Weaver CH, Carson K, Buckner CD, A randomized trial of once vs twice daily administration of intravenous granisetron with dexamethasone in patients receiving high-dose cyclophosphamide, thiotepa and carboplatin [In Process Citation]. *Bone Marrow Transplant* 1998; **22**:685–8.

31. Noble A, Bremer K, Goedhals L et al, A double-blind, randomised, crossover comparison of granisetron and ondansetron in 5-day fractionated chemotherapy: assessment of efficacy, safety and patient preference. The Granisetron Study Group. *Eur J Cancer* 1994; **8**:1083–8.

32. Italian Group of Antiemetic Research, Ondansetron versus granisetron, both combined with dexamethasone, in the prevention of cisplatin-induced emesis. *Ann Oncol* 1995; **6**:805–10.

33. Gralla RJ, Navari RM, Hesketh PJ et al, Single-dose oral granisetron has equivalent antiemetic efficacy to intravenous ondansetron for highly emetogenic cisplatin-based chemotherapy. *J Clin Oncol* 1998; **16**:1568–73.

34. Spector JI, Lester EP, Chevlen EM et al, A comparison of oral ondansetron and intravenous granisetron for the prevention of nausea and emesis associated with cisplatin-based chemotherapy. *Oncologist* 1998; **3**:432–8.

35. Roila F, Tonato M, Cognetti F et al, Prevention of cisplatin-induced emesis: a double-blind multicenter randomized crossover study

comparing ondansetron and ondansetron plus dexamethasone. *J Clin Oncol* 1991; **9**:675–8.

36. Smyth JF, Coleman RE, Nicolson M et al, Does dexamethasone enhance control of acute cisplatin induced emesis by ondansetron? *BMJ* 1991; **303**:1423–6.

37. Ahn MJ, Lee JS, Lee KH et al, A randomized double-blind trial of ondansetron alone versus in combination with dexamethasone versus in combination with dexamethasone and lorazepam in the prevention of emesis due to cisplatin-based chemotherapy. *Am J Clin Oncol* 1994; **17**:150–6.

38. Chevallier B, Marty M, Paillarse JM, Methylprednisolone enhances the efficacy of ondansetron in acute and delayed cisplatin-induced emesis over at least three cycles. Ondansetron Study Group. *Br J Cancer* 1994; **70**:1171–5.

39. Hesketh PJ, Harvey WH, Harker WG et al, A randomized, double-blind comparison of intravenous ondansetron alone and in combination with intravenous dexamethasone in the prevention of high-dose cisplatin-induced emesis. *J Clin Oncol* 1994; **12**:596–600.

40. Joss RA, Bacchi M, Buser K et al, Ondansetron plus dexamethasone is superior to ondansetron alone in the prevention of emesis in chemotherapy-naive and previously treated patients. Swiss Group for Clinical Cancer Research (SAKK). *Ann Oncol* 1994; **5**:253–8.

41. Latreille J, Stewart D, Laberge F et al, Dexamethasone improves the efficacy of granisetron in the first 24 h following high-dose cisplatin chemotherapy. *Support Care Cancer* 1995; **3**:307–12.

42. Handberg J, Wessel V, Larsen L et al, Randomized, double-blind comparison of granisetron versus granisetron plus prednisolone as antiemetic prophylaxis during multiple-day cisplatin-based chemotherapy. *Support Care Cancer* 1998; **6**:63–7.

43. Kleisbauer JP, Garcia-Giron C, Antimi M et al, Granisetron plus methylprednisolone for the control of high-dose cisplatin-induced emesis. *Anticancer Drugs* 1998; **9**:387–92.

44. Italian Group for Antiemetic Research, Double-blind, dose-finding study of four intravenous doses of dexamethasone in the prevention of cisplatin-induced acute emesis. *J Clin Oncol* 1998; **16**:2937–42.

45. Hacking A. Oral granisetron – simple and effective: a preliminary report. The Granisetron Study Group. *Eur J Cancer* 1992; **28A**:S28–32.

46. Bleiberg HH, Spielmann M, Falkson G, Romain D, Antiemetic treatment with oral granisetron in patients receiving moderately emetogenic chemotherapy: a dose-ranging study. *Clin Ther* 1995; **17**:38–51.

47. Stewart A, McQuade B, Cronje JD et al, Ondansetron compared with granisetron in the prophylaxis of cyclophosphamide-induced emesis in out-patients: a multicentre, double-blind, double-dummy, randomised, parallel-group study. Emesis Study Group for Ondansetron and Granisetron in Breast Cancer Patients. *Oncology* 1995; **52**:202–10.

48. Ettinger DS, Eisenberg PD, Fitts D et al, A double-blind comparison of the efficacy of two dose regimens of oral granisetron in preventing acute emesis in patients receiving moderately emetogenic chemotherapy. *Cancer* 1996; **78**:144–51.

49. Massidda B, Ionta MT, Prevention of delayed emesis by a single intravenous bolus dose of 5-HT3-receptor-antagonist in moderately emetogenic chemotherapy. *J Chemother* 1996; **8**:237–42.

50. Davidson NG, Paska W, Van Belle S et al, Ondansetron suppository: a randomised, double-blind, double-dummy, parallel-group comparison with oral ondansetron for the prevention of cyclophosphamide-induced emesis and nausea. The Ondansetron Suppository emesis study group. *Oncology* 1997; **54**:380–6.

51. Grote TH, Pineda LF, Figlin RA et al, Oral dolasetron mesylate in patients receiving moderately emetogenic platinum-containing chemotherapy. Oral Dolasetron Dose Response Study Group. *Cancer J Sci Am* 1997; **3**:45–51.

52. Rubenstein EB, Gralla RJ, Hainsworth JD et al, Randomized, double blind, dose–response trial across four oral doses of dolasetron for the prevention of acute emesis after moderately emetogenic chemotherapy. Oral Dolasetron Dose–Response Study Group. *Cancer* 1997; **79**:1216–24.

53. Beck TM, York M, Chang A et al, Oral ondansetron 8 mg twice daily is as effective as 8 mg three times daily in the prevention of nausea and vomiting associated with moderately emetogenic cancer chemotherapy. S3A-376 Study Group [see comments]. *Cancer Invest* 1997; **15**:297–303.

54. Perez EA, Hesketh P, Sandbach J et al, Comparison of single-dose oral granisetron versus intravenous ondansetron in the prevention of nausea and vomiting induced by moderately emetogenic chemotherapy: a multicenter, double-blind, randomized parallel study. *J Clin Oncol* 1998; **16**:754–60.

55. Perez EA, Lembersky B, Kaywin P et al, Comparable safety and antiemetic efficacy of a brief (30-second bolus) intravenous granisetron infusion and a standard (15-minute) intravenous ondansetron infusion in breast cancer patients receiving moderately emetogenic chemotherapy. *Cancer J Sci Am* 1998; **4**:52–8.

56. Fauser AA, Duclos B, Chemaissani A et al, Therapeutic equivalence of single oral doses of dolasetron mesilate and multiple doses of ondansetron for the prevention of emesis after moderately emetogenic chemotherapy. European Dolasetron Comparative Study Group. *Eur J Cancer* 1996; **32A**:1523–9.

57. Lofters WS, Pater JL, Zee B et al, Phase III double-blind comparison of dolasetron mesylate and ondansetron and an evaluation of the additive role of dexamethasone in the prevention of acute and delayed nausea and vomiting due to moderately emetogenic chemotherapy. *J Clin Oncol* 1997; **15**:2966–73.

58. Carmichael J, Bessel EM, Harris AL et al, Comparison of granisetron alone and granisetron plus dexamethasone in the prophylaxis of cytotoxic-induced emesis [published erratum appears in *Br J Cancer* 1995 May; **71**:1123]. *Br J Cancer* 1994; **70**:1161–4.

59. The Italian Group for Antiemetic Research, Dexamethasone, granisetron, or both for the prevention of nausea and vomiting during chemotherapy for cancer [see comments]. *N Engl J Med* 1995; **332**:1–5.

60. Kirchner V, Aapro M, Terrey JP, Alberto P, A double-blind crossover study comparing prophylactic intravenous granisetron alone or in combination with dexamethasone as antiemetic treatment in controlling nausea and vomiting associated with chemotherapy. *Eur J Cancer* 1997; **33**:1605–10.

61. Roila F, Baschetti E, Tonato M et al, Predictive factors of delayed emesis in cisplatin-treated patients and antiemetic activity and tolerability of metoclopramide or dexamethasone. A randomized, single-blind study. *Am J Clin Oncol* 1991; **14**:238–42.

62. Gandara DR, Harvey WH, Monaghan GG et al, Delayed emesis following high-dose cisplatin: a double-blind randomised comparative trial of ondansetron (GR 38032F) versus placebo. *Eur J Cancer* 1993; **29A**: S35–8.

63. Esseeboom EU, Rojer RA, Borm JJ, Statius van Eps LW, Prophylaxis of delayed nausea and vomiting after cancer chemotherapy. *Neth J Med* 1995; **47**:12–17.

64. Navari RM, Madajewicz S, Anderson N et al, Oral ondansetron for the control of cisplatin-induced delayed emesis: a large, multicenter, double-blind, randomized comparative trial of ondansetron versus placebo. *J Clin Oncol* 1995; **13**:2408–16.

65. Matsui K, Fukuoka M, Takada M et al, Randomised trial for the prevention of delayed emesis in patients receiving high-dose cisplatin. *Br J Cancer* 1996; **73**:217–21.

66. Olver I, Paska W, Depierre A et al, A multicentre, double-blind study comparing placebo, ondansetron and ondansetron plus dexamethasone for the control of cisplatin-induced

delayed emesis. Ondansetron Delayed Emesis Study Group. *Ann Oncol* 1996; 7:945–52.

67. Latreille J, Pater J, Johnston D et al, Use of dexamethasone and granisetron in the control of delayed emesis for patients who receive highly emetogenic chemotherapy. National Cancer Institute of Canada Clinical Trials Group. *J Clin Oncol* 1998; **16**:1174–8.

68. Goedhals L, Heron JF, Kleisbauer JP et al, Control of delayed nausea and vomiting with granisetron plus dexamethasone or dexamethasone alone in patients receiving highly emetogenic chemotherapy: a double-blind, placebo-controlled, comparative study. *Ann Oncol* 1998; 9:661–6.

69. The Italian Group for Antiemetic Research, Ondansetron versus metoclopramide, both combined with dexamethasone, in the prevention of cisplatin-induced delayed emesis. *J Clin Oncol* 1997; 15:124–30.

70. Kris MG, Gralla RJ, Tyson LB et al, Controlling delayed vomiting: double-blind, randomized trial comparing placebo, dexamethasone alone, and metoclopramide plus dexamethasone in patients receiving cisplatin. *J Clin Oncol* 1989; 7:108–14.

71. Kaizer L, Warr D, Hoskins P et al, Effect of schedule and maintenance on the antiemetic efficacy of ondansetron combined with dexamethasone in acute and delayed nausea and emesis in patients receiving moderately emetogenic chemotherapy: a phase III trial by the National Cancer Institute of Canada Clinical Trials Group. *J Clin Oncol* 1994; **12**:1050–7.

72. Koo WH, Ang PT, Role of maintenance oral dexamethasone in prophylaxis of delayed emesis caused by moderately emetogenic chemotherapy. *Ann Oncol* 1996; 7:71–4.

73. Pater JL, Lofters WS, Zee B et al, The role of the 5-HT3 antagonists ondansetron and dolasetron in the control of delayed onset nausea and vomiting in patients receiving moderately emetogenic chemotherapy. *Ann Oncol* 1997; 8:181–5.

74. Razavi D, Delvaux N, Farvacques C et al, Prevention of adjustment disorders and anticipatory nausea secondary to adjuvant chemotherapy: a double-blind, placebo-controlled study assessing the usefulness of alprazolam. *J Clin Oncol* 1993; 11:1384–90.

SECTION 8: Prognostic/Predictive Factors

Section Editor: J Hugh

28

Histological prognostic factors in invasive breast cancer

Sarah E Pinder, Ian O Ellis, Andrew HS Lee, Christopher W Elston

Historically, the role of the histopathologist in the treatment of patients with breast cancer lay solely in providing the correct diagnosis on excision biopsy material, with or without frozen section. Examination of locoregional lymph nodes for the presence or absence of metastases may also have been performed, but it was unusual for any other prognostic information to be requested by clinical colleagues and therefore it was not supplied. In the last few decades, the treatment of breast cancer has changed dramatically; a wide variety of possible therapeutic options is now available and choices have to be made regarding both local and systemic treatments for each patient. However, none of the possible adjuvant treatments presently available is without side effects or morbidity. It has therefore become increasingly important to assess prognosis for each patient and to devise an appropriate therapeutic plan. The determination of predictive factors, as opposed to prognostic factors, is also becoming increasingly recognized as a role of the histopathologist. These features can be used to identify particular tumors that are likely to respond to specific treatments.

A large number of factors have been proposed as being of prognostic significance in patients with invasive breast cancer. Many have been reported to be of value in series when univariate analysis has been performed, but have not withstood multivariate analysis. We describe below those that are of greatest importance.

TUMOR SIZE

Tumour size is, at least in part, a time-dependent factor which has been shown to influence prognosis in many series of patients with invasive breast carcinoma.[1-5] Patients with small tumors have a better long-term survival than those with extensive invasive disease. For example, in the long-term study from the Memorial–Sloan Kettering Cancer Centre,[6] the projected relapse-free survival rates 20 years after initial treatment were: < 10 mm – 88%; 11–13 mm – 73%; 14–16 mm – 65%; 17–22 mm – 59%. The inherent strength of tumor size as a prognostic factor is confirmed in series where local rather than central review pathologists have carried out the measurement of tumors. Even then strong correlations with prognosis are seen.[2,3,5]

Clinical measurement of tumor size is notoriously inaccurate; if an estimate of tumor size is required for therapeutic planning it should be performed by ultrasonography. For accurate assessment, however, the size of a breast cancer should be assessed on the excised pathological specimen. Size of the surgically excised tumor is measured in the histopathology laboratory to the nearest millimetre in three planes. This is performed initially in the fresh state, confirmed after fixation, and size is finally checked on the histological section using the stage micrometer of the microscope. The greatest dimension of the invasive component is taken as the final tumor size, although the total dimension of invasive carcinoma plus ductal carcinoma in situ (DCIS) is also recorded. The confirmation of size from the histological sections is particularly important for DCIS or tumors with a large in situ component and also for small lesions, such as those measuring less than 1 cm in size. It is, however, clear that as size decreases, the risk of errors in measurement increases and inconsistencies between histopathologists' measurements from tissue sections have been reported.[7,8]

It is vital that pathologists measure tumor dimensions as accurately as possible in order to provide accurate data for audit. Tumor size is an important quality assurance measure for breast screening programmes[9-11] and is utilized to confirm the ability of radiologists to detect impalpable invasive carcinomas mammographically. Thus, a target in the UK National Health Service Breast Screening Programme (NHSBSP) (prevalent round) is for 50% of invasive cancers to measure less than 15 mm in size.[11]

LYMPH NODE STAGE

Involvement of locoregional lymph nodes in invasive breast cancer is well recognized as a most important prognostic factor. Patients who have metastatic deposits in locoregional lymph nodes have a significantly poorer prognosis than those without nodal disease.[1,2,12-16] The 10 year survival rate is reduced from 75% for node-negative patients to 25–30% for those with nodal disease. The clinical assessment of the presence of disease in axillary lymph node is not accurate and in particular is not sufficiently robust for therapeutic decision-making.[17] The accurate evaluation of node stage must be based on careful and thorough histological examination of excised lymph nodes.

As well as the simple presence of metastatic disease in the lymph nodes, it is clear that outcome of patients with invasive breast carcinoma is also related to the number and the level of lymph nodes involved. The greater the number of nodes involved, the poorer the patient survival.[3,18] Thus, for therapeutic purposes three groups of patients can be defined, based on the number of nodes involved: those with no nodal disease, those with one to three positive nodes and those with four or more containing metastatic deposits. Metastatic disease in lymph nodes in the higher levels of the axilla (specifically the apex), also carries a worse prognosis[16,19] as do metastatic deposits in the internal mammary nodes.[19]

The extent of axillary surgery in patients with breast cancer is, however, controversial. Strong arguments in favor of both axillary sampling and axillary clearance have been made.[20-25] Sentinel node biopsy for patients with invasive breast cancer has also been widely advocated in the last few years and the concept has now been validated.[26-30] The basis of the concept is that the first nodal deposit of metastatic disease will be dictated by the lymphatic system draining any individual tumor. If the sentinel lymph node contains metastatic tumor further axillary surgery or radiotherapy can be undertaken. If it is not involved, the remaining lymph nodes in that area should be free of metastatic disease. Early series have confirmed that if only one node contains metastatic carcinoma, it is almost always the sentinel node. However, a weakness of many of the series published to date is that the sentinel node has often been examined more intensively than the other lymph nodes. Metastases in 'non-sentinel' nodes may therefore have been missed.[31–33] Cases have been reported where the sentinel lymph node is negative but metastases have been found elsewhere in the axilla; to date, this varies in the literature from 1% to 11%.[29,31–35]

There is at present debate about the most appropriate technique for examination of excised sentinel nodes in order to obtain the optimum prognostic information. The methodology is of vital importance because the historical prognostic data on axillary nodal status is largely based on series in which one slice from each lymph node has been examined, using only routinely stained sections. Clinical decisions are routinely based on this information from the world literature.

Other techniques can increase the sensitivity of detection of metastatic disease by examining a greater surface area of any individual lymph node. This may be done simply by embedding all of the node in multiple slices or by examining multiple levels (serial sections) through a lymph node.[36–38] It is also clear that the use of immunohistochemistry increases detection of small deposits of metastatic tumor,[38–40] partly by again increasing the surface area of the node examined and partly by making the deposits easier to recognize histologically. Both immunohistochemistry and serial sections increase the detection of metastases in sentinel lymph node biopsies.[16,41] Use of the more sensitive reverse transcriptase polymerase chain reaction (RT-PCR) has been proposed by some.

The role of these more sensitive methods to detect deposits is unclear. As described above, many of the prognostic data in the literature on node status are based on less extensive histological examination. The prognostic implications of smaller deposits identified by new techniques remains unclear; although there is some evidence that the size of the deposit in lymph nodes is of prognostic significance,[38,40–44] there is neither an agreed definition for these small deposits nor a universal methodology for their detection. Definitions of 'occult' or 'micrometastases' have included a variety of lesions:

- Metastases that are less than a given size such as 2 mm.
- Metastases found on review that were initially missed.
- Deposits shown only in deeper histological sections.
- Metastases shown with immunohistochemistry for cytokeratins.

As a result of the different definitions and criteria used for these deposits of metastatic disease, comparison of published results is at present impossible and their significance is thus uncertain.

Many of the larger studies have, nevertheless, shown a poorer prognosis for patients with 'micrometastases' compared with node-negative patients in univariate analysis.[36,38–40,45] The effect is clearer for disease-free survival than for overall survival. There are also conflicting data about whether the position of the metastatic deposit, i.e. in the marginal sinus or parenchyma, is important.[36,37,46,47] Further series with strict adherence to well-described protocols and definitions are urgently required to clarify the optimum methodology for detecting disease and to determine the significance of small metastatic deposits in sentinel lymph nodes.

In our view, routine use of frozen sections for perioperative examination of lymph nodes has an unacceptably high false-negative rate. This ranges from approximately 10% to 30%.[33,48–50] Frozen section may be appropriate in a few cases, e.g. if the node clinically contains tumor. If the presence of disease can be confirmed histologically, immediate axillary surgery can be undertaken. Time-consuming, labor-intensive and expensive intraoperative assessment with serial sections and immunohistochemistry have also been described but are not widely performed. Intraoperative imprint cytology has been advocated by some groups, who have found acceptably low false-negative rates of 2–3%,[30,48] but many have not been able to achieve this level of accuracy. The authors' current routine practice is based on pragmatism;[51] axillary lymph nodes are in general cut into slices about 3 mm thick perpendicular to the long axis (thus maximizing the assessment of the marginal sinuses). Each node is examined in a single cassette. The vast majority of nodes can be completely embedded, although larger nodes may have only alternate slices examined. Very large, obviously involved nodes have only one section taken.

Extranodal spread

The prognostic significance of extranodal spread of carcinoma into adipose tissue in the axilla surrounding the lymph nodes is uncertain. This feature has been described as carrying a poor prognosis,[52] particularly in patients with up to three nodes involved, but not in those with four or more involved nodes.[53] Other groups have found that extranodal disease confers no additional information to lymph-node disease[54] and has no intrinsic prognostic significance.[55,56]

LYMPHOVASCULAR INVASION

Lymphovascular invasion is, not surprisingly, strongly related to locoregional lymph node involvement,[57–59] with some groups claiming that it can provide prognostic information as powerful as lymph node stage.[60] Others have confirmed that the presence of vascular invasion predicts for both recurrence[20,60,61] and survival.[62–64,77] Conversely, some earlier series found no correlation between lymphovascular invasion and prognosis.[65,66] Such discrepancies may, in part, be explained by the wide variation in the frequency of vascular invasion in the literature (20–54%).

Tumor emboli are sought histologically within thin-walled vascular channels. It is impossible to determine reliably whether such spaces are capillaries, venules or lymphatic spaces, and the broad term 'vascular invasion' is used. Muscular blood vessels are only rarely involved. The wide variety in frequency of vascular invasion reported might itself be partly explained by the difficulty in distinguishing true vessels from artefactual soft tissue spaces, especially in suboptimally fixed specimens. Both DCIS and shrinkage artefact may be misinterpreted as vascular invasion.[57,58] However, when strict criteria are used, the feature can be assessed reproducibly.[3,57,67]

Vascular invasion is related to long-term survival, an effect that is independent of lymph node stage.[57] There is also a correlation between the presence of vascular invasion and early recurrence in lymph node-negative patients.[60,61,68] However, the most important clinical application of vascular invasion lies in its power as a predictor of local recurrence after conservation therapy[20,57,61,68] and of flap recurrence after mastectomy.[69]

DIFFERENTIATION

Lymph-node stage and tumor size are, at least in part, time-dependent factors. In addition, histological features can be assessed to establish the aggressiveness of an individual invasive breast carcinoma. Historically, histological classification of mammary cancer was restricted to in situ or invasive breast carcinoma. It is now evident that the latter group of invasive carcinomas can be further subdivided according to their differentiation. This may be performed in two ways, by examination of (1) histological grade and (2) histological type.

Histological grade

The first study of histological grading of invasive breast cancer to be recognized was performed by Greenhough over 70 years ago.[70] Eight morphological features were examined (in a somewhat subjective way) and showed an association with 'cure'. Greenhough's method was reassessed by Scarff and colleagues who found that only three factors – tubule formation, nuclear pleomorphism and hyperchromatism – were of importance.[71] Most subsequent grading systems for invasive breast cancer have been based on this technique. Some use multiple features of the tumor histology;[3,72–76] others include only an assessment of nuclear appearances.[77–79] A very large number of studies have demonstrated the significant association between grade and survival of breast cancer patients, despite these many methods used. Histological grade has been convincingly proved to be associated with prognosis; life-table analysis of over 1800 patients in Nottingham with long-term follow-up shows survival worsens with increasing (higher) grade.[76]

Histological grading must be carried out by trained histopathologists working to an agreed protocol; one of the fundamental problems with systems used in previous studies was the lack of strictly defined written criteria. Bloom and Richardson[74] made a highly valuable contribution to Patey and Scarff's method by adding numerical scoring.[71] They did not, however, define clear criteria for cut-off points and additional modifications to their method have been made subsequently to introduce greater objectiv-

ity.[76] The features assessed are tubule formation, nuclear pleomorphism and mitotic count, as described in Patey and Scarff's original work, but each is scored from 1 to 3 based on strictly defined criteria. The amendments are both qualitative and quantitative.

Despite clear evidence that histological grade determined by this modified, more objective methodology is of prognostic value, acceptance of the technique into routine practice has been slow. This has resulted largely from lack of clinical demand. In the past, there was also a perception that grading was of poor reproducibility and consistency.[80] However, a significant number of studies have now reported acceptable levels of observer variability.[81–85] The method has now been adopted for use in the pathological data sets of the UK National Coordinating Group for Breast Screening Pathology,[86] the rest of Europe[87] and in the USA.[88]

In addition to being of prognostic value, histological grade is a predictive factor that can be used to predict response to chemotherapy. We have found that patients with lymph node-positive disease who had grade 3 tumors obtained a significant overall and disease-free survival benefit from prolonged compared with perioperative chemotherapy, whereas those with grade 1 and grade 2 primary tumors did not.[89]

Histological type

In addition to histological grade, the widely varied histological appearances of invasive mammary carcinoma may be subgrouped by means of large numbers of histological types.[14,90,91] This information also provides prognostic information.[90] The criteria for diagnosis of different histological types of invasive breast carcinoma have been described in detail,[51,90,91] but it should be recognized that there is a subjective element to histological typing and there is as yet no universal agreement. For example, in the UK

NHSBSP pathology quality assurance scheme, the consistency of diagnosis of histological type has been disappointingly low,[7] suggesting that pathologists adhere poorly to criteria in protocols for typing. Histological type is not used to determine clinical management and it may be that histopathologists concentrate their efforts on features that they perceive to have greater clinical implications.

This relatively poor reproducibility of histological type may in part explain the widely varying proportions of types in the literature. Although there are relatively few long-term, comprehensive, follow-up studies addressing survival of patients with different subtypes of invasive breast carcinoma, it is well established that certain histological types have a good prognosis. Tubular[92–94] and invasive cribriform carcinoma,[95] medullary carcinoma,[96,97] mucinous carcinoma,[98,99] infiltrating lobular carcinoma[100] and tubulo-lobular carcinoma[101] have all been reported to have a better prognosis than carcinomas of ductal/no special type (NST).[65] Papillary carcinomas have been subsequently added to those types found among long-term survivors with breast cancer.[102] It is also evident that there is a relative excess of these 'special-type' tumors in cancers detected in the prevalent round of mammographic breast screening.[103,104]

Patients with invasive carcinoma of the breast can be stratified into broad prognostic groups according to their histological type.[105] The excellent (> 80% 10-year survival rate) prognosis group comprises mucinous, tubular, invasive cribriform and tubulo-lobular carcinomas. The good (60–80% 10-year survival rate) prognosis group is composed of mixed ductal/NST in association with a special-type element, tubular mixed and also alveolar lobular carcinomas. The average prognosis group (50–60% 10-year survival rate) includes classic lobular, invasive papillary, medullary and atypical medullary carcinomas. The poor prognosis group (< 50% 10 year survival rate) is composed of ductal/NST, mixed ductal and lobular, solid lobular and lobular mixed carcinomas.

The authors believe that subtyping adds to our understanding of the biology of breast carcinoma, while adding relatively little prognostic information to histological grade. It is clear that some subtypes of carcinoma are likely to express certain markers or infiltrate in a particular fashion. For example, the pattern of metastatic spread is different in breast cancers of infiltrating lobular type[106,107] and these lesions are also more frequently estrogen receptor (ER)-positive than tumors of ductal/NST.[108] Similarly the identification of a relative excess of carcinomas of ductal/NST with medullary features in patients with *BRCA1* compared with *BRCA2* mutations is adding to our knowledge of tumor biology and genetics.[109–111]

OTHER HISTOLOGICAL FACTORS

A variety of other morphological features has been proposed in the literature from time to time as potential prognostic factors. In the authors' experience, these are of relatively less importance than those discussed above. These proposed factors include: extent of DCIS, stromal fibrosis, stromal elastosis and tumor necrosis.

The extent of DCIS identified in association with an invasive tumor is extremely variable. The assessment of its degree is also subjective; however, it has been suggested that a prominent DCIS component within an invasive carcinoma conveys a better prognosis for the patient and a decreased frequency of nodal metastases.[112,113] An extensive DCIS component may be of greater clinical importance in the management of patients undergoing breast-conserving therapy. It has been suggested that the principal risk factor for disease relapse after breast-conserving surgery is a large residual tumor burden, and the main source of this burden may be an extensive in situ component (EIC).[114] EIC has been defined as the presence of DCIS in an invasive breast cancer that occupies 25% or more of the overall tumor, extending beyond the confines of the main invasive element.[115] Invasive breast carcinomas with EIC have been reported to have a considerably higher local recurrence rate than those without EIC disease. The Boston group have, more recently, reported that the most powerful predictor of local recurrence was assessment of excision margins and that EIC was not important if complete excision was achieved.[116] They found that EIC did, however, predict the likelihood of margin involvement.

Stromal fibrosis is common, in varying amounts, in invasive breast carcinoma. It is reported to be associated with a poorer survival,[117,118] a favorable prognosis[119] and to have no effect on outcome.[65] This is almost certainly because an association with tumor type confounds the data. There are similarly conflicting data on the prognostic significance of stromal elastosis, which is also a feature of many breast lesions but which may be seen diffusely through a tumor or in a periductal distribution.[120] Some studies have indicated that its presence is associated with an improved prognosis,[121,122] but this has not been universally reported.[123,124] Tumor necrosis is a relatively common feature in invasive breast cancers, particularly high-grade lesions, but its prognostic value has been addressed in only a few studies. Its presence has been reported to be related to poor outcome and early treatment failure.[3,117,125] However, a precise definition is not included in many of the studies in which it is reported, and terms such as 'extensive' have been utilized, making reassessment impossible.

NOTTINGHAM PROGNOSTIC INDEX

Research into prognostic features in invasive breast cancer has grown exponentially in the last decade. Many of the histological features described above have been examined in very large numbers of series. It is now clear that use of prognostic factors can be made in order to select the most appropriate treatment for an individual invasive breast cancer patient. In particular, women with an excellent prognosis (comparable to those without breast cancer) can avoid the unnecessary side effects and morbidity of systemic adjuvant treatment and those with a poor prognosis can appropriately receive more aggressive therapies.[126]

Although lymph-node stage is the most commonly proposed prognostic factor in mammary cancer, it is a relatively poor discriminator when used alone. A group of patients with an almost 100% survival rate cannot be defined and one with an almost 100% mortality rate cannot be identified based on node stage. Similarly, histological grade is a complex morphological result of the losses and gains of a multitude of molecular markers, but it is also not sufficiently discriminatory on its own on which to base definitive therapy.

The features that are of greatest prognostic import in multivariate analysis are histological grade, lymph-node stage and tumor size. These have been combined into the Nottingham Prognostic Index (NPI),[15] with appropriate weighting. This is calculated as:

NPI = tumor size × 0.2 (in cm) + lymph node stage (1–3) + histological grade (1–3).

The NPI has been confirmed prospectively[12] in studies from Nottingham as providing robust information for women aged 70 or under with operable primary invasive breast carcinoma. Other groups have validated the findings in series of large numbers of patients.[127,128] Cut-off points of 3.4 and 5.4 are used to group the patients into three categories for management purposes. Women with an NPI of 3.4 or less have a good survival and receive no adjuvant systemic treatment. Those patients with a score greater than this have systemic adjuvant treatment and receive hormone therapy if their tumor is ER-positive (see below).

PREDICTIVE FACTORS

Steroid hormones have been known to affect the growth of some tumors, particularly breast and prostatic cancer, since the late nineteenth century.[129] Previously, cytosol assays were used for determining hormone receptor levels in tumors, but these required significant amounts of tissue and were affected by endogenous hormones in premenopausal women. Monoclonal antibodies raised to the nuclear ER[130–132] allow in situ localization of receptors by immunocyto-chemistry. Immunohistochemical determination of ER status is now routinely performed on formalin-fixed, paraffin-embedded material.[133,134] A semiquantitative scoring of the proportion and intensity of nuclear immunoreactivity is undertaken.[131] Conversely, a simple categorical scoring system can be used.[135] The authors have not, however, found that assessment of ER status is of independent prognostic significance because it is associated closely with histological grade. ER status is, however, a predictive factor. Although about 30% of unselected patients with breast carcinoma will respond to hormone therapies, ER assays allow more accurate prediction, with 50–60% of ER-positive tumors responding.[136] None of the systems for predicting response to hormone therapies is, however, completely specific or sensitive; a small proportion of ER-negative tumors will respond to hormone manipulation[137,138] and approximately 30% of apparently ER-positive tumors will develop progression of disease.[134]

Other possible 'predictive' factors are emerging in conjunction with new therapies such as the humanized anti-c-ErbB-2 monoclonal antibody, trastuzumab (Herceptin). Patients suitable for this treatment require preselection by determination of overexpression of the c-ErbB-2 oncoprotein by immunohistochemistry or amplification of the gene by fluorescent in situ hybridization. Which of these techniques is better is under investigation. In multivariate analyses, molecular markers such as c-ErbB-2 protein expression,[139] epidermal growth factor receptor (EGFR) expression[140] and epithelial mucin immunohistochemistry[141] have not achieved significance as independent *prognostic* factors when included with histological grade, tumor size and lymph-node stage. The future may prove, however, at least some additional molecular markers to be *predictive* factors.

Histological grading is derived by combining the appearance of various morphological features and mitotic figure frequency.[142] It thus provides a summation of a variety of tumor-related variables and, in essence, gives an overview of various molecular events affecting morphological appearance. It is not surprising therefore that a single molecular event cannot compete with histological grade in multivariate analysis for survival. It would indeed be fortunate if a single molecular event could offer analogous information to thorough histological evaluation of an invasive breast cancer. The traditional histopathological factors are dependent on a host of complex variables, including the time a tumor has been present (size and lymph-node stage), differentiation (grade and type), proliferation (grade) and metastatic potential (lymph node stage and vascular invasion).

CONCLUSION

In conclusion, the most important prognostic factors in invasive breast cancer are the main traditional histological features of histological grade, lymph node stage and tumor size. Once prognosis has been indicated by a combination of these features, a decision regarding the appropriateness of adjuvant therapy can be made. Then assessment of predictive factors including histological grade, ER and c-ErbB-2 status enables the prediction of the probable response to specific treatments and the optimum therapy can be selected.

REFERENCES

1. Cutler SJ, Black MM, Mork T et al, Further observations on prognostic factors in cancer of the female breast. *Cancer* 1969; **24**:653–7.
2. Elston CW, Gresham GA, Rao GS et al, The Cancer Research Campaign (Kings/Cambridge) trial for early breast cancer – pathological aspects. *Br J Cancer* 1982; **45**:655–69.
3. Fisher ER, Sass R, Fisher B et al, Pathologic findings from the National Surgical Adjuvant Project for breast cancer (protocol no 4). Discrimination for tenth year treatment failure. *Cancer* 1984; **53**:712–23.
4. Carter GL, Allen C, Henson DE, Relation of tumour size, lymph node status, and survival in 24,740 breast cancer cases. *Cancer* 1989; **63**:181–7.
5. Neville AM, Bettelheim R, Gelber RD et al, Predicting treatment responsiveness and prognosis in node-negative breast cancer. *J Clin Oncol* 1992; **10**:696–705.
6. Rosen PP, Groshen S, Factors influencing survival and prognosis in early breast carcinoma (T1N0M0–T1N1M0). Assessment of 644 patients with median follow up of 19 years. *Surg Clin North Am* 1990; **70**:937–62.
7. Sloane JP, National Co-ordinating Group for Breast Screening Pathology, Consistency of histopathological reporting of breast lesions detected by screening: findings of the UK National External Quality Assessment (EQA) Scheme. *Eur J Cancer* 1994; **30**:1414–19.
8. Beahrs OH, Shapiro S, Smart C et al, Summary report of the Working Group to review the National Cancer Institute–American Cancer Society Breast Cancer Demonstration Detection Projects. *J Natl Cancer Inst* 1979; **62**:641–709.
9. Hartman WH, Minimal breast cancer: an update. *Cancer* 1984; **53**:681–4.
10. Tabar L, Duffy SW, Krusemo UB, Detection method, tumour size and node metastases in breast cancers diagnosed during a trial of breast cancer screening. *Eur J Cancer Clin Oncol* 1987; **23**:959–62.
11. Royal College of Radiologists, *Quality Assurance Guidelines for Radiologists.* January 1997. NHSBSP Publications no 15, 1997.
12. Galea MH, Blamey RW, Elston CW et al, The Nottingham Prognostic Index in primary breast cancer. *Breast Cancer Res Treat* 1992; **22**:207–19.
13. Ferguson DJ, Meier P, Karrison T et al, Staging of breast cancer and survival rates: an assessment based on 50 years of experience with radical mastectomy. *JAMA* 1982; **248**:1337–41.
14. Fisher ER, Gregorio RM, Fisher B, The pathology of invasive breast cancer. A syllabus derived from findings of the National Surgical Adjuvant Breast Cancer Project (protocol no 4). *Cancer* 1975; **36**:144–56.
15. Haybittle JL, Blamey RW, Elston CW et al, A prognostic index in primary breast cancer. *Br J Cancer* 1982; **45**:361–6.
16. Veronesi U, Galimberti V, Zurrida S et al, Prognostic significance of number and level of axillary node metastases in breast cancer. *Breast* 1993; **2**:224–8.
17. Barr LC, Baum M, Time to abandon TNM staging of breast cancer? *Lancet* 1992; **339**:915–17.
18. Nemoto T, Vana J, Bedwani RN, Management

and survival of female breast cancer: results of a national survey by the American College of Surgeons. *Cancer* 1980; **45**:2917–24.

19. Handley RF, Observations and thoughts on carcinoma of the breast. *Proc R Soc Med* 1972; **65**:437–44.

20. Locker AP, Ellis IO, Morgan DAL et al, Factors influencing local recurrence after excision and radiotherapy for primary breast cancer. *Br J Surg* 1989; **76**:890–4.

21. Steele RJC, Forrest APM, Gibson T, The efficacy of lower axillary sampling in obtaining lymph node status in breast cancer: a controlled randomized trial. *Br J Surg* 1985; **72**:368–9.

22. Dixon JM, Dillon P, Anderson TJ, Chetty U, Axillary sampling in breast cancer: an assessment of its efficacy. *Breast* 1998; **7**:206–8.

23. Kutianawala MA, Sayed M, Stotter A et al, Staging the axilla in breast cancer: an audit of lymph-node retrieval in one UK regional centre. *Eur J Surg Oncol* 1998; **24**:280–2.

24. O'Dwyer PJ, Editorial. Axillary dissection in primary breast cancer; the benefits of node clearance warrant reappraisal. *BMJ* 1992; **302**:360–1.

25. Cabanes PA, Salmon RJ, Vilcoq JR et al, Value of axillary dissection in addition to lumpectomy and radiotherapy in early breast cancer. *Lancet* 1992; **339**:1245–8.

26. Albertini JJ, Lyman GH, Cox C et al, Lymphatic mapping and sentinel node biopsy in the patient with breast cancer. *JAMA* 1996; **276**:1818–22.

27. Giuliano AE, Kirgan DM, Guenther JM, Morton DL, Lymphatic mapping and sentinel lymphadenectomy for breast cancer. *Ann Surg* 1994; **220**:391–401.

28. Giuliano AE, Sentinel lymphadenectomy in primary breast carcinoma: an alternative to routine dissection. *J Surg Oncol* 1996; **62**:75–7.

29. Nwariaku FE, Euhus DM, Beitsch PD et al, Sentinel lymph node biopsy, an alternative to elective axillary dissection for breast cancer. *Am J Surg* 1998; **176**:529–31.

30. Rubio IT, Korourian S, Cowan C, Krag DN, Colvert M, Klimberg VS, Sentinel lymph node biopsy for staging breast cancer. *Am J Surg* 1998; **176**:532–5.

31. Borgstein P, Pijpers R, Comans EF, vanDiest PJ, Boom RP, Meijer S, Sentinel lymph node biopsy in breast cancer: Guidelines and pitfalls of lymphoscintigraphy and gamma probe detection. *J Am Coll Surg* 1998; **186**:275–83.

32. Giuliano A, Jones R, Brennan M, Statman R, Sentinel lymphadenectomy in breast cancer. *J Clin Oncol* 1997; **15**:2345–50.

33. Veronesi U, Paganelli G, Viale G et al, Sentinel lymph node biopsy and axillary dissection in breast cancer: Results in a large series. *J Natl Cancer Inst* 1999; **91**:368–73.

34. Krag D, Weaver D, Ashikaga T et al, The sentinel node in breast cancer – A multicenter validation study. *N Engl J Med* 1998; **339**:941–6.

35. Miltenburg DM, Miller C, Brunicardi FC, Meta-analysis of sentinel lymph node biopsy in breast cancer. *J Surg Res* 1999; **84**:138–42.

36. International Breast Cancer Study Group, Prognostic importance of occult axillary lymph node micrometastases from breast cancers. *Lancet* 1990; **335**:1565–8.

37. Wilkinson EJ, Hause LL, Hoffman RG et al, Occult axillary lymph node metastases in invasive breast carcinoma: characteristics of the primary tumor and significance of the metastases. *Pathol Ann* 1982; **17**:67–91.

38. Nasser IA, Lee AKC, Bosari S et al, Occult axillary lymph node metastates in 'node-negative' breast carcinoma. *Hum Pathol* 1993; **24**:950–7.

39. Hainsworth PJ, Tjandra JJ, Stillwell RG et al, Detection and significance of occult metastases in node-negative breast cancer. *Br J Surg* 1993; **80**:459–63.

40. McGuckin MA, Cummings MC, Walsh MD et al, Occult axillary node metastases in breast cancer: their detection and prognostic significance. *Br J Cancer* 1996; **73**:88–95.

41. Cserni G, Metastases in axillary sentinel

lymph nodes in breast cancer as detected by intensive histopathological work-up. *J Clin Pathol* 2000; in press.

42. Fisher ER, Palekar A, Rockette H et al, Pathologic findings from the National Surgical Adjuvant Breast Project (protocol no 4). V. Significance of axillary nodal micro and macro metastases. *Cancer* 1978; **42**:2032–8.

43. Huvos AG, Hutter RVP, Berg JW, Significance of axillary macrometastases and micrometastases in mammary cancer. *Ann Surg* 1971; **173**:441–61.

44. Rosen PP, Saigo PE, Braun DW et al, Axillary micro- and macrometastases in breast cancer. *Ann Surg* 1981; **194**:585–91.

45. de Mascarel I, Bonichon F, Coindre JM, Trojani M, Prognostic significance of breast cancer axillary lymph node micrometastases assessed by two special techniques: re-evaluation with longer follow-up. *Br J Cancer* 1992; **66**:523–7.

46. Friedman S, Bertin F, Mouriesse H et al, Importance of tumor cells in axillary sinus margins ('clandestine' metastases) discovered by serial sectioning in operable breast cancer. *Acta Oncol* 1988; **27**:483–7.

47. Hartveit F, Lilleng PK, Breast cancer: two micrometastatic variants in the axilla that differ in prognosis. *Histopathology* 1996; **28**:241–6.

48. Fisher CJ, Boyle S, Burke M, Price AB, Intraoperative assessment of nodal status in the selection of patients with breast cancer for axillary clearance. *Br J Surg* 1993; **80**:457–8.

49. Galimberti V, Zurrida S, Zucali P, Luini A, Can sentinel node biopsy avoid axillary dissection in clinically node-negative breast cancer patients? *Breast* 1998; **7**:8–10.

50. van Diest PJ, Torrenga H, Borgstein PJ et al, Reliability of intraoperative frozen section and imprint cytological investigation of sentinel lymph nodes in breast cancer. *Histopathology* 1999; **35**:14–18.

51. Royal College of Pathologists National Group for Breast Screening, *Pathology Reporting in Breast Cancer Screening*, 2nd edn. NHS BSP Publications No 3, Sheffield, 1995.

52. Cascinelli N, Greco M, Bufalino R et al, Prognosis of breast cancer with axillary node metastases after surgical treatment only. *Eur J Cancer Clin Oncol* 1987; **23**:795–9.

53. Mambo NC, Gallager HS, Carcinoma of the breast. The prognostic significance of extranodal extension of axillary disease. *Cancer* 1977; **39**:2280–5.

54. Fisher ER, Gregorio RM, Redmond C et al, Pathologic findings from the National Surgical Adjuvant Breast Project (protocol no 4). III. The significance of extranodal extension of axillary metastases. *Am J Clin Pathol* 1976; **65**:439–44.

55. Hartveit F, Paranodal tumour in breast cancer: extranodal extension versus vascular spread. *J Pathol* 1984; **144**:253–6.

56. Donegan WL, Stine SB, Samter TG, Implications of extracapsular nodal metastases for treatment and prognosis of breast cancer. *Cancer* 1993; **72**:778–82.

57. Pinder SE, Ellis IO, O'Rourke S et al, Pathological prognostic factors in breast cancer. III. Vascular invasion: relationship with recurrence and survival in a large series with long-term follow-up. *Histopathology* 1994; **24**:41–7.

58. Örbo A, Stalsberg H, Kunde D, Topographic criteria in the diagnosis of tumor emboli in intramammary lymphatics. *Cancer* 1990; **66**:972–7.

59. Davis BW, Gelber R, Goldhirsh A et al, Prognostic significance of peritumoral vessel invasion in clinical trials of adjuvant therapy for breast cancer with axillary node metastases. *Hum Pathol* 1985; **16**:1212–18.

60. Bettelheim R, Penman HG, Thornton-Jones H et al, Prognostic significance of peritumoral vascular invasion in breast cancer. *Br J Cancer* 1984; **50**:771–7.

61. Roses DF, Bell DA, Fotte TJ et al, Pathologic predictors of recurrence in stage 1 (T1N0M0 and T2N0M0) breast cancer. *Am J Clin Pathol* 1982; **78**:817–20.

62. Nime FA, Rosen PP, Thaler HT et al, Prognostic significance of tumour emboli in intramammary lymphatics in patients with mammary carcinoma. *Am J Surg Pathol* 1977; 1:25–30.

63. Nealon TF, Nkongho A, Grossi CE et al, Treatment of early cancer of the breast (T1N0M0 and T2N0M0) on the basis of histologic characteristics. *Surgery* 1981; 89:279–89.

64. Dawson PJ, Karrison T, Ferguson DJ, Histologic features associated with long-term survival in breast cancer. *Hum Pathol* 1986; 17:1015–21.

65. Dawson PJ, Ferguson DJ, Karrison T, The pathologic findings of breast cancer in patients surviving 25 years after radical mastectomy. *Cancer* 1982; 50:2131–8.

66. Sears HF, Janus J, Levy W et al, Breast cancer without axillary metastases. Are there subpopulations? *Cancer* 1982; 50:1820–7.

67. Gilchrist KW, Gould VE, Hirschl S et al, Interobserver variation in the identification of breast carcinoma in intramammary lymphatics. *Hum Pathol* 1982; 13:170–2.

68. Rosen PP, Saigo PE, Brown DW et al, Predictors of recurrence in stage 1 (T1N0M0) breast carcinoma. *Ann Surg* 1981; 193:15–25.

69. O'Rourke S, Galea MH, Euhus D et al, An audit of local recurrence after simple mastectomy. *Br J Surg* 1994; 81:386–9.

70. Greenhough RB, Varying degrees of malignancy in cancer of the breast. *J Cancer Res* 1925; 9:452–63.

71. Patey DH, Scarff RW, The position of histology in the prognosis of carcinoma of the breast. *Lancet* 1928; i:801–4.

72. Bloom HJG, Prognosis in carcinoma of the breast. *Br J Cancer* 1950; 4:259–88.

73. Bloom HJG, Further studies on prognosis of breast carcinoma. *Br J Cancer* 1950; 4:347–67.

74. Bloom HJG, Richardson WW, Histological grading and prognosis in breast cancer. A study of 1409 cases of which 359 have been followed for 15 years. *Br J Cancer* 1957; 11:359–77.

75. Contesso G, Mouriesse H, Friedman S et al, The importance of histologic grade in long-term prognosis of breast cancer: a study of 1010 patients, uniformly treated at the Institut Gustave-Roussy. *J Clin Oncol* 1987; 5:1378–86.

76. Elston CW, Ellis IO, Pathological prognostic factors in breast cancer. I. The value of histological grade in breast cancer: experience from a large study with long-term follow-up. *Histopathology* 1991; 19:403–10.

77. Hartveit F, Prognostic typing in breast cancer. *BMJ* 1971; 4:253–7.

78. Black MM, Barclay THC, Hankey BR, Prognosis in breast cancer utilizing histologic characteristics of the primary tumor. *Cancer* 1975; 36:2048–55.

79. Le Doussal V, Tubiana-Hulin M, Friedman S et al, Prognostic value of histologic grade nuclear components of Scarff Bloom Richardson (SBR). An improved score modification based on a multivariate analysis of 1262 invasive ductal breast carcinomas. *Cancer* 1989; 64:1914–21.

80. Gilchrist KW, Kalish L, Gould VE et al, Interobserver reproducibility of histopathological features in stage II breast cancer. An ECPG study. *Br Cancer Res Treat* 1979; 5:3–10.

81. Fisher ER, Redmond C, Fisher B, Histologic grading of breast cancer. *Pathol Annu* 1980; 15:239–51.

82. Hopton DS, Thorogood T, Clayden AD et al, Observer variation in histological grading of breast cancer. *Eur J Surg Oncol* 1989; 15:21–3.

83. Robbins P, Pinder S, de Klerk N et al, Histological grading of breast carcinomas. A study of interobserver agreement. *Hum Pathol* 1995; 26:873–9.

84. Frierson HF, Wolber RA, Berean KW et al, Interobserver reproducibility of the Nottingham modification of the Bloom and Richardson histological grading scheme for infiltrating ductal carcinoma. *Am J Clin Pathol* 1995; 105:195–8.

85. Dalton LW, Page DL, Dupont WD, Histologic grading of breast carcinoma: a reproducibility study. *Cancer* 1994; **73**:2765–70.

86. National Coordinating Group for Breast Screening Pathology, *Pathology Reporting in Breast Screening Pathology*, 2nd edn. NHSBSP Publications, no 3 1997. Sheffield: HNSBSP.

87. European Commission, *European Guidelines for Quality Assurance in Mammography Screening*, 2nd edn. Luxembourg: Office for Official Publications of the European Communities, 1996.

88. Connolly JL, Fechner RE, Kempson RL et al, Recommendations for the reporting of breast carcinoma. *Hum Pathol* 1996; **27**:220–4.

89. Pinder SE, Murray S, Ellis IO et al, The importance of histological grade in invasive breast carcinoma and response to chemotherapy. *Cancer* 1998; **83**:1529–39.

90. Ellis IO, Galea M, Broughton N et al, Pathological prognostic factors in breast cancer. II. Histological type. Relationship with survival in a large study with long-term follow-up. *Histopathology* 1992; **20**:479–89.

91. Page DL, Anderson TJ, *Diagnostic Histopathology of the Breast*. Edinburgh: Churchill Livingstone, 1987.

92. McDivitt RW, Boyce W, Gersell D, Tubular carcinoma of the breast. *Am J Surg Pathol* 1982; **6**:401–11.

93. Cooper HS, Patchefsky AS, Krall RA, Tubular carcinoma of the breast. *Cancer* 1978; **42**:2334–42.

94. Carstens PHB, Greenberg RA, Francis D, Lyon H, Tubular carcinoma of the breast. A long-term follow-up. *Histopathology* 1985; **9**:271–80.

95. Page DL, Dixon JM, Anderson TJ et al, Invasive cribriform carcinoma of the breast. *Histopathology* 1983; **7**:525–36.

96. Bloom HJC, Richardson WW, Field JR, Host resistance and survival in carcinoma of the breast: a study of 104 cases of medullary carcinoma in a series of 1411 cases of breast cancer followed for 20 years. *BMJ* 1970; **ii**:181–8.

97. Ridolfi RL, Rosen PP, Port A et al, Medullary carcinoma of the breast – a clinicopathologic study with a ten year follow-up. *Cancer* 1977; **40**:1365–85.

98. Lee BJ, Hauser H, Pack GT, Gelatinous carcinoma of the breast. *Surg Gynecol Obstet* 1934; **59**:841–50.

99. Clayton F, Pure mucinous carcinomas of the breast: morphologic features and prognostic correlates. *Hum Pathol* 1986; **17**:34–8.

100. Haagensen CD, Lane N, Lattes R, Bodian C, Lobular neoplasia (so-called lobular carcinoma in situ) of the breast. *Cancer* 1978; **42**:737–67.

101. Fisher ER, Gregorio RM, Redmond C et al, Tubulolobular invasive breast cancer: A variant of lobular invasive cancer. *Hum Pathol* 1977; **8**:679–83.

102. Dixon JM, Page DL, Anderson TJ et al, Long term survivors after breast cancer. *Br J Surg* 1985; **72**:445–8.

103. Anderson TJ, Lamb J, Donnan P et al, Comparative pathology of breast cancer in a randomised trial of screening. *Br J Cancer* 1991; **64**:108–13.

104. Ellis IO, Galea MH, Locker A et al, Early experience in breast cancer screening: Emphasis on development of protocols for triple assessment. *Breast* 1993; **2**:148–53.

105. Pereira H, Pinder SE, Sibbering DM et al, Pathological prognostic factors in breast cancer. IV: Should you be a typer or a grader? A comparative study of two histological prognostic features in operable breast carcinoma. *Histopathology* 1995; **27**:219–26.

106. Lamovec J, Bracko M, Metastatic pattern of infiltrating lobular carcinoma of the breast: an autopsy study. *J Surg Oncol* 1991; **48**:28–33.

107. Harris M, Howell A, Chrissohou M, A comparison of the metastatic pattern of infiltrating lobular carcinoma and infiltrating duct carcinoma of the breast. *Br J Cancer* 1984; **50**:23–30.

108. Domagala W, Markiewski M, Kubiak R et al, Immunohistochemical profile of invasive

lobular carcinoma of the breast: predominantly vimentin and p53 protein negative, cathepsin D and oestrogen receptor positive. *Virchows Arch Pathol Anat Histopathol* 1993; 423:497–502.

109. Breast Cancer Linkage Consortium, Pathology of familial breast cancer: differences between breast cancer in carriers of BRCA1 or BRCA2 mutations and sporadic cases. *Lancet* 1997; 349:1505–10.

110. Marcus JN, Watson P, Page DL et al, Hereditary breast cancer. Pathobiology, prognosis and BRCA1 and BRCA2 gene linkage. *Cancer* 1996; 77:697–709.

111. Lakhani SR, Jacquemier J, Sloane JP et al, Multifactorial analysis of differences between sporadic breast cancers and cancers involving BRCA1 and BRCA2 mutations. *J Natl Cancer Inst* 1998; 90:1138–45.

112. Matsukuma A, Enjoji M, Toyoshima S, Ductal carcinoma of the breast. An analysis of the proportion of intraductal and invasive components. *Pathol Res Prac* 1991; 187:62–7.

113. Silverberg SG, Chitale AR, Assessment of the significance of the proportion of intraductal and infiltrating tumor growth in ductal carcinoma of the breast. *Cancer* 1973; 32:830–7.

114. Van Dongen JA, Fentiman IS, Harris JR et al, In situ breast cancer: the EORTC consensus meeting. *Lancet* 1989; ii:25–7.

115. Schnitt SJ, Connelly JL, Harris JR et al, Pathologic predictors of early local recurrence in stage I and stage II breast cancer treated by primary radiation therapy. *Cancer* 1984; 53:1049–57.

116. Gage I, Schnitt SJ, Nixon AJ et al, Pathologic margin involvement and the risk of recurrence in patients treated with breast-conserving therapy. *Cancer* 1996; 78:1921–8.

117. Parham DM, Hagen N, Brown RA, Morphometric analysis of breast carcinoma: association with survival. *J Clin Pathol* 1988; 41:173–7.

118. Black R, Prescott R, Bers K et al, Tumour cellularity, oestrogen receptors and prognosis in breast cancer. *Clin Oncol* 1983; 9:311–18.

119. Sistrunk WE, MacCarty WC, Life expectancy following radical amputation for carcinoma of the breast – a clinical and pathological study of 218 cases. *Ann Surg* 1922; 75:61–9.

120. Parfrey NA, Doyle CT, Elastosis in benign and malignant breast disease. *Hum Pathol* 1985; 16:674–6.

121. Shivas AA, Douglas JG, The prognostic significance of elastosis in breast carcinoma. *J R Coll Surg Edinb* 1972; 17:315–20.

122. Masters JR, Millis RR, King RJB, Rubens RD, Elastosis and response to endocrine therapy in human breast cancer. *Br J Cancer* 1979; 39:536–9.

123. Robertson AJ, Brown RA, Cree IA et al, Prognostic value of measurement of elastosis in breast carcinoma. *J Clin Pathol* 1981; 34:738–43.

124. Rasmussen BB, Pederson BV, Thorpe SM, Rose C, Elastosis in relation to prognosis in primary breast carcinoma. *Cancer Res* 1985; 45:1428–30.

125. Carter D, Elkins RC, Pipkin RD et al, Relationship of necrosis and tumor border to lymph node metastases and 10 year survival in carcinoma of the breast. *Am J Surg Pathol* 1978; 2:39–46.

126. Clark GM, Do we really need prognostic factors for breast cancer? *Breast Cancer Res Treat* 1994; 30:117–26.

127. Brown JM, Benson EA, Jones M, Confirmation of a long-term prognostic index in breast cancer. *Breast* 1993; 2:144–7.

128. Balslev I, Axelsson CK, Zedelev K et al, The Nottingham Prognostic Index applied to 9,149 patients from the studies of the Danish Breast Cancer Cooperative Group (DBCG). *Breast Cancer Res Treat* 1994; 32:281–90.

129. Beatson JT, Treatment of inoperable cases of carcinoma of the mamma: suggestions for a new method of treatment with illustrative cases. *Lancet* 1896; ii:104–7.

130. King WJ, Greene GL, Monoclonal antibodies localize oestrogen receptor in nuclei of target cells. *Nature* 1984; 307:745–7.

131. McCarty Jr KS, Miller LS, Cox EB et al, Estrogen receptor analyses: Correlation of biochemical and immunohistochemical methods using monoclonal antireceptor antibodies. *Arch Pathol Lab Med* 1985; **109**:716–21.

132. Greene GL, Nolan C, Engler JP et al, Monoclonal antibodies to human estrogen receptor. *Proc Natl Acad Sci USA* 1980; **77**:5115–19.

133. Snead DJR, Bell JA, Dixon AR et al, Methodology of immunohistochemical detection of oestrogen receptor in human breast carcinoma in formalin fixed paraffin embedded tissue: a comparison with frozen section morphology. *Histopathology* 1993; **23**:233–8.

134. Goulding H, Pinder S, Cannon P et al, A new method for the assessment of oestrogen receptor status on routine formalin-fixed tissue samples. *Hum Pathol* 1995; **26**:291–4.

135. Barnes DM, Millis RR, Oestrogen receptors: the history, the relevance and the methods of evaluation. In:. Kirkham N, Lemoine NR, eds. *Progress in Pathology*. Edinburgh: Churchill Livingstone, 1995: 89–114.

136. NIH Consensus Development Conference. Steroid receptors in breast cancer. *Cancer* 1980; **46**:2759–963.

137. Robertson JFR, Bates K, Pearson D et al, Comparison of two oestrogen receptor assays in the prediction of the clinical course of patients with advanced breast cancer. *Br J Cancer* 1992; **65**:727–30.

138. McClelland RA, Berger U, Miller LS et al, Immunocytochemical assay for oestrogen receptor in patients with breast cancer. Relationship to biochemical assay and to outcome of therapy. *J Clin Oncol* 1986; **4**:1171–6.

139. Lovekin C, Ellis IO, Locker A et al, c-erbB-2 oncoprotein expression in primary and advanced breast cancer. *Br J Cancer* 1990; **63**:439–43.

140. Lewis S, Locker A, Todd JH et al, Expression of epidermal growth factor receptor in breast carcinoma. *J Clin Pathol* 1990; **43**:385–9.

141. Ellis IO, Bell J, Todd J et al, Evaluation of immunoreactivity with monoclonal antibody NCRC-II in breast carcinoma. *Br J Cancer* 1987; **56**:295–9.

142. Elston CW. Grading of invasive carcinoma of the breast. In: Page DL, Anderson TJ, eds. *Diagnostic Histopathology of the Breast*. Edinburgh: Churchill Livingstone, 1987: 300–11.

29

Predictive factors in breast cancer

Ann D Thor

Randomized clinical trials have provided important data that allow comparison of chemotherapeutic strategies for adjuvant, neoadjuvant, palliative or preventive treatments. Tissues acquired from patients enrolled on these randomized trials have become an important resource for correlative studies, allowing analysis of tumor markers for prognosis, prediction of therapeutic benefit or molecular epidemiologic studies. Prognostic factors have been defined as 'clinical, pathologic and biologic features of cancer patients and their tumors that forecast clinical outcome'. Predictive factors, in contrast, are 'clinical, pathologic and biologic features that are used to estimate the likelihood of a response to a particular type of adjuvant therapy'.[1] Knowing which therapeutic options to choose for a given patient, in what order and in what combination provide the challenge that drives predictive marker studies. Increased emphasis will be placed on predictive factors as the pathways of tumor biology and chemotherapy responsiveness are better defined and targeted by specific molecular or genetic therapeutics.

Estimates of the magnitude of predictive interactions provide guidance about the relative value of each marker and allow comparability between markers and test systems. As reported in a breast cancer consensus panel overview:[2]

> ...the P value only indicates the strength of evidence against a null hypothesis and is not a measure of the magnitude of treatment effect. Consequently, a factor that appears to distinguish responders from non-responders on the basis of the calculated P values may, in fact, predict a quantitative difference in response that is positive for all sub-populations.

A much better understanding of the relationship of the marker with outcome or treatment response can be acquired when it is tested in the 'presence' of other well-established factors (i.e. multivariate analyses). It is important when this analysis is performed to include the most powerful clinical, histologic and other markers in the model. Failure to do so may cause a new marker to appear important, when in reality it lacks independent value. Testing for treatment interactions often involves the utilization of bivariate factors, which include both the marker and treatment in the statistical analyses of outcomes.

STEROID RECEPTOR ANALYSES

Prognosis
Estrogen and progesterone receptors (ER and PgR) have been routinely determined on surgically

resected primary breast cancers since the late 1970s.[3] Receptor-containing tumors have a better short-term prognosis, although the magnitude of this difference (and hence the prognostic value of ER) is relatively small (8–10% difference in recurrence rate for node-negative patients at 5 years).[4,5] Long-term relapse and survival rates for receptor-positive and receptor-negative tumor patients tend to merge with time.[6–8]

Testing

Steroid receptor analyses generally include determination of both ER and PgR. 'Positive' tumors are generally defined by laboratory testing using ligand-binding or immunohistochemical methods. It is important to note that the definition of positivity (cut-off point, intensity or percentage of positive cells) is often institutionally defined; reporting of the level of expression and method of testing is important for comparability but is often not provided in the test report. Immunohistochemical testing will not be affected by concurrent tamoxifen therapy, whereas falsely low data may result if ligand-binding assays are utilized for these patients. Ligand-binding assays may also generate falsely low data if the tumor : stroma ratio is low. They may give falsely high scores if the tumor : benign epithelial ratio is low; macrodissection may minimize these problems. Immunohistochemical tests are the most widely performed and can use routinely fixed, paraffin-embedded tissues or cytology samples. These are often performed on sections of the primary cancer. Repeat receptor assays on tumor metastases or progressive disease may be useful if there is reason to suspect clonal progression to an ER-negative phenotype. Recent data suggest that, to optimize ER data for prognostic or predictive value, assay cut-off points may vary.[8] Methodologic issues that may affect ER assays are critical, because patients may be denied a powerful and potentially life-saving therapy if a 'negative' result is reported. Methodology issues have been discussed elsewhere in greater detail,[1,8] and a task force convened by the College of American Pathologists has recently issued guidelines for steroid receptor testing.[9]

Prediction

Hormone receptor positivity predicts response to tamoxifen, a commonly utilized anti-breast-cancer therapeutic. Meta-analysis of randomized trials that started before 1990 of adjuvant tamoxifen versus no tamoxifen before recurrence, including 37 000 women from 55 trials (87% of the worldwide evidence) are compelling and provide level I evidence for the predictive value of ER data for response to tamoxifen.[10] Of the 18 000 women with 'ER-positive' tumors and the almost 12 000 women with untested tumors (of which about 8000 should have been ER-positive), the proportional recurrence reductions in mortality as a result of tamoxifen during about 10 years of follow-up for 1, 2 and 5 years were 21% (standard deviation (SD) of 3), 29% (SD 2) and 47% (SD 3), respectively. In the almost 8000 women with low or no ER measured in their primary tumor, the effect of tamoxifen was small (corresponding proportional mortality reductions were 12% (SD 3), 17% (SD 3) and 26% (SD 4), respectively, for 1, 2 and 5 years).[10]

HUMAN erbB-2 (HER2/neu)

The human erbB-2 gene (also known as HER2/neu), located on chromosome 17, encodes a 185-kDa transmembrane protein, ErbB-2, with structural homology to the epidermal growth factor receptor (EGFR). Although encoded by individual genes, ErbB-2, EGFR and two other family members, ErbB-3 and ErbB-4, are highly homologous. Each possesses an extracellular ligand-binding domain (although a selective ligand for ErbB-2 has not yet been identified) and may be altered in breast cancers.

Mechanisms of *erb*B-2 gene amplification and protein overexpression and activation (via phosphorylation) are complex. Amplification is often associated with protein overexpression, which occurs in approximately one-third of invasive and up to two-thirds of in situ carcinomas.

Prognosis

Alterations of *erb*B-2 have been associated with nodal metastases, high histologic grade, steroid receptor negativity, younger patient age and a poorer prognosis in breast cancer patients. Although *erb*B-2 has been used as a marker of poor outcome in breast cancer patients, the value of *erb*B-2 to predict therapeutic response has become the most commonly cited reason for clinical testing.

Testing for *erb*B-2

All normal cells and most breast cancer cells bear two copies of the *erb*B-2 gene and produce low levels of the encoded protein ErbB-2. Assays to evaluate *erb*B-2 generally measure either gene copy number (Southern blot, fluorescence in situ hybridization (FISH) or protein expression (western blot, immunohistochemistry). Abnormal *erb*B-2 can be defined as protein expression at levels above normal cells *or* gene copy number greater than two. Assay systems for *erb*B-2 must be specific (and not recognize homologous proteins or genes), sensitive and discriminatory (to separate abnormal from normal). Laboratory variance in methodology or reagents may increase or decrease the sensitivity, specificity or discrimination of *erb*B-2 testing (no matter what procedure is utilized). False negatives or positives in particular are clinically problematic, because they may result in inappropriate, inadequate or different applications of chemotherapy regimens. Commercially supplied 'kits' to detect *erb*B-2 overexpression (by immunohistochemistry) or gene amplification (by FISH) are avail-

able and have been approved by the US Food and Drug Administration for distinct purposes. Some laboratories continue to use non-kit-based commercial primary reagents for both immunohistochemistry and FISH, and a serum *erb*B-2 test kit is also available. A superior reagent/method has not yet been widely accepted. Intratumoral heterogeneity of *erb*B-2 gene copy number and chromosome 17 centromeric copy number are common.[11] Further methodologic discussion is beyond the scope of this chapter.

USE OF *erb*B-2 AS A PREDICTIVE MARKER IN BREAST CANCER

Molecular and immunohistochemical *erb*B-2 data have now been generated on patient samples from a number of randomized clinical breast cancer trials. Many of these studies were retrospective, and differences in methodology, reliability, validity and incidence have been reported. There are several agents for which *erb*B-2 data have reported predictive value, including doxorubicin (by dose), tamoxifen, methotrexate, Herceptin (discussed elsewhere) and taxanes.

Doxorubicin and *erb*B-2

The first study to report a significant interaction between *erb*B-2 data and response to dose of CAF (cyclophosphamide, doxorubicin and 5-fluorouracil (5-FU)) was a companion study of the Cancer and Leukemia Group B (CALGB) 8541, which evaluated selected cases from nearly 1000 stage II breast cancers randomized to the three-arm trial.[12-14] Patients whose tumors had amplified or overexpressed *erb*B-2 in general had a worse outcome (i.e. *erb*B-2 served as a poor prognostic marker). However, for patients treated with dose-intensive CAF, a significantly better survival was observed in patients with *erb*B-2-altered tumors when compared with those without *erb*B-2 abnormalities.[12,14] This effect appeared linear (continuous), with stronger interactions in patients with a higher percentage of invasive breast cancer cells overexpressing *erb*B-2 or with increasing amounts of the *erb*B-2 gene copy. Unfortunately, for this trial, cases were split for correlative testing by early[12] and late[14] enrollment on to the clinical trial. Statistical analysis of the *erb*B-2 × dose interaction was also affected by failure of randomization to the low-dose arm, and a drift in the population of breast cancer patients who were entered on to the trial over time (from a worse to a better prognosis). Statistical associations were observed in all patients as well as the first subset; however, the second set required statistical correction to make the patient groups comparable on the low-dose arm.[14] Not all were convinced that true level II evidence was at hand on the basis of this study alone.

Interactions between *erb*B-2 and response to CAF or trends that suggest interaction have also been reported in other trials as well, including CALGB 8082,[14] National Surgical Adjuvant Breast and Bowel Project (NSABP) B-15[15] and B-11,[16] and the Intergroup Trial 102.[17] Most importantly, the similarity of magnitude and direction of data in these trials is close, providing level II evidence that the interaction is real.[18] Some important controversies remain, including the best way to test for *erb*B-2 alteration (although the CALGB data suggest that for prediction immunohistochemistry is similar to FISH, which is similar to molecular assays), and whether or not *erb*B-2 data are a surrogate for drug sensitivity or identify only those patients who will benefit from dose intensification. It is unclear, based on the current data, whether or not there is benefit from doxorubicin if a patient's tumor is *erb*B-2-negative; perhaps the chemotherapeutic response is just less.

Methotrexate and *erb*B-2

Breast cancer with altered *erb*B-2 may be less likely to respond to non-doxorubicin, alkylating-agent-based chemotherapies, such as CMF (cyclophosphamide, methotrexate and 5-FU) or PF (melphalan and 5-FU) in the adjuvant setting.[19–21] The International (Ludwig) Breast Cancer Study Group Trial V[20] demonstrated that, for node-positive patients, the effect of prolonged-duration therapy (CMFP) on disease-free survival (DFS) was greater for patients without *erb*B-2 expression compared with those with immunopositivity. For node-negative patients, the effect of perioperative chemotherapy on DFS was greater for patients without *erb*B-2 expression compared with those with *erb*B-2 alterations.[20] A subgroup of patients from the Intergroup Trial 0011 (*n* = 231) treated with CMFP also showed significantly longer DFS if their cancer was *erb*B-2-negative, compared with *erb*B-2-positive cases.[21] These two early level II–III studies suggest that patients with *erb*B-2-negative tumors gain substantially more benefit from CMF than *erb*B-2-positive patients. However, these studies were retrospective in nature and included only a fraction of the entire randomized patient population in the analysis. A more extensive discussion of the statistical limitations can be found in Pegram et al.[15] Three further studies (level of evidence, (LOE) II–III) also support the notion that patients with *erb*B-2-positive tumors may not gain much from CMF-like adjuvant therapies.[22–24] Recent trials, however, fail to support the interaction. Data from the original Milan CMF adjuvant trial do not confirm that *erb*B-2-positive patients will not respond to CMF (LOE II). Those results suggest that patients with *erb*B-2-positive breast cancers may gain more benefit from CMF on a relative scale compared with patients whose tumors are *erb*B-2-negative but, in fact, both subgroups show therapeutic benefit.[25]

In summary, there is conflicting level II–III evidence regarding interactions between *erb*B-2 and response or lack thereof to CMF adjuvant therapy. Given the lack of compelling evidence to use *erb*B-2 data as a marker of resistance to CMF, clinical implementation is not well justified.

Tamoxifen and *erb*B-2

Some reports have suggested resistance of ER-positive, *erb*B-2-positive or EGFR-positive tumor patients to endocrine therapy.[26,27] The first report linking *erb*B-2 and EGFR alterations to tamoxifen resistance was by Nicholson in 1990.[28] This retrospective study included 61 patients who were treated with tamoxifen at the time of first relapse. Of these, only one of the *erb*B-2-positive patients responded to tamoxifen. In a follow-up report of the same cases, the *erb*B-2 expression reduced the response rate of ER-positive patients from 48% to 20%, and that of ER-negative cases from 27% to 0%.[11] Similar data in early and late stage breast cancer patients were also published by Borg et al,[29] who reported that the response to tamoxifen was considerably less in early stage *erb*B-2-positive patients from a cohort of 445. An additional patient group also supported the *erb*B-2/tamoxifen interaction (126 patients with metastatic breast cancer cases, of whom 23 were *erb*B-2 gene-amplified).[29] Each of the above studies was retrospective, included relatively few *erb*B-2-positive cases and was not designed to test the interaction (level III).

The first randomized trial to consider the issue of interactions between the receptor tyrosine kinase receptors (*erb*B-2/EGFR) and response to adjuvant tamoxifen was reported in 1996. Node-negative breast cancer cases from the Gruppo Universitario Napoletano 1 (GUN-1) trial were examined for *erb*B-2 expression to determine interactions between *erb*B-2 and tamoxifen response; 145 cases randomized to receive tamoxifen for 2 years were compared with untreated cases.[30] For *erb*B-2-negative cases, tamoxifen significantly prolonged DFS. For *erb*B-2-positive cases, tamoxifen did not affect DFS and may have been detrimental to overall survival (OS).[30] A recent 20-year follow-up of these patients confirmed the interaction (level II evidence[31]). In a recently reported Swedish study of 312 consecutive primary breast cancers from Uppsala, *erb*B-2 immunopositivity was identified by CB-11 in 19%. For the 47 node-positive patients treated with adjuvant tamoxifen and local radiotherapy, striking differences in the 5-year OS were observed (13% for *erb*B-2-positive and 75% for *erb*B-2-negative), providing level III evidence.[32]

An interaction between *erb*B-2 and tamoxifen has not been observed in some important later trials that compared tumor *erb*B-2 data with tamoxifen response. Data from CALGB 8541, a three-armed trial of dose/dose intensity of CAF in stage II breast cancer patients, described above, demonstrated no level II evidence of interaction between ER positivity and *erb*B-2 (as determined by immunohistochemistry, molecular or FISH methods)[33] (Berry D, personal communication, 1999). Similar but less compelling level II data were reported by Elledge et al,[34] who studied 205 tamoxifen-treated patients with metastatic breast cancer from the Southwest Oncology Group (SWOG) Study 8228. Patient tumors were analyzed for *erb*B-2 expression using antibody Tab 250. Using data based on one scoring system, no differences in response rates, time to failure or OS were observed in the *erb*B-2-positive subgroup. Re-analysis of data from another pathologist using a different scoring system, however, showed a somewhat worse outcome for *erb*B-2-positive cases,[34] making conclusions from these data somewhat difficult. Most recently, data from the NSABP B-14 trial of 2800 node-negative patients randomized to tamoxifen or placebo were evaluated for the erbB-2 interaction. Based on the data from approximately 900 patients, no interaction has yet been observed[35] (Paik S, personal communication, 1999).

In summary, interactions between erbB-2 and response to tamoxifen have been demonstrated by some, but not most, trials in which interactions have been investigated. Methodologic testing issues may, at least in part, contribute to these discrepancies. As noted in a recent review, erbB-2 testing and interaction data are complex, and results may depend to some extent on how positivity for ER and erbB-2 were defined and by which methods/reagents erbB-2 was analyzed.[15]

Taxanes and erbB-2

Clinical and preclinical level II–IV data regarding interactions between paclitaxel and erbB-2 overexpression/amplification have been contradictory and controversial,[36–38] and, therefore, clinical testing of erbB-2 before taxane use is not indicated at this time.

CONCLUSIONS

Steroid hormone receptors (ER and PgR) should be considered positive predictive markers of response (category A) to hormonal therapies based on level I evidence from large meta-analyses. Alterations of erbB-2 (HER2/neu) (including gene amplification and increased protein expression) provide negative prognostic data and appear to predict a positive response to dose-intensive, doxorubicin-containing, chemotherapeutic regimens based on level II (category B) evidence from several recent trials. Meta-analyses have not yet been performed. There is continued controversy over interactions between erbB-2 and response to tamoxifen. Although ER and erbB-2 receptors tend to be inversely expressed, co-expression does occur,

and in those cases some studies suggest less, if any, response to tamoxifen. Levels of expression may be important, but have not been well considered in studies to date. Interactions between erbB-2 and CMF are less compelling, because recent trials have not supported a significant interaction. Interactions between erbB-2 and taxanes are the least certain, and will need to be defined in further randomized clinical trials. In summary, only steroid receptors and erbB-2 appear to be useful predictive markers in breast cancer at this time.

REFERENCES

1. Allred DC, Harvey JM, Bernardo M, Clark GM, Prognostic and predictive factors in breast cancer by immunohistochemical analysis. *Mod Pathol* 1998; **11**:155–68.
2. Goldhirsch A, Wood WC, Senn H-J, Glick JH, Gelber RD, Meeting highlights: International Consensus Panel on the Treatment of Primary Breast Cancer. *J Natl Cancer Inst* 1995; **87**: 1441–5.
3. Jordan VC, *Tamoxifen: A Guide for Clinicians and Patients*. Huntington, NY: PRR Publishers, 1996.
4. Clark GM, Prognostic and predictive factors. In: Harris JR, Hellman S, Lippman M, Morrow M, eds. *Diseases of the Breast*. Philadelphia: Lippincott-Raven, 1996: 461–85.
5. Clark GM, McGuire WL, Steroid receptors and other prognostic factors in primary breast cancer. *Semin Oncol* 1988; **15**:20.
6. Hirshaut Y, Pressman P, *Breast Cancer: The Complete Guide*. New York: Bantam, 1996.
7. Early Breast Cancer Trialists' Collaborative Group, I. Systematic treatment of early breast cancer by hormonal, cytotoxic, or immune therapy: 133 randomised trials involving 31,000 recurrences and 24,000 deaths among 75,000 women. *Lancet* 1992; **339**:1–15, 71–85.
8. Elias JM, Masood S, Estrogen receptor assay: Are we all doing it the same way? A survey. *J Histotechnol* 1995; **18**:95–6.

9. Fitzgibbons PL, Page DL, Weaver D et al, Prognostic factors in breast cancer, College of American Pathologists Consensus Statement 1999. *Arch Pathol Lab Med* 2000; in press.

10. Early Breast Cancer Trialists' Collaborative Group, Tamoxifen for early breast cancer: An overview of the randomized trials. *Lancet* 1998; **351**:1451–67.

11. Wright C, Nicholson S, Angus B et al, Relationship between c-erbB-2 protein product expression and response to endocrine therapy in advanced breast cancer. *Br J Cancer* 1992; **65**:118–21.

12. Muss HB, Thor AD, Berry DA et al, c-erbB-2 expression and response to adjuvant therapy in women with node-positive early breast cancer. *N Engl J Med* 1994; **330**:1260–6.

13. Thor AD, Budman DR, Berry DA et al, Selecting patients for higher dose adjuvant CAF: c-erbB-2, p53, dose and dose intensity in Stage II, node positive breast cancer. *Proc Am Soc Clin Oncol* 1997; **16**:128a.

14. Thor AD, Berry DA, Budman DR et al, ErbB-2, p53 and efficacy of adjuvant therapy in lymph node-positive breast cancer. *J Natl Cancer Inst* 1998; **90**:1346–60.

15. Pegram MD, Konecny G, Slamon DJ, Use of HER2 for predicting response to breast cancer therapy. In: Harris JR, Lippman ME, eds. *Diseases of the Breast Updates*. New Jersey: Lippincott Williams & Wilkins Healthcare, 1999: Vol 3, No. 3, 1–9.

16. Paik S, Bryant J, Park C et al, erbB-2 and response to doxorubicin in patients with axillary lymph node-positive, hormone receptor-negative breast cancer. *J Natl Cancer Inst* 1998; **90**:1361–70.

17. Ravdin PM, Green S, Albain KS et al, Initial report of the SWOG Biological Correlative Study of c-erbB-2 expression as a predictor of outcome in a trial comparing adjuvant CAF T with tamoxifen (T) alone. *Proc Am Soc Clin Oncol* 1998; **17**:97a.

18 Clark GM, Should selection of adjuvant chemotherapy for patients with breast cancer be based on erbB-2 status? [Editorial] *J Natl Cancer Inst* 1998; **90**:1320–1.

19. Ravdin PM, Chamness GC, The c-erbB-2 proto-oncogene as a prognostic and predictive marker in breast cancer: A paradigm for the development of other macromolecular markers – A review. *Gene* 1995; **159**:19–27.

20. Gusterson BA, Gelber RD, Goldhirsch A et al, Prognostic importance of c-erbB-2 expression in breast cancer. *J Clin Oncol* 1992; **10**:1049–56.

21. Allred DC, Clark GM, Tandon AK et al, HER-2/neu in node-negative breast cancer: prognostic significance of overexpression influenced by the presence of in situ carcinoma. *J Clin Oncol* 1992; **10**:599–605.

22. Tetu B, Brisson J, Prognostic significance of HER-2/neu oncoprotein expression in node-positive breast cancer. The influence of the pattern of immunostaining and adjuvant therapy. *Cancer* 1994; **73**:2359–65.

23. Giai M, Roagna R, Ponzone R et al, Prognostic and predictive relevance of c-erbB-2 and ras expression in node positive and negative breast cancer. *Anticancer Res* 1994; **14**:1441–50.

24. Stal O, Sullivan S, Wingren S et al, c-erbB-2 expression and benefit from adjuvant chemotherapy and radiotherapy of breast cancer. *Eur J Cancer* 1995; **31A**:2185–90.

25. Menard S, Valagusa P, Pilotti S et al, Benefit of CMF treatment in lymph node-positive breast cancer overexpressing HER-2. *Proc Am Soc Clin Oncol* 1999; **18**:69a.

26. Leitzel K, Teramoto Y, Konrad D et al, Elevated serum c-erbB-2 antigen levels and decreased response to hormone therapy of breast cancer. *J Clin Oncol* 1995; **13**:1129–35.

27. Benz CC, Scott GK, Sarup JC et al, Estrogen-dependent, tamoxifen-resistant tumorigenic growth of MCF-7 cells transfected with HER2/neu. *Breast Cancer Res Treat* 1993; **24**:85–95.

28. Nicholson S, Wright C, Sainsbury JR et al, Epidermal growth factor receptor (EGFR) as a

marker for poor prognosis in node-negative breast cancer patients: neu and tamoxifen failure. *J Steroid Biochem Mol Biol* 1990; 37:811–14.

29. Borg A, Baldetorp B, Ferno M et al, ErbB-2 amplification is associated with tamoxifen resistance in steroid-receptor positive breast cancer. *Cancer Lett* 1994; **81**:137–44.

30. Carlolomagno C, Perrone F, Gallo C et al, c-erbB-2 overexpression decreases the benefit of adjuvant tamoxifen in early-stage breast cancer without axillary lymph node metastases. *J Clin Oncol* 1996; **14**:2702–8.

31. Biano AR, DeLaurentiis M, Carlomagno C et al, 20 year update of the Naples GUN Trial of Adjuvant Breast Cancer Therapy: Evidence of interaction between c-erbB-2 expression and tamoxifen efficacy. *Proc Am Soc Clin Oncol* 1998; **17**:373.

32. Sjogren S, Inganas M, Lindgren A et al, Prognostic and predictive value of c-erbB-2 overexpression in primary breast cancer, alone and in combination with other prognostic markers. *J Clin Oncol* 1998; **16**:462–9.

33. Muss H, Berry D, Thor A et al, Lack of interaction of tamoxifen use and erbB-2/HER-2/neu expression in CALGB 8541: A randomized adjuvant trial of three different doses of cyclophosphamide, doxorubicin and fluorouracil (CAF) in node-positive primary breast cancer. *Proc Am Soc Clin Oncol* 1999; **18**:68a.

34. Elledge RM, Green S, Ciocca D et al, HER-2 expression and response to tamoxifen in estrogen receptor-positive breast cancer: A Southwest Oncology Group Study. *Clin Cancer Res* 1998; **4**:7–12.

35. Nelson NJ, Can HER2 status predict response to cancer therapy? *J Natl Cancer Inst* 2000; **92**:366–7.

36. Baselga J, Seidman AD, Rosen PP, Norton L, HER2 overexpression and paclitaxel sensitivity in breast cancer: therapeutic implications. *Oncology* 1997; **11**:43–8.

37. Seidman A, Baselga J, Yao T-J et al, HER-2/neu over-expression and clinical taxane sensitivity: A multivariate analysis in patients with metastatic breast cancer. *Proc Am Soc Clin Oncol* 1996; **15**:104a.

38. Gianni L, Capri G, Mezzelani A et al, HER-2/neu amplification and response to doxorubicin/paclitaxel (AT) in women with metastatic breast cancer. *Proc Am Soc Clin Oncol* 1997; **16**:139a.

PART III
Integration of New Therapies into Breast Cancer Management

SECTION 9: Special Issues in Metastatic Breast Cancer

Metastatic breast cancer is usually treated with hormonal therapy, chemotherapy or both in sequence. Nowadays, patients who are positive for ErbB-2 have, in addition, the option for trastuzumab, which after hormonal treatments, is the newest gene-based directed therapy. More gene therapies are being tested and will be used routinely in the coming years. Of course many patients also need radiation treatment, especially for bone disease and for emergencies such as spinal cord compression. In addition, we are increasingly using drugs such as bisphosphonates and other supportive therapy, such as the cytokines, to mitigate the side effects either of therapy or of the disease process itself.

These therapies are covered in Part II, where the authors have discussed in detail the most recently available treatments. This section does not recapitulate all these data, but focuses on two important issues – care of the elderly patient and quality of life.

30
Breast cancer in elderly patients

Matti S Aapro

The ageing population in most areas in the world means that we are facing an increasing problem, termed a 'time-bomb' in an editorial a few years ago (http://www.who.org/ageing/overview.html).[1] One-third of all breast cancers occur in women aged over 70, who have often been excluded from breast cancer trials. Although justified by many bad reasons, such an exclusion is difficult to understand, because women aged 70 have a median life expectancy of 15.5 years, i.e. half of them will live much longer. Older and younger women with operable breast cancer have a similar prognosis, but older women are more likely to have metastatic disease at diagnosis, and to die from intercurrent disease.[2] In a study evaluating 9228 patients, of whom 2919 were aged 65 and over, Clark demonstrated that elderly women have a higher frequency of hormone receptor-positive tumors (84% estrogen receptor [ER]-positive vs 67% in younger patients). In another study, 58% (compared with 50%) were diagnosed with node-negative disease, although 20% had tumors larger than 5 cm, vs 13% in those aged under 65.[3] This illustrates that elderly patients may have a different biology of disease when compared with younger women. It is therefore crucial for us to undertake studies in this population of patients.

MAMMOGRAPHY SCREENING IN ELDERLY WOMEN

In spite of some recent controversy,[4] mammography screening is a most efficient early detection method for breast cancer. The efficacy of mammography is well established for women between the ages of 50 and 69 years, but very little information exists about the value of mammography in women older than 70 years. In 1991, a Forum on Breast Cancer Screening in Older Women, sponsored by the National Institute of Cancer (NCI),[5] concluded in favor of breast cancer screening in elderly women. Although there is no direct evidence about breast cancer screening efficacy in women aged over 65, several important factors supported its extension to elderly women: rising incidence until the eighth decade; breast changes with age from a prevalent glandular pattern to a fatty pattern, which is easier to interpret with mammography; and fewer non-cancerous causes of abnormal mammograms in older women.

In an effort to validate the use of screening mammography in elderly women, a decision analysis and cost-effectiveness analysis using a Markov model have recently been presented. The analysis compared three strategies: (1) biennial mammography from age 65 to 69 years; (2) biennial mammography from age 65 to 69 years, with measurement of distal radial bone mineral density (BMD) at 65 years, discontinuing screening at 69 years in women in the lowest BMD quartile for age, and continuing biennial mammography to 79 years in those in the top three quartiles of distal radius BMD; and (3) biennial mammography from age 65 to 79 years. This analysis suggested that continuing mammography screening after the age of 69 results in a small gain in life expectancy and is moderately cost-effective in those with high BMD and more costly in those with low BMD.[6] A cost–utility analysis has been conducted using a computer model that simulated the demography, epidemiology and natural history of breast carcinoma, to estimate expected life-years gained, extra incidence, extra life-years with disease, and costs incurred by different breast carcinoma screening programs in the general population. The results suggested that a 3-year interval could be justified in elderly women.[7] Finally, another evaluation has suggested that extending breast cancer screening to the age of 74 would be more effective than cervical screening at any age.[8]

PATIENT EVALUATION

The number of coexisting illnesses increases with advancing age and these co-morbid conditions have an influence on treatment in individual patients.[9] The correct assessment of a cancer patient is a key step in the treatment process. In elderly patients with breast cancer, this assessment entails not only the patient's basic medical history and standard cancer staging, but also a much more comprehensive evaluation of the various facets of the patient's health and environment. Patient fitness for elective surgery, radiation therapy and chemotherapy has to be considered using scientifically validated methods.

Operative risk assessment

Although operating on elderly, and even very elderly, patients for orthopaedic or cardiovascular diseases is increasingly accepted, there is continued reluctance to recommend adequate interventions for breast cancer. Careful evaluation of renal and cardiorespiratory function is essential and will lead to adapted drug doses and specific types of anesthesia and pre- and post-operative care.[10] Although acute surgery remains a major cause of perioperative death in elderly people, elective operations are a well-controlled procedure, with costs similar to those for younger patients.[11] Older women tolerate breast surgery well,[12] but may have operative mortality rates of between 1% and 2%.[13,14]

Radiation therapy

Older women also tolerate breast radiation[15,16] and should be offered the option of breast preservation because body image and loss are important issues regardless of age. A possible problem for the elderly patient treated with radiotherapy is the need, five times a week, to be in a radiotherapy center under conditions necessary for treatment, such as immobilization or adopting a supine position for prolonged periods. Patient transportation often depends on family or partner support, community support or the availability of public transportation, and immobilization may be difficult for many elderly patients. In one study in women aged 70, who were given the choice of breast conservation or mastectomy, more women chose breast conservation.[17]

Chemotherapy

Tolerance of chemotherapy varies among patients, and co-morbidity and decreased bodily functions complicate the issue in elderly people. Recent studies have, however, shown that elderly people who are carefully screened for any possible disease have less function loss than reported traditionally.[18] Changes in renal and hepatic function, as well as modifications of lean body mass and bone marrow reserves are important to consider when chemotherapy is contemplated. It is recommended that calculation is made of the actual creatinine clearance in a particular patient using, for example, the formula of Cockroft and Gault,[19] which is more reliable in this population than an evaluation based on standard 24-hour

urine collections. Hepatic function is modified in several aspects by aging: decreased blood flow, decreased albumin production and decreased cytochrome P450 function.[20,21] Another factor to be considered is that elderly people often use several non-oncological drugs concomitantly. This polypharmacy may lead to changes in cytochrome P450 function and unpredictably affect the metabolism of cytotoxic agents such as oxazaphosphorines (cyclophosphamide, ifosfamide). Finally, the neurotoxicity of vinca alkaloids, taxoids and platinum derivatives means that an elderly person may be considerably handicapped by the loss of peripheral sensitivity, as well as by what may prove to be clinically significant hearing loss.[22]

ASSESSING CO-FACTORS

A multidimensional assessment is a key part of the approach to older cancer patients. Co-morbidity, functional status, depression, cognitive impairment, nutritional status and insufficient social support have all been demonstrated to affect survival of elderly and/or cancer patients, with relative risks of death often in the two to four times range, with an even higher figure for co-morbidity.[23]

Several well-defined and validated scales for measuring co-morbidity (Charlson, Cumulative Illness Rating Scale – Global (CIRS-G)) have been shown to correlate with outcomes such as mortality, hospitalization duration or disability in various populations outside geriatric oncology.[23,24] The Charlson scale focuses on a short list of selected diseases, and is aimed at simplicity. It is based on the 1-year mortality of patients admitted to a medical hospital service. The CIRS-G is aimed at comprehensiveness, and allows rating of all diseases encountered. The CIRS-G has a structure analogous to the WHO or the NCI toxicity scales, well known to medical and radiation oncologists. This scale classifies co-morbidities into 14 organ systems, and grades each condition from 0 (no problem) to 4 (severely incapacitating or life-threatening condition). Scores may be summarized in different ways, with comparable results. The scale encompasses both potentially lethal and non-lethal co-morbid conditions.

TAMOXIFEN OR AROMATASE INHIBITORS AS PRIMARY TREATMENT

Early studies suggested that tamoxifen as the sole treatment was effective in elderly patients with breast cancer, with response rates in an unselected population being as high as 73%. Further follow-up has shown that tamoxifen alone does not provide long-term local control of disease in two-thirds of patients.[25] Two major published randomized trials have examined the effect of surgery in addition to tamoxifen.[26,27] In the Cancer Research Campaign (CRC) trial, surgery was necessary in 35 patients treated with tamoxifen alone compared with 15 ($p = 0.001$) local recurrences in patients receiving tamoxifen combined with surgery.[26] Similar data were reported in the other trial. These studies did not select patients on the basis of ERs. Much higher response and long-term local control rates are reported if patients are selected on the basis of ERs.[28] Survival data in the combined analysis of the GRETA (Group for Research on Endocrine Therapy in the Elderly) and CRC studies[29] as well as in the unpublished European Organization for Research and Treatment of Cancer (EORTC) 10891 and 10892 studies show that surgery is an important factor and reduces the hazard ratio to 0.66.

Studies with tamoxifen or aromatase inhibitors have shown that, in ER-positive patients, between 75% and 92%[30,31] respond to neoadjuvant endocrine therapy. After such treatment, breast cancers can be reduced in volume over a 3-month period to a size at which breast conservation is possible. Patients who do not respond to endocrine treatments within the first 3 months should be considered for non-conservative surgery.

ADJUVANT THERAPY

The 1998 Overview has shown the benefits of adjuvant tamoxifen therapy in women aged 70 years or older,[32] and this benefit seems restricted to ER-positive patients. The proportional reductions in breast cancer relapse and mortality are similar for women with node-negative and those with node-positive disease. Unfortunately, the adjuvant chemotherapy trials[33] included only 600 women aged 70 years or older and the sample size was insufficient to determine the benefits of chemotherapy at this age. However, the proportional benefits of chemotherapy in patients aged over 70 without major co-morbidity are unlikely to be significantly different from those in women aged 50–60 years. In postmenopausal women the proportional risk reductions after mainly CMF (cyclophosphamide, methotrexate, 5-fluoro-uracil)-like chemotherapy were 20% for recurrence and 11% for overall mortality rates. The 1998 St Gallen consensus suggested that adjuvant hormonal therapy with tamoxifen should be considered for all postmenopausal women with hormone receptor-positive tumors. Only older women with a very low risk of distant metastases (<10%) or severe co-morbid conditions should not be offered tamoxifen.[34] The consensus suggested that adjuvant systemic chemotherapy could be considered for ER-negative elderly women who are fit and whose risk of systemic relapse is high.

METASTATIC DISEASE

Endocrine therapy is the standard primary treatment for women with hormone receptor-positive metastatic disease. Hormone treatment can be considered in elderly patients with hormone receptor-negative, slowly progressive or non-life-threatening, metastatic breast cancer. The use of chemotherapy in elderly patients with metastatic breast cancer should be considered for patients with symptomatic disease who have progression on endocrine therapy or are truly ER zero.

All the potential benefits and caveats discussed above for chemotherapy would be expected to apply in elderly patients with metastatic disease. In addition, quality-of-life issues may be different in this population than in younger women. Issues surrounding benefits and risks of aggressive treatment need to be discussed openly with these patients as they are for younger women. As such a large proportion of our patients are currently aged over 70 years, we should be entering these patients on to relevant clinical trials. In this way we will gather information on the most appropriate treatment strategies for this growing population of individuals.

REFERENCES

1. Boyle P, Trends in cancer mortality in Europe. *Eur J Cancer* 1992; **28**:7–8.
2. Castiglione M, Gelber RD, Goldhirsch A, Adjuvant systemic therapy for breast cancer in the elderly: competing causes of mortality. International Breast Cancer Study Group. *J Clin Oncol* 1990; **8**:519–26.
3. Clark GM, The biology of breast cancer in older women. *J Gerontol* 1992; **47**:19–23.
4. Gotzsche PC, Olsen O, Is screening for breast cancer with mammography justifiable? *Lancet* 2000; **355**:129–34.
5. Costanza ME, Breast cancer screening in older women. Synopsis of a Forum. *Cancer* 1992; **69**:1925–31.
6. Kerlikowske K, Salzmann P, Phillips KA et al, Continuing screening mammography in women aged 70 to 79 years: impact on life expectancy and cost-effectiveness. *JAMA* 1999; **282**:2156–63.
7. Boer R, de Koning HJ, van der Maas PJ, A longer breast carcinoma screening interval for women age older than 65 years? *Cancer* 1999; **86**:1506–10.
8. Law MR, Morris JK, Wald NJ, The importance of age in screening for cancer. *J Med Screen* 1999; **6**:16–20.
9. Extermann M, Aapro M, Assessment of the older cancer patient. *Hematol Oncol Clin North Am* 2000; **14**:63–77.
10. Yeager M, Glass D, Neff R, Brinck-Johnsen T, Epidural anesthesia and analgesia in high-risk surgical patients. *Anesthesiology* 1987; **66**:729–36.
11. Audisio RA, Cazzaniga M, Robertson C, Veronesi P, Andreoni B, Aapro MS, Elective surgery for colorectal cancer in the aged: a clinical–economical evaluation. *Br J Cancer* 1997; **76**:382–4.
12. Wazer DE, Erban JK, Robert NJ et al, Breast conservation in elderly women for clinically negative axillary lymph nodes without axillary dissection. *Cancer* 1994; **74**:878–83.
13. Amsterdam E, Birkenfeld S, Gilad A, Krispin M, Surgery for carcinoma of the breast in women over 70 years of age. *J Surg Oncol* 1987; **35**:180–5.
14. Svastics E, Sulyok Z, Besznyak I, Treatment of breast cancer in women older than 70 years of age. *J Surg Oncol* 1989; **41**:19–24.
15. Lindsey AM, Larson PJ, Dodd MJ, Brecht ML, Packer A, Comorbidity, nutritional intake, social support, weight and functional status over time on older cancer patients receiving radiotherapy. *Cancer Nurs* 1994; **17**:113–19.
16. Wyckoff J, Greenberg H, Sanderson R, Wallach P, Balducci L, Breast irradiation in the older women: a toxicity study. *J Am Geriatr Soc* 1994; **42**:150–6.
17. Sandison AJ, Gold DM, Wright P, Jones PA, Breast conservation or mastectomy: treatment choice of women aged 70 years and older. *Br J Surg* 1996; **83**:994–6.

18. Lindeman RD, Tobin JD, Shock NW, Longitudinal studies on the rate of decline in renal function with age. *J Am Geriatr Soc* 1985; **33**:278–85.

19. Cockroft DW, Gault MH, Prediction of creatinine clearance from serum creatinine. *Nephron* 1976; **16**:31–41.

20. Russell RM, Changes in gastrointestinal function attributed to aging. *Am J Clin Nutr* 1992; **55**:1203–7.

21. Durnas C, Loi C, Cusack BJ, Hepatic drug metabolism and aging. *Clin Pharmacokin* 1990; **17**:236–63.

22. Hussain M, Neurotoxicity of antineoplastic agents. *Crit Rev Oncol Hematol* 1993; **14**:61–75.

23. Extermann M, Overcash J, Lyman GH, Parr J, Balducci L, Comorbidity and functional status are independent in older cancer patients. *J Clin Oncol* 1998; **16**:1582–7.

24. Extermann M, Measurement and impact of comorbidity in older cancer patients. *Crit Rev Oncol Hematol* 2000; in press.

25. Horobin JM, Preece PE, Dewar JA, Wood RAB, Cuschieri A, Long-term follow up of elderly patients with loco-regional breast cancer treated with tamoxifen only. *Br J Surg* 1991; **78**:213–17.

26. Bates T, Riley DL, Houghton J, Fallowfield L, Baum M, Breast cancer in elderly women: a Cancer Research Campaign trial comparing treatment with tamoxifen and optimal surgery with tamoxifen alone. The Elderly Breast Cancer Working Party. *Br J Surg* 1991; **78**:591–7.

27. Mustacchi G, Milani S, Plunchinotta A, De Matteis A, Rubagotti A, Perrota A, Tamoxifen or surgery plus tamoxifen as primary treatment for elderly patients with operable breast cancer: the G.R.E.T.A. trial. Group for Research on Endocrine Therapy in the Elderly. *Anticancer Res* 1994; **14**:2197–200.

28. Gaskell DJ, Hawkins RA, Sangster K, Chetty U, Forrest APM, Relation between immunocytochemical estimate of estrogen receptor in elderly patients with primary breast cancer in response to tamoxifen. *Lancet* 1989; **i**: 2197–203.

29. Mustacchi G, Latteier J, Milani S, Bates T, Houghton J, Tamoxifen versus surgery plus tamoxifen as primary treatment for elderly patients with breast cancer. Combined data from the GRETA and CRC trials. *Proc Am Soc Clin Oncol* 1998; **17**:383.

30. Keen JC, Dixon JM, Miller EP et al, The expression of Ki-S1 and BCL-2 and the response to primary tamoxifen therapy in elderly patients with breast cancer. *Breast Cancer Res Treat* 1997; **44**:123–33.

31. Dixon JM, Love CDB, Tucker S et al, Letrozole as primary medical therapy for locally advanced and large operable breast cancer. *Breast Cancer Res Treat* 1997; **46**(suppl):54.

32. Anonymous, Tamoxifen for early breast cancer: an overview of the randomised trials. Early Breast Cancer Trialists' Collaborative Group. *Lancet* 1998; **351**:1451–7.

33. Anonymous, Polychemotherapy for early breast cancer: an overview of the randomised trials. Early Breast Cancer Trialists' Collaborative Group. *Lancet* 1998; **352**:930–49.

34. Goldhirsch A, Glick JH, Gelber RD, Senn H-J, Meeting highlights: International Consensus Panel on the treatment of primary breast cancer. *J Natl Cancer Inst* 1998; **90**:1601–4.

31

Quality of life data interpretation: Key issues in advanced breast cancer

Andrew Bottomley

INTRODUCTION

Health-related quality of life (HRQOL), a multi-dimensional construct, is generally regarded as encompassing clinical subjective perceptions of positive and negative aspects of cancer patient domains, including physical, emotional, social and cognitive functions, and, importantly, disease symptoms and treatment.[1]

Some 20 years ago, scant literature reporting quality of life in cancer research existed. However, over recent years, a significant increase has been noted in studies reporting the assessment of HRQOL in peer-reviewed publications. A recent review of the published literature indicates that the number of HRQOL studies supports this substantial increase. Further, at present some 10% of all randomized cancer clinical trials include HRQOL as a main endpoint.[2]

However, introducing HRQOL into the medical arena has not been without numerous difficulties. There are several conceptual, methodological, practical, and attitudinal explanations for the challenges that have faced HRQOL researchers.[3–5] Today, many of these are being slowly overcome.[6,7] While researchers are increasingly faced with situations where patients may not gain benefits in terms of traditional end-points, such as survival or disease-free survival, it is possible to see significant changes in HRQOL.[8]

While there is a greater use of HRQOL in clinical trials, clinicians remain faced with challenges. In particular, these challenges can limit HRQOL study integration and can influence results. Realizing the subjective nature of HRQOL studies generates barriers to acceptance by clinicians.[8] Further, as Moinpour[9] points out, the high number of and unfamiliarity with HRQOL measures available presents a serious challenge to clinicians' awareness of interpretation, and subsequent understanding of the conclusions.

The purpose of this chapter is to aid clinicians in the interpretation of HRQOL data from reported studies in advanced breast cancer. This is particularly important because the treatment of advanced breast cancer remains mainly palliative, and, while it is possible to see high response rates and sometimes modest increases in survival, these can be associated with treatment-related toxicity.[10,11] However, unlike early breast cancer, where a significant number of HRQOL studies have been published,[12–15] in advanced breast cancer, Carlson[16] and Overmoyer[17] suggest that only a limited number of studies are available. Fossati et al[18] confirmed this when they reported the results of a systematic review of published literature on medical interventions used in the treatment of advanced breast cancer. Between 1975 and 1997, a total of 189 studies were identified, treating 31 510 patients. However, only 9% (2995) of these patients were reported to have been involved in any quality of life assessment. Perhaps this low figure represents the difficulty when dealing with a population where treatment is mainly palliative and thus studies can be fraught with difficulties in design and implementation.

DESIGN AND ANALYSIS INFLUENCES ON HRQOL DATA INTERPRETATION

Analysis of HRQOL data is difficult, and represents a significant challenge to researchers.[19] If researchers are to report on evidence-based studies, it is essential when producing (or reviewing) the results that attention be given to matters of appropriate design and analysis. It is essential to determine that certain precautions have been taken to ensure a well-designed trial.

One key issue that is frequently raised concerns the appropriateness of measures used. In many cases, if well-validated instruments have not been used in the correct manner, for example, appropriate populations, timing, and place of assessment, there is already an issue of concern regarding appropriate interpretation.[19] If the HRQOL instrument is not well known, it needs to be examined in detail to ensure that its psychometric properties of reliability and validity are suitable before any useful interpretation of the results can be made. Kong and Gandhi[20] note that, of 265 articles reviewed reporting the assessment of HRQOL in clinical trials, only 23% provided reliability data, and only 21% provided validity data. Unfortunately, many of the studies in advanced breast cancer have not published such data, including those by Bernhard et al[21] and Seidman et al.[22]

Given the multidimensional nature of HRQOL data, it is important that researchers provide information on all measures used, including the domain investigated, even if not significant. One early study conducted by Priestman and Baum[23] serves as an example of problems of not using robust measures and failing to include the data on the psychometric properties of the measures. In this study, the researchers examined 29 women undergoing two different chemotherapy regimes, assessed using a linear analogue self-assessment (LASA) technique. This method simply required patients to mark, on a line, a point that most accurately describes their symptoms or views, ranging from the best (e.g. no pain) to the worst (e.g. extremely severe pain). While this type of assessment can be valuable, Priestman and Baum apparently self-selected the questions for the LASA (e.g. feelings of well-being, mood, anxiety, appetite, social activities) without any explicit rationale. This can have serious implications for interpretation of the results: as the researchers could have been assessing certain aspects of HRQOL that they believe to be important, it is also possible that other issues that patients believe to be important (e.g. spirituality, social support. symptoms such as hair loss) might not be assessed.[24,25] If we are to ensure evidence-based practice in HRQOL studies, researchers should ensure that they provide as much detail as possible regarding the development of the measures to avoid such criticisms.

Fayers et al[26] suggest that HRQOL data analysis can be classified into two broad categories: confirmatory and descriptive/exploratory. If confirmatory data analysis is used, then specifically defined questions are asked to test the statistical significance differences as specified in the protocol. One key issue is the selection of the pre-trial hypotheses. This proposes the key HRQOL domains to be investigated, to avoid the problem of significant results from multiple significance testing.[27]

However, several studies of advanced breast cancer have not followed this approach. One example is the Seidman et al[22] phase II study, where 30 metastatic breast cancer patients underwent quality of life evaluation with no rationale for selecting which quality of life domains were presented. Tannock et al[28] investigated the effects of two dose levels (high and low) of CMF in a sample of 133 metastatic breast cancer patients. Only a subset of 49 patients completed a LASA 34 item scale, since compliance was limited by the 'availability of personnel to monitor completion of the quality of life measures'. In addition, an unspecified number of patients completed the Profile of Mood States. While it is clearly very difficult to make any interpretation based on such methodological limitations, it is surprising to see no prior HRQOL hypothesis in such a study.

Similarly, Bishop et al[29] report the results of a study with metastatic breast cancer patients where 209 patients were randomized to receive either intravenous paclitaxel or standard cyclophosphamide. HRQOL results were presented after analyzing data from the QOL Linear Analogue Scale and by clinicians using the Spitzer QOL Index.[30] While overall no significant differences were seen on any of the domains of physical well-being, mood, pain, nausea, appetite, overall QOL, or physical-related QOL, the authors conclude that, 'with the exception of pain, patients on the paclitaxel arm experienced slightly better QOL for each parameter during treatment than patients on the CMFP arm'. Because the researchers proposed no prior hypothesis it is clearly problematic to undertake repeated analysis without a clear idea of the influence on which HRQOL domain one is looking for.

However, failure to state a prior hypothesis is not always the case. Some researchers demonstrate clarity. Bernhard et al[31] compared breast cancer patients who underwent two second-line endocrine treatments. Patients were randomized into formestane and megestrol acetate groups. Given that the aims were a comparison of global HRQOL between the two groups, the methodology clearly justified the use of a global HRQOL score as a prior hypothesis. Osoba and Burchmore[32] also reported a well-designed randomized phase III study with 469 metastatic breast cancer patients. In this study, patients were allocated into two arms of either trastuzumab (Herceptin) combined with chemotherapy or chemotherapy alone. A clear priori was selected of four domains (global quality of life, physical role, social functioning, and fatigue) on the validated EORTC QLQ-C30,[33] and the results suggested that those patients on the combined treatment had a higher HRQOL than chemotherapy alone.

After this confirmatory analysis, in both the Bernhard et al and Osoba and Burchmore studies, it was possible to undertake exploratory analysis on subscale and domains. This type of analysis is used to explore, clarify, describe, and, more importantly, help interpret HRQOL data. While such analysis can often reveal important information about the data and can help interpretation, one needs to be aware that results are often generated after multiple testing and analysis, and, as Douglas[34] points out, often significant influences can be seen under such circumstances. In essence, while exploratory/descriptive analysis can help in interpreting the data, ideally this should serve the later testing of hypotheses.

When interpreting HRQOL results, it is vital that attention be given to incomplete data. Although the assessment of HRQOL is critical in cases of advanced breast cancer, it is affected by the problems of rapidly diminishing patient numbers. Frequently, this is due to so few patients completing a set of assessments in the weeks/days immediately preceding death. One example is the study reported by Kramer and colleagues,[35] who investigated the effects of HRQOL on patients with advanced breast cancer. In this prospective randomized phase II/III crossover study, 166 patients were assigned to treatment with paclitaxel and 165 to treatment with doxorubicin. However, less than two-thirds of patients completed baseline assessment, and compliance rates deteriorated continually thereafter.

This is not the only study with such poor rates of compliance. For example, the investigation of HRQOL in advanced breast cancer by Coates et al[36] reports that only 44% of patients (133 of 305) were available for analysis after three cycles of chemotherapy. Similarly, in the study by Richards et al,[37] patients with advanced breast cancer underwent two different schedules of doxorubicin; this demonstrated only 71% with data at baseline and at the end of the third cycle three months later. Therefore, failure to take missing data into consideration when interpreting HRQOL results can lead to incorrect conclusions. For example, treatment differences may be biased if large numbers of patients fail to complete the questionnaire, and several studies have failed to consider these issues (e.g. those by Bishop et al[29] and Priestman and Baum[23]).

In some studies, such as that reported by Harper-Wynne et al,[38] the quality of the HRQOL information collected has been so limited by missing data that the planned analysis could not be performed. In other studies, such as that reported by Kristensen et al,[39] the results are so plagued with missing data that the analysis could only be undertaken on the initial two assessments, allowing limited follow-on. Clearly, these problems limit the extent to which we can make any reasonable interpretations of the data; thus it is imperative that robust methods be adopted to ensure that high-quality data are collected and appropriately analyzed.[27]

CLINICAL SIGNIFICANCE

Experience in medicine has led to an understanding that certain clinical events are related to health outcomes. A classical example, often cited in the literature, concerns a blood pressure reading of 110/60 mmHg being normal for a healthy, young adult but dangerously low for a trauma victim. A change of 2 or 3 mmHg in blood pressure probably has little or no clinical significance, but a 10 mmHg could indicate shock or hypertension, depending on the situation. However, while this is a well-established fact, this level of clarity in the interpretation of HRQOL scores has not been achieved.[19] For clinicians, it must be stressed that what constitutes clinical significance on many of these standard, objective measures is based on years of experience and learning and contact with a large numbers of patients over time – something that researchers and clinicians have yet to gain to a substantial degree of accuracy in HRQOL assessment.

As clinicians continue to gain more experience, this leads to greater awareness of how to relate scores to meaning of and events in life. However, questions must be asked: What do scores of 20 or 40 or whatever mean clinically? What degree of change is needed for a clinically meaningful change? While a four-point difference on a HRQOL scale may be statistically significant, is this clinically relevant to patients or society? Can these scores actually reflect the need to use or to recommend non-continuance of a treatment? Perhaps what is considered meaningful really depends on who is looking at the results of the studies. It is often relatively easy to conduct large-scale studies that could, under correct procedures, give statistically significant results even when there are only small differences in scores. When epidemiologists, policy makers or statisticians view the results, they may appear valuable simply because they are statistically significant. Perhaps, from a clinician's point of view, the most important aspect of understanding the results is to make them meaningful in terms of the patient.

Often researchers refer to what is called *minimal clinical importance difference*, noted as the smallest difference in a score in a domain of interest that a patient perceives as beneficial. This indicates, in the absence of adverse scale effects, a change in patient treatment and care.[40]

However, even with such a useful definition, clinicians can face difficulty in interpreting data in accordance with this.[41] For example, when simply comparing mean score differences between two groups, some difficult interpretations could easily arise. That is, while it is intuitive to look for a mean difference, it is important to be aware that such a group mean could easily mask certain patients in the sample by ignoring the distribution about the mean. Indeed, when examining most reported studies of advanced breast cancer, interpretation is generally focused on changes in mean scores as opposed to using other techniques of interpretation.[22,29,31]

Perhaps this is understandable, since clinicians have a long way to go in understanding the clinical significance of HRQOL scores. Fortunately, several methods have been proposed to help interpretation. Perhaps the most common approach is to *anchor* the changes seen in disease-specific questions to a global rating question – one that asks about overall HRQOL changes, such as 'In general, how would you rate your quality of life?' Then, researchers would look at changes in answers to such a global HRQOL question over time and compare these with changes seen on the disease-specific questionnaire.[42] In effect, the changes in the disease-specific measures are thus *anchored* to reported changes in overall health status. Also, it is possible to use time as an anchor – or, for that matter, changes in therapy. Changes in therapy or time can help in interpreting HRQOL scores. However, while these anchor-based interpretations can help clinicians to understand a little more about the meaning of HRQOL, it is important to recognize that they only reflect changes in HRQOL; they do not reflect score distribution.

Osoba et al[43] investigated this issue using a subjective significance questionnaire, asking patients about perceived changes in physical, emotional, social functioning, and global HRQOL using the EORTC QLQ-C30.[33] The patients were receiving chemotherapy for metastatic breast cancer or extensive-disease small cell lung cancer. Osaba et al found it possible to rate, on the seven-point subjective significance question, the significance of the changes in QLQ-C30 scores, from *much worse* to *much better*.

From the data, Osoba et al were able to interpret changes on the QLQ-C30 as meaningful, to the point of proposing, on a scale of 1–100, a difference of 5–10 as *little change*; patients who fell in the 10–20 range experienced a *moderate change*; and those with a 20+ change reported *very much change*. It is also important to bear in mind that, in using anchoring, the degree of change perceived to be clinically significant could well differ from population to population and from patient to patient.

Another common method used to interpret HRQOL data is the norm-based approach. Here clinicians compare particular individual or group scores with the distribution of the instrument scores in different populations using known criteria, including a general population, gender, age, diagnosis, and clinical populations. For example, the EORTC QLQ-C30 is used extensively not only with different cancer populations[44] but also in the general population.[26,45,46] Thus it becomes possible to explore, compare, and interpret these data with other groups.[47,48] However, while some authors have used reference data to help in the interpretation of HRQOL scores, a few studies of patients with advanced breast cancer have used this approach. It should also be noted that while reference data are often very useful, as in the case of the EORTC QLQ-C30 data, collection took place in the framework of a cancer clinical trial. In such cases, there are clear subject-recruitment selection procedures;[21] therefore, it is essential that such reference data be used carefully, ensuring that it is representative of the group(s) under study.

PREDICTIVE VALUE OF HRQOL

Belief in the growing body of evidence suggests that, in the near future, clinicians can begin to interpret the HRQOL scores as measures in context, predicting both survival rates and the effectiveness of the HRQOL during treatment. While a number of studies in other cancer sites report that HRQOL predicts survival rates,[49,50] few have been reported in advanced breast cancer. Coates[51] found that baseline scores in women who underwent chemotherapy for advanced cancer were interpreted to indicate a prognostic factor. Kramer et al[35] also found, in patients undergoing chemotherapy, that scores on the EORTC QLQ-C30 were predictive of survival outcome. It is possible that, if results continue to be generated in support of this prognostic value, then it will be possible to interpret HRQOL scores and use them as factors in important prognostic considerations, replacing the more conventional performance scales. Indeed such scores may eventually help to identify patients eligible for clinical trials, thus ensuring appropriate stratification.

WHETHER TO AGGREGATE SCORES OR USE DOMAINS IN INTERPRETATION

Some researchers argue for the aggregation of scores of various HRQOL domains as a way of expressing and interpreting overall HRQOL. The advantage of this is single-number representation. This can be easily understood and compared with other single-number representations, and can be useful in some other cases, such as calculating quality-adjusted years of life.[41] However, while it is intuitive to have a single number, there are ongoing questions, including whether it is realistic to expect that a single number can adequately reflect the various domains of HRQOL. Many assumptions are made. For example, when summed together, do these complex domains make such an accurate, global interpretation? Clinicians assume that the various domains added have equal weight or importance. This is not necessarily true, and is not supported by any evidence. It is highly possible, given the subjective nature of HRQOL, that some patients place greater weight on the HRQOL physical rather than psychological domains. While there will be individual weighting of such concerns, it is likely that there is not only this variation but also a variation over time. In addition, such interpretation is difficult, since a single score lacks any detailed information about how the various domains are influenced by the disease and treatment. As such, it is possible that certain effects of the disease and the treatment are hidden. These would not be hidden had domain scores been examined.

One way to address this limitation is the method adopted by the EORTC Quality of Life Study Group, where researchers ensure that they are able to obtain both a single global score and detailed knowledge of the various domains.[33] Here not only does the EORTC QLQ-C30 collect details on the domains, but also assessment of two global HRQOL items gives additional indication of global HRQOL, independently of the domain scores. This advantage avoids making assumptions about the weighting of domains and drawing conclusions.

While global quality of life items have the advantage of being easy to interpret by clinicians, they can have disadvantages.[52] Specifically, while the use of a global quality of life item is valuable for detecting change in general, this provides somewhat limited information; it is impossible for clinicians to identify the nature of the HRQOL change. Global items also represent an interpretative difficulty, because it is difficult to know how people are relating the change in global HRQOL to specific HRQOL issues. In advanced breast cancer patients, it is possible that patients focus on limited physical functioning and possibly spiritual or psychological issues when their condition becomes more serious.[11]

LIMITATIONS AND CHALLENGES ON HRQOL INTERPRETATION

Given the potential difficulties faced by researchers in HRQOL studies, it is understandable that there are a number of potential limitations influencing the interpretation.[53] There are the general and actual difficulties that must be considered by authors reporting HRQOL research results. As already mentioned, these include the following: making sure that the researchers have selected appropriate, valid, and reliable instruments; ensuring that analysis of data is robust, taking into account the problem of missing data; and making sure that researchers are aware of potential bias from social desirability of cancer patients (the tendency to put oneself in a favorable light and endorse questionnaire statements), and that demographic factors are considered.[27]

It is important that particular attention be paid, specifically in cancer clinical trials, to the potential problems of cultural bias; results of treatment to one group may not have the same weight or value in another culture.[54] Indeed, even if cultural differences are reported in multinational trials, it is essential that researchers consider, for example, patient characteristics and institutional participation, to avoid creating an ecological fallacy whereby results are misinterpreted as cultural differences in HRQOL, when in reality they could simply be differences in patient selection in different cultural populations.[55] In addition, clinicians are increasingly aware that patterns of response to HRQOL assessment do vary with marital status, education, income, and race,[56] with geography,[57] and with a host of other extraneous psychological factors that need to be increasingly monitored when reporting HRQOL results.[42,58,59]

SUMMARY

HRQOL data can be invaluable for assessing various interventions when used with patients suffering from advanced breast cancer. Despite this, unfortunately only a limited number of studies have been published, and many of these have suffered from methodological problems that limit the interpretation of the results. Adopting basic scientific principles of effective design and analysis of new studies will ensure that researchers collect reliable and robust data for accurate evidence-based interpretation. This will ensure that HRQOL assessment in the field of advanced breast cancer acquires a stronger scientific basis and thus could be used to a greater degree in treatment decision making.

REFERENCES

1. Teplege A, Hunt S, The problem of quality of life in medicine. *JAMA* 1997; **278**:47–50.

2. Sanders C, Egger M, Donovan J et al, Reporting on quality of life in randomised controlled trials: bibliographic study. *BMJ* 1998; 317:1191–4.

3. Detmar SB, Aaronson NK, Quality of life assessment in daily clinical oncology practice: a feasibility study. *Eur J Cancer* 1998; 34:1181–6.

4. Feld R, Endpoints in cancer clinical trials: Is there a need for measuring quality of life? *Support Care Cancer* 1995; 3:23–7.

5. Muldoon MF, Barger SD, Flory JD, Manuck SB, What are quality of life measurements measuring? *BMJ* 1998; 316:542–5.

6. Osoba D, Lessons Learned from measuring health-related quality of life in oncology. *J Clin Oncol* 1994; 12:608–16.

7. Young T, Maher J, Collecting quality of life data in EORTC clinical trials – What happens in practice? *Psycho-oncology* 1999; 8:260–3.

8. Velikova G, Stark D, Selby P, Quality of life instruments in oncology. *Eur J Cancer* 1999; 35:1571–80.

9. Moinpour CM, Do quality of life assessments make a difference in the evaluation of cancer treatments? *Control Clin Trials* 1997; 18:311–17.

10. Bull AA, Meyerowitz BE, Hart S et al, Quality of life in women with recurrent breast cancer. *Breast Cancer Res Treat* 1999; 54:47–57.

11. Groenvold M, Methodological issues in the assessment of health-related quality of life in palliative care trials. *Acta Anaesthesiol Scand* 1999; 43:948–53.

12. Fisher B, Bauer M, Margolese R et al, Five year results of a randomised clinical trial comparing total mastectomy and segmental mastectomy with or without radiation in the treatment of breast cancer. *N Engl J Med* 1985; 312:665–73.

13. Levy SM, Herberman RB, Lee JK et al, Breast conservation versus mastectomy: distress sequelae as a function of choice. *J Clin Oncol* 1989; 7:367–75.

14. Shimozuma K, Ganz PA, Petersen L, Hirji K,

Quality of life in the first year after breast cancer surgery: rehabilitation needs and patterns of recovery. *Breast Cancer Res Treat* 1999; 56:45–57.

15. Pusic A, Thompson TA, Kerrigan CL et al, Surgical options for the early-stage breast cancer: factors associated with patient choice and postoperative quality of life. *Plast Reconstr Surg* 1999; 104:1325–33.

16. Carlson RW, Quality of life issues in the treatment of metastatic breast cancer. *Oncology (Huntingt)* 1998; 12(3 Suppl 4):27–31.

17. Overmoyer BA, Chemotherapeutic palliative approaches in the treatment of breast cancer. *Semin Oncol* 1995; 22(2 Suppl 3):2–9.

18. Fossati R, Confalonieri C, Torri V et al, Cytotoxic and hormonal treatment for metastatic breast cancer: a systematic review of published randomized trials involving 31,510 women. *J Clin Oncol* 1998; 16:3439–60.

19. Green SB, Does assessment of quality of life in comparative cancer trials make a difference? A discussion. *Control Clin Trials* 1997; 18:306–10.

20. Kong SX, Gandhi SK, Methodologic assessments of quality of life measures in clinical trials. *Ann Pharmacother* 1997; 31:830–6.

21. Bernhard J, Hurny CDT, Coates A et al, Applying quality of life principles in international cancer clinical trials. In: Spilker B, ed. *Quality of Life and Pharmacoeconomics in Clinical Trials*, 2nd edn. Philadelphia: Lippincott-Raven, 1996.

22. Seidman AD, Hudis CA, Norton L, Memorial Sloan-Kettering Cancer Center experience with paclitaxel in the treatment of breast cancer: from advanced disease to adjuvant therapy. *Semin Oncol* 1995; 22:3–8.

23. Priestman TJ, Baum M, Evaluation of quality of life in patients receiving treatment for advanced breast cancer. *Lancet* 1976; i:899–900.

24. Calkins DR, Rubenstein LV, Cleary PD et al, Failure of physicians to recognise functional disability in ambulatory patients. *Ann Intern Med* 1991; 114:451–4.

25. Nelson E, Conger B, Douglass R et al, Func-

tional health status levels of primary care patients. *JAMA* 1983; **249**:3331–8.

26. Fayers PM, Machin D, Summarizing quality of life data using graphical methods. In: Staquet MJ, Hays RD, Fayers PM, eds. *Quality of Life Assessment in Clinical Trials: Methods and Practice*. Oxford: Oxford Medical Publications, 1998.

27. Staquet M, Berzon R, Osoba D, Machin D, Guidelines for reporting results of quality of life assessments in clinical trials. *Qual Life Res* 1996; **5**:496–502.

28. Tannock IF, Boyd NF, DeBoer G et al, A randomized trial of two dose levels of cyclophosphamide, methotrexate, and fluorouracil chemotherapy for patients with metastatic breast cancer. *J Clin Oncol* 1988; **6**:1377–87.

29. Bishop JF, Dewar J, Toner GC et al, Initial paclitaxel improves outcome compared with CMFP combination chemotherapy as frontline therapy in untreated metastatic breast cancer. *J Clin Oncol* 1999; **17**:2355–64.

30. Spitzer WO, Dobson AJ, Hall J et al, Measuring the quality of life of cancer patients: a concise QL-index for use by physicians. *J Chronic Dis* 1981; **34**:585–97.

31. Bernhard J, Thurlimann B, Schmitz S et al, Defining clinical benefit in postmenopausal patients with breast cancer under second-line endocrine treatment: does quality of life matter? *J Clin Oncol* 1999; **17**:1672–9.

32. Osoba D, Burchmore M, Health-related quality of life in women with metastatic breast cancer treated with trastuzumab (Herceptin). *Semin Oncol* 1999; **26**(4 Suppl 12):84–8.

33. Aaronson NK, Ahmedzai S, Bergman B et al, The European Organization for Research and Treatment of Cancer QLQ-C30: a quality-of-life instrument for use in international clinical trials in oncology. *J Natl Cancer Inst* 1993; **85**:365–76.

34. Douglas JA, Item response models for longitudinal quality of life data in clinical trials. *Stat Med* 1999; **18**:2917–31.

35. Kramer J, Curran D, Parridaens R, Quality of

36. Coates A, Gebski V, Stat M et al, Improving the quality of life during chemotherapy for advanced breast cancer: a comparison of intermittent and continuous treatment strategies. *N Engl J Med* 1987; **317**:1490–5.

37. Richards MA, Hopwood P, Ramirez AJ et al, Doxorubicin in advanced breast cancer: influence of schedule on response, survival and quality of life. *Eur J Cancer* 1992; **28A**:1023–8.

38. Harper-Wynne C, English J, Meyer L et al, Randomized trial to compare the efficacy and toxicity of cyclophosphamide, methotrexate and 5-fluorouracil (CMF) with methotrexate and mitoxantrone (MM) in advanced carcinoma of the breast. *Br J Cancer* 1999; **81**:316–22.

39. Kristensen B, Ejlertsen B, Groenvold M et al, Oral clodronate in breast cancer patients with bone metastases: a randomized study. *J Intern Med* 1999; **246**:67–74.

40. Juniper EF, Guyatt GH, Willan A, Griffith LE, Determining a minimal important change in a disease-specific quality of life questionnaire. *J Clin Epidemiol* 1994; **47**:81–7.

41. Smith KW, Avis NE, Assmann SF, Distinguishing between quality of life and health status in quality of life research: a meta-analysis. *Qual Life Res* 1999; **8**:447–59.

42. Koller M, Heitmann K, Kussmann J, Lorenz W, Symptom reporting in cancer patients II: relations to social desirability, negative affect, and self-reported health behaviors. *Cancer* 1999; **86**:1609–20.

43. Osoba D, Rodrigues G, Myles J et al, Interpreting the significance of changes in health-related quality-of-life scores. *J Clin Oncol* 1998; **16**:139–44.

44. Hjermstad MJ, Fayers PM, Bjordal K, Kaasa S, Using reference data on quality of life – the importance of adjusting for age and gender, exemplified by the EORTC QLQ-C30 (+3). *Eur J Cancer* 1998; **34**:1381–9.

45. Hjermstad M, Holte H, Evensen S et al, Do

patients who are treated with stem cell transplantation have a health-related quality of life comparable to the general population after 1 year? *Bone Marrow Transplant* 1999; 24:911–18.

46. King MT, Dobson AJ, Hernett PR, A comparison of two quality-of-life questionnaires for cancer clinical trials: the functional living index–cancer (FLIC) and the quality of life questionnaire core module (QLQ-C30). *J Clin Epidemiol* 1996; 49:21–29.

47. Ringdal GI, Ringdal K, Testing the EORTC Quality of Life Questionnaire on cancer patients with heterogeneous diagnosis. *Qual Life Res* 1993; 2:129–40.

48. Ringdal K, Ringdal GI, Kaasa S et al, Assessing the consistency of psychometric properties of the HRQoL scales within the EORTC QLQ-C30 across populations by means of the Mokken Scaling Model. *Qual Life Res* 1999; 8:25–43.

49. Ganz PA, Lee JJ, Siau J, Quality of life assessment. An independent prognostic variable for survival in lung cancer. *Cancer* 1991; 67:3131–5.

50. Kassa S, Mastekassa A, Lund E, Prognostic factors for patients with inoperable non-small cell lung cancer, limited disease. The importance of patients' subjective experience of disease and psychosocial well-being. *Radiother Oncol* 1989; 15:235–42.

51. Coates A, Porzsolt F, Osoba D, Quality of life in oncology practice: prognostic value of EORTC QLQ-C30 Scores in patients with advanced malignancy. *Eur J Cancer* 1997; 33:1025–30.

52. Mozes B, Maor Y, Shmueli A, Do we know what global ratings of health-related quality of life measure? *Qual Life Res* 1999; 8:269–73.

53. Ware JF Jr, Keller SD, Interpreting general health measures. In: Spilker B, ed. *Quality of Life and Pharmacoeconomics in Clinical Trials*, 2nd edn. Philadelphia: Lippincott-Raven, 1996.

54. Browman GP, Science, language, intuition and the many meanings of quality of life. *J Clin Oncol* 1999; 17:1651–3.

55. Padilla GV et al, Quality of Life – Cancer. In: Spilker B, ed. *Quality of Life and Pharmacoeconomics in Clinical Trials*, 2nd edn. Philadelphia: Lippincott-Raven, 1996.

56. Juarez G, Ferrell B, Borneman T, Cultural considerations in education for cancer pain management. *J Cancer Educ* 1999; 14:168–73.

57. Wahl A, Moum T, Hanestad BR, Wiklund I, The relationship between demographic and clinical variables, and quality of life aspects in patients with psoriasis. *Qual Life Res* 1999; 8:319–26.

58. Bucquet C, Guillemin F, Briancon S, Non-specific effects in longitudinal studies: impact on quality of life measures. *J Clin Epidemiol* 1996; 49:15–20.

59. van Dam FS, Schagen SB, Muller MJ et al, Impairment of cognitive function in women receiving adjuvant treatment for high risk breast cancer: high-dose versus standard dose chemotherapy. *J Natl Cancer Inst* 1998; 90:210–18.

SECTION 10: Treatment of Early Stage Breast Cancer

32.1
Adjuvant treatment: Node-negative breast cancer

Miguel Martín

Node-negative breast cancer (NNBC) is progressively increasing in incidence in developed countries relative to node-positive disease. This has occurred as a result of screening mammography campaigns in at-risk populations and increased health education programs for women. At present, it is estimated that, in Spain, more than 40% of women with breast cancer are diagnosed before node involvement occurs, and it is hoped that this level of detection increases in the next decade. In North America, 61% of women present with NNBC and 30% with regional nodes.[1] As such, it is not unreasonable to believe that NNBC will be the predominant form of presentation of the disease throughout the Western World (in the near future). Despite this, knowledge of prognostic and predictive factors and therapeutic guidelines are more limited in patients with NNBC than in those with node-positive breast cancer. Hence, it is increasingly important that clinical studies be conducted in this subgroup of patients to evaluate prognostic and predictive factors and to determine optimum therapies using cytotoxic drugs, hormones and, more recently, biological response modifiers such as trastuzumab (Herceptin) that, with fewer side effects, may offer an important risk–benefit ratio in NNBC.

Traditionally, NNBC, as opposed to node-positive breast cancer, has been considered a disease with good prognosis and, in the great majority of cases, curable with local treatment. In 1985, the NIH Consensus Conference on Adjuvant Therapy of Breast Cancer concluded that the routine administration of systemic adjuvant therapy in node-negative patients could not be recommended at that time. However, by May 1988, the National Cancer Institute published a 'clinical alert' describing the preliminary results from three major node-negative studies, and concluded: 'adjuvant hormonal or cytotoxic chemotherapy can have a meaningful impact on the natural history of node-negative breast cancer patients'.[2]

There are certain crucial points that need to be taken into account when deciding the most appropriate treatment for an individual patient with NNBC:

- With local treatment alone, 60–70% of all NNBC patients will remain disease-free at 10 years.
- About two-thirds of patient with NNBC, therefore, would not benefit from any systemic adjuvant postsurgical therapy.
- Those patients at high risk of recurrence

require an adjuvant therapy that needs to be as aggressive as for patients with node-positive cancer, because patients with NNBC who have a relapse will die exactly as those with node-positive cancer.

- The relative benefit of adjuvant therapy is the same in women with NNBC as in those with node-positive disease. However, the absolute benefit is less in the former group because of the lower risk of recurrence, and this needs to be taken into account at the time of assessing the risk–benefit balance of treatment.

Clinical investigation of postsurgical adjuvant therapy for NNBC poses specific problems. The definition of the patient selection criteria (especially the criteria for high risk) is of crucial importance because it facilitates comparisons between studies and meta-analyses. Another relevant issue that has logistic and economic implications is the necessity for protracted follow-up before differences in disease-free survival (DFS) and, especially, overall survival (OS) between study treatments becomes evident. Alternatively, validated surrogate endpoints for DFS and OS must be used.

PROGNOSTIC/PREDICTIVE FACTORS AND DETERMINATION OF RISK OF RECURRENCE

Given that only one in three patients with NNBC presents with recurrence after local treatment,[3,4] it is fundamental to assess the prognostic factors capable of predicting recurrence of the disease.

Tumor size is, without doubt, one of the most studied prognostic factors and constitutes a variable that is independent of the rest of the other prognostic factors. Risk of recurrence increases progressively with the size of the tumor. A classic study[4] indicated that the rate of recurrence over 20 years in patients with NNBC of less than 1 cm in size is 14%, rising to 31% in patients with tumors of 1–2 cm and to 39% in patients with tumors of 3–5 cm. A tumor size of 2 cm has commonly been used as a cut-off point in considering a patient with NNBC as having a high risk of recurrence based on this factor alone.

Pathological criteria such as histological and/or nuclear grade constitute other independent prognostic factors in NNBC. For some authors, the nuclear grade is a more potent prognostic factor than the histological grade, but both appear to possess independent prognostic capacities. The limitation of grade as an efficient prognostic factor rests in its subjectivity. There are few problems of concordance for criteria between pathologists when dealing with well-differentiated or clearly undifferentiated tumors, but discrepancies can arise in intermediate grades.

Hormone receptors are prognostic and predictive factors that have been extensively investigated in women with NNBC. The presence of hormone receptors is usually associated with good histological differentiation and less aggressive clinical behavior. In the most extensive series in the clinical literature, patients with NNBC and positive receptors had an OS and DFS greater than those who did not express receptors (although the absolute difference did not reach 10%). In addition, hormone receptors constitute a clear example of a predictive factor in the response to adjuvant treatment with tamoxifen. However, the value of studies of estrogen receptors/progesterone receptors (ER/PgR) to discriminate outcome of groups of patients appears to decrease over time, and almost disappears by 10 years of follow-up.

Histological subtype has also been investigated as a prognostic factor. Tubular and papillary carcinomas appear to have a less aggressive course than invasive ductal and lobular carcinomas.

Table 32.1.1   Risk groups in women with NNBC

Prognostic factor	Low risk	Intermediate risk	High risk
Tumor size	<1 cm	1–2 cm	>2 cm
Hormonal receptors	Positive	Positive	ER and PR negative
Grade	1	1–2	2–3
Age	>35 years		≤35 years

Colloid and medullar carcinomas have an intermediate prognosis. Some investigators exclude carcinomas of good prognosis (tubular and papillary) from adjuvant studies in NNBC (unless the size exceeds 3 cm), but this criterion is not as yet supported by conclusive data.

The age of the patient has been recognized, more recently, as a potentially important prognostic factor. Women aged less than 35 years at diagnosis are considered, by some, to be at high risk[5] for relapse. Whether age is truly an independent prognostic factor remains to be determined by further studies.

Among the various biological factors, aneuploidy and a high fraction of cells in S phase have been suggested as being factors that determine poor prognosis, although these have not always appeared as independent variables in multivariate studies. A similar situation exists with respect to cathepsin D levels and c-erbB-2 status. Overexpression of c-erbB-2 is found in 20% of NNBC patients, and appears to be associated with a poorer outcome.[6]

Recently, markers of tumor angiogenesis and proteolysis have been reported as having independent prognostic value with respect to survival in NNBC,[7,8] but these preliminary results need to be confirmed in further studies.

Based on the most comprehensive evaluation of the literature, the St Gallen Consensus Conference of 1998[8] defined three groups of risk of recurrence in women with NNBC (Table 32.1.1). According to the St Gallen criteria, more than half of all the patients with NNBC can be included in the high-risk group. Aggressive adjuvant therapy is justified in this group because the accumulated rate of recurrence at 10 years is around 40–50%. As a result of the low probability of recurrence, adjuvant therapy is not recommended in the low-risk group, although the use of tamoxifen is acceptable. The best adjuvant treatment for the intermediate-risk group is more difficult to define, although both tamoxifen and chemotherapy may have a certain value (see later). The 1998 guidelines have changed from those issued in 1995.[9] The current recommendation is that patients with less than a 10% chance of relapse within 10 years should not receive routine adjuvant systemic therapy. In 1995, the wording used was mortality within 10 years rather than recurrence.

The panel felt that nodal status and number of nodes remain the most important factor with respect to estimation of risk. Within NNBC, tumour size, histological plus nuclear grade, receptor status, lymphatic and/or vascular invasion, and age are factors that define groups with differential prognosis and can be used for treatment selection.

Two new strategies were discussed by the panel at St Gallen as having great potential for altering risk estimation, but both of these require further study. The first is sentinel node biopsy and the second the use of preoperative systemic therapy, which leads to assessment of pathological features using only one biopsy. Preoperative systemic therapy is likely to modify the characteristics of the primary tumor plus axillary nodes. However, use of preoperative treatment gives the clinician the unique opportunity to determine the clinical and pathological response to therapy, which also influences risk assessment.

There continues to be difficulty in assigning node-negative status. This is true using established surgical dissection of level I and II nodes, and is made more complex by the use of sentinel node evaluation. The latter usually requires a level of expertise by the surgeon, and it is usual for the pathologist to examine the sentinel node with special care, checking multiple levels and utilizing techniques such as immunohistochemical staining to rule out node-positivity. These techniques are not considered routine when axillary dissection is performed. Thus, the assignation of NNBC and subclassification into high-, intermediate- and low-risk categories continues to change with the evolution of new technologies. Our interventional strategies need to keep pace with these new developments.

SYSTEMIC ADJUVANT THERAPY IN NNBC

As commented earlier, NNBC had been considered, historically, as having a good prognosis with local treatment alone. However, a survey of the clinical literature indicates a recurrence rate of approximately 30% at 10 years, which has prompted the conduct of controlled clinical trials with chemotherapy and tamoxifen. What follows are brief highlights of the most relevant studies on adjuvant therapy of NNBC published so far.

Adjuvant hormone therapy

The B-14 study of the North American National Surgical Adjuvant Breast and Bowel Project (NSABP) constitutes the most important trial of adjuvant hormonotherapy in NNBC because of its appropriate methodology and sample size.[10] The study included 2843 patients with NNBC with positive ER who were randomized to receive tamoxifen 20 mg/day or placebo over a period of 5 years. The patients treated with tamoxifen had a DFS at 4 years that was statistically greater than for those treated with placebo (83% versus 77%), although the difference in OS was not statistically significant at the time of the first communication of the results. The authors concluded that this benefit due to tamoxifen, despite its small impact on DFS, constituted a notable advance in the treatment of such patients and, as such, warranted further studies to improve the outcome of patients. In a subsequent extension of the study, the patients who were disease-free after 5 years of treatment with tamoxifen were re-randomized to continue with tamoxifen or with placebo for a further 5 years. No additional benefit was observed by extending treatment with tamoxifen to 10 years.[11] The survival analysis at 10 years of follow-up demonstrated maintenance of benefits in DFS in favor of tamoxifen compared with placebo (69% versus 57%) and at the same time showed a statistically significant benefit in OS in favour of hormonal treatment (80% versus 76%).

The meta-analysis of the Early Breast Cancer Trialists' Collaborative Group (EBCTCG) reported in 1998 demonstrated that adjuvant tamoxifen increased OS at 10 years by 5.6% (standard deviation 1.3) with respect to the no-treatment group of women with NNBC.[12] The benefit was clear in women with positive or unknown ER, but not in those with negative receptors. According to the data of this meta-analysis, the improvement in DFS observed with tamoxifen was produced, essentially, in the first 5 years, although the improvement in OS was over the longer term of 10 years. This is exactly the same result that the NSABP B-14 generated.

Adjuvant chemotherapy

Various studies have assessed different protocols of adjuvant chemotherapy compared with observation-only in patients with NNBC at high risk of relapse. The great majority of these studies demonstrated a benefit in DFS and OS with chemotherapy, except when the protocols used were those that, today, would be considered suboptimal with respect to dose intensity. This is the case of the study by the West Midlands Oncology Association in which 574 patients with NNBC were randomized to receive oral LMF (chlorambucil, methotrexate and 5-fluorouracil (5-FU)) or observation alone, and no differences in DFS or OS were encountered.[13]

Chemotherapy versus no treatment

The Ludwig Breast Cancer Study Group randomized 1275 patients with NNBC to receive either a single cycle of CMF (cyclophosphamide, methotrexate and 5-FU) immediately postoperatively or no treatment (Ludwig V trial). The chemotherapy produced a small, albeit statistically significant, benefit in DFS at 4 years (77% versus 73%).[14]

The B-13 protocol of the NSABP randomized 679 patients with NNBC and negative ER to receive either chemotherapy treatment with MFL (methotrexate, 5-FU and folinic acid) or no treatment. At 4 years of follow-up, the DFS was significantly better in the group of patients who received chemotherapy (80% versus 71%).[15]

Similarly, the North American Intergroup (Eastern Cooperative Oncology Group (ECOG), Southwest Oncology Group (SWOG) and Cancer and Leukemia Group B (CALGB)) conducted a study in 536 women with NNBC and with criteria of high risk of recurrence (ER-negative or ER-positive plus tumor size > 3 cm) in which the patients were randomized to receive either six cycles of CMFP (CMF plus prednisone) or no treatment. The DFS and OS rates at 10 years were 73% and 81%, respectively, among patients who received chemotherapy, compared with 58% and 71% in the observation group.[16,17]

The Instituto Nazionale Tumori of Milan initiated a study in women with NNBC and negative ER in 1980;[18] 90 patients were included in the study and randomized to receive either 12 cycles of intravenous CMF or no treatment. The DFS rate at 12 years was significantly greater in the group that received chemotherapy (71% versus 43%), as was the OS rate (80% versus 50%).

Anthracyclines versus non-anthracycline-based chemotherapy

The role of anthracyclines as adjuvant therapy in patients with NNBC has been explored by the American Intergroup (Protocol INT 0102).[19] A total of 2691 patients who were stage N0 but high-risk (ER- and PgR-negative, tumors of ≥ 2 cm, or a high S-phase fraction) were randomized to receive CAF (oral cyclophosphamide, doxorubicin and 5-FU) or CMF (with oral cyclophosphamide) with or without 5 years of tamoxifen. DFS as well as OS were statistically greater with CAF, although the benefit was slight (absolute increase of 2% in OS and DFS at 5 years). The inclusion of tamoxifen showed an additional positive effect on DFS and OS only in receptor-positive patients.

The Spanish group GEICAM (Spanish Group for Investigation in Breast Cancer) initiated, in 1987, a randomized trial comparing CMF (cyclophosphamide 600 mg/m^2 i.v., methotrexate 60 mg/m^2 i.v., 5-FU 500 mg/m^2 i.v., on day 1 every 3 weeks × 6 cycles) with FAC (5-FU 500 mg/m^2 i.v., doxorubicin 50 mg/m^2 i.v., cyclophosphamide 500 mg/m^2 i.v., day 1 every

3 weeks × 6 cycles) in women with operable breast cancer. Both regimens were found to be equi-myelotoxic.[20] The patients were prospectively stratified with respect to nodal status. In the group of 416 patients with NNBC, with a median follow-up of 73 months, FAC was statistically superior to CMF in terms of DFS and OS (73% versus 60%, 83% versus 75%, respectively, at 10 years).

The results of polychemotherapy studies were analysed in a meta-analysis by the EBCTCG in 1998.[21] In women with NNBC, adjuvant chemotherapy significantly improved DFS and OS compared with no treatment in all age subgroups. The magnitude of benefit was clinically relevant (e.g. the OS rate at 10 years increased from 71% to 78%). The benefit in DFS was observed in the first 5 years, whereas the benefit in OS appeared in the longer term of 10 years. The combinations that included anthracyclines were moderately better than those without anthracyclines (absolute increment of 3% at 10 years).

Taxanes versus non-taxanes

Various studies in the USA and Europe are currently being conducted to assess the role of taxanes in adjuvant therapy in NNBC patients at high risk. The GEICAM group, for example, began the TARGET 0 study in July 1999 to compare their standard therapy (FAC) × 6 cycles with TAC × 6 cycles (docetaxel, doxorubicin, cyclophosphamide all given intravenously) as postoperative adjuvant therapy in women with NNBC and at high risk as defined by the 1998 St Gallen Consensus Conference.

Adjuvant chemo/hormonal therapy

The B-20 protocol of the NSABP[22] investigated the effect of the combination of chemotherapy (methotrexate plus 5-FU or CMF) plus tamoxifen versus tamoxifen alone in 2036 patients with NNBC and positive ER. The two chemo/hor-

monal combinations were better than tamoxifen alone (DFS rate at 5 years of 89–90% versus 85%), and this benefit was apparent in all the age subgroups.

CONCLUSIONS

NNBC will constitute, without doubt, one of the epidemics of the next century. Adjuvant treatment for women with NNBC poses specific problems that are different to those that apply to women with node-positive breast cancer. For example, although the relative benefits of adjuvant treatments are similar, the absolute benefits are quantitatively less in the case of NNBC. As such, it is necessary to calculate the risk–benefit ratio and to define precisely the subgroups of risk. For the moment, we know that adjuvant chemotherapy benefits the NNBC patient at high and intermediate risk in terms of DFS and OS and that tamoxifen, administered over 5 years, benefits women with positive ER. We know, as well, that chemotherapy protocols should be used at optimum doses, and there is solid evidence that the regimens that include anthracyclines have a small additional benefit compared with regimens without them. Despite this, there are no general consensus guidelines with respect to standard adjuvant chemotherapy in women with NNBC. In the author's opinion, the option of an anthracycline-containing regimen should be offered to all high-risk NNBC patients who do not present with contraindications to their use. It has been demonstrated that most women are likely to accept a higher risk of toxicity if, in exchange, they can obtain a therapeutic benefit, however small. As shown before, even with the best current chemotherapy or chemo/hormonal therapy, at least 10–30% of women with intermediate- and high-risk NNBC, respectively, will continue to present with recurrence of their disease (Table 32.1.2), and, as such, the need to

Table 32.1.2   Disease-free survival after adjuvant chemotherapy or chemohormonal therapy in NNBC[a]

Reference	Hormonal status	Adjuvant therapy	DFS (%)	OS (%)
Intergroup[17] (n = 536)	ER-negative or ER-positive + T > 3 cm	CMFP vs No treatment	73 at 10 years vs 58	81 71
Istituto Nazionale Tumori[18] (n = 90)	ER-negative	CMF vs No treatment	71 at 12 years vs 43	80 50
NSABP B-13[15] (n = 679)	ER-negative	MFL vs No treatment	80 at 4 years vs 71	NA NA
Intergroup INT 0102[19] (n = 2091)	ER-negative plus PR-negative or ER/PR-positive + T > 2 cm/HSPF	CAF+ tamoxifen vs CMF + tamoxifen	87 at 5 years vs 85	NA NA
GEICAM 8701 (unpublished) (n = 416)	All	FAC vs CMF	73 at 10 years vs 60	83 75
Ludwig V (n = 1275)[14]	ER-positive or -negative or unknown	CMF vs No treatment	77 at 4 years vs 73	
NSABP B-20[22] (n = 2036)	ER-positive	MF or CMF+ tamoxifen vs Tamoxifen	89–90 at 5 years vs 85	NA NA

[a] Results of the best arm of randomized studies.
HSPF, high S-phase fraction; T, tumor size; NA, not available.
For details of chemotherapy regimens, see text.

investigate potentially more active regimens continues. Undoubtedly, the taxanes are the next generation of pharmacological agents whose efficacy needs to be intensively explored. Trastuzumab (Herceptin), an anti-c-ErbB-2 monoclonal antibody, is a new biological response modifier whose efficacy as adjuvant therapy for NNBC patients with c-*erb*B-2 overexpression warrants investigation. This therapy might be particularly appropriate because of its low side-effect profile, which would make the risk–benefit ratio especially attractive in women with NNBC.

REFERENCES

1. Ries Lag, Kosary CL, Hankey BF et al, eds. *SEER Cancer Statistics Review 1973–95.* Bethesda, MD: National Cancer Institute, 1998.

2. Anonymous, Treatment Alert issued for node-negative breast cancer. *J Natl Cancer Inst* 1998; 8:550–1.

3. Husbey RA, Ownby HE, Frederick J et al, Node-negative breast cancer treated by modified radical mastectomy without adjuvant therapies: Variables associated with disease recurrence and survivorship. *J Clin Oncol* 1988; 6:83–8.

4. Rosen PP, Groshen S, Kinne DW, Prognosis in T2N0M0 stage I breast carcinoma. A 20-year follow-up study. *J Clin Oncol* 1991; 9:1650–61.

5. Nixon NJ, Neuberg D, Hayes DF et al, Relationship of patient age to pathologic features of the tumor and prognosis for patients with stage I or II breast cancer. *J Clin Oncol* 1994; 12:888–94.

6. Andrulis IL, Bull SB, Blackstein ME et al, Neu/erbB-2 amplification identifies a poor-prognosis group of women with node-negative breast cancer. *J Clin Oncol* 1998; 16:1340–9.

7. Linderholm B, Tavelin B, Grankvist K, Heriksson R, Vascular endothelium growth factor is of high prognostic value in node-negative breast carcinoma. *J Clin Oncol* 1998; 16:3121–8.

8. Eppenberger U, Keung W, Schlaeppi JM et al, Markers of tumor angiogenesis and proteolysis independently define high- and low-risk subsets of node-negative breast cancer. *J Clin Oncol* 1998; 16:3129–36.

9. Goldhirsch A, Glick JH, Gelber RD, Senn HJ, Meeting highlights: International Consensus Panel on the Treatment of Primary Breast Cancer. *J Natl Cancer Inst* 1998; 90:1601–8.

10. Fisher B, Constantino J, Redmond C et al, A randomized clinical trial evaluating tamoxifen in the treatment of patients with node-negative breast cancer who have estrogen-receptor-positive tumors. *N Engl J Med* 1989; 320:479–84.

11. Fisher B, Digman J, Bryant J et al, Five versus more than five years of tamoxifen therapy for breast cancer patients with negative lymph nodes and estrogen-receptor-positive tumors. *J Natl Cancer Inst* 1996; 88:1529–34.

12. Early Breast Cancer Trialists' Collaborative Group, Tamoxifen for early breast cancer: An overview of the randomised trials. *Lancet* 1998; 351:1451–67.

13. Morrison JM, Kelly KA, Howell A, West Midlands Oncology Association Trial on adjuvant chemotherapy in node-negative breast cancer. *Natl Cancer Inst Monogr* 1992; 11:85–8.

14. The Ludwig Breast Cancer Study Group. Prolonged disease-free survival after one course of perioperative adjuvant chemotherapy for node-negative breast cancer. *N Engl J Med* 1989; 320:491–6.

15. Fisher B, Redmond C, Dimitrov NV et al, A randomized clinical trial evaluating sequential methotrexate and fluorouracil in the treatment of patients with node-negative breast cancer who have estrogen-receptor-negative tumors. *N Engl J Med* 1989; 320:473–8.

16. Mansour EG, Gray R, Shatila AH et al, Efficacy of adjuvant chemotherapy in high-risk node-negative breast cancer. *N Engl J Med* 1989; 320:485–90.

17. Mansour EG, Gray R, Shatila AH et al, Survival advantage of adjuvant chemotherapy in high-

risk node-negative breast cancer: Ten-year analysis: An Intergroup study. *J Clin Oncol* 1998; **16**:3486–92.

18. Zambetti M, Valagussa P, Bonadonna G. Adjuvant cyclophosphamide, methotrexate and fluorouracil in node-negative and estrogen receptor-negative breast cancer. *Ann Oncol* 1996; **7**:481–5.

19. Hutchins L, Green S, Ravdin P et al, CMF versus CAF with and without tamoxifen in high-risk node-negative breast cancer patients and a natural history follow-up study in low-risk node-negative patients: First results of Intergroup trial INT 0102. *Proc Am Soc Clin Oncol* 1998; **17**:2.

20. Martín M, Villar A, Solé-Calvo et al, A randomized trial comparing CMF with FAC in breast cancer adjuvant treatment. Toxicity analysis. *Ann Oncol* 1994; **5**(Suppl 8):21.

21. Early Breast Cancer Trialists' Collaborative Group, Polychemotherapy for early breast cancer: An overview of the randomised trials. *Lancet* 1998; **352**:930–43.

22. Fisher B, Digman J, Wolmark N et al, Tamoxifen and chemotherapy for lymph node-negative, estrogen receptor-positive breast cancer. *J Natl Cancer Inst* 1997; **89**:1673–82.

32.2

Adjuvant treatment: Node-positive breast cancer

Caroline Lohrisch, Martine J Piccart

ENDOCRINE THERAPY

The principle of adjuvant endocrine (or hormonal) therapy is to minimize exposure of any residual foci of breast cancer cells (after surgical removal of the primary) to estrogen, which may stimulate cellular proliferation. Approximately two-thirds of breast cancers have nuclear receptors for estrogen (ER) and/or progesterone (PgR). Binding of estrogen and progesterone to their respective receptors results in molecular activation and secondary cell signalling. The final result of this multistep pathway is upregulation of cell cycling through activation of nuclear transcription factors. There are various ways to inhibit activation of this pathway, including removing circulating estrogens (ovarian ablation in premenopausal women, aromatase inhibitors in postmenopausal women), and introducing drugs such as tamoxifen and novel anti-estrogens, which compete with estrogen for receptor binding, but do not fully activate the second-messenger cascade. These therapeutic approaches are effective in only a minority of patients with tumors that do not express ER or PgR, and so the following discussion is almost entirely focused on evidence from patients with ER-positive or ER-negative/PgR-positive disease.

Tamoxifen

The most comprehensive synthesis of data on tamoxifen in early breast cancer trials comes from the Early Breast Cancer Trialists' Collaborative Group (EBCTCG) overview, last updated for trials initiated before 1990 and comprising data finalized in 1995–96.[1] This systematic overview analyzed outcomes of 37 000 individual patients enrolled in 55 randomized clinical trials (RCTs) of adjuvant tamoxifen compared with no adjuvant hormonal intervention, with an average follow-up of 10 years. Data were unavailable for eight trials, consisting of approximately 5700 women, 4200 of whom were enrolled in three large trials of 5 years of tamoxifen. ER status was positive in 18 000, negative in 8000 and unknown in about 12 000 women. Analysis was divided according to whether tamoxifen was given for 1, 2 or about 5 years, each compared with no hormonal therapy, and the primary outcomes of interest were recurrence and death from breast cancer. Using an intention-to-treat analysis, log-rank observed minus expected values were calculated for each study (tamoxifen versus control) and combined for an estimate of overall effect.

The use of tamoxifen was associated with a highly significant decrease in both recurrence and death, and there was a significant trend of increased benefit with longer duration of therapy. Overall, with 5 years of tamoxifen use, the relative risk reduction (RRR) was 47% (two-sided p, $2p < 0.00001$) for recurrence, and 26% ($2p < 0.00001$) for death. The greatest benefit in mortality was observed in node-positive (NP) disease ($n = 2210$, 92% ER-positive), with an RRR of 43% for recurrence and 28% for death with 5 years of tamoxifen. This is equivalent to an absolute 10-year survival improvement of 10.9% (from 50.5% for no hormonal therapy to 61.4%; $2p < 0.00001$). For 1 and 2 years of tamoxifen use, the absolute 10-year survival benefits were 4.5% and 7.2%, respectively.

The benefit of tamoxifen was observed irrespective of age, menopausal status, daily dose (which in most cases was 20 mg/day) and additional chemotherapy received. For women aged under 50 years (661 treated and 666 control patients), RRRs for recurrence and mortality were 45% and 32%, respectively. RRRs for recurrence and mortality in women aged 50–59 (1285 treated, 1251 controls) were 37% and 11%, respectively (confidence intervals crossed unity for mortality but not recurrence), and for women aged 60–69 (1606 treated, 1568 controls) 54% and 33%, respectively. The number of women older than 70 enrolled in trials was much smaller (tamoxifen 186, control 204); however, a benefit of 5 years of tamoxifen was still observed, with an RRR of 54% in recurrence and 34% in mortality.

Of note, the benefit of tamoxifen after chemotherapy in premenopausal women is still debated, despite significant overall positive results from the EBCTCG overview. This issue is addressed in the chemoendocrine section of this chapter.

Duration of therapy

It is clear from the Oxford overview that the benefits of adjuvant tamoxifen are cumulatively improved with 5 years of use compared with 1 or 2 years. Two large trials have recently finished recruiting patients to comparisons of 2 versus 5 years (Cancer Research Campaign or CRC trial, target $n = 4000$) and 1 versus 2 years (Danish Breast Cancer Group, DBCG 89C trial, target $n = 2000$), and their results may further confirm these observations.

There is a debate about whether more than 5 years of adjuvant therapy provides additional protective benefit against breast cancer recurrence or death, or is associated with lower survival as a result of cumulative serious adverse events. Thus far, no additional benefit has been observed with more than 5 years of tamoxifen therapy. In an extension of two trials (Eastern Cooperative Oncology Group (ECOG) E4181 (premenopausal) + E5181 (postmenopausal), and the Scottish tamoxifen trial), women who had completed 5 years of adjuvant tamoxifen were offered re-randomization to stop or continue tamoxifen.[2,3] The ECOG study found no difference in relapse-free survival (RFS) rate (85% and 73%; $p = 0.10$) or overall survival (OS) rate (86% and 89%; $p = 0.52$), in continued and discontinued users, respectively, with 5 years of follow-up. In the Scottish trial, with 6.2 years of median follow-up from the second randomization, the relapse rates were 22.5% and 16.2% ($p = $ NS) in those who stopped ($n = 169$) or continued ($n = 173$) tamoxifen, respectively. In a trial of similar design with 4 years of follow-up, the National Surgical Adjuvant Breast and Bowel Project (NSABP) also found no difference in OS between node-negative (NN) patients continuing ($n = 583$) or stopping ($n = 570$) tamoxifen after 5 years (96% and 94%, respectively).[4] In both the Scottish and NSABP trials, there was a higher incidence of endometrial cancer (but no endometrial cancer deaths) in continuing users.

Given that, in NP disease, most relapses occur

within the first 5 years of diagnosis, it is not surprising that little further reduction in recurrence rates occurs after 5 years of tamoxifen use. Any additional survival benefit (reduction in breast cancer and cardiovascular deaths) may be offset by the cumulative risks of endometrial cancer and thromboembolic events, which persist with continued use. Nevertheless, proponents of continuous tamoxifen use argue that studies that have compared 5 and more than 5 years of use are underpowered to detect small differences in outcome. The Adjuvant Tamoxifen Longer Against Shorter (ATLAS) trial is attempting to settle the issue definitively by randomizing approximately 20 000 women (about 5000 thus far) to continue for 5 more years or stop tamoxifen after completion of 5 years. However, at present, adjuvant tamoxifen for longer than 5 years cannot be recommended based on available level I evidence.

Other benefits
Contralateral breast cancer
The EBCTCG overview estimated a 47% RRR in the incidence of contralateral breast cancer with 5 years of tamoxifen. This is similar to the relative risk estimate of 0.61 derived from (some of the same) RCTs of tamoxifen versus control.[5]

Lipids and cardiovascular mortality
Studies have demonstrated a reduction in serum low-density lipoprotein cholesterol, total serum cholesterol and lipoprotein(a), and an increase in apolipoprotein B levels with tamoxifen therapy.[6,7] This probably contributes to the significant reduction in deaths from coronary heart disease observed in tamoxifen-treated breast cancer patients compared with untreated controls.[1,8,9]

Osteoporosis
By increasing bone mineral density, tamoxifen is protective against osteoporosis in postmenopausal women.[10–15] In premenopausal

women treated with tamoxifen, bone mineral density decreases. However, studies have concluded that the rate of loss is similar for breast cancer patients treated with tamoxifen or placebo.[11,16] The incidence of clinical osteoporosis in premenopausal breast cancer patients taking tamoxifen compared with no tamoxifen has been examined only in small prospective trials.

Negative impact
An analysis of survival impact with the use of adjuvant tamoxifen was accomplished by MEDLINE and CANCERlit searches for RCTs of tamoxifen versus no tamoxifen, which specifically recorded non-breast-cancer deaths.[5] The relative risk of dying of contralateral breast cancer, cardiovascular disease, endometrial cancer and thromboembolic events was calculated for tamoxifen users versus non-users. Over 10 years, the relative risk of contralateral breast cancer (0.61) and cardiovascular deaths (0.75) favored tamoxifen users, and the relative risk of death from endometrial cancer (7.5) and thromboembolic events (7.0) favored non-users. The 10-year summed deaths for all four endpoints favored tamoxifen use in all age groups examined, with net mortality differences (number of deaths per 1000 women in tamoxifen users − non-users) of −5.0, −2.7, −10.1 and −43.0 for women aged 50, 60, 70 and 80 years at diagnosis, respectively.

The NSABP B-14 trial ($n = 2843$, NN, ER-positive breast cancer randomized to placebo or 5 years of tamoxifen 20 mg/day) reported an annual hazard rate of endometrial cancer of 1.6/1000 (23 cases) and 0.2/1000 (2 cases) in tamoxifen and placebo users, respectively.[17] The EBCTCG overview estimated the excess incidence of endometrial cancer over 10 years to be fourfold, and excess endometrial cancer deaths of 1–2/1000 with 5 years of tamoxifen.[1] Excluding deaths from endometrial and breast cancers, the relative risk of death was 0.99, suggesting that the risk of death from other causes is neither increased nor decreased by the use of tamoxifen.

Aromatase inhibitors and novel anti-estrogens

Although tamoxifen is still the gold-standard hormonal therapy for postmenopausal women with ER-positive breast cancer, numerous new hormonal agents have been developed and are in advanced stages of clinical evaluation. New avenues of investigation are exploring the value, if any, of switching to peripheral aromatase inhibitors (AIs) or selective estrogen receptor modifiers (SERMs) after adjuvant tamoxifen, replacing tamoxifen by these newer endocrine agents up front, or combining tamoxifen with new AIs (Table 32.2.1). The rationale is that the different mechanisms of action of these drugs may inhibit the emergence of hormone-insensitive clones. In addition, hormone-suppressing drugs with fewer side effects and lower risks of serious sequelae, such as venous thromboembolic disease and endometrial cancer, may be preferable to tamoxifen if equivalence is established.

Aminoglutethimide

Aromatase is an enzyme found in peripheral adipose tissue and breast cancer cells, which converts androstenedione to estrone, and testosterone to estradiol, both active estrogens. Inhibition of aromatase effectively suppresses circulating estrogen levels in postmenopausal women, because this is the major source of estrogen production after the menopause. A large trial of an early AI, aminoglutethimide 250 mg/day with hydrocortisone 20 mg/day for 2 years, versus placebo in NP postmenopausal women, showed improved DFS and OS for the aminoglutethimide group for up to, but not beyond, 4

years of follow-up.[18] An RCT comparing tamoxifen (20 mg/day × 5 years) with tamoxifen and aminoglutethimide (250 mg twice daily × 2 years) in 2021 postmenopausal women with ER-positive, NP (38%) or NN breast cancer found no difference in either RFS rate (86%, 86%) or OS rate (94%, 95%) for the tamoxifen or combination arms, respectively, with 49 months of median follow-up.[19] No subset analysis was performed for the NP group. Given the need for concurrent hydrocortisone as a result of adrenal suppression, and other significant toxicities, coupled with the emergence of new peripheral AIs with significantly improved side-effect profiles, the further production and sale of this drug were recently discontinued in North America.

New aromatase inhibitors

The new-generation steroidal and non-steroidal AIs act peripherally, and thus do not suppress adrenal function as aminoglutethimide does. The most frequently cited side effect is nausea, and the risk of thromboembolic events is substantially lower than with tamoxifen.[20] By irreversibly (exemestane, formestane) or reversibly (anastrozole, letrozole) inhibiting peripheral and tumor aromatase, these drugs effectively reduce levels of circulating estrogens, thereby removing a growth stimulus for hormone-sensitive tumors. Adjuvant efficacy trials comparing tamoxifen, peripheral AIs and the combination are ongoing, but no results are available (Table 32.2.1). Given their tolerability and previously established efficacy in hormone-sensitive metastatic breast cancer, these agents are likely to play an increasingly prominent role in adjuvant therapy. Until adjuvant trial results are mature, however, their routine use in the adjuvant setting cannot be recommended outside clinical trials.

Table 32.2.1   Ongoing and planned adjuvant RCTs of aromatase inhibitors and tamoxifen in node-positive breast cancer[27]

Trial/group	Accrual target/ actual to data	Population	Comparison arms
ATAC	9100 closed	Post local therapy Postmenopausal NN/NP	(1) Tamoxifen (2) Tamoxifen + anastrozole (3) Anastrozole
GABG-IV C ARNO	1300/324	RFS after 2 y of adjuvant tamoxifen Postmenopausal and age ≤70 y NN or NP (0–9) ER+	(1) Tamoxifen 30 mg/d × 3 y (2) Anastrozole 1 mg/d × 3 y
ABCSG 06A	1700/2021	RFS after 5 y of adjuvant tamoxifen ± aminoglutethimide Postmenopausal NN and NP, ER+	(1) No further therapy (2) Anastrozole 1 mg/d × 3 y
NCIC-CTG MA.17 and BIG 01-97	2380/564	RFS after 5 y of adjuvant tamoxifen	(1) Letrozole 2.5 mg/d × 5 y (2) Placebo
ICCG and BIG 02-97	2206/1315	RFS after 2–3 y of adjuvant tamoxifen	(1) Tamoxifen 20 mg/d × 2–3 y (2) Exemestane 25 mg/d × 2–3 y

IBCSG 18-98 and BIG 01-98	4-arm 3500/51
	 2-arm 1680/1788
		ER+	(1) Tamoxifen × 5 y (2-arm)
			 (2) Letrozole × 5 y (2-arm)
			 (3) Tamoxifen × 2 y →
			     Letrozole × 3 y
			 (4) Letrozole × 2 y →
			     Tamoxifen × 3 y

ABCSG 12	1250/38	Premenopausal
		 NN and NP
		 ER+
			(1) OA (goserelin)
			     + tamoxifen × 3 y
			 (2) OA (goserelin)
			     + anastrozole × 3 y

GABG, German Adjuvant Breast Cancer Group; ABCSG, Austrian Breast Cancer Study Group; NCIC-CTG, National Cancer Institute of Canada Clinical Trials Group; BIG, Breast International Group; ATAC, Adjuvant Tamoxifen Anastrozole Comparison; IBCSG, International Breast Cancer Study Group; NN, node-negative; NP, node-positive; ER, estrogen receptor; RFS, relapse-free survival; OA, ovarian ablation.

Novel anti-estrogens

Novel anti-estrogens have been developed with fewer or no estrogen agonist properties, to eliminate the proliferative stimulus on the endometrium seen with tamoxifen (Table 32.2.2).[21] One of these drugs, raloxifene, has already demonstrated significant preventive benefits against osteoporosis, and favorable modulation of serum cholesterol, although the risk of venous thromboembolic complications persists, as with tamoxifen.[22] The efficacy of raloxifene against breast cancer is unknown; however, a new prevention trial is comparing it with tamoxifen in women with risk factors for breast cancer (STAR trial). This was prompted by the MORE (Multiple Outcome of Raloxifene Evaluation) trial results, which suggested reduced breast cancer incidence with raloxifene compared with placebo, although patients in this trial were not randomized or stratified by breast cancer risk factors.[23] Although efficacy in the realm of primary prevention does not constitute proof of recurrence reduction in women with established breast cancer, encouraging results from prevention trials may lead to subsequent investigation of raloxifene and similar drugs in established disease.

Other novel anti-estrogens are already being compared with tamoxifen in adjuvant RCTs of early breast cancer. In a Finnish study, the anti-estrogen toremifene is being compared with tamoxifen in postmenopausal NP breast cancer patients.[24] The study is powered to demonstrate equivalence with endpoints of DFS, OS and recurrence rate, and accrual of 1480 patients was completed in July 1999. An interim analysis, performed after randomization of the first 900 patients, showed a balanced distribution of patient and tumor characteristics, and no difference in recurrence (25.9% tamoxifen versus 23.3% toremifene, $p = 0.39$), or serious toxicity with 3.3 years of follow-up.[25] In two RCTs

(target accruals 1140 and 850), the International Breast Cancer Study Group (IBCSG) is comparing toremifene (60 mg/day × 5 years) with tamoxifen (20 mg/day × 5 years) in peri- and postmenopausal NP patients who are also receiving either AC (doxorubicin, cyclophosphamide) or AC followed by CMF (cyclophosphamide, methotrexate, 5-fluorouracil (5-FU)).[24] Results of all three trials should be available in the next 2–5 years.

The European Organization for Research and Treatment of Cancer (EORTC) is examining the potential benefit of preoperative Faslodex (ICI 182,780), a pure anti-estrogen, compared with placebo, in a randomized, blinded trial. The target accrual is 3500 women with operable breast cancer, and they will be followed by endpoints of DFS, OS and toxicity.[27] The study hopes to demonstrate any inhibitory effect that Faslodex may have on the development of new, or growth of pre-existing, metastases. Various new SERMs are being actively investigated in the metastatic setting, and are likely to shift into the adjuvant arena in the coming years.

Other hormonal therapies

Estrogen is the most well-studied hormonal stimulus for growth of breast cancer microsatellites that may give rise to future recurrences. However, as understanding of cell signalling, growth factors, growth factor receptors and transcription regulation increases, modulation of some of these factors may provide complementary protection against breast cancer recurrence. Examples under current clinical investigation include octreotide and retinoids, and others are likely to follow.

Octreotide, a somatostatin analogue, inhibits production of insulin-like growth factor, known to regulate cellular proliferation, and thus may provide additive or synergistic activity to tamoxifen. The National Cancer Institute of Canada

Table 32.2.2   Comparison of novel anti-estrogens[21]

Drug	Class	Biological characteristics compared with tamoxifen	Metastatic breast cancer studies
Toremifene	Triphenylethylene (tamoxifen analogue) Cross-resistance with tamoxifen	ER affinity: lower Endometrial effects: same Cytotoxic: by apoptosis $t_{\frac{1}{2}} = 5$ d; steady state 14 d Some LH/FSH ↓; SHBG ↑	Phase II, 1st line ER+, RR 48–68% dose 60 and 240 mg/d (3 trials) Randomized II, 1st line, (3 trials) RR inferior, better, equivalent to tamoxifen 40 mg/d III: 1st line, ER +/?, $n = 648$, RR 19% vs 21%; median OS 32 mo vs 38 mo (tamoxifen vs toremifene 60 mg/d)
Droloxifene[a]	Triphenylethylene (tamoxifen analogue) Cross-resistance with tamoxifen	ER affinity: 10 × higher Cytotoxic: G_0/G_1 arrest, Induces TGF-β $t_{\frac{1}{2}}$ short; steady state 5 h No long-term accumulation LH/FSH ↓; SHBG ↑	Phase II: pretreated pts, dose range 30–200 mg/d; RR 0–70%. No dose–response effect II: 1st line, $n = 369$, 268 assessable, doses of 20, 40, 100 mg/d, RR 30%, 47%, 44%. Well tolerated (hot flashes, nausea, fatigue)
Idoxifene	Triphenylethylene (tamoxifen analogue) Cross-resistance with tamoxifen	ER affinity: 2 × higher $t_{\frac{1}{2}} = 15$ h (3 × longer) Modest ↓ LH/FSH; no SHBG ↑	Phase II: 2nd line, $n = 20$, ER +/? PR 14%; NC 29% (1.4−14 mo); mild toxicity
TAT-59	Triphenylethylene (tamoxifen analogue) Cross-resistance with tamoxifen	ER affinity: higher ++ Metabolized to active drug	No available data
ICI 182, 780 (Faslodex)	Pure anti-estrogen Potential use after refractory to tamoxifen	Receptor affinity: competitive inhibitor of estradiol binding Destroys ER No agonist effect on endometrium LH/FSH, SHBG no effect	Neoadjuvant $n = 56$; 6 mg ($n = 21$) or 18 mg ($n = 16$) or none ($n = 19$) d1–7 i.m. ↓ in Ki67, PgR, ER in tumors compared with control Phase II, $n = 19$, tamoxifen-resistant, PR 37%, NC 32% (250 mg/m^2 i.m.), mild toxicity

Continued

Table 32.2.2 Continued			
Drug	Class	Biological characteristics compared with tamoxifen	Metastatic breast cancer studies
Raloxifene	Targeted anti-estrogen (agonist on bone, CVS; antagonist on endometrial, breast tissues)	ER affinity = estradiol affinity No endometrial agonist effect ↓ LDL cholesterol, maintains BMD	Phase III: 1st line, ER+, postmenopausal Ongoing, no results Primary prevention: phase III vs tamoxifen underway (MORE trial suggested benefit)[23]

[a]Being developed primarily for use in osteoporosis prevention.
ER, estrogen receptor; PgR, progesterone receptor; LH, luteinizing hormone; FSH, follicle-stimulating hormone; SHBG, sex-hormone-binding globulin; TGF-β, transforming growth factor β; RR, response rate; PR, partial response; NC, no change; ?, unknown; $t_{\frac{1}{2}}$, half-life; i.m., intramuscular; CVS, cardiovascular; LDL, low-density lipoprotein; BMD, bone mineral density.

Clinical Trials Group (NCIC-CTG) is examining the value of combining tamoxifen and octreotide in postmenopausal women with NN and NP breast cancer (trial MA.14). Target accrual is 850 patients with endpoints of RFS, OS and quality of life.

Preclinical data have suggested synergy of fenretinide, a vitamin A analogue, with tamoxifen.[28] Retinoic acid is an endogenous compound that induces cellular differentiation, thus reducing the capacity of cells to proliferate. Various synthetic retinoids, including fenretinide, are being explored for their anticancer activity. An American Intergroup trial (INT 0151) is addressing the value of 5 years of fenretinide added to tamoxifen (20 mg/5 years) compared with tamoxifen alone in NP, ER-positive postmenopausal breast cancer patients.[27]

Finally, the question of whether tamoxifen provides additional benefit in premenopausal NP breast cancer patients who have received either adjuvant ovarian ablation (OA) or chemotherapy remains unanswered. A discussion of tamoxifen in combination with chemotherapy can be found in the chemoendocrine section of this chapter. The combination of OA and tamoxifen is discussed below.

Ovarian ablation

Ovarian ablation is associated with a significant protective effect against recurrence and breast cancer mortality in premenopausal women.[29] By ablating ovarian function, hormone-sensitive breast tumors lose a hormonal stimulus for growth. It is logical to anticipate that the value of such treatment, if any, would be seen in a population whose hormonal milieu changes most significantly as a result of ablation, and whose tumors are most likely to be stimulated by hormones, i.e. in premenopausal women with ER- or PgR-positive disease. Since the first example of

OA for early breast cancer was reported in *The Lancet* in 1896, numerous randomized trials have addressed the role of OA in this disease.[30]

The EBCTCG meta-analysis comprehensively reviewed RCTs beginning before 1990, which compared OA with no hormonal manoeuvre, and for which at least 15 years of follow-up were available.[29] Data were retrieved for 12 trials, all of which began before 1980 and induced OA surgically or by irradiation, corresponding to 96% of patients randomized in such studies (data were unavailable for one trial of 143 women, and for four more recent trials that used luteinizing-hormone-releasing hormone (LHRH) agonists to suppress ovarian function). Age (< 50 and ⩾ 50) was used as a surrogate for menopausal status, because not all trials indicated menopausal status at randomization. Log-rank observed minus expected values were calculated for RFS and OS in each trial, and these were combined to determine an overall effect.

For women under 50 years or premenopausal

A summary of the trials that have compared OA with control or chemotherapy can be found in Table 32.2.3. The EBCTCG trial found that, for women aged under 50 years ($n = 2102$), the absolute risk reductions in recurrence and survival were 6% ($2p = 0.0007$) and 6.3% ($2p = 0.001$), respectively, and the corresponding numbers needed to treat (NNT) to avoid one recurrence and one death were about 17 and 16 women, respectively. Given that cytotoxic therapy frequently suppresses ovarian function, it is expected that the magnitude of benefit of OA would be lower in women who also received chemotherapy. In four trials, both the control and ablation groups received a common chemotherapy regimen, and, in one additional trial, a factorial design was used to randomize for both OA and chemotherapy. The incremental survival benefit of OA in the presence of chemotherapy was found to be smaller than when OA was the sole adjuvant therapy given; however, these observations were based on small numbers. Current trials are specifically addressing the value of combining OA and chemotherapy, compared with either alone.

The benefit of OA in axillary NP disease was addressed only in trials with no routine chemotherapy ($n = 696$, NP/unknown). The proportional risk reductions for recurrence and death were similar to those observed in the NN subset. The RFS rate was 24% in the control and 37.4% in the ablation groups ($2p = 0.0002$), a difference of 3.8 events per 100 women treated: NNT 7.5. The OS rate at 15 years was 29.2% in the control and 41.7% in the ablation groups ($2p = 0.0007$), a difference of 3.9 deaths per 100 women: NNT 8. No difference in the incidence of non-breast-cancer deaths was noted between the control and ablation groups.

The use of an untreated control arm limits the application of these findings because the current standard in NP breast cancer is to give some form of systemic adjuvant therapy. A more relevant question is whether OA is an equivalent, inferior or superior treatment to chemotherapy in premenopausal women. This has been the subject of more recent RCTs (Table 32.2.3); however, interpretation is somewhat limited by the immaturity of the results.

Thus far, neither therapeutic approach has proved superior. A Scandinavian trial randomized 732 women to OA or CMF between 1990 and 1998.[31] A preliminary analysis showed no difference in endpoints, with 101 and 103 events in the OA and CMF groups, and 79 and 66 deaths, respectively ($p = NS$). It is important to note that 68% of women in the CMF group developed amenorrhea, which may confound the value of chemotherapy independent of inducing hormone suppression.

Table 32.2.3   Results of RCTs of ovarian ablation (OA) control, or chemotherapy in women younger than 50

Trial	Population	n	Comments	Comparison arms	DFS (%)	p-value	OS (%)	p-value
EBCTCG[29]	Age <50 y	2012	Pooled results[a]	OA Control	61 55	2p 0.0007	53.9 47.6	2p 0.001
	NP or N unknown	696	Pooled results[a]	OA Control	24 37.4	2p 0.0002	41.7 29.2	2p 0.0007
Scandinavia[31]	NP or tumor > 5 cm Premenopausal	732	Preliminary results	OA CMF d1 q21d × 9	67 66	NS	78 82	NS
ABCSG 5[32]	NN/NP (54%) ER+ Premenopausal	1045	Preliminary results	OA (goserelin) + tamoxifen × 5 y CMF d1,8 q28d × 6	– –	– <0.02	– –	NS
CRC, Sweden, Italy[33]	NN/NP (44%) Premenopausal (43% had chemotherapy)	2631	Preliminary results	OA OA + tamoxifen Tamoxifen Control	0.77[b]	p 0.001 (95%CI 0.66–0.90)	0.85[b]	p 0.12 (95%CI 0.67–1.02)

[a]Results for DFS and OS are for 15 years.
[b]Hazard ratio for OA versus no-OA arms with 95% confidence intervals (95%CI).
DFS, disease-free survival rate; OS, overall survival rate; NP, node-positive; NN, node-negative; ER, estrogen receptor; CMF, cyclophosphamide, methotrexate and 5-FU.

Table 32.2.4   Ongoing adjuvant RCTs of ovarian ablation (OA) versus chemotherapy in node-positive (NP) breast cancer

Trial/group	Accrual target/actual	Population	Arms
GABG-ZEBRA	1600/1550	Pre-perimenopausal Age <50 y NP	OA (goserelin × 2 y) 6 CMF
IBCSG 11-93	760/116	Premenopausal NP	OA + Tamoxifen × 5 y OA + 4 AC + Tamoxifen × 5 y
DBCG 89B, CSB II-2	800/650	Premenopausal NP, ER+	OA 9 CMF
CRC	1000/1119 closed	Age <50 y	Control Tamoxifen Goserelin (LHRH agonist) + tamoxifen Goserelin
GFEA 06	430/332 closed, low accrual	Premenopausal 1–3 NP, ER+	OA (triptorelin) + tamoxifen × 3 y 6 FEC

DBCG, Danish Breast Cancer Cooperative Group; CRC, Cancer Research Campaign; GFEA, Groupe Français d'Etude Adjuvante. ER, estrogen receptor; CMF, cyclophosphamide, methotrexate and 5-FU; AC, doxorubicin and cyclophosphamide; LHRH, luteinizing-hormone-releasing hormone; FEC, 5-FU, epirubicin and cyclophosphamide.

Early results of an Austrian Breast Cancer Study Group (ABCSG) RCT comparing Bonadonna's CMF with the combination of OA (using goserelin, an LHRH agonist, 3.6 mg s.c. every 28 days × 3 years) and tamoxifen (20 mg/day × 5 years) in ER-positive breast cancer patients (1045 randomized, 157 recurrences, 56 deaths) also showed no difference in OS, with a median follow-up of 42 months, despite better RFS ($p < 0.02$) in the OA group.[32] Subset analysis of the NP population at the time of study maturity may provide some insight into the relative benefits of these therapies in NP disease.

Finally, a combined Cancer Research Campaign (CRC), Swedish and Italian group reported results of an RCT of OA (goserelin monthly for 26 months), OA and tamoxifen 20 mg/day × 2 years, tamoxifen alone or no hormonal intervention, using a 2 × 2 factorial design.[33] From the available data, it is not clear whether chemotherapy, which was given to 43% of the patients, was equally distributed. There were 261 and 330 events in the two groups that received OA and the two groups with no OA, respectively, and 140 and 165 deaths. The hazard ratio for RFS favored OA (0.77, 95%CI 0.66–0.90, $p = 0.001$), but was not significant for OS (0.85, 95%CI 0.67–1.02, $p = 0.12$) with 4.3 years of follow-up.

Several randomized trials comparing OA and chemotherapy are still accruing (Table 32.2.4). A definitive position on the value of OA compared with chemotherapy must be deferred until mature results from these comparative trials are available. Consideration of side effects and adverse sequelae of these therapeutic modalities must also enter the equation when comparing their benefits.

Negative impact

Ovarian ablation can be achieved through irradiation, surgical oophorectomy or the use of an LHRH agonist. Apart from a small mortality risk associated with any surgical procedure, these procedures do not carry risk of life-threatening complications. Sequelae related to early menopause are the only significant long-term morbidities. In contrast, a 1% mortality risk is generally accepted with chemotherapy. In addition, significant, although usually short-lived, morbidities are common with chemotherapy, including alopecia, nausea, vomiting, fatigue, infection, stomatitis, diarrhoea, neuropathy and various others, depending on the regimen. Serious long-term sequelae include the risk of alkylator- and anthracycline-induced leukaemias, anthracycline-induced cardiotoxicity and premature menopause. These are discussed in more detail in the chemotherapy section of this chapter.

Estrogen is cardioprotective, and thus women with prematurely induced menopause have increased risk of cardiac disease compared with premenopausal age-matched controls. However, with 15 years of follow-up, the OS benefit, which takes into account death from all causes (including breast cancer and cardiovascular causes), continues to favor OA and chemotherapy over no adjuvant therapy.[29] Longer follow-up may demonstrate a late convergence in the survival curves attributable to higher incidence of cardiovascular events in the treated groups.

Premature menopause is also associated with an increased risk of osteoporosis. The incidence of osteoporosis in older trials is hard to interpret in light of the currently available preventive measures, including supplemental calcium and bisphosphonates, which substantially reduce the risk of osteoporosis in postmenopausal women.[34,35]

In summary, the EBCTCG meta-analysis demonstrated clear benefits in RFS and OS for premenopausal women with NP breast cancer treated with OA compared with controls. Thus far, the comparison of OA with chemotherapy has not demonstrated a superior modality; however, mature results of some relevant trials are not available. The benefits of OA in the presence of chemotherapy can be estimated only from trials that randomized women who had chemotherapy to OA versus no OA. These are discussed in the chemoendocrine section of this chapter.

Women over 50 years

The EBCTCG overview examined the value of OA in the subset of women aged over 50.[29] No significant differences in RFS or OS were observed between the OA and control groups among the 1354 randomized patients (1018 deaths and 48 additional recurrences without death). This is not surprising given that the estrogen levels in this predominantly perimenopausal and postmenopausal age group are likely to be similar to castrate levels before OA takes place.

CHEMOTHERAPY

There are many active cytotoxic drugs against breast cancer, used singly and in combination. The adjuvant regimens currently in common use are CMF and anthracycline-based combinations. The oral Bonadonna schedule of CMF consists of oral cyclophosphamide 100 mg/m^2 on days 1–14, intravenous methotrexate 40 mg/m^2 on days 1 and 8, and intravenous 5-FU 600 mg/m^2 on days 1 and 8 every 28 days. In many patients, cyclophosphamide (600 mg/m^2) is given intravenously on days 1 and 8, to minimize nausea and improve compliance, although equivalence of the two regimens has never been established. Anthracycline-containing regimens in current use include AC (doxorubicin 60 mg/m^2 and intravenous cyclophosphamide 600 mg/m^2 on day 1 every 21 days), FAC/CAF (5-FU 500 mg/m^2, doxorubicin 50–60 mg/m^2, cyclophosphamide 500–600 mg/m^2 either every 21 days or days 1, 8 every 28 days), EC (epirubicin 60–75 mg/m^2 and cyclophosphamide 500–600 mg/m^2 i.v. on day 1 every 21 days), and FEC/CEF (5-FU 500–600 mg/m^2 either every 21 days or days 1, 8 every 28 days), epirubicin 60–120 mg/m^2, cyclophosphamide 500–600 mg/m^2). Many centres in Europe give several cycles of doxorubicin (75 mg/m^2) followed by CMF, according to a schedule developed by Bonadonna.

The EBCTCG systematic overview of polychemotherapy provides a comprehensive review of RCTs in adjuvant breast cancer therapy.[36] It summarizes results from 18 000 women in 47 trials of prolonged polychemotherapy versus no chemotherapy, 6000 women in 11 trials of anthracycline-containing regimens compared with CMF, and 6000 women in 11 trials of shorter versus longer chemotherapy. For the entire group, mortality was significantly reduced for women younger than 50 (27% RRR, $2p < 0.00001$) and older than 50 (11% RRR, $2p = 0.0001$). The improvement in 10-year OS for women with NP disease was greater for those younger than 50 – 11% absolute improvement (26% relative; from 42% to 53%) – but was also significant for women aged 50–69 – 3% absolute improvement (6.5% relative; from 46% to 49%). These benefits were irrespective of ER status, menopausal status and the added use of tamoxifen.

In the relatively few trials that compared polychemotherapy for 6 or less months with longer duration of the same regimens, there was a non-significant improvement in recurrence (7%, $2p = 0.06$) but no improvement in survival (−1%, NS) with longer therapy regardless of age group examined (<50 years old and all ages).

In randomized comparisons of anthracycline-containing and CMF regimens, most women (70%) were aged under 50 years. Anthracycline-containing chemotherapy was superior in reducing recurrence (12% greater relative reduction, $2p = 0.006$) and death (11% greater relative reduction, $2p = 0.02$); however, the 99% confidence interval for this observation reached zero, and results from some large comparative trials were not available. Two of these trials have since been reported in abstract form. An advantage of anthracyclines (CAF) over CMF, albeit marginal, was demonstrated in 4406 randomized, NN, breast cancer patients.[37] As well, comparison of CMF (600/40/600 mg/m^2 i.v. on day 1 for 21 days) and FEC (600/60/600 mg/m^2 i.v. on day 1 every 21 days) in 1195 patients, demonstrated OS superiority for FEC in the subset of premenopausal women with NN high-risk disease (CMF 83%, FEC 93%, $p < 0.01$), or with either high-risk NN or ER-negative NP disease (CMF 69%, FEC 76%, $p = 0.01$), but not for postmenopausal NP women.[38] However, a criticism of this study is the use of an inferior comparative CMF regimen. Several trials comparing CMF and anthracycline regimens are still ongoing (Table 32.2.5). As they are relatively small, they may not, however, show a significant difference between the two regimens if that difference is small, as suggested by current evidence.

Taxanes are a relatively new class of cytotoxic drugs that act by inhibiting disassembly of the microtubule complex during mitosis, and by inhibiting phosphorylation of Bcl-2, which is involved in anti-apoptosis.[39,40] They have

Table 32.2.5   Ongoing or recently completed RCTs of CMF versus anthracycline-containing regimens in adjuvant breast cancer therapy

Group/trial[a]	Accrual target/actual to date	Population	Comparison arms[b]
GEICAM 8701	998 closed	Early breast cancer	(1) 6 FAC (500/50/500 q21d) (2) 6 CMF (600/60/600 q21d)
GOIRC SANG 2B	480/446	NP 1–3 NN, T2, 3 or T1c high risk	(1) 6 CMFEV alternating (epirubicin 40 d1,8; vincristine 1.4 d1) (2) 6 CMF (i.v. d1,8 q28d)
ICCG C/6/89	–/861	NN high risk	(1) 6 FEC (600 d1,8/60 d1/600 d1/8 q28d) (2) 6 CMF (600 d1,8/40 d1/600 d1,8 q28d)
DBGC 89D CSB II-2	1200/1148 closed	Premenopausal NP, ER–	(1) 9 FEC (2) 9 CMF
UK	2000		(1) AC or EC (2) CMF
Hutchins[37]	4406	NN	(1) CAF (2) CMF
DiLeo[52]	777	NP	(1) CMF (2) EC (60/500 d1 q21d) (3) EC (100/830 d1 q21d)

[a]Where a reference is given, the study has been reported in abstract form.
[b]CMFEV, cyclophosphamide 600 cycle 1,2,4,5, methotrexate 40 cycle 1,3,4,6, 5-FU 600 cycle 2,3,5,6, epirubicin 40 cycle 1–6 (all d1,8), and vincristine 1.4 d1 cycle 1–6; see text for other chemotherapy regimen abbreviations; all doses are in mg/m^2.
GEICAM, Grupo Español de Investigación en Cáncer de Mama; GOIRC, Italian Oncology Group for Clinical Research; ICCG, International Collaboration Cancer Group; NP, node-positive; NN, node-negative; ER, estrogen receptor.

established activity in breast cancer and different side effects from anthracyclines, with no cardiotoxicity, but potentially significant neurotoxicity. Large adjuvant RCTs are now under way, comparing taxane- with anthracycline-based regimens, and with the combination of both either concurrently or sequentially.

Interim results from the collaborative trial (CALGB 9344) of the CALGB, ECOG, SWOG and NCIC-CTG suggest improved DFS rate (90%, 86%, $p = 0.008$) and OS rate (97%, 95%, $p = 0.04$) for patients randomized to AC followed by four cycles of paclitaxel (175 mg/m^2 every 21 days) compared with AC alone.[41] These results are clearly encouraging, based on 540 events and 22 months of median follow-up in 3170 randomized patients, and they have recently been confirmed at 30 months of follow-up. Nevertheless, they are still somewhat immature, and by no means provide level I evidence for the routine use of taxanes in adjuvant therapy.

A wealth of evidence about the efficacy of taxanes should be available within the next decade, as results mature in ongoing adjuvant and neoadjuvant paclitaxel and docetaxel RCTs (Table 32.2.6). Metastatic trials suggest better response with single-agent docetaxel than with single-agent doxorubicin, and with anthracycline–taxane combinations than with AC.[42,43] If this proves to be the case in the adjuvant setting, a substantial change in adjuvant chemotherapy practice is likely to follow. However, adjuvant taxanes remain within the experimental arena for the time being.

Recent evidence suggests that women with tumors that overexpress c-ErbB-2 – a transmembrane tyrosine kinase with sequence homology to the epidermal growth factor receptor – may have inferior outcome with chemotherapy regimens that do not contain anthracyclines.[44–46] However, the results from different trials are conflicting, and the role of c-ErbB-2 in predicting response to chemotherapy remains controversial. Trastuzumab (Herceptin), a humanized monoclonal antibody directed against c-ErbB-2, has been shown to improve efficacy of chemotherapy regimens and survival in metastatic disease among women with c-ErbB-2 overexpressing tumors (25–30% of breast cancers).[47,48] An unexpected finding was a higher incidence of cardiotoxicity in the Herceptin/AC arm than in the AC arm. In the pivotal metastatic trial of Herceptin given as a single agent, six cases (2.8%) of symptomatic cardiotoxicity were observed; all of these patients had previous anthracyclines or significant antecedent cardiac history.[49] Although the mechanism remains unknown, Herceptin may have a cardiotoxic effect, and this would limit its utility in the adjuvant setting. However, if a reduction in or elimination of the excess relapse risk associated with c-ErbB-2 overexpression can be achieved with Herceptin, its use in this population may be worth the potential cardiac risk, even in the adjuvant setting. Carefully designed and monitored adjuvant clinical trials are now starting, with the aim of evaluating the risk–benefit ratio associated with the use of this innovative anticancer agent in early breast cancer.

Negative impact

In the EBCTCG overview, there was no excess of non-breast-cancer deaths in the comparison of trials of polychemotherapy versus no chemotherapy: death ratio 0.89 ($p = \text{NS}$). This was true for both vascular (death hazard ratio 0.99) and other neoplastic (death hazard ratio 0.75) deaths. Among women younger than 50, the number of deaths from causes other than breast cancer was low and there was no significant difference in the incidence according to adjuvant chemotherapy versus none. Although small (less than 1% with conventional doses), there is a risk of secondary leukemia with both anthracycline- and alkylator-based chemotherapy, and this risk increases with dose escalation.[50,51] Moreover, other long-term sequelae include cardiotoxicity and early menopause, with its attendant symptoms, increased coronary heart disease and osteoporosis risks. Although these may not have an impact on overall mortality, they may significantly alter long-term quality of life, and must be considered alongside the expected benefits in any discussion of adjuvant chemotherapy.

Although the benefit of chemotherapy in NP breast cancer is clearly evident for women younger than 50 (11% mortality reduction), it is more modest in women aged 50–69 years (3% absolute mortality reduction). There is an upper age limit for most trials, so the magnitude of

Table 32.2.6   Ongoing adjuvant RCTs with taxanes in node-positive breast cancer[27]

Group/trial	Accrual target/actual to date	Population	Comparison arms[a]
BIG 02-98	2200/800	NP	(1) 4 A (75 q21d) → 3 CMF (B) (2) 4 AC (60/600) → 3 CMF (B) (3) 3 A → 3 Doce (100 q21d) → 3 CMF (B) (4) 4 A Doce (50/75 q21d) → 3 CMF (B)
FNCLCC + Belgium	1600/700	NP	(1) 6 FEC 100 (500/100/500 q21d) (2) 3 FEC 100 → 3 Doce (100 q21d)
GABGV	1000/79	T2–3, N0–2, M0	(1) 4 A + Doce + tamoxifen → Surgery (2) 4 A + Doce → (3) 24-week AC–Doce + tamoxifen → Surgery
GONO MIG 5	1000/735	NP	(1) 6 CEF (600/60/600 q21d) (2) 4 ET (90/175 q21d)
ICCG	800/130	NP postmenopausal	(1) 6 E (50 d1,8 d28d) (2) 4 E → 3 Doce (100 q21d)
NCIC-CTG MA.21	1200/not open	NP, high-risk NN Age <60 y	(1) CEF (2) EC + G-CSF → T (3) AC → T
Intergroup S9623	???	4–9 NP	(1) 3 A → 3 T → 3 C (2) 4 AC → High dose with SCT
NSABP B-26	Closed	–	(1) 4 AC (2) 4 AC → 4 T
NSABP B-28	2450/500	NP	(1) 4 AC (60/600) (2) 4 AC → 4 T (225/3 h/q21d)
NSABP B-27	2400/1900+ closes 04/00	Neoadjuvant Operable	(1) 4 AC (60/600) → Surgery/tamoxifen (2) 4 AC → 4 Doce → Surgery/tamoxifen (3) 4 AC → Surgery → 4 Doce/tamoxifen
ECTO	1250/583	Neoadjuvant Tumor > 2 cm, operable	(1) Surgery → 4 A → 4 CMF (2) Surgery → 4 AT → 4 CMF (3) 4 AT → 4 CMF → Surgery
GABG V	200/250 closed pRR is endpoint	Neoadjuvant Tumor ≥ 3 cm, operable	(1) A + Doce high dose → Surgery (2) A + Doce standard dose → Surgery
BCIRG TAX 316	1000/1500 closed	NP, <65 years	(1) Doce–AC × 6 (2) FAC × 6

[a]A, doxorubicin; Doce, docetaxel; E, epirubicin; T, paclitaxel; G-CSF, granulocyte colony-stimulating factor; SCT, stem cell transplantation; ET, E 90 + T175 (over 3 h) d1 q21d × 4 cycles; AT, doxorubicin + T (doses not available); see text for other chemotherapy regimen abbreviations; (B), Bonadonna. Doses are mg/m².
FNCLCC, Fédération Nationale des Centres de Lutte contre le Cancer; GONO MIG, Gruppo Oncologico Nord Ovest–Mammella Intergruppo; ECTO, European Cooperative Trial in Operable Breast Cancer; pRR, pathological response rate; NP, node-positive; NN, node-negative.

benefit and toxicity observed in these trials cannot be easily generalized to women older than 69. Given the low absolute benefit in women aged 50–69, and an estimated 1% mortality risk of chemotherapy, coupled with substantial short-term morbidity, the decision to give chemotherapy to these women must include consideration of individual risk, which can be estimated by examining well-established prognostic factors.

Women aged 50–65 with relatively high risk of relapse, and women with ER-negative tumors, who are unlikely to derive significant benefit from adjuvant tamoxifen, can expect a higher relative benefit from chemotherapy. In these individuals, the potential sequelae of chemotherapy are more justifiable. In contrast, for older women with relatively low-risk features, such as grade I, ER-positive and low lymph-node burden cancers, the added benefit of chemotherapy to tamoxifen, if any, may be too low to justify the attendant toxicity. For women older than 65, competing causes of death become more significant, and tolerance to chemotherapy tends to decline. These factors should be strongly weighed against prognostic factors in the consideration to offer chemotherapy to elderly women.

For younger and premenopausal women, the decision to offer CMF or anthracycline-based chemotherapy should also take into account absolute relapse risk. Mounting evidence suggests a small but real benefit of anthracycline-containing chemotherapy over CMF. Keeping in mind the toxicity differences between anthracyclines and CMF at conventional doses, particularly cardiac, patients with NP disease should be offered anthracycline-containing chemotherapy (in the absence of pre-existing cardiac disease or significant cardiac risk factors), given their high risk of relapse. Prospective evaluation of c-ErbB-2 and other predictive factors may define a population for which anthracyclines are definitively superior, and thus enable individual tailoring of

chemotherapy options. Furthermore, mature results of adjuvant taxane and Herceptin trials may dramatically change the standard of adjuvant chemotherapy, and may tip the risk–benefit ratio more strongly in favor of routine chemotherapy in older women.

CHEMOENDOCRINE THERAPY

The essential question in considering combined therapy for NP breast cancer is whether, in women with strong indications for chemotherapy (namely pre- and postmenopausal women with ER-negative tumors or high-risk features), the addition of hormonal therapy further improves outcome, and whether chemotherapy adds further benefits in women for whom adjuvant hormonal therapy is indicated (postmenopausal women with ER-positive tumors and other low-risk features for relapse, and premenopausal women with ER-positive tumors who have chosen ovarian ablation).

The EBCTCG overview of polychemotherapy demonstrated a highly significant improvement in 10-year OS for women younger than 50 who received chemotherapy, compared with controls, for NP breast cancer (11% absolute, 26% relative). For older women, the risk reduction was still significant, but of a modest magnitude (3% absolute, 6.5% relative).[36] In a separate EBCTCG meta-analysis, tamoxifen was associated with an 11% absolute gain in 10-year OS among women (all ages) with NP disease, again irrespective of ER status and adjuvant chemotherapy.[1] These results suggest that the activities of chemotherapy and hormonal therapies are complementary.

Postmenopausal women
ER-positive and low-risk tumors
The EBCTCG overviews found that, for older women, the small survival gain with chemotherapy and the larger gain seen with tamoxifen adju-

vant therapy were independent of ER status, menopausal status and combination with another systemic therapy. However, as a result of the heterogeneity of different studies, and the loss of power associated with subset analyses, this overview was unable to address the benefit of chemoendocrine therapy reliably in specific risk groups, such as postmenopausal ER-positive NP and ER-negative NP women.

A large body of level I evidence supports the use of adjuvant tamoxifen for a significant reduction in both recurrence and death in postmenopausal women with ER-positive NP breast cancer. In contrast, large RCTs comparing adjuvant chemotherapy or hormonal therapy with chemoendocrine therapy have consistently failed to demonstrate a survival advantage for either arm in this population (Table 32.2.7). Only four trials enrolled a pure population of postmenopausal, NP, ER-positive breast cancer patients, and in none was there a difference between the two arms, despite the fact that in only one was tamoxifen given for 5 years.[53] For completeness, all trials of tamoxifen versus chemotherapy/tamoxifen that included postmenopausal women are described below (all in NP disease unless otherwise indicated).

The largest recent study, conducted by the IBCSG, was a 2×2 design that accrued 1266 (1212 evaluable) women between 1986 and 1993.[54] All patients received tamoxifen (5 years), and randomization was to no additional therapy (group A, $n = 306$), early CMF (group B, $n = 302$), delayed CMF (group C, $n = 308$) or early plus delayed CMF (group D, $n = 296$). Analysis of DFS and OS was carried out using the ITT principle after 60 months of median follow-up. Chemotherapy-related toxicity of common toxicity criteria (CTC) grade > 2 was 11%. There was no significant difference in 5-year OS ($p = 0.70$ for the comparison of all four groups), despite better DFS for the comparisons of any

chemotherapy (groups B, C, D) and early chemotherapy (groups B + D) versus tamoxifen alone (group A). Among patients who had ER-positive disease (77%), compared with tamoxifen alone, there was a RRR for recurrence of 33% (hazard ratio 0.67, 95%CI 0.50–0.91) for early chemotherapy, and 21% (hazard ratio 0.78, 95%CI 0.58–1.04) for late chemotherapy, suggesting that any benefit of adding chemotherapy is maximized when it is given early. However, the lack of OS improvement in this large RCT suggests that the actual benefit is small and may not warrant the attendant toxicity.

A 3-arm study of similar magnitude compared 5 years of tamoxifen ($n = 361$) with tamoxifen plus six cycles of CAF (100 mg/m² days 1–14, 30 mg/m² days 1–8, 500 mg/m² days 1 and 8 every 28 days) with the tamoxifen beginning either with (CAFT, $n = 546$) or after (CAF + T, $n = 563$) chemotherapy.[55] Results were reported in 1997, when an interim analysis demonstrated a significantly better DFS for CAFT compared with tamoxifen. For the two chemotherapy arms, the combined 4-year DFS rate was 79%, compared with 72% for the tamoxifen arm ($p = 0.001$); however, a survival advantage has not yet been demonstrated (85% versus 86%, $p = 0.84$). Follow-up is short, and the full publication of mature data is awaited.

The NCIC-CTG compared CMF and tamoxifen (30 mg/days for 2 years) with tamoxifen in an RCT of 705 postmenopausal ER- or PR-positive patients stratified according to local therapy received, number of positive nodes, level of hormone-positivity and time since menopause.[56] Of the 353 chemotherapy-randomized patients 84% completed the six cycles of intravenous CMF (day 1 every 21 days). No differences in 5-year DFS rate (64% and 61%, $p = 0.8$), locoregional RFS rate (56% and 49%, $p = 0.72$) or OS rate (82% and 80%, $p = 0.94$) were observed between the chemotherapy/tamoxifen and

Table 32.2.7   Adjuvant RCTs of tamoxifen versus tamoxifen plus chemotherapy in postmenopausal ER-positive and -negative, node-positive breast cancer

Trial/group	n	ER status	Intervention[a] A (tamoxifen)	B (chemotherapy + tamoxifen)	5-year DFS (%) A	B	5-year OS (%) A	B
NCIC-CTG[56] 1997	705	+	Tamoxifen 30 mg/d × 2 y	6 CMF i.v. day 1 q21d + tamoxifen 30 mg/d × 2 y	61	64 p 0.80	80	82 p 0.94
ICCG[58] 1999	604	±	Tamoxifen 20 mg/d × 4 y	6 Epirubicin 50 d1,8 i.v. q4w + tamoxifen 20 mg/d × 4 y	73.7	62.1 p 0.02	80.6	77 p 0.46
INT100[55]	1558 (1470)[b]	+	Tamoxifen 20 mg/d × 5 y	CAF + paclitaxel CAF → paclitaxel	72 p 0.001	79 p 0.84	85	86
IBCSG[54] 1997	1266	±	A: tamoxifen 20 mg/d × 5 y B: tamoxifen + CMF months 1,2,3	C: tamoxifen + CMF months 9,12,15 D: tamoxifen + CMF months 1,2, 3,9,12,15	A: 55 B: 64 C: 59 D: 63	p NA	A: 77 B: 74 C: 74 D: 76	p 0.70
Gelber meta-analysis[53] 1996	323	±	Tamoxifen × 12 months + prednisone	12 CMF + tamoxifen × 12 months + prednisone	33.5	44.8 p 0.02	44.9	55.1 p NS
	72	±	Tamoxifen × 24 months	8 AC + tamoxifen × 24 months	35.1	45.7 p NA	51.3	54.3 p NA
	91	±	Tamoxifen × 36 months	12 CMFVP + tamoxifen × 36 months	53.2	68.2 p 0.04	59.6	75.0 p 0.11
	59	+	Tamoxifen × 12 months	6 CMF + tamoxifen × 12 months	62.0	46.6 p NA	65.5	60.0 p NA
	593	+	Tamoxifen × 12 months	12 CMFVP + tamoxifen × 12 months	66.8	68.7 p NS	77.0	74.1 p NS
	113	±	Tamoxifen × 24 months	24 CMF + tamoxifen × 24 months	38.8	50.0 p NS	71.6	58.7 p 0.06
	210	+	Tamoxifen × 60 months	6 CMF, 4 epirubicin + tamoxifen × 60 months	76.0	80.0 p 0.10	89.4	90.6 p 0.70
	1233	±	Tamoxifen × 12 months	8 CMF + tamoxifen × 12 months	60.2	67.9 p NA	75.0	76.4 p NA
	1226	<60 y+ >60 y±	Tamoxifen × 60 months	4 AC or 17 PF or 17 PAF all with tamoxifen × 60 months	79.7	88.0 p 0.0004	91.4	94.2 p 0.04

[a]PF, melphalan 4 p.o. d1–5 + 5-FU 300 d1–5 q6wk × 17 cycles; PAF, as PF + doxorubicin 30 d1, 21 q6wk to maximum of 300 mg/m²; see text for chemotherapy regimen abbreviations; all doses are in mg/m² unless stated otherwise.

[b]Results from interim analysis on 1470 patients; 4-year DFS and OS figures.

ER, estrogen receptor; DFS, disease-free survival rate; OS, overall survival rate; NA, not available; NS, not significant.

tamoxifen arms, respectively. Two toxic deaths occurred in the combination arm. Although the CMF regimen used in this trial has been shown to be inferior to the oral Bonadonna–CMF regimen in metastatic disease, they have never been directly compared in adjuvant therapy.[57] Nevertheless, proponents of chemoendocrine therapy might argue that the lack of superiority of the combination arm may be related to delivery of an inferior chemotherapy regimen.

A multicenter RCT, conducted by the International Collaborative Cancer Group (ICCG), compared low-dose epirubicin plus tamoxifen ($n = 301$) with tamoxifen alone ($n = 303$) in postmenopausal patients.[58] Analysis of RFS and OS was performed using ITT, with a median follow-up of 4.8 years. Of the patients 75% had ER-positive (50%) or ER-unknown disease, 38% had four to nine positive axillary nodes, and 58% had more than nine positive nodes. Among patients randomized to the combination, 79% completed all cycles of epirubicin, with a 95% total dose density; 31 patients received no chemotherapy. Non-significant trends favoring the combination were observed in 5-year RFS rate (73.7% and 62.1%) and OS rate (80.6% and 77%). There was no subset analysis according to number of involved nodes. Toxicity was higher in the combination arm: one sudden death; two congestive heart failures; eight of the nine thromboembolic complications; and five hematological malignancies (two acute myelogenous leukemia (AML), three other).

In 1996, a systematic overview reviewed the available data from earlier RCTs of tamoxifen alone versus chemotherapy plus tamoxifen in women aged over 50 who had axillary NP breast cancer.[53] Nine trials, comprising 3920 women with an average follow-up of 7 years, were analysed using Q-TWiST (quality-adjusted time without symptoms or toxicity) for RFS and OS. Four trials were restricted to ER-positive

tumors, and four included both ER-negative and ER-positive tumors. No difference in quality-adjusted survival time was found. Patients treated with chemotherapy/tamoxifen gained 5.4 months of RFS and 2 months of OS ($p = $ NS); however, this was at the expense of 2–24 months of chemotherapy. Although, in five of these trials, tamoxifen was given for only 1 or 2 years (which we know from the EBCTCG overview is inferior to longer therapy), a significant difference was still not apparent, strengthening the argument that chemotherapy might not provide significant additional benefit in ER-positive postmenopausal women who receive tamoxifen.

Several RCTs have included both pre- and postmenopausal women. One such multicenter study randomized 613 women with ER-positive disease to tamoxifen (20 mg/day $\times$ 2 years) or tamoxifen plus one cycle of chemotherapy (doxorubicin 20 mg/m^2 and vincristine 1 mg/m^2 day 1, cyclophosphamide 300 mg/m^2, methotrexate 25 mg/m^2 and 5-FU 600 mg/m^2 day 36, all intravenously).[59] Using ITT analysis, the respective 5-year RFS and OS rates were 62% and 64.4% for the tamoxifen arm, and 60% and 61% for the combination arm ($p = $ NS). A subset analysis in postmenopausal women was not carried out.

The IBCSG Trials I–IV enrolled pre- and postmenopausal NP women in four different trials comparing different combinations of CMF and hormonal therapy (tamoxifen in postmenopausal women, OA in premenopausal women).[60] For the comparison of observation versus tamoxifen/prednisone (Pr) versus CMF/tamoxifen/Pr, 10-year OS rates were 45%, 53% and 61% ($p = 0.04$) for patients with one to three positive nodes ($n = 86$, 83, 89 for the three treatment arms, respectively), and 25%, 26% and 35% ($p = 0.27$) for four or more positive nodes ($n = 70$, 70, 65). There was insufficient power to make separate statistical comparisons between the hormone and hormone/chemotherapy arms.

A few trials in postmenopausal NP breast cancer have compared chemoendocrine therapy with chemotherapy alone, rather than hormonal therapy.[61,62] These studies show borderline improved outcome for the combination arm, or no difference. In a subset of 259 women aged 50 years or more with high-risk breast cancer (one to three NP and ER-negative, or four or more NP) from an RCT of the German Gynecological Adjuvant Breast Group (GABG), superior DFS ($p = 0.01$) and a trend towards improved survival were observed in the AC/tamoxifen arm compared with AC alone.[61] However, for the entire study population ($n = 471$), no significant difference was observed in either endpoint. Similarly, in the IBCSG I–IV trials, there was no significant difference in 10-year OS rate for CMFPr ($n = 112$) versus CMFPr/hormonotherapy ($n = 125$): 37% and 45%, respectively ($p = 0.34$) among women older than 40.

Taken together, outcome and toxicity evidence from meta-analyses and individual trials support the conclusion that, for postmenopausal women with hormone-sensitive NP tumors, adjuvant therapy should include at least a hormonal agent, and that the magnitude of the added benefit of chemotherapy is small. Although no survival advantage has been conclusively demonstrated, large comparative trials with an anthracycline-based regimen have consistently shown improved DFS over tamoxifen alone, whereas CMF-containing trials of similar magnitude have not. Studies that enrolled patients with four or more positive nodes were not sufficiently powered to allow subset analyses in ER-positive high-node-burden disease, a group that might derive the largest relative benefit from combined-modality therapy. Nevertheless, in this setting, the addition of anthracycline-based chemotherapy to tamoxifen may be preferable. Several postmenopausal NP chemoendocrine versus hormone studies are still ongoing (Table 32.2.8),

and they will, it is hoped, contribute sufficient patient numbers to reach a confident conclusion about the value of combined therapy in this latter group.

ER-negative and high-risk tumors

In postmenopausal women with ER-negative, NP disease, which carries a high risk of relapse, systemic therapy is indicated to reduce recurrence and breast cancer death. Tamoxifen is not effective as single therapy in ER-negative tumors, and the incremental value of adding it to chemotherapy is likely to be negligible. Although some comparative studies addressing this question have included ER-negative patients, analysis of these subsets involves small numbers and unreliable statistical comparisons.[54,58,62]

In the IBCSG 2×2 trial (tamoxifen versus tamoxifen plus three different CMF schedules), the DFS rate was lower for patients with ER-negative compared with ER-positive tumors in all groups (ER-negative: 51%, 51%, 38%, 42%; ER-positive: 57%, 69%, 64%, 70% for groups A, B, C, D, respectively).[54] For the comparison of early chemotherapy (B and D) and no early chemotherapy (A and C), the recurrence hazard ratio for ER-negative tumors was 0.85 (95%CI 0.61–1.17). This non-significant benefit is most probably the result of subset analysis with small numbers. Similarly, in the ICCG study (tamoxifen versus tamoxifen/epirubicin), the number of ER-negative patients was too small (82 epirubicin/tamoxifen, 75 tamoxifen) to provide a meaningful statistical comparison in this subgroup.[58]

In the comparison of three and six cycles of CMF (500/40/600 mg/m^2 i.v. days 1 and 8 every 28 days), with ($n = 184$) and without ($n = 189$) tamoxifen (30 mg/day $\times$ 2 years), the proportion of ER-negative tumors was 37% and 39%, respectively.[62] Accrual fell short of the planned 1500 patients (actual 473) and 240 events (actual 187

Table 32.2.8   Ongoing adjuvant RCTs of chemoendocrine therapy in node-positive postmenopausal breast cancer[27]

Group/trial	Accrual target/actual to date	Population	Comparison arms[a]
ABCSG 09	660/165	ER+ NN, NP; grade 3	Tamoxifen 20 mg × 5 y Tamoxifen + 4 EC (60/600 q21d)
EORTC 10901	1816/1526	NN, NP	Chemotherapy[b] + tamoxifen 20 mg × 3 y Chemotherapy[b] only [b]6 CMF/FAC/CAF/CEF or 4 AC/EC
GABG IVD	950/730	ER−; age ≤70 y NN, 1–3 NP ER−; age ≤70 y 4–9 NP	3 CMF 3 CMF + tamoxifen × 5 y 4 EC → 3 CMF 4 EC → 3 CMF → Tamoxifen × 5 y
IKA-IKMN	500/110 closed, low accrual	NP	Tamoxifen 30 mg × 3 y 4 EC + tamoxifen × 3 y
NCIC-CTG MA-12	800/659	Pre- and perimenopausal NP, high-risk NN	Chemotherapy + tamoxifen Chemotherapy + placebo
UKCCCR-ABC	2000/1241	NP and NN	Tamoxifen Tamoxifen + chemotherapy
GFEA 07	546/334	1–3 NP, age <65 y, ER+	Tamoxifen 30 mg/d × 3 y 6 FEC (500/50/500 q21d) + tamoxifen
GFEA 08	534/321	NP, age >65 y, ER+	Tamoxifen 30 mg/d × 3 y Tamoxifen + epirubicin 30 weekly × 2 q3w × 8 cycles
GEICAM 9401	1000/380	NP Sequential vs concomitant	4 EC → Tamoxifen (20 mg/d × 5 y) 4 EC + tamoxifen

[a]See text for chemotherapy regimen abbreviations; all doses are in mg/m^2 unless stated otherwise.
EORTC, European Organization for the Research and Treatment of Cancer; IKA, Integraal Kanker Amsterdam; UKCCCR, United Kingdom Co-ordinating Committee on Cancer Research; ER, estrogen receptor; NN, node-negative; NP, node-positive.

recurrences, 130 deaths) and there were non-significant 5-year hazard ratios for RFS (0.85; 95%CI 0.62–1.17, $p = 0.32$) and OS (0.97; 95%CI 0.67–1.41, $p = 0.89$) favoring tamoxifen. No subset analysis according to ER status was reported.

In ER-negative NP disease, there is insufficient comparative evidence of chemotherapy versus chemotherapy/tamoxifen to make conclusions about the added value of tamoxifen. However, given that there is no substrate (ER and PgR) for tamoxifen to exert its main mode of action, it is likely that the added benefit of tamoxifen to chemotherapy in preventing recurrence is negligible and does not warrant the side effects, however small. Nevertheless, the observed reduction in contalateral breast cancer with adjuvant tamoxifen may change this approach.

For postmenopausal women with high relapse risk for reasons other than negative hormone receptors, such as high positive node burden or high grade, available data do not demonstrate superiority of chemoendocrine therapy using standard chemotherapy doses. However, the trials described above, many of which included women with up to nine positive nodes, were not powered to detect small differences in outcome in nodal subsets. Many of them did stratify for the number of positive nodes, however, and therefore pooled results from similar trials may provide a clue as to the value of chemoendocrine therapy for this population.

In the GBSG four-arm trial, there was a survival trend favoring the chemotherapy/tamoxifen arm for women with PgR-positive, one to three NP disease (low risk), but no difference for the group with PgR-negative, more than three NP (high-risk) disease.[62] Although the GABG trial of AC/tamoxifen versus AC demonstrated better DFS ($p = 0.01$) and an OS trend favoring the combination in a subset of women aged 50 or over with ER-negative, one to three NP and more

than 4 NP breast cancer, no significant difference was observed in either endpoint for the study population as a whole.[61]

Despite the lack of evidence supporting the superiority of chemoendocrine therapy in postmenopausal women with high nodal burden, high-grade or large primary tumors, the toxicity associated with chemotherapy is more acceptable in the light of their excessive risk of relapse. It must be remembered that lack of evidence supporting the combination may be the result of insufficiently powered studies, or inferior chemotherapy regimens, rather than lack of efficacy. Given that tamoxifen is associated with a larger magnitude of benefit than chemotherapy in postmenopausal women, until evidence suggests otherwise, the treatment plan for postmenopausal women with high risk of relapse should always include a hormonal agent if the ER status is positive. Consideration to add chemotherapy should be made for each individual on the basis of absolute risk, keeping in mind the added toxicity and uncertain magnitude of benefit. In ER-negative disease, chemotherapy alone should be given, because the addition of tamoxifen is unlikely to influence the outcome.

Premenopausal women

In premenopausal women, randomized comparisons of adjuvant chemotherapy and OA have thus far demonstrated equivalence in NP disease. The value of combined hormonal and cytotoxic drugs has also been extensively examined.

Tamoxifen and chemotherapy

On the basis of the EBCTCG findings, many oncologists routinely prescribe tamoxifen to premenopausal women after adjuvant chemotherapy. However, the overview examined the benefit of tamoxifen (independent of chemotherapy) in younger women of all risks (NP and NN), and individual studies of chemotherapy versus chemotherapy/tamoxifen in NP disease have failed to demonstrate an advantage for the combination. The volume of mature evidence is small, and several large studies addressing the value of tamoxifen in premenopausal women after chemotherapy are still accruing patients and were not included in the overview. Thus, future results of trials such as the NCIC-CTG MA-12 (placebo or tamoxifen after adjuvant chemotherapy in pre- and perimenopausal, high-risk, NN and NP breast cancer), the EORTC 10901 (CT followed by tamoxifen or observation) and ICCG C/9/91 (FEC 50 or 75 followed by hormone or no hormone therapy) may provide more reliable estimates of benefit.

Ovarian ablation and chemotherapy

The EBCTCG overview of OA examined the value of OA in trials that combined OA and chemotherapy.[29] For women aged under 50 years (NP and NN), the benefit attributable to OA compared with control was 10% and 8% for DFS and OS, respectively, in patients who had both OA and chemotherapy, compared with 25% and 24%, respectively, for OA alone. Both treatment approaches were statistically better than their respective control arms ($2p < 0.001$). This suggests that some of the benefit of chemotherapy derives from induction of transient or permanent ovarian suppression. The overview did not address the benefits of combined therapy in NP disease specifically, but several trials have examined this population.

SWOG compared adjuvant CMFVP ($n = 140$; cyclophosphamide 60 mg/m^2 per day for 1 year, methotrexate 15 mg/m^2, 5-FU 400 mg/m^2 i.v. weekly $\times$ 1 year, vincristine 0.625 mg/m^2 i.v. weekly for 10 weeks, and prednisone in decreasing doses from 30 mg/m^2 per day for 10 weeks) with CMFVP plus surgical OA ($n = 148$) in premenopausal, NP, ER-positive breast cancer patients.[63] Stratification was according to the number of involved nodes and type of primary surgery. With a median follow-up of 7.7 years, and a power to detect a 15% difference in relapse and death using ITT, the OS rate was 71% and 73% ($p = 0.70$) for the chemotherapy and combination arms (43 and 38 deaths), respectively, with no significant difference in toxicity.

The IBCSG II trial enrolled 327 premenopausal women with four or more positive nodes in an RCT of CMFPr versus CMFPr + oophorectomy, and found no OS difference with 10 years of follow-up.[60] For the subset of 107 ER-positive patients, there was a non-significant OS trend favoring the combination (combination 41%, CMFPr 30%, $p = 0.12$).

In a three-arm RCT, ECOG compared chemotherapy alone (CAF, 100 mg/m^2 p.o. days 1–14 30/500 mg/m^2 i.v. days 1 and 8 every 28 days $\times$ 6) with CAF + OA (goserelin 3.6 mg s.c. every 28 days $\times$ 5 years), and with CAF, OA + tamoxifen (20 mg/days $\times$ 5 years) in premenopausal women with ER-positive, NP breast cancer.[64] Fifty-nine percent of the patients had one to three nodes, and 29% had four or more nodes involved. With 6 years of median follow-up, no difference in 5-year OS rate has been observed (85%, 86%, 86%, respectively) among 1504 randomized patients.

In summary, for premenopausal women who have ER-positive, NP breast cancer associated with a non-extreme recurrence risk (up to 10 involved nodes, low grade, small size tumor, etc.), either OA or chemotherapy can be recommended, given that cumulative evidence from several large studies suggests equivalence. Chemotherapy may be preferable in women with a higher nodal burden, given a higher absolute risk of recurrence, and the cytotoxic activity against micrometastases characteristic of chemotherapy. Several large ongoing trials (Table 32.2.9) may provide more definitive consensus about the value of combining chemother-

Table 32.2.9   Ongoing adjuvant RCTs of ovarian ablation (OA) versus ovarian ablation + chemotherapy in premenopausal node-positive breast cancer[27]

Group/trial	Target/ actual accrual	Population	Comparison arms
UKCCCR-ABC	4000/2569	Pre/perimenopausal NP and NN	Tamoxifen Tamoxifen + chemotherapy Tamoxifen + OA Tamoxifen + chemotherapy + OA
FNCLCC	1000/950	After adjuvant chemotherapy NP and NN	OA (RT/LHRH agonist/surgery) Control
GABG IVB	950/657	NN, ER− 1–3 NP, ER+ 4–9 NP	3 CMF 3 CMF + OA (goserelin × 2 y) 4 EC → CMF OA (goserelin) + 4 EC → CMF
IBCSG 11-93	760/174	NP	OA → Tamoxifen × 5 y OA → 4 AC → Tamoxifen × 5 y

NP, node-positive; NN, node-negative; ER, estrogen receptor; RT, radiotherapy; LHRH, luteinizing-hormone-releasing hormone; see text for chemotherapy regimen abbreviations.

apy and hormonal therapy (OA or tamoxifen). Given that this is still an unsettled issue, whenever possible, women with high-risk disease should be considered for a therapeutic randomized trial.

Premenopausal women with ER-negative tumors should not be offered OA as an equivalent alternative to chemotherapy, for the same reasons that tamoxifen is not adequate in postmenopausal women with ER-negative disease.

DOSE-INTENSIVE/DOSE-DENSE CHEMOTHERAPY

Although adjuvant chemotherapy and hormonal therapy reduce recurrence of and death from NP

breast cancer, relapses still occur with unacceptably high frequency. Whether escalating drug doses (increasing dose intensity) and/or reducing the interval between cycles (increasing dose density) is associated with improved outcome has been subject of numerous RCTs.[65]

In many early trials, the 'high-dose' arms contained what are currently considered 'conventional' chemotherapy doses, whereas the low-dose arms had inferior, or suboptimal, doses (Table 32.2.10). These studies effectively demonstrated that there is a threshold dose and intensity below which DFS and OS are compromised.[41,65–70]

The CALGB 8541 study compared three dose intensities of CAF and found inferior DFS and

Table 32.2.10 Reported adjuvant RCTs of conventional versus low-dose chemotherapy, and of dose-intense or dose-dense versus conventional-dose chemotherapy for node-positive breast cancer

Trial/group	Population	n	Drug intensified	Comparative doses	5-year DFS (%)	p-value	OS (%)	p-value
Low-dose vs conventional-dose chemotherapy								
CALGB 8541[66]	NP	1550	Doxorubicin	30 mg/m² d1 q28d × 6 (1) 60 mg/m² d1 q28d × 4 (2) 40 mg/m² d1 q28d × 6 (3)	56 61 66	1 vs 2/3 <0.0001 2 vs 3 0.85	72 77 78	1 vs 2/3 0.04 2 vs 3 0.11
FASG[67]	NP Premenopausal	595	Epirubicin	50 mg/m² d1 q21d × 6 (1) 50 mg/m² d1 q21d × 3 (2) 75 mg/m² d1 q21d × 3 (3)	64.2 55.6 55.2	1 vs 2/3 0.03 2 vs 3 NS	82.6 74.9 79.5	1 vs 2/3 NS 2 vs 3 NS
FASG[70]	≥4 NP or 1–3 NP and ER– Premenopausal	565	Epirubicin	50 mg/m² d1 q21d × 6 100 mg/m² d1 q21d × 6	58.5 70.0	0.01	70 80	0.002
Dose-dense or dose-intense vs conventional-dose chemotherapy								
CALGB 8541[66]	NP	1023	Doxorubicin	60 mg/m² d1 q28d × 4 40 mg/m² d1 q28d × 6	61 66	0.85	77 78	0.11
Intergroup 72	NP and ER–	646	Doxorubicin 5FU	Doxorubicin 15 mg/m²/wk 5-FU 250 mg/m²/wk Doxorubicin 20 mg/m²/wk 5-FU 600 mg/m²/wk	62.7[a] 67.5[a]	2p 0.19 p 0.09	71.4[b] 78.1[b]	2p 0.10 p 0.05
Intergroup 41	NP	3170	Doxorubicin	60 mg/m² d1 q21d × 4 75 mg/m² d1 q21d × 4 90 mg/m² s1 q21d × 4	– – –	NS	– – –	NS
NSABP B-22[73]	NP	2305	Cyclophosphamide	600 mg/m² × 4 1200 mg/m² × 2 1200 mg/m² × 4	62 60 64	0.3	78 77 77	0.95

Trial	Menopausal status	N	Drug	Regimen		p		p
NSABP B-25[74]	NP	—	Cyclophosphamide	1200 mg/m² × 4	62	NS^c	81	NS^c
				2400 mg/m² × 2	66		80	
				2400 mg/m² × 4	70		82	
NCIC[76]	NP Premenopausal	716	Epirubicin	CMF (Bonadonna) × 6	53	0.009	70	0.03
				CEF (E 60 mg/m² d1,8 q28d) × 6	63			
Belgian[52]	NP	777	Epirubicin (E) and cyclophosphamide (C)	CMF (Bonadonna) (1)	71^d	1 vs 2 vs 3	85	1 vs 2 vs 3
				E 60 mg/m² d1 q21d (2)	64^d	NS	78	NS
				C 500 mg/m² d1 q21d		2 vs 3	86	2 vs 3
				E 100 mg/m² d1 q21d (3)	74^d	0.03		0.04
				C 830 mg/m² d1 q21d				

[a]4-year recurrence-free survival.
[b]4-year overall survival.
[c]Interim analysis results.
[d]Event-free survival.
NP, node-positive; ER, estrogen receptor; see text for chemotherapy regimen abbreviations.

OS in the low-dose arm compared with the moderate- and high-dose arms at 9 years of follow-up.[66] By today's standards, the low-dose arm had suboptimal doses of all three drugs and the other two arms had doses within the 'conventional' range. The French Adjuvant Study Group (FASG) found a trend towards superior outcome with six versus three cycles of FEC_{50} (the subscript denotes the dose of epirubicin in mg/m^2) and three cycles of FEC_{75}.[67] In another study from the same group, six cycles of FEC_{50} was inferior to six cycles of FEC_{100}.[70] Thus, below a certain threshold, anthracycline dose can be associated with inferior outcome. A trial in metastatic disease, which compared the Bonadonna CMF schedule with intravenous CMF given on day 1 every 21 days, suggests that cyclophosphamide is also associated with a minimum effective dose density.[57]

Since the advent of colony-stimulating growth factors, which shorten the absolute nadir and duration of neutropenia, delivery of higher drug doses, with shorter intervals, has become more feasible.[71] Nevertheless, any additional benefit observed with dose-dense and dose-intense therapies must be viewed in the light of increased short- and long-term toxicity. True dose-dense and dose-intense RCTs have addressed the benefit of increased doses of anthracyclines or cyclophosphamide (Table 32.2.10).

Anthracyclines

The high-dose arm of the CALGB 8541 trial contained the same total dose of doxorubicin but increased dose intensity compared with the moderate-dose arm.[66] No difference in DFS and OS was observed between these arms, although both arms were still within the 'conventional' dose range. Grade IV leukopenia was substantially higher in the high-dose than in the moderate-dose arm (66% and 17%, respectively), but the frequency of other toxicities was similar.

An Intergroup RCT (ECOG, CALGB and SWOG) compared CAF with a dose-dense, optimized, 16-week schedule of weekly chemotherapy.[72] In the 16-week regimen, total doses of doxorubicin and 5-FU were 13% and 60% respectively, higher than in CAF, and two additional drugs (methotrexate and vincristine) were given. The dose intensity was slightly higher for doxorubicin and substantially higher for 5-FU in the 16-week schedule. With 3.9 years of follow-up, 4-year RFS and OS were similar for both groups. The 16-week schedule was superior to CAF in women with one to three positive nodes (RFS rate: CAF 73.6%; 16-week 82.1%, $2p = 0.085$; OS rate: CAF 77.7%, 16-week 86.8%, $2p = 0.052$) but not in women with more than three positive nodes. Treatment-related morbidities were different, including three toxic deaths in the CAF arm, and the 16-week schedule was substantially more complicated to deliver.

Another collaborative RCT (CALGB 9344) compared three different doses of doxorubicin (60, 75 or 90 mg/m^2 i.v. on day 1 every 21 days) in four cycles of AC, followed by a second randomization in each arm with four cycles of paclitaxel versus no further treatment.[41] Although only interim analysis results are available, based on 540 events, no difference in DFS or OS has been observed when analyzed according to doxorubicin dose received.

Cyclophosphamide

The NSABP B-22 trial compared regimens that were dose-intense, dose-intense plus dose-dense, and standard doses of cyclophosphamide in adjuvant AC.[73] Patients were stratified by age (< 50 versus $\geq$ 50 years), as well as number of positive nodes, ER level and type of surgery. With 5 years of follow-up, no OS or DFS differences were observed for the three groups, or for subsets of patients with one to three NP (55% of study population), four to nine NP (30% of study population), or more than 10 NP (14% of study population) disease. Toxicity, in particular severe infection, septic episodes and vomiting, was higher in the arm with both dose intensity and dose density, as might be expected. The frequency of AML and myelodysplastic syndrome (MDS) after chemotherapy was similar in all arms (one, three and two cases, respectively). A subsequent NSABP trial (B-25) has thus far reported no differences in DFS and OS between three higher than conventional cyclophosphamide doses, also in combination with doxorubicin; however, only interim analysis results are available.[74] Sixteen cases of AML and MDS have occurred in this trial (incidence 0.87%, similar frequency in each arm), with cytogenetics typical of post-alkylator and post-topoisomerase II-inhibitor leukemia in six and three cases, respectively.[75]

Anthracyclines versus CMF

Finally, there are a few trials that have compared high-dose anthracyclines with CMF. The NCIC-CTG reported a 19% RRR in mortality (OS rate 77% and 70% for CEF and CMF, respectively, $p = 0.03$), and 29% RRR in recurrence for dose-intense epirubicin in CEF compared with Bonadonna CMF.[76] Median follow-up was 59 months, and the actual dose intensities of epirubicin and methotrexate were 77% (608 mg/m^2) and 88% (470 mg/m^2), respectively. Although there were no treatment-related deaths, hospitalization for febrile neutropenia was higher in the CEF arm (8.5%) than in the CMF arm (1.1%), despite antibiotic prophylaxis given throughout the CEF. Four fatal cases of AML have occurred in the CEF arm, although classic post-topoisomerase II-inhibitor cytogenetics were observed only in one case. There was a non-significant lower survival rate in the women with more than three positive nodes who received CMF (CMF 58%, CEF 70%, p = NS), but no difference for women with one to three NP (CMF 78%, CEF 82%). In contrast, a Belgian three-arm study of similar size ($n = 777$), which randomized among Bonadonna CMF × 6, EC × 8 and high-dose EC × 8, found no difference in OS between CMF and the high-dose EC arm (85% and 86%, respectively) with 50 months of median follow-up; however, the 'high-dose' was superior to the 'low-dose' EC arm.[52] Three cases of AML, all in the high-dose EC arm, have been reported.

Whether the superiority of the CEF schedule in the NCIC trial is a result of the increased dose intensity of anthracyclines compared with standard dose, or the substitution of methotrexate for epirubicin, remains unanswered. The EBCTCG overview found an improved DFS ($2p = 0.006$) and OS ($2p = 0.02$) for anthracycline-containing chemotherapy over CMF, although confidence intervals approached zero. A subsequent RCT ($n = 4406$) demonstrated a marginal advantage of CAF over CMF in NN breast cancer.[37] It appears that, at standard doses, anthracyclines are slightly superior, but, at high doses, the question remains unanswered.

It is clear from the above trials that suboptimal doses of cytotoxic drugs produce inferior outcomes. Furthermore, studies that have compared conventional and high-dose cyclophosphamide or anthracyclines have failed to show an improvement in OS for the dose-intense/dense schedules. They are, however, associated with substantially increased serious toxicity, of which infection, cardiotoxicity and secondary leukemia are of particular concern. Future trials that address dose intensity will undoubtedly need to include taxanes in the comparison, because this class of drugs is likely to move into the adjuvant setting in the next few years. Other scientific approaches of interest include optimizing the duration of exposure to cytotoxic drugs, selecting the most promising drug combinations, and targeting the population most likely to benefit from dose intensification.

Based on the available evidence, for premenopausal women with NP disease, conventional-dose anthracyclines probably offer a small advantage over CMF regimens, and should be offered in the absence of pre-existing cardiac dysfunction or other contraindications. The added survival benefit of anthracyclines in postmenopausal women has not been established, and they are best offered in the setting of extreme relapse risk, to balance the cardiac toxicity, which tends to increase with age. Of note, at least one trial suggested that AC was better tolerated than CMF when global toxicity was considered.[77] Until the efficacy of dose-intense regimens has been confirmed, they should be used judiciously, preferably in a controlled trial setting, given the increased toxicity. Several large ongoing trials (Table 32.2.11) may establish superior efficacy of dose-intense and dose-dense over conventional-dose chemotherapy, but at present it cannot be recommended as routine therapy, even in very high-risk disease.

HIGH-DOSE TREATMENT AND STEM CELL TRANSPLANTATION

The risk of breast cancer relapse after adjuvant systemic therapy increases with increasing number of positive nodes at diagnosis.[78] In an attempt to ameliorate this adverse risk, investigators have explored the role of high-dose chemotherapy with hematopoietic stem cell harvest and rescue reinfusion ('stem cell transplantation': SCT) in women with multiple positive nodes. RCTs comparing high-dose regimens with SCT with less myeloablative doses of chemotherapy drugs are still accruing patients, or have provided only immature data so far (Table 32.2.12). Given the higher potential treatment-related mortality and long-term sequelae, high-dose chemotherapy with SCT cannot

currently be recommended outside an experimental setting, preferably an RCT.

Results from three RCTs were presented at the 1999 American Society of Clinical Oncology meeting.[79–81] The combined groups of the CALGB, SWOG and NCIC-CTG compared high-dose alkylating agents plus SCT with intermediate doses of the same drugs after four cycles of CAF in women with 10 or more positive nodes (CALGB 9082).[79] The median number of involved nodes was 14, and 19% had more than 20 involved. Patients ($n = 783$) were randomized to high-dose CPB (cyclophosphamide, cisplatin, carmustine (BCNU)) with SCT or intermediate-dose CPB with transplantation allowed at the time of relapse. With 37 months of median follow-up, the actuarial 5-year event-free survival rates were 68% and 64% ($p = 0.7$), and the OS rates were 78% and 80% ($p = 0.1$), for the high- and intermediate-dose arms, respectively. The lower number of relapses in the high-dose arm was balanced by higher treatment-related mortality (29 of 394 deaths; 3% within 100 days of transplantation). These results are immature, because only 60% of the expected events have occurred, and an additional 3 years of follow-up are planned.

The Scandinavian Breast Cancer Study Group (SBG) randomized 525 patients with high-risk NP breast cancer (> 70% risk of relapse within 5 years) to tailored FEC with granulocyte colony-stimulating factor (G-CSF) and prophylactic antibiotics, or to conventional FEC and stem cell mobilization, followed by high-dose chemotherapy (cyclophosphamide 6 g/m^2, thiotepa 0.5 g/m^2 and carboplatin 0.8 g/m^2) with SCT.[80] All patients received locoregional radiotherapy and tamoxifen for 5 years. With a median follow-up of 20.2 months, there were 133 relapses, 40 deaths (two treatment-related in the SCT arm) and seven cases of AML/MDS (all in the non-SCT arm). No difference in recurrence or OS has been observed so far, but, again, results are immature.

Table 32.2.11   Ongoing adjuvant RCTs of dose-dense or -intense chemotherapy in node-positive breast cancer[27]

Trial/group	Accrual target/actual to date	Population	Comparative arms
ABCSG 10	400/97	Pre-/postmenopausal NN and NP	4 EC (60/600 mg/m^2 q21d) $\rightarrow$ 3 CMF $\rightarrow$ Tamoxifen 4 EC + uromitexan + G-CSF $\rightarrow$ 4 CMF $\rightarrow$ Tamoxifen
GABG IVE	400/–	Postmenopausal, age <70 y >10 NP	4 EC ⟶ 3 CMF 4 E (120 mg/m^2)
OCSGL	380/51	>10 NP 2–3 NP, high risk	6 FEC (E 50 mg/m^2 q28d) 6 FEC (E 60 mg/m^2 d1,8 q28d) 6 EC, G-CSF (E 120 mg/m^2 C 830 mg/m^2 q21d)
INT 0137	3000/1956	Pre-/postmenopausal 1–3 NP NN high risk	6 AC (54 mg/m^2/1.2 g/m^2 q21d) + G-CSF 4 A (81 mg/m^2 q21d) + G-CSF $\rightarrow$ 3 C 2.4 g/m^2 q21d + G-CSF
GONO MIG 1	1200/1214 closed	NP NN high risk	6 FEC (600/60/600 mg/m^2 d1,8 q28d) 6 FEC q14d + G-CSF.

OCSGL, Oncological Center Study Group in Lodz; NN, node-negative; NP, node-positive; G-CSF, granulocyte colony-stimulating factor; E, epirubicin; C, cyclophosphamide; A, doxorubicin; see text for chemotherapy regimen abbreviations.

Table 32.2.12   Ongoing adjuvant RCTs of high-dose chemotherapy with SCT in node-positive breast cancer[27]

Trial/group	Accrual target/actual to date	Population	Comparison arms[a]	Comments
Dutch[82]	97	>10 NP	(1) 4 FEC + RT + tamoxifen (2) 4 FEC → STAMP V + SCT	Results negative for DFS and OS ($p = 0.8$)
MDA[83,84]	78 closed early, low accrual	>10 NP	(1) 8 FAC (2) 8 FAC → High-dose chemotherapy × 2 with SCT	Results negative 62%, 48% DFS ($p = 0.35$) 77%, 58% OS ($p = 0.23$)
Intergroup (CALGB 9082)[79]	783/713 extended	≥10 NP stage II, III	(1) CAF (600/60/1200) → C 1.9 g/m^2 × 3 d, CDDP 55 × 3 d, BCNU 600 + SCT + tamoxifen + RT (2) 1 CAF → C 300 × 3 d, CDDP 30 × 3 d, BCNU 90 + tamoxifen + RT	Preliminary results negative
SBG 9401[80]	525	>70% relapse risk and NP	(1) 9 FEC individual dose (5-FU 600/E 38–120/C 450–1800 mg/m^2) with G-CSF (2) 3 FEC → C 1.5 g/m^2, thio 125, carbo 200 d1–4 + SCT + RT + tamoxifen	Preliminary results negative
South Africa[81]	154	≥10 NP ≥7 NP and Tumor >5 cm high risk	(1) C 4.4 g/m^2 + mitox 45 + VP16 1.5 g/m^2 + SCT (2) CAF (600/50/600) or CEF (600/70/600)	Results positive for high-dose arm
IBCSG 15-95	210/329	Age ≤65 y and ≥10 NP or ≥5 NP and ER− or ≥5 NP and T3	(1) EC (200/4 g/m^2) → SCT, tamoxifen (2) 4 AC (50/600) or EC (90/600) q3w → 3 CMF + tamoxifen	No results

PEGASE 01	240/280	≥8 NP	(1) 3FEC$_{100}$ (500/100/600) (2) 3FEC$_{100}$ + SC harvest → Mitox 45 C 200 × 2 d, mel 140 + SCT	No results
GABG-IV EH-93	420/159	≥9 NP	(1) 4 EC (90/900) → 3 CMF (2) 4 EC (90/900) → C 6 g/m², thio 0.6 g/m², mitox 40 + SCT	No results
MCG	390 closed 9/98	≥3 NP	(1) 3E (120) + 6 CMF (2) C 7 g/m², harvest → Vcr; MTX 8 g/m² E 120 → Mel 140 + thio 0.6 g/m² + SCT	No results
ICCG	230/256	???	(1) 6 FEC (2) 3 FEC → C 6 g/m²/thio 500/carbo 800 4d IVCI + SCT	No results
ACCOG 1	600/605 closed	>4 NP	(1) 4 A → 8 CMF (2) 4 A → C 6 mg/m²/thio 800 + SCT	No results
ACCOG II	300/4	After neoadjuvant AC or AT NP	(1) 8 CMF (2) C 6 g/m² + thio 800 + SCT	No results
ABCSG	240/74	NP, NN high risk	(1) 6 ET (90/200 q21d) + G-CSF + tamoxifen 20 mg/5 y (2) 3 ET (90/200) + C 1500/thio 125/carbo 1500 d −7 to −4 + uromitexan 1500 d −7 to −3 + SCT + tamoxifen	No results
GABG-IMA	300/57	Age ≤50 y and ≥10 NP and stage III	(1) 3 EC (45/500 d1,2 q15d) → C 2 g/m²; carbo 500 thio 200; mitox 20 d1–3 + SCT (2) 3 EC → 3 CMF (Bonadonna IV)	No results
GABG-IMA	320/60	Age ≤60 y and ≥10 NP and Stage II	(1) VIPE (VP16 500; ifos 4 g/m²; CDDP 50; E 50 d1) → HD-VIC (VP16 500; ifos 4 g/m²; carbo 500 d1–3) (2) 4 EC (90/600 q21d) → 3 CMF (500/40/600 d1,8 q28)	No results

Continued

Table 32.2.12 Continued

Trial/group	Accrual target/actual to date	Population	Comparison arms[a]	Comments
INT 0121	429/338	NP Stage II, III	(1) CAF (100 p.o. d1–14/30 d1,8/500 d1,8) (2) CAF → C 6 g/thio 800 i.v. 96 h + SCT	No results
INT S9623	1000/–	4–9 NP	(1) A 80 d1,15,29 + T 200/24 h d43,57,71 + C 3 g/m² d85,99,113 + G-CSF (2) AC (80/600) d1,22,43,64 → STAMP I or V + SCT	No results
NWSAT	800/–	≥4 NP II, III	(1) 5 FEC (2) 4 FEC → C 6 g/m², thio 0.48 g/m², carbo 1.6 g/m² SCT	No results, closed

[a]Doses are in mg/m² unless otherwise indicated. E, epirubicin; A, doxorubicin; C, cyclophosphamide; CDDP, cisplatin; BCNU, carmustine; mitox, mitoxantrone; mel, melphalan; Vcr, vincristine; thio, thiotepa; carbo, carboplatin; ifos, ifosfamide; MTX, methotrexate; T, paclitaxel; MCG, Michelangelo Cooperative Group; IVCI, intravenous continuous infusion; SCT, chemotherapy with hematopoietic stem cell harvest and rescue reinfusion; VP16, etoposide; HD-VIC, high-dose VP16, ifos and carbo; STAMP I, C 1875 d −1 to −4, CDDP, 55 mg/m²/d over 24 h d −6 to −4, BCNU 600 d −3; STAMP V, C 6000 + carbo 1600 + thio 480 IVCI over d −7 or −4; RT, radiotherapy; G-CSF, granulocyte colony-stimulating factor. See text for other chemotherapy regimens. MDA, MD Anderson; ACCOG, Anglo-Celtic Cooperative Oncology Group; IMA, Interdisziplinäre Mammakarzinom-Arbeitsgruppe; INT, Intergroup; NWSAT, Netherlands Working Party for Autotransplantation in Solid Tumors; NP, node-positive; NN, node-negative; ER, estrogen receptor.

The smallest transplantation trial reported had the longest follow-up and was positive.[81] In this RCT, 154 women were randomized to two cycles of high-dose chemotherapy with SCT, or to standard-dose CAF or CEF. All women had 10 or more involved nodes, or tumor less than 5 cm in size with seven to nine positive nodes plus one other adverse prognostic factor. With a median follow-up of 69 months, the relapse and death rates were, respectively, 25.3% and 10.6% for the high-dose group and 65.8% and 35.4% for the standard-dose group ($p < 0.001$ for relapse, $p < 0.01$ for death). Unfortunately, recent independent investigation suggests serious misconduct of this trial, which would invalidate the results.

Two smaller trials, from MD Anderson and the Netherlands, have also failed to show a superior outcome for the women treated with high-dose therapy and SCT compared with conventional-dose anthracycline-based chemotherapy.[82–84]

A recommendation for routine, adjuvant, high-dose chemotherapy with SCT cannot be made on the basis of one small flawed positive trial and four additional immature or small trials that demonstrate equivalence. However, this is an active area of investigation and, within a few years, mature results from large pivotal trials will be available (Table 32.2.12). It is hoped that together these data will provide a definitive conclusion about the value of this kind of therapy for multiple NP breast cancer.

PREDICTIVE/PROGNOSTIC FACTORS

Prognostic factors help to assess relapse and death risk in breast cancer, whereas predictive factors forecast response to therapy. A myriad of clinical, histological and molecular factors have been evaluated for their prognostic and predictive potential.

Prognostic factors

The presence of axillary node invasion remains the most significant prognostic factor in early breast cancer.[85] In NP disease, there is a progressive increase in the risk of relapse and death as the number of involved lymph nodes increases.[85–87] Accordingly, in most NP breast cancer trials, participants are stratified according to the number of involved nodes, usually one to three, four to nine, and over nine. In addition, studies of high-dose therapies, which carry increased treatment-related mortality, have so far targeted the subset of NP patients with more than three or more than nine positive nodes and, therefore, the highest relapse risk. Unfortunately, we have not yet identified systemic therapies that are superior to conventional regimens for women with extreme risk. Whether high-dose therapy is of value in this population awaits maturity of ongoing trials.

Independent of nodal burden, there is a linear relationship between relapse risk and tumor size.[86–88] In a subset of 620 tumor and lymph-node samples from patients in the NSABP B-04 trial, which compared surgery and regional radiotherapy to the axilla for clinically NP patients (with no systemic therapy); nodal status, tumor size and nipple involvement were the only independent prognostic factors for survival among 15 pathological and 5 clinical putative factors examined.[86] Nodal status was most significant, with the relative risk of death (using NN disease as unity reference) of 1.63, 2.78, and 3.92 for one to three, four to nine, and more than nine positive nodes, respectively ($p = 0.0004$, 0.0001, 0.0001). Compared with tumors smaller than 2 cm, the relative risk of death for tumors sized 2.1–4 cm was 1.39 ($p = 0.13$), and for tumors over 4.0 cm it was 1.73 ($p = 0.0003$). Nipple involvement was associated with a relative risk of 1.42 ($p = 0.013$). Factors notably absent in the multivariate analysis, which might have altered the independent significance of these three factors, were hormone receptor status, ploidy, S phase and c-ErbB-2 status. It is not known whether tumor size and nipple involvement would remain independent in the presence of systemic adjuvant therapy, which is known to affect outcome independently.[1,29,36]

The relationship between 5-year survival, nodal status and tumor size was examined in a cohort of 24 740 patients with non-metastatic breast cancer registered with the SEER (Surveillance, Epidemiology and End Results) program between 1978 and 1982, and for whom tumor size and at least eight lymph nodes were examined.[89] For each tumor size category, survival decreased as the number of positive nodes increased. Similarly, for a given number of positive nodes, the survival decreased as the tumor size increased. For example, 5-year survival rates for patients with tumors smaller than 2 cm were 87.4% and 66.0% with one to three and more than four positive nodes, respectively; for 2–5 cm tumors, the corresponding survival rates were 79.9% and 58.7%. These observations were made on 9387 NP patients, so, although p-values were not given, even small differences are likely to be significant.

In the Naples GUN trial, women (n = 941) who were premenopausal received chemotherapy and postmenopausal women were given tamoxifen.[90] In a retrospective review of prognostic factors, the number of involved nodes, tumor size, skin and/or fascia involvement, nipple invasion, and adjuvant therapy were independent on multivariate analysis.

Rate of locoregional failure (LRF) with or without simultaneous distant failure (DF) was examined by ECOG in patients with T1–3, NP breast cancer enrolled in four RCTs of chemotherapy versus chemoendocrine therapy, and of short and longer chemotherapy regimens.[88] The tumor size and number of involved nodes were found to be independently associated with increased risk of LRF ± DF. At 10 years, the risk of LRF ± DF was 12.9% and 28.7% for one to three and four or more positive nodes, respectively. In the one to three NP group, the 10-year risk was 12.4%, 12.1% and 31.4% for patients with T1, T2 and T3 tumors, whereas in the four to seven NP group, the corresponding 10-year risks of LRF ± DF were 19.9%, 26.7% and 44.8%.

Recent reports suggest that tumors located in the medial quadrants of the breast have a lower survival, perhaps as a result of occult spread to the internal mammary nodes, a region not routinely given local therapy in many centers.[91,92] Currently, open RCTs from the EORTC and NCIC-CTG are prospectively examining the value of irradiation of the internal mammary node regions.[27]

Since in the presence of positive axillary nodes, the benefit of adjuvant systemic therapy is clearly evident, other traditionally significant 'St Gallen' prognostic factors, including tumor grade (using the Scarff–Bloom–Richardson grading system), presence of tumor emboli within the lymphatic, vascular and/or neural spaces of the tumor specimen, and hormone receptor status, assume less importance in making adjuvant therapy decisions.[93,94] However, they are still taken into consideration when assessing individual recurrence risk.

In recent years, our understanding of the cell cycle and its regulation has mushroomed. Integral to this has been the development of techniques that allow detection and cloning of numerous genes, whose gene products are thought to be involved in the genesis or progression of cancer, or which might be associated with more aggressive phenotypes. In breast cancer, numerous factors appear to have prognostic and/or predictive potential, including overexpression of c-erbB-2, bcl-2, uPAI, PAI-1, mutation of *p53*, indices indicative of high proliferation (including Ki67 and S phase) and DNA ploidy, to name a few. The degree to which these are independently predictive in NP disease is currently a hotbed of investigation. As our understanding of them increases, the upregulation, mutation or downregulation of these various molecular markers may come to negate the independent significance of some of the traditional 'St Gallen' risk factors.

Predictive factors

A very real limitation in establishing the predictive value of molecular markers is in standardizing the method of measurement or detection. A prototypical example is the measurement of c-ErbB-2 overexpression. Several different commercial antibodies are available for detection, each with different sensitivities and specificities. Moreover, different laboratories use different cut-off and scoring systems to label a test as 'positive', producing a range of results for the same samples. Although in the USA attempts have been made to minimize this variability by approving only one, the HercepTest, this kit has been shown to have a low specificity.[95]

The most scientifically sound method of evaluating putative factors is prospective; however, few factors have been investigated in this way. Retrospective evaluation limits interpretation of the true value of various factors, primarily because the patient cohorts receive a variety of adjuvant systemic therapies, which are known to alter prognosis significantly.[1,29,36]. Although investigators have tried to overcome this problem by studying women enrolled in clinical trials of uniform adjuvant therapy, invariably data and tumor block sets are incomplete. In addition, in virtually all cases, stratification for the factor in question is missing. These methodological limitations lead to significant imbalances in known prognostic factors and/or small sample sizes, which in turn lead to unreliable observations. Another problem is failure to include all known prognostic or predictive variables in multivariate analyses, which is the only way of reliably eliminating confounding bias. Nevertheless, in the absence of prospective data, retrospective analyses on large patient groups that received similar therapy and standard follow-up are the best alternative.

An important source of prognostic information comes from women enrolled in older studies that did not employ routine adjuvant systemic therapy. These cohorts allow exploration of the natural history of early breast cancer, and the relationship of various factors to relapse and survival. However, they cannot address the predictive value of such factors in patient populations that are now routinely offered systemic therapy, such as NP breast cancer patients, because the therapy may eliminate or substantially reduce the negative prognostic impact of some factors. These limitations must be kept in mind whenever one is evaluating reports of prognostic and predictive factors, no matter how large the sample size.

One well-accepted predictive factor of poor response to hormone therapy is lack of expression of hormone receptors, ER and PgR.[96] As a result, assays for these receptors at diagnosis are done as a matter of course in most centers, and chemotherapy is used in preference to hormone therapy in patients whose tumors do not have ER or PgR.

Recent retrospective evidence suggests that women with tumors that overexpress c-ErbB-2 – a transmembrane tyrosine kinase with sequence homology to the epidermal growth factor receptor – have higher relapse risk, and may be resistant to some chemotherapy and hormonal therapies.[44–46,97–105] In a multivariate analysis of a subset of patients in an RCT of three different anthracycline dose intensities (CALGB 8541), c-ErbB-2 overexpression (defined as > 50% cell staining using polyclonal antibody OA-11-854) was a significant predictor of shorter RFS and OS, along with number of positive nodes, larger tumor size and premenopausal status.[99] Hormone receptor status, *p53* mutation and S-phase fraction, among others, were not predictive. Retrospective analyses from other adjuvant trials have supported this association, although others still have refuted it.[46,97,98] Similar controversy exists about whether c-ErbB-2 overexpression correlates with resistance to tamoxifen.[99-105]

At present, most, but not all, of the literature supports the value of c-ErbB-2 overexpression in predicting lower survival, but its value in predicting response to various therapies remains unresolved.[106] This is not surprising given the low specificity of the HercepTest, and the retrospective nature of the studies that have examined the predictive value of c-ErbB-2. Prospective evaluation and stratification for c-ErbB-2 status is needed to satisfy this controversy definitively. This is of particular importance, because the determination of c-ErbB-2 status at the time of primary tumor diagnosis is becoming more routine, and specific therapies that modulate the excess risk of c-ErbB-2 overexpression, such as Herceptin, may soon enter the adjuvant realm.[47,48]

One factor that has been examined prospectively is the presence of individual tumor cells within the bone marrow at diagnosis.[107] Two hundred and sixty breast cancer patients underwent bone marrow biopsies at diagnosis. There were 22 (22 of 81, or 27%) relapses and 10 deaths in the bone marrow-positive group, and four (4 of 130, or 3%) relapses with five deaths in the bone marrow-negative group during the 24-month follow-up period. Using Cox's regression analysis to control for nodal status, PR, EgR, menopausal state, stage and grade, bone marrow positivity was independently correlated with

relapse at any site ($p < 0.0005$) and bone relapse ($p < 0.004$). Nodal and PgR (but not ER) status were also independent predictors for relapse. The follow-up in this study was too short to determine whether marrow positivity predicts for increased rate of, or just earlier, relapse. Moreover, this is the only study of its kind, so the conclusions that can be drawn from it are limited.

A more comprehensive discussion of prognostic and predictive factors is beyond the scope of this chapter. As our understanding of the molecular and genetic changes that occur in breast cancer increases, the prognostic factors that we use today may lose some of their current relevance. There is no question that they assist the clinician in evaluating the individual risk of patients and, consequently, what systemic adjuvant therapies are best for them. Eventually, we may be able to examine the unique molecular and genetic changes in each breast cancer, and thus assess more accurately the absolute risk, so that we can tailor treatment of the individual patient accordingly. However, our current understanding of factors that predict for poor response to various therapies in the adjuvant setting is limited, and application of this knowledge in routine clinical practice, with the exception of ER and PgR, may be premature.

REFERENCES

1. Early Breast Cancer Trialists' Collaborative Group, Tamoxifen for early breast cancer: An overview of the randomised trials. *Lancet* 1998; **351**:1451–67.
2. Stewart HJ, Forrest AP, Everington D et al, Randomised comparison of 5 years of adjuvant tamoxifen with continuous therapy for operable breast cancer. *Br J Cancer* 1996; 74:297–9.
3. Tormey DC, Gray R, Falkson HC, Postchemotherapy adjuvant tamoxifen therapy beyond five years in patients with

lymph node-positive breast cancer. *J Natl Cancer Inst* 1996; **88**:1828–33.

4. Fisher B, Dignam J, Bryant J et al, Five versus more than five years of tamoxifen therapy for breast cancer patients with negative lymph nodes and estrogen receptor-positive tumors. *J Natl Cancer Inst* 1996; **88**:1529–42.

5. Ragaz J, Coleman A, Survival impact of adjuvant tamoxifen on competing causes of mortality in breast cancer survivors, with analysis of mortality from contralateral breast cancer, cardiovascular events, endometrial cancer, and thromboembolic episodes. *J Clin Oncol* 1998; **16**:2018–24.

6. Love RR, Wiebe DA, Feyzi JM et al, Effects of tamoxifen on cardiovascular risk factors in postmenopausal women after 5 years of treatment. *J Natl Cancer Inst* 1994; **86**:1534–9.

7. Gotto AM, Results of recent large cholesterol-lowering trials and implications for clinical management. *Am J Cardiol* 1997; **79**:1663–6.

8. McDonald CC, Stewart HJ, Fatal myocardial infarction in the Scottish Adjuvant Tamoxifen trial. The Scottish Breast Cancer Committee. *BMJ* 1991; **303**:435–7.

9. Rutqvist LE, Mattsson A, Cardiac and thromboembolic morbidity among postmenopausal women with early-stage breast cancer in a randomized trial of adjuvant tamoxifen. The Stockholm Breast Cancer Study Group. *J Natl Cancer Inst* 1993; **85**:1398–406.

10. Powles TJ, Hickish T, Kanis J, Tidy A, Ashley S, Effect of tamoxifen on bone mineral density measured by dual-energy x-ray absorptimometry in healthy premenopausal and postmenopausal women. *J Clin Oncol* 1996; **14**:78–84.

11. Love RR, Mazess RB, Tormey DC et al, Bone mineral density in women with breast cancer treated with adjuvant tamoxifen for at least two years. *Breast Cancer Res Treat* 1988; **12**:297–301.

12. Love RR, Mazess RB, Barden HS et al, Effects of tamoxifen on bone mineral density in postmenopausal women with breast cancer. *N Engl J Med* 1992; **326**:852–6.

13. Fornander T, Rutquist LE, Sjoberg HE et al, Long-term adjuvant tamoxifen in early breast cancer: effect on bone mineral density in postmenopausal women. *J Clin Oncol* 1990; **8**:1019–24.

14. Turken S, Siris E, Seldin D, Effect of tamoxifen on spinal bone density in women with breast cancer. *J Natl Cancer Inst* 1989; **81**:1086–8.

15. Ryan WG, Wolter J, Bagdade JD, Apparent beneficial effect of tamoxifen on bone mineral content in patients with breast cancer: A preliminary study. *Osteoporosis Int* 1992; **2**:39–41.

16. Gotfredsen A, Christiansen C, Palshof T et al, The effect of tamoxifen on bone mineral content in premenopausal women with breast cancer. *Cancer* 1984; **53**:853–7.

17. Fisher B, Costantino JP, Redmond CK et al, Endometrial cancer in tamoxifen-treated breast cancer patients: findings from the National Surgical Adjuvant Breast and Bowel Project (NSABP B-14). *J Natl Cancer Inst* 1994; **86**:527–37.

18. Jones AL, Powles TJ, Law M et al, Adjuvant aminoglutethimide for postmenopausal patients with primary breast cancer: analysis at 8 years. *J Clin Oncol* 1992; **10**:1547–52.

19. Samonigg H, Jakesz R, Hausmaninger D et al, Tamoxifen versus tamoxifen plus aminoglutethimide for stage I and II receptor-positive postmenopausal node-negative or node-positive breast cancer patients: Four-year results of a randomized trial of the Austrian Breast Cancer Study Group (ABCSG). *Proc Am Soc Clin Oncol* 1999; **18**:68a (Abst 253).

20. Nabholtz JM, Bonneterre J, Buzdar AU et al, Preliminary results of two multi-center trials comparing the efficacy and tolerability of Arimidex (anastrozole) and tamoxifen in postmenopausal women with advanced breast cancer. *Breast Cancer Res Treat* 1999; **57**:31 (Abst 27).

21. Gradishar WJ, Jordan VC, Clinical potential

of new antiestrogens. *J Clin Oncol* 1997; **15**:840–52.

22. Ettinger B, Black DM, Mitlak BH et al, Reduction of vertebral fracture risk in postmenopausal women with osteoporosis treated with raloxifene: results from a 3-year randomized clinical trial. Multiple Outcomes of Raloxifene Evaluation (MORE) Investigators. *JAMA* 1999; **282**:637–45.

23. Cummings SR, Eckert S, Krueger KA et al, The effect of raloxifene on risk of breast cancer in postmenopausal women: results from the MORE randomized trial Multiple Outcome of Raloxifene Evaluation. *JAMA* 1999; **281**:2189–97.

24. Holli K, Adjuvant trials of toremifene vs tamoxifen: The European experience. *Oncology* 1998; **5S**:23–7.

25. Mäenpää J, Toremifene: Where do we stand? Second Biennial International Meeting of the Flemish Gynaecological Oncology Group, December 3–4 1999, Brussels, Belgium. Oral presentation.

26. Ratko TA, Detrisac CJ, Dinger NM et al, Chemopreventive efficacy of combined retinoid and tamoxifen treatment following surgical excision of a primary mammary cancer in female rats. *Cancer Res* 1989; **49**:4472–6.

27. Piccart MJ, Goldhirsch A, *An Overview of Recent and Ongoing Adjuvant Clinical Trials for Breast Cancer*, 2nd edn. EORTC and BIG, 2000.

28. Awada A, Piccart M, *New Agents in Development for Cancer Therapy*. Consultant Series No. 18. Cheshire: Gardiner-Caldwell Communications, 1997: 71.

29. Early Breast Cancer Trialists' Collaborative Group, Ovarian ablation in early breast cancer: Overview of the randomised trials. *Lancet* 1996; **348**:1189–96.

30. Beatson GT, On the treatment of inoperable cases of carcinoma of the mamma: Suggestions for a new method of treatment, with illustrative cases. *Lancet* 1896; **ii**:104–7.

31. Ejlertsen B, Dombernowsky P, Mouridsen HT et al, Comparable effect of ovarian ablation and CMF chemotherapy in premenopausal hormone receptor positive breast cancer patients. *Proc Am Soc Clin Oncol* 1999; **18**:66a (Abst 248).

32. Jakesz R, Hausmaninger H, Samonigg H et al, Comparison of adjuvant therapy with tamoxifen and goserelin versus CMF in premenopausal stage I and II hormone-responsive breast cancer patients: four-year results of Austrian Breast Cancer Study Group (ABCSG). *Proc Am Soc Clin Oncol* 1999; **18**:67a (Abst 250).

33. Rutqvist LE, Zoladex and tamoxifen as adjuvant therapy in premenopausal breast cancer: a randomised trial by the Cancer Research Campaign Breast Cancer Trials Group, the Stockholm Breast Cancer Study Group, the South-East Sweden Breast Cancer Group and the Gruppo Interdisciplinare Valutazione Interventi in Oncologia. *Proc Am Soc Clin Oncol* 1999; **18**:67a (Abst 251).

34. Filipponi P, Pedetti M, Fedeli L et al, Cyclical IV clodronate in postmenopausal osteoporosis: results of a long-term clinical trial. *Bone* 1996; **18**:179–84.

35. Reid IR, Watti DJ, Evans MC et al, Continuous therapy with pamidronate, a potent bisphosphonate, in postmenopausal osteoporosis. *J Clin Endocrinol Metab* 1994; **79**:1595–9.

36. EBCTCG, Polychemotherapy for early breast cancer: An overview of the randomised trials. *Lancet* 1998; **352**:930–42.

37. Hutchins L, Green S, Ravdin P et al, CMF versus CAF with and without tamoxifen in high-risk node-negative breast cancer patients and a natural history follow-up study in low-risk node-negative patients: first results of Intergroup trial INT 0102. *Proc Am Soc Clin Oncol* 1998; **17**:1a.

38. Mouridsen HT, Andersen J, Anderson M et al, Adjuvant anthracycline in breast cancer. Improved outcome in premenopausal patients

following substitution of methotrexate in the CMF combination with epirubicin. *Proc Am Soc Clin Oncol* 1999; **18**:68a.

39. O'Leary J, Volm M, Wasserheit C, Muggia F, Taxanes in adjuvant and neoadjuvant therapies for breast cancer. *Oncology (Huntingt)* 1998; **12**(Suppl 1):23–7.

40. Moos PJ, Fitzpatrick FA, Taxanes propagate apoptosis via two cell populations with distinctive cytological and molecular traits. *Cell Growth Differ* 1998; **9**:687–97.

41. Henderson IC, Berry D, Demetri G et al, Improved disease-free and overall survival from the addition of sequential paclitaxel but not from the escalation of doxorubicin dose level in the adjuvant chemotherapy of patients with node-positive primary breast cancer. *Proc Am Soc Clin Oncol* 1998; **17**:101a (Abst 390a).

42. Nanbholtz JM, Falkso C, Campos D et al, Doxorubicin and docetaxel (AT) is superior to standard doxorubicin and cyclophosphamide as 1st line CT for MBC: Randomized phase III trial. *Breast Cancer Res Treat* 1999; **57**:84 (Abst 330).

43. Di Leo A, Piccart MJ, Paclitaxel activity, dose, and schedule: Data from phase III trials in metastatic breast cancer. *Semin Oncol* 1999; **26**(3 Suppl 8):27–32.

44. Stal O, Sullivan S, Wingren S et al, C-erbB-2 expression and benefit from adjuvant chemotherapy and radiotherapy of breast cancer. *Eur J Cancer* 1995; **31**A:2185–90.

45. Allred DC, Clark GM, Tandon AK et al, HER-2/neu in node-negative breast cancer: prognostic significance of overexpression influenced by the presence of in situ carcinoma. *J Clin Oncol* 1992; **10**:599–605.

46. Menard S, Valagussa P, Pilotti S et al, Benefit of CMF treatment in lymph node-positive breast cancer overexpressing HER2. *Proc Am Soc Clin Oncol* 1999; **18**:69a (Abst 257).

47. Slamon D, Leyland-Jones B, Shak S et al, Addition of Herceptin (humanized anti-her2 antibody) to first line chemotherapy for her2 overexpressing metastatic breast cancer markedly increases anticancer activity: a randomized multinational controlled phase III trial. *Proc Am Soc Clin Oncol* 1998; **17**:98a (Abst 377).

48. Norton L, Slamon D, Leyland-Jones B et al, Overall survival advantage to simultaneous chemotherapy plus the humanized anti-HER2 monoclonal antibody Herceptin in HER2-overexpressing metastatic breast cancer. *Proc Am Soc Clin Oncol* 1999; **18**:127a (Abst 483).

49. Cobleigh MA, Vogel CL, Tripathy D et al, Efficacy and safety of Herceptin (humanized anti-her2 antibody) as a single agent in 222 women with her2 overexpression who relapsed following chemotherapy for metastatic breast cancer. *Proc Am Soc Clin Oncol* 1998; **17**:97a (Abst 376).

50. Tucker MA, Meadows AT, Boice JD Jr et al, Leukemia after therapy with alkylating agents for childhood cancer. *J Natl Cancer Inst* 1987; **78**:459–64.

51. Chambers SK, Chopyk RL, Chambers JT, Schwartz PE, Duffy TP, Development of leukemia after doxorubicin and cisplatin treatment for ovarian cancer. *Cancer* 1989; **64**:2459–61.

52. Di Leo A, Larsimont D, Beauduin A et al, CMF or anthracycline-based chemotherapy for node-positive breast cancer patients: 4 year results of a Belgian randomised clinical trial with predictive markers analysis. *Proc Am Soc Clin Oncol* 1999; **18**:69a.

53. Gelber RD, Cole BF, Goldhirsch A et al, Adjuvant chemotherapy plus tamoxifen compared with tamoxifen alone for postmenopausal breast cancer: meta-analysis of quality-adjusted survival. *Lancet* 1996; **347**:1066–71.

54. International Breast Cancer Study Group, Effectiveness of adjuvant chemotherapy in combination with tamoxifen for node positive postmenopausal breast cancer patients. International Breast Cancer Study Group. *J Clin Oncol* 1997; **15**:1385–94.

55. Albain K, Green S, Osborne K et al, Tamoxifen (T) versus cyclophosphamide, Adriamycin® and 5-FU plus either concurrent or sequential T in postmenopausal, receptor (+), node (+) breast cancer: A Southwest Oncology Group phase III Intergroup trial (SWOG-8814, INT-0100). *Proc Am Soc Clin Oncol* 1997; **16**:128a (Abst 450).

56. Pritchard KI, Paterson AHG, Fine S et al, Randomized trial of cyclophosphamide, methotrexate, and fluorouracil chemotherapy added to tamoxifen as adjuvant therapy in postmenopausal women with node-positive estrogen and/or progesterone receptor-positive breast cancer: A report of the National Cancer Institute of Canada Clinical Trials Group. *J Clin Oncol* 1997; **15**:2302–11.

57. Engelsman E, Klijn JCM, Rubens RD et al, 'Classical' CMF versus a 3-weekly intravenous CMF schedule in postmenopausal patients with advanced breast cancer. *Eur J Cancer* 1991; **27**:966–70.

58. Wils JA, Bliss JM, Marty M et al, Epirubicin plus tamoxifen versus tamoxifen alone in node positive postmenopausal patients with breast cancer. A randomized trial of the International Collaborative Cancer Group. *J Clin Oncol* 1999; **17**:1988–98.

59. Jakesz R, Hausmaninger H, Haider K et al, Randomized trial of low-dose chemotherapy added to tamoxifen in patients with receptor-positive and lymph node-positive breast cancer. *J Clin Oncol* 1999; **17**:1701–9.

60. Castiglione-Gertsch M, Johnsen C, Goldhirsch A et al, The International (Ludwig) Breast Cancer Study Group Trials I–IV: 15 years of follow-up. *Ann Oncol* 1994; **5**:717–24.

61. Kaufmann M, Jonat W, Abel U et al, Adjuvant randomized trials of doxorubicin/cyclophosphamide versus doxorubicin/cyclophosphamide/tamoxifen and CMF chemotherapy versus tamoxifen in women with node-positive breast cancer. *J Clin Oncol* 1993; **11**:454–60.

62. Schumacher M, Bastert G, Bojar H et al, Randomized 2×2 trial evaluating hormonal treatment and the duration of chemotherapy in node-positive breast cancer patients. *J Clin Oncol* 1994; **12**:2086–93.

63. Rivkin SE, Green S, O'Sullivan J et al, Adjuvant CMFVP versus adjuvant CMFVP plus ovariectomy for premenopausal, node-positive, and estrogen receptor-positive breast cancer patients: A Southwest Oncology Group study. *J Clin Oncol* 1996; **14**:46–51.

64. Davidson N, O'Neill A, Vukov A et al, Effect of chemohormonal therapy in premenopausal, node positive, receptor positive breast cancer: An Eastern Cooperative Oncology Group phase III Intergroup trial. *Proc Am Soc Clin Oncol* 1999; **18**:67a (Abst 249).

65. Biganzoli L, Piccart MJ, The bigger the better? . . . or what we know and what we still need to learn about anthracycline dose per course, dose density and cumulative dose in the treatment of breast cancer [editorial]. *Ann Oncol* 1997; **8**:1177–82.

66. Budman DR, Berry DA, Cirrincione CT et al, Dose and dose intensity as determinants of outcome in the adjuvant treatment of breast cancer. *J Natl Cancer Inst* 1998; **90**:1205–11.

67. Bremond A, Kerbrat P, Fumoleau P et al, Five year follow-up results of a randomized trial testing the role of the dose intensity and duration of chemotherapy in node positive premenopausal breast cancer patients. *Proc Am Soc Clin Oncol* 1996; **15**:113.

68. Bonadonna G, Valagussa P, Dose–response effect of adjuvant chemotherapy in breast cancer. *N Engl J Med* 1981; **304**:10–15.

69. Hryniuk W, Levine MN, Analysis of dose intensity for adjuvant chemotherapy trials in stage II breast cancer. *J Clin Oncol* 1986; **4**:1162–70.

70. Bonneterre J, Roche H, Bremond A et al, Results of a randomized trial of adjuvant chemotherapy with FEC 50 vs FEC 100 in high risk node-positive breast cancer patients. *Proc Am Soc Clin Oncol* 1998; **17**:124a.

71. Del Mastro L, Garrone O, Setoli MR et al, A pilot study of accelerated cyclophosphamide, epirubicin and 5-fluorouracil plus granulocyte colony stimulating factor as adjuvant therapy in early breast cancer. *Eur J Cancer* 1994; **30A**:606–10.

72. Fetting JH, Gray R, Fairclough DL et al, Sixteen-week multidrug regimen versus cyclophosphamide, doxorubicin, and fluorouracil as adjuvant therapy for node-positive, receptor-negative breast cancer: an Intergroup study. *J Clin Oncol* 1999; **16**:2382–91.

73. Fisher B, Anderson S, Wickerham DL et al, Increased intensification and total dose of cyclophosphamide in a doxorubicin–cyclophosphamide regimen for the treatment of primary breast cancer: Findings from National Surgical Adjuvant Breast and Bowel Project B-22. *J Clin Oncol* 1997; **15**:1858–69.

74. Sledge GW, Adjuvant chemotherapy: Shifting rules, shifting roles. Educational lecture. *Proc Am Soc Clin Oncol Educational Book* 1999: 208–10.

75. DeCillis A, Anderson S, Bryant J et al, Acute myeloid leukemia and myelodysplastic syndrome on NSABP B-25: An update. *Proc Am Soc Clin Oncol* 1997; **16**:130a.

76. Levine MN, Bramwell VH, Pritchard KI et al, Randomized trial of intensive cyclophosphamide, epirubicin, and fluorouracil chemotherapy compared with cyclophosphamide, methotrexate, and fluorouracil in premenopausal women with node-positive breast cancer. *J Clin Oncol* 1998; **16**:2651–8.

77. Fisher B, Brown AM, Dimitrov NV et al, Two months of doxorubicin–cyclophosphamide with and without interval reinduction therapy compared with 6 months of cyclophosphamide, methotrexate, and fluorouracil in node-positive breast cancer patients with tamoxifen-nonresponsive tumors: Results from the National Surgical Adjuvant Breast and Bowel Project B-15. *J Clin Oncol* 1990; **8**:1483–96.

78. Fisher B, Bauer M, Wickerman DL et al, Relation of number of positive axillary nodes to the prognosis of patients with primary breast cancer. An NSABP update. *Cancer* 1983; **52**:1551–7.

79. Peters W, Rosner G, Vredenburgh J et al, A prospective, randomized comparison of two doses of combination alkylating agents as consolidation after AC in high-risk primary breast cancer involving ten or more axillary lymph nodes: Preliminary results of CALGB 9082/SWOG 9114/NCIC MA-13. *Proc Am Soc Clin Oncol* 1999; **18**:1a.

80. The Scandinavian Breast Cancer Study Group 9401, Results from a randomized adjuvant breast cancer study with high dose chemotherapy with CTCb supported by autologous bone marrow stem cells versus dose escalated and tailored FEC therapy. *Proc Am Soc Clin Oncol* 1999; **18**:2a.

81. Bezwoda WR, Randomised, controlled trial of high dose chemotherapy versus standard dose chemotherapy for high risk, surgically treated, primary breast cancer. *Proc Am Soc Clin Oncol* 1999; **18**:2a.

82. Rodenhuis S, Richel DJ, van der Wall E et al, Randomised trial of high-dose chemotherapy and haemopoietic progenitor-cell support in operable breast cancer with extensive axillary lymph-node involvement. *Lancet* 1998; **352**:515–21.

83. Hortobagyi GN, Buzdar AU, Champlin R et al, Lack of efficacy of adjuvant high-dose tandem combination chemotherapy for high-risk primary breast cancer – A randomized trial. *Proc Am Soc Clin Oncol* 1998; **17**:123a (Abst 471).

84. Hortobagyi GN, Buzdar AU, Theriault RL et al, Randomized trial of high-dose chemotherapy and blood cell autografts for high-risk primary breast carcinoma. *J Natl Cancer Inst* in press.

85. Dent DM, Axillary lymphadenectomy for breast cancer. *Arch Surg* 1996; **131**:1125–7.

86. Soonmyoung P, Hazan R, Fisher ER et al,

Pathologic findings from the National Surgical Adjuvant Breast and Bowel Project: Prognostic significance of cerbB-2 protein overexpression in primary breast cancer. *J Clin Oncol* 1990; **8**:103–12.

87. Jatoi I, Hilsenbeck SG, Clark GM, Osborne CK, Significance or axillary lymph node metastases in primary breast cancer. *J Clin Oncol* 1999; **17**:2334–40.

88. Recht A, Gray R, Davidson NE et al, Locoregional failure 10 years after mastectomy and adjuvant chemotherapy with or without tamoxifen without irradiation: Experience of the Eastern Cooperative Oncology Group. *J Clin Oncol* 1999; **17**:1689–700.

89. Carter CL, Allen C, Henson DE, Relation of tumor size, lymph node status, and survival in 24,740 breast cancer cases. *Cancer* 1989; **63**:181–7.

90. Perrone F, Carlomagno C, Lauria R et al, Selecting high-risk early breast cancer patients: What to add to the number of metastatic nodes? *Eur J Cancer* 1996; **32A**:41–6.

91. Zucali R, Mariani L, Marubini E et al, Early breast cancer: Evaluation of the prognostic role of the site of the primary tumor. *J Clin Oncol* 1998; **16**:1363–6.

92. Lohrisch C, Jones A, Jackson J et al, The relationship between tumor location and relapse in 6,781 women with invasive breast cancer. *J Clin Oncol* 2000; in press.

93. Elston CW, Willis IO, Pathological prognostic factors in breast cancer. The value of histological grade in breast cancer: Experience from a large study with long-term follow-up. *Histopathology* 1991; **19**:403–10.

94. Goldhirsch A, Wood WC, Senn HJ et al, Fifth International conference on adjuvant therapy of breast cancer, St Gallen, March 1995. International Consensus Panel on the Treatment of Primary Breast Cancer. *Eur J Cancer* 1995; **31A**:1754–9.

95. Jacobs TW, Gown AM, Yaziji H, Barnes MJ, Schnitt ST, Specificity of HercepTest in determining Her-2/neu status of breast cancer using the United States Food and Drug Administration – Approved Scoring System. *J Clin Oncol* 1999; **17**:1983–7.

96. Early Breast Cancer Trialists' Collaborative Group, Systemic treatment of early breast cancer by hormonal, cytotoxic, or immune therapy. *Lancet* 1992; **339**:1–15.

97. Sjogren S, Inganas M, Lindgren A et al, Prognostic and predictive value of c-erbB2 overexpression in primary breast cancer, alone and in combination with other prognostic markers. *J Clin Oncol* 1998; **16**:462–9.

98. Gusterson BA, Gelber RD, Goldhirsch A et al, Prognostic importance of c-erbB2 expression in breast cancer. International (Ludwig) Breast Cancer Study Group. *J Clin Oncol* 1992; **10**:1049–56.

99. Muss H, Berry D, Thor A et al, Lack of interaction of tamoxifen use and erbB-2/Her-2/Neu expression in CALGB 8541: A randomized adjuvant trial of three different doses of cyclophosphamide, doxorubicin and fluorouracil (CAF) in node-positive primary breast cancer. *Proc Am Soc Clin Oncol* 1999; **18**:68a.

100. Bianco AR, De Laurentiis M, Carlomagno C et al, 10 year update of the Naples GUN trial of adjuvant breast cancer therapy: evidence of interaction between c-erbB2 expression and tamoxifen efficacy. *Proc Am Soc Clin Oncol* 1998; **17**:97a.

101. Borg A, Baldetorp B, Ferno M et al, ERBB2 amplification in associated with tamoxifen resistance in steroid-receptor positive breast cancer. *Cancer Lett* 1994; **81**:137–44.

102. Stal O, Ferno M, Borg A et al, ErbB2 expression and the benefit from 5 versus 2 years of adjuvant tamoxifen for postmenopausal stage II breast cancer patients. *Breast Cancer Res Treat* 1997; **46**:32 (Abst 112).

103. Newby JC, Johnston SR, Smith IE, Dowsett M, Expression of epidermal growth factor receptor and c-erbB2 during the development of tamoxifen resistance in human breast cancer. *Clin Cancer Res* 1997; **3**:1643–51.

104. Leitzel K, Teramoto Y, Konrad K et al, Elevated serum c-erbB2 antigen levels and decreased response to hormone therapy of breast cancer. *J Clin Oncol* 1995; **13**:1129–35.

105. Elledge RM, Green S, Ciocca D et al, Her-2 expression and response to tamoxifen in estrogen receptor-positive breast cancer: A Southwest Oncology Group Study. *Clin Cancer Res* 1998; **4**:7–12.

106. Ross J, Fletcher JA, The Her-2/Neu oncogene in breast cancer: Prognostic factor, predictive factor, and target for therapy. *Oncologist* 1998; **3**:237–52.

107. Diel KJ, Kaufmann R, Goerner R, Costa SD, Kaul S, Bastert G, Detection of tumor cells in bone marrow of patients with primary breast cancer: a prognostic factor for distant metastasis. *J Clin Oncol* 1992; **10**:1534–9.

33

Predictive molecular markers: A new window of opportunity in the adjuvant therapy of breast cancer

Angelo Di Leo, Denis Larsimont, David Gancberg,
Antonio Fabiano Ferreira Filho, Fatima Cardoso, Martine J Piccart

The results of important and large randomized clinical trials and the conclusions of the Oxford meta-analysis have had a major impact on treatment recommendations for patients with early breast cancer.[1-7] Today, adjuvant medical therapy is offered to the vast majority of node-negative breast cancer patients.[1,4-6] An international panel of experts on adjuvant therapy met in St Gallen in February 1998. They concluded that only node-negative patients aged 35 years or older, with tumors of small size (<1 cm), well differentiated and positive for both the estrogen and progesterone receptors (ER and PgR), might be spared adjuvant therapy because of their minimal risk of relapse. All other subgroups are considered to benefit from adjuvant medical therapy.[8]

According to these recent guidelines, most early breast cancer patients receive treatment, and the main challenge becomes the identification of predictive factors, which may help in selecting the optimal adjuvant therapy for each individual patient. The accomplishment of this ambitious aim would most probably translate into a substantial increase of the absolute benefit associated with adjuvant therapy.

PREDICTIVE FACTORS: DEFINITION AND GENERAL CONCEPTS

The main difference between predictive and prognostic factors is illustrated in Figure 33.1. Although a prognostic factor will influence the disease outcome, whatever adjuvant therapy is used (Figure 33.1a), a predictive factor will interfere with disease outcome only when a specific treatment is given (Figure 33.1b, c). Figure 33.1b shows how the outcome of treatment A is positively influenced by the predictive factor under study, which has no impact on the efficacy of treatment B. A predictive factor can also influence the outcome of two alternative adjuvant therapies in different ways, as illustrated in Figure 33.1(c). This latter scenario would be the ideal situation, because one single factor might clearly select between two different forms of adjuvant therapy, one being the most active and the second being of very limited efficacy.

The identification of predictive factors demands great effort and so far there are only a few parameters that can be reliably defined. Prospective studies in which two different treatments are compared in two different patient subgroups, identified according to the putative predictive factor, have not been reported to date.

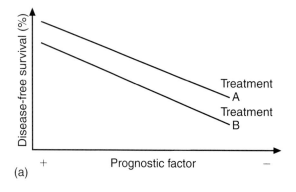

(a)

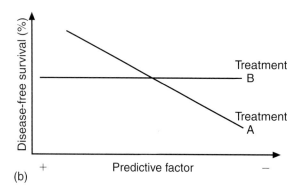

(b)

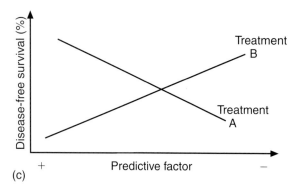

(c)

Figure 33.1

Prognostic and predictive factors: (a) prognostic factors; (b) predictive factors interacting with only one treatment; (c) predictive factors interacting with two different treatments.

The main advantage of these studies would be that the predictive marker hypothesis and the anticipated benefit would be formulated before study initiation and the study sample size would be calculated to reach an adequate number of patients in the two different subgroups, to demonstrate the anticipated difference statistically.

The lack of prospective studies has drawn the attention of the scientific community towards retrospective studies, which will be discussed later. These studies have, along with the limit of being retrospective studies, some other difficulties. These include the number of patients analyzed in the predictive marker study not accounting for the whole clinical trial population, because of problems with the retrospective collection of tumor samples, and the often suboptimal quality of collected tumor tissue for performing immunohistochemistry, which is the most commonly used technique for predictive marker studies. An effort has recently been made to ameliorate the credibility of the last generation of retrospective studies: by collecting tumour samples from patients entered into the clinical trial on an ongoing basis, rather than at the end of the clinical study, as was done for the first generation of retrospective studies. This effort might allow collection of tumor samples from the largest number of patients entered into the clinical trial. This measure will certainly lead to an improved quality and interpretation of retrospective studies, and will allow exhaustive tissue banks to be created, which might contribute in the generation of new hypotheses about future predictive and prognostic factors. Nevertheless, in the authors' opinion, the ultimate validation and transfer into clinical practice of potential predictive markers will require well-designed prospective studies, and now is the time to set these trials in motion on both sides of the Atlantic.

As a principle, the most interesting and

Table 33.1   ER as a predictive factor for tamoxifen – trials of adjuvant tamoxifen for about 5 years

ER status (no. of patients)	Reduction in			
	Recurrence rate		Death rate	
	(%)	(SD)	(%)	(SD)
ER-poor (922)	6	11	−3	11
ER-positive (5869)	50	4	28	5
ER < 100 fmol/mg	43	5	23	6
ER ≥ 100 fmol/mg	60	6	36	7

Adapted from EBCTCG.[9]

promising predictive marker should have the following features: it should be highly reproducible across different laboratories, and should be a simple technique and limited costs for assessment. A marker that could be evaluated on formalin-fixed, paraffin-embedded tissue would have the advantage of being potentially assessable by virtually any laboratory, and collection of tumor samples for the predictive marker assessment would certainly be facilitated, although the latter could be a major issue if the marker evaluation requires frozen tissue.

In the next section, an overview of the different predictive markers tested to date or under evaluation in patients with early breast cancer is presented. The overview concentrates first on those factors that predict the activity of adjuvant tamoxifen and second, on data about markers that predict chemotherapy, which is summarized.

PREDICTIVE MARKERS FOR ADJUVANT TAMOXIFEN

Table 33.1 summarizes the data available about the predictive power of ER when the efficacy of 5 years of adjuvant tamoxifen is evaluated. These results are part of the last meta-analysis on tamoxifen published by the Oxford group.[9]

From these data, it may be concluded that the activity of tamoxifen is strictly dependent on the results of ER assessment. There is also a correlation between the level of ER positivity and the efficacy of tamoxifen. The same report emphasizes the predictive role of PgR in the evaluation of tamoxifen efficacy.[9] Nowadays, ER and PgR are the most firmly established and consolidated factors known to predict the efficacy of adjuvant tamoxifen.

At the 1998 meeting of the American Society for Clinical Oncology (ASCO), two different groups presented results of retrospective studies in which the activity of adjuvant tamoxifen was correlated with the expression of c-erbB-2 (Table 33.2).[10,11] Both studies concluded that tumors overexpressing the c-ErbB-2 protein, measured by immunohistochemistry, were less responsive to tamoxifen. The authors of the American Intergroup study emphasized that their results needed to be interpreted cautiously because of several factors that might have influenced them. These

Table 33.2   c-_erbB_-2 and hormone sensitivity

Group	Study arms	No. of patients	Percentage with c-_erb_B-2 measured	Results
Naples[11]	Tamoxifen No tamoxifen	433	57	c-_erb_B-2 is a strong predictor of adjuvant tamoxifen failure independent of ER
American Intergroup[10]	Tamoxifen CAF + tamoxifen CAF → tamoxifen	1470	40	In patients with c-_erb_B-2 overexpression, CAFT > T

CAF, cyclophosphamide + doxorubicin + 5-fluorouracil.

included a low percentage of patients entered into the clinical study who could be evaluated in the companion study, the percentage of patients defined as c-_erb_B-2-positive, which was somewhat lower than expected from previous experience, and the limited number of patients evaluated in the tamoxifen-alone arm as a result of a one-to-three unbalanced randomization. These two studies have nevertheless the merit to have stimulated an intensive debate on the value of c-_erb_B-2 assessment in patients considered to be candidates for tamoxifen. The results of these two trials came to the same conclusion and, interestingly, they are supported by biological data.[12] The main difficulties in translating this observation into clinical practice are: (1) their retrospective nature; and (2) the lack of standardization of c-_erb_B-2 measurements across different laboratories. This issue is extensively discussed in the section dealing with chemotherapy and c-_erb_B-2.

PREDICTIVE MARKERS FOR ADJUVANT CHEMOTHERAPY

Recently reported trials have clearly shown that chemotherapy combined with tamoxifen is superior to tamoxifen alone as adjuvant treatment of node-negative, ER-positive patients or of node-positive, ER-positive postmenopausal patients.[1–3] According to these results, the vast majority of early breast cancer patients should be treated with adjuvant chemotherapy followed by tamoxifen. In this setting, the most powerful panel of predictive markers should be able to identify the optimal chemotherapy regimen to be given to each individual patient. Those putative predictive factors that have been the subject of a series of retrospective studies in patients with early breast cancer treated with adjuvant chemotherapy are dealt with below.

c-*erb*B-2 as a predictive marker for CMF and anthracycline-based regimens

Only recent trials have convincingly shown the superiority of an anthracycline-based regimen over CMF (cyclophosphamide, methotrexate, 5-fluorouracil (5-FU)) in the adjuvant treatment of premenopausal node-positive breast cancer patients.[13] The benefit is, however, modest and associated with a definite increase in toxicity. This is the typical clinical situation where the use of a predictive marker might help in selecting those patients in whom the benefit related to the more aggressive treatment might be substantial and justify the increased toxicity. c-*erb*B-2 has been investigated in this setting, and its behavior as a predictive factor seems to be quite similar to that presented in Figure 33.1(c). Data suggesting that c-*erb*B-2-positive tumors might be resistant to an adjuvant treatment with CMF (plus prednisone: CMFP) come from two different retrospective studies. In both trials, when patients were divided into two subgroups according to the expression of c-*erb*B-2 measured by immunohistochemistry on primary tumor samples, it was observed that adjuvant CMFP was more effective than no adjuvant treatment only in the subset of c-*erb*B-2-negative patients.[14,15] In a study recently reported by the Milan group, c-*erb*B-2 failed to show any predictive activity in a population of node-positive breast cancer patients randomly allocated to receive CMF or no treatment.[16] The results of this retrospective study, albeit obtained on a limited number of patients, contradict those in the previously reported studies.

Recently, the NSABP (National Surgical Adjuvant Breast and Bowel Project) group and the Belgian Adjuvant Study Group have reported the results of three retrospective studies (Table 33.3).[17-19] These reports suggest reduced CMF efficacy in patients overexpressing the c-ErbB-2 oncoprotein, and all three studies agree in defining the c-*erb*B-2-positive subgroup as the most

sensitive one to anthracycline-based adjuvant chemotherapy. Do the results of these trials authorize the clinician to use c-*erb*B-2 in the standard clinical practice for choosing between CMF or anthracycline-based chemotherapy? The answer is 'no' for at least three reasons:

1. All three studies are retrospective, with all the limits of retrospective studies, which have already been discussed.
2. The most suitable technique for c-*erb*B-2 assessment remains unknown. In the three studies mentioned, immunohistochemistry has been used. However, the NSABP group evaluated the c-ErbB-2 oncoprotein by a 'cocktail technique', consisting of concomitant staining with two different antibodies (the monoclonal TAB-250 plus the polyclonal p-Ab1).[17,18] The Belgian study used two different monoclonal antibodies (CB11 and 4D5) directed towards two different epitopes of the c-ErbB-2 protein.[19] The cocktail technique of the American study allowed the identification of a higher percentage of c-*erb*B-2-positive patients, compared with the monoclonal antibodies evaluated in the Belgian study. The Belgian group has also presented some results suggesting that the positivity rate for c-*erb*B-2 may increase if more sophisticated techniques are evaluated (fluorescence in situ hybridization, FISH).[20] From these data, it may be concluded that the positivity rate for c-*erb*B-2 can change according to the technique. The question raised is whether the most sensitive techniques (FISH or cocktail immunohistochemistry) are capable of identifying all the patients who may benefit from anthracycline-based chemotherapy or whether they introduce, within the so-called 'c-*erb*B-2-positive subgroup' a certain number of patients who have a clinical behavior that does not belong to the classic c-*erb*B-2-positive category.

Table 33.3   c-*erb*B-2 as a predictive marker for anthracycline-based adjuvant chemotherapy

Group	Study arms	No. of patients	Percentage of patients with c-*erb*B-2 measurement	Findings

NSABP[17]	PF
	PAF
		682	94	DFS c-*erb*B-2-negative:
				  PF vs PAF, RR = 0.96
				DFS c-*erb*B-2-positive:
				  PF vs PAF, RR = 0.60

NSABP[18]	CMF AC AC → CMF	2338	87	AC > CMF if c-*erb*B-2-positive

Belgian[19]	CMF
	EC
	High-dose EC
	(HEC)
		777	62	4-year DFS c-*erb*B-2-negative:
				  CMF 78%, EC 67%, HEC 74%
				4-year DFS c-*erb*B-2-positive:
				  CMF 54%, EC 53%, HEC 81%

P, melphalan; F, 5-fluorouracil; A, doxorubicin; C, cyclophosphamide; E, epirubicin.
DFS, disease-free survival; RR, relative risk.

3. The best cut-off value for defining a tumor as c-*erb*B-2-positive or -negative remains unknown. In the three studies presented, all tumors with at least 1% of cells showing positivity for c-*erb*B-2 were considered as c-*erb*B-2-positive. The rationale behind this policy relies on data that indicate that, in snap-frozen sections, c-*erb*B-2 expression is generally present in either none or almost all cells. In formalin-fixed, paraffin-embedded, tumor samples, the percentage of cells staining positively seems to be correlated more with fixation defects, leading to a certain loss of c-ErbB-2 antigenicity.[21] This phenomenon has already been well documented, and a direct correlation has been found between loss of antigenicity and time elapsed between preparation of the formalin-fixed, paraffin-embedded sample and time of marker assessment.[22] According to these data, the selection of a cut-off point that is different from 1% might be problematic, particularly in a retrospective study in which the quality of tumor samples, and therefore of c-ErbB-2 antigenicity, might be compromised. Along with the best cut-off value, another issue remains open and so far not entirely explored: the staining intensity. What would be the clinical behavior of those tumors with a high percentage of positive cells and low-intensity staining? So far, the intensity score has not been evaluated in any of the studies.

Markers predicting the activity of anthracycline-based regimens

Markers belonging to this category appear to have behavior similar to that illustrated in Figure 33.1(b): they may predict the outcome of an anthracycline-based regimen, but they do not interfere with treatment efficacy when other chemotherapy regimens are evaluated.

Topoisomerase IIα is perhaps the most representative and promising marker of this specific category. The interest in topoisomerase IIα is related to the fact that this enzyme is inhibited by anthracyclines and seems to be the main target of these drugs. Preclinical data indicate that intratumoral topoisomerase IIα levels may explain some forms of resistance to anthracyclines observed in vitro systems.[23] Data on human breast cancer samples show a good level of correlation between topoisomerase IIα levels and c-erbB-2 overexpression: high levels of the enzyme are found in tumors overexpressing the c-ErbB-2 oncoprotein.[24] According to these findings, it is tempting to postulate that c-erbB-2 would be a predictive marker for patients receiving an anthracycline-based regimen, in view of the correlation with topoisomerase IIα levels.

The Belgian group has evaluated topoisomerase IIα levels by immunohistochemistry on 481 archival primary tumor samples from node-positive breast cancer patients randomly allocated to receive adjuvant therapy with CMF or epirubicin plus cyclophosphamide.[19] The evaluation of this marker presented some technical difficulties (i.e. non-specific staining outside the nucleus of tumor cells), leading to a high rate of tumors with unknown topoisomerase IIα levels (27%). Interestingly, in those cases where the topoisomerase IIα status was evaluable, it was observed that topoisomerase IIα-positive tumors had a better outcome with the anthracycline-based regimen than with CMF, although equivalence between the two regimens was found in the subgroup of c-erbB-2-negative tumors. Nevertheless, no formal statistical significance was found when an interaction test was performed in order to evaluate the predictive role of topoisomerase IIα. The same group is now evaluating, in collaboration with Tampere University, Finland, the impact of topoisomerase IIα gene amplifications and deletions on the efficacy of anthracycline-based regimens.

Drug-efflux pumps such as P-glycoprotein (PGP) and multidrug-resistance-related protein (MRP) have been implicated in some forms of resistance to anthracyclines, taxanes, etoposide and vinblastine.[25,26] They might show predictive activity in clinical studies. The hypothesis has not been tested to date; nevertheless, these markers will not show any specificity for anthracyclines, given their involvement in multidrug resistance.

Markers predicting the activity of taxane-based regimens

Some retrospective studies in the metastatic or neoadjuvant setting have suggested that tumours overexpressing c-erbB-2, or with p53 mutations, might be more sensitive to paclitaxel than to an anthracycline-based regimen.[27,28] Nevertheless, these observations are based on the analysis of response rates in phase II studies in which no more than 50 patients have been evaluated. No formal randomization between a taxane-based and an anthracycline-based regimen has been done, and other reports from different trials have drawn the opposite conclusions.[29] The IDBBC branch of the EORTC (European Organization for Research and Treatment of Cancer) Breast Group will soon publish the results of a retrospective predictive markers study, in which 331 patients with advanced breast cancer were randomized to receive a first-line treatment with paclitaxel or doxorubicin. Samples of the primary tumor have been collected for almost

Table 33.4   Docetaxel: predictive factors[a]

Marker:	Mβ4-tubulin	Tau	α-Tubulin
Material:	mRNA	mRNA	Protein
Technique:	PCR	PCR	Immunohistochemistry
Resistant tumors:	=	=	=
Sensitive tumors:	↑	↑↑	↑↑

[a]Murine model; mammary and pancreatic tumors tested.
Adapted from Veitia et al.[30]

half of these patients, and some markers, such as c-erbB-2, p53 and bcl-2, have been retrospectively correlated with clinical outcome. Unfortunately none of these markers showed any predictive activity.

Probably the most attractive markers, as far as taxane treatment is concerned, are the microtubule-associated proteins (MAP) (Table 33.4). These are a specific target for taxanes because these drugs interact with microtubules. Preclinical data suggest that mammary and pancreatic tumors showing a remarkable level of sensitivity to docetaxel in vitro models have the highest expression of the Tau protein, which belongs to the MAP-2 family.[30] The 'good news' regarding this marker is that the assessment of MAP-2 expression by immunohistochemistry on paraffin-embedded samples is feasible, allowing activation of retrospective studies that correlate MAP-2 levels and docetaxel activity in both the metastatic and the adjuvant settings. These studies are ongoing at the Jules Bordet Institute.

Markers predicting the activity of 5-FU-based regimens

The relevance of such markers for the clinician comes from two recent observations: some regimens based on the administration of protracted 5-FU infusion have shown outstanding activity in the neoadjuvant setting;[31] and some 5-FU prodrugs, such as capecitabine, administered orally to advanced breast cancer patients, retain an appreciable level of anti-tumor activity after anthracyclines and taxanes, with the obvious advantage of avoiding protracted 5-FU infusion.[32]

Thymidylate synthase (TS) seems to be the most interesting predictive marker for 5-FU and its derivatives. The enzyme is normally inhibited by 5-FU, and, in gastrointestinal malignancies, it has already been shown that high TS levels predict a poor response rate to a 5-FU-based regimen.[33] At least three different techniques are available for TS assessment, although the polymerase chain reaction seems to be the most reliable.[33] In breast cancer patients, TS levels have already been investigated, but as a prognostic rather than a predictive factor.[34] No data correlating the activity of 5-FU-based chemotherapy with TS levels have been reported so far in breast cancer.

Implicated in the same metabolic pathway is another potential predictive marker: thymidine phosphorylase (TP). This has been investigated by immunohistochemistry on a series of 328 early breast cancer specimens. The population of TP-positive patients showed a significant survival benefit when treated with CMF in the adjuvant setting.[35] Further data are needed in this area to clarify the predictive role of both TS and TP when the activity of 5-FU or 5-FU-based regimens is evaluated.

Markers predicting the activity of 'high-dose' chemotherapy

The first published predictive marker study has been presented in this specific area and belongs to the Cancer and Leukemia Group B (CALGB) group.[36] This well-known study demonstrated that a dose-intensive CAF (cyclophosphamide, doxorubicin, 5-FU) regimen was more effective than two other CAF regimens, of intermediate- and low-dose intensity, in only the subgroup of node-positive breast cancer patients with c-*erb*B-2 overexpression, measured by immunohistochemistry on formalin-fixed, paraffin-embedded, primary tumor samples. The first results, presented with a 4-year median follow-up, have recently been confirmed by a second report with a 9-year median follow-up.[37] This is the only trial suggesting that c-*erb*B-2-positive tumors might be more sensitive to dose-intensive regimens. No other dose-intensive regimens have been evaluated so far, and therefore these data, although of considerable interest, cannot be translated into clinical practice yet.

CONCLUSIONS

An increasing number of early breast cancer patients receive a form of systemic adjuvant therapy. As a consequence, the main challenge for the oncology community becomes the identi-fication of predictive markers that may assist the clinician in selecting, from the different forms of medical therapies currently available, the one that is the best for an individual patient. The assessment of ER and PgR expression remains the 'gold standard' to predict the efficacy of adjuvant tamoxifen. A growing number of putative markers have been proposed to help with the selection of the different chemotherapy regimens. Among them, c-*erb*B-2 is probably the one for which the largest volume of data has been gathered. The main difficulties with the published literature are the lack of prospective studies, which are needed for definite clarification of the merits of the investigated marker, and a certain loss of reproducibility across different laboratories when each single marker is evaluated. Therefore, to date, no single putative predictive marker has been fully validated for routine clinical use.

Nevertheless, the significant amount of clinical research that has been carried out in the last 5 years in this field has been useful because it has led to the generation of some fascinating hypotheses. It is now the time to test these hypotheses in a new generation of predictive marker prospective studies, which will give great impetus to this field and may radically modify the strategic approach to the treatment of early breast cancer in the coming years.

REFERENCES

1. Fisher B, Dignam J, Wolmark N et al, Tamoxifen and chemotherapy for lymph node-negative, estrogen receptor-positive breast cancer. *J Natl Cancer Inst* 1997; **89**:1673–82.

2. International Breast Cancer Study Group, Effectiveness of adjuvant chemotherapy in combination with tamoxifen for node-positive postmenopausal breast cancer patients. *J Clin Oncol* 1997; **15**:1385–94.

3. Wils J, Bliss JM, Coombes RC et al, A multi-

centre randomized trial of tamoxifen vs. tamoxifen plus epirubicin in postmenopausal women with node-positive breast cancer. *Proc Am Soc Clin Oncol* 1996; **15**:109 (Abst 101).

4. Fisher B, Dignam J, Mamounas EP et al, Sequential methotrexate and fluorouracil for the treatment of node-negative breast cancer patients with estrogen receptor-negative tumors: Eight-year results from National Surgical Adjuvant Breast and Bowel Project (NSABP) B-13 and first report of findings from NSABP B-19 comparing methotrexate and fluorouracil with conventional cyclophosphamide, methotrexate, and fluorouracil. *J Clin Oncol* 1996; **14**:1982–92.

5. Mansour EG, Gray R, Shatila AH et al, Survival advantage of adjuvant chemotherapy in high-risk node-negative breast cancer: Ten-year analysis. An Intergroup study. *J Clin Oncol* 1998; **16**:3486–92.

6. Fisher B, Costantino J, Redmond C et al, A randomized clinical trial evaluating tamoxifen in the treatment of patients with node-negative breast cancer who have estrogen receptor positive tumors. *N Engl J Med* 1989; **320**:479–84.

7. Early Breast Cancer Trialist's Collaborative Group, Polychemotherapy for early breast cancer: An overview of the randomized trials. *Lancet* 1998; **352**:930–42.

8. Goldhirsch A, Glick JH, Gelber RD et al, Meeting highlights: international consensus panel on the treatment of primary cancer. *J Natl Cancer Inst* 1998; **90**:1601–8.

9. Early Breast Cancer Trialist's Collaborative Group, Tamoxifen for early breast cancer: An overview of the randomized trials. *Lancet* 1998; **351**:1451–67.

10. Ravdin PM, Green S, Albain KS et al, Initial report of the SWOG biological correlative study of c-erbB2 expression as a predictor of outcome in a trial comparing adjuvant CAF T with tamoxifen alone. *Proc Am Soc Clin Oncol* 1998; **17**:97a (Abst 374).

11. Bianco AR, De Laurentis M, Carlomagno C et

al, 20 year update of the Naples GUN trial of adjuvant breast cancer therapy: Evidence of interaction between c-erb B2 expression and tamoxifen efficacy. *Proc Am Soc Clin Oncol* 1998; **17**:97a (Abst 373).

12. Heintz NH, Leslie KO, Rogers LA et al, Amplification of the c-erb B2 oncogene in prognosis of breast adenocarcinoma. *Arch Pathol Lab Med* 1990; **114**:160–3.

13. Levine MN, Bramwell VH, Pritchard KI et al, Randomized trial of intensive cyclophosphamide, epirubicin, and fluorouracil chemotherapy in premenopausal women with node-positive breast cancer. *J Clin Oncol* 1998; **16**:2651–8.

14. Allred DC, Clarck GM, Tandon AK et al, HER-2/neu node-negative breast cancer: prognostic significance of overexpression influenced by the presence of in-situ carcinoma. *J Clin Oncol* 1992; **10**:599–605.

15. Gusterson BA, Gelber RD, Goldhirsch A et al, Prognostic importance of c-erb B2 expression in breast cancer. *J Clin Oncol* 1992; **10**: 1049–56.

16. Menard S, Valagussa P, Pilotti S et al, Benefit of CMF treatment in lymph-node positive breast cancer overexpressing HER2. *Proc Am Soc Clin Oncol* 1999; **18**:69a (Abst 257).

17. Paik S, Bryant J, Park C et al, erb B2 and response to doxorubicin in patients with axillary lymph node-positive, hormone receptor-negative breast cancer. *J Natl Cancer Inst* 1998; **90**:1361–70.

18. Paik S, Bryant J, Wolmark N, ERB-B2 overexpression and response to chemotherapy – NSABP study. *Proceedings of the 21st Annual San Antonio Breast Cancer Symposium* 1998: 231 (Abst 18).

19. Di Leo A, Larsimont D, Beauduin M et al, CMF or anthracycline-based adjuvant chemotherapy for node-positive breast cancer patients: 4-year results of a Belgian randomized clinical trial with predictive marker analysis. *Proc Am Soc Clin Oncol* 1999; **18**:69a (Abst 258).

20. Gancberg D, Lespagnard L, Rouas G et al, Routine evaluation of HER-2/NEU amplification and overexpression in breast cancer: correlation with grade, proliferation and E-cadherin expression. *Am J Clin Pathol* 2000; in press.

21. Slamon DJ, Godolphin W, Jones LA et al, Studies of the HER-2/neu proto-oncogene in human breast and ovarian cancer. *Science* 1989; **244**:707–12.

22. Jacobs TW, Prioleau JE, Stillman IE et al, Loss of tumor marker-immunostaining intensity on stored paraffin slides of breast cancer. *J Natl Cancer Inst* 1996; **88**:1054–9.

23. Nitiss JI, Beck WT, Anti-topoisomerase drug action and resistance. *Eur J Cancer* 1996; **32A**:958–66.

24. Jarvinen TAH, Kononen J, Pelto-Huikko M et al, Expression of topoisomerase IIα is associated with rapid cell proliferation, aneuploidy, and c-erb B2 overexpression in breast cancer. *Am J Pathol* 1996; **148**:2073–82.

25. Endicott JA, Ling V, The biochemistry of P-glycoprotein-mediated multidrug resistance. *Annu Rev Biochem* 1989; **58**:137–71.

26. Loe DW, Deeley RG, Lole SPC, Biology of the multidrug resistance-associated protein, MRP. *Eur J Cancer* 1996; **32A**:945–57.

27. Gianni L, Capri G, Mezzelani A et al, HER-2/neu amplification and response to doxorubicin/paclitaxel in women with metastatic breast cancer. *Proc Am Soc Clin Oncol* 1997; **16**:139a (Abst 491).

28. Kandioler D, Taucher S, Steiner B et al, p-53 genotype and major response to anthracycline or paclitaxel based neoadjuvant treatment in breast cancer patients. *Proc Am Soc Clin Oncol* 1998; **17**:102a (Abst 392).

29. Stender MJ, Neuberg D, Wood W et al, Correlation of circulating c-erb B2 extracellular domain (HER-2) with clinical outcome in patients with metastatic breast cancer. *Proc Am Soc Clin Oncol* 1997; **16**:154a (Abst 541).

30. Veitia R, Bissery MC, Martinez C et al, Tau expression in model adenocarcinomas correlates with docetaxel sensitivity in tumour-bearing mice. *Br J Cancer* 1998; **78**:871–7.

31. Smith IE, Walsh G, Jones A et al, High complete remission rates with primary neoadjuvant infusional chemotherapy for large early breast cancer. *J Clin Oncol* 1995; **13**:424–9.

32. Blum JL, Buzdar AU, Lorusso PM et al, A multicenter phase II trial of Xeloda (capecitabine) in paclitaxel-refractory metastatic breast cancer. *Proc Am Soc Clin Oncol* 1998; **17**:125a (Abst 476).

33. Lenz HJ, Leichman CG, Danenberg KD et al, Thymidylate synthase mRNA level in adenocarcinoma of the stomach: a predictor for primary tumor response and overall survival. *J Clin Oncol* 1995; **14**:176–82.

34. Pestalozzi BC, Peterson HF, Gelber RD et al, Prognostic importance of thymidylate synthase expression in early breast cancer. *J Clin Oncol* 1997; **15**:1923–31.

35. Fox SB, Engels K, Comley M et al, Relationship of elevated tumor thymidine phosphorylase in node-positive breast carcinomas to the effects of adjuvant CMF. *Ann Oncol* 1997; **8**:271–5.

36. Muss HB, Thor AD, Berry DA et al, C-erbB2 expression and response to adjuvant therapy in women with node-positive early breast cancer. *N Engl J Med* 1994; **330**:1260–6.

37. Thor AD, Berry DA, Budman DR et al, erb-B2, p-53, and efficacy of adjuvant therapy in lymph node-positive breast cancer. *J Natl Cancer Inst* 1998; **90**:1346–60.

34

p53 as a potential predictive factor of response to chemotherapy: From bench to bedside

Hervé Bonnefoi, Richard Iggo, Caroline Lohrisch

INTRODUCTION

Prognostic factors define the natural history of a tumor, thus guiding the selection of patients who require adjuvant systemic treatment (e.g. chemotherapy) according to their risk of relapse. There are numerous well-characterized prognostic factors in routine clinical use, and many more putative ones are being explored. Predictive factors permit individualization of systemic treatment by providing estimates about the likelihood of response or resistance to a given therapy. The best studied and most widely used predictive factor in breast cancer is the presence or absence of steroid hormone receptors, which determine whether hormonal therapy is likely to be of any therapeutic value. Unfortunately, factors predictive of response to chemotherapy are virtually non-existent. Overexpression of c-ErbB2, a transmembrane tyrosine kinase receptor, has been extensively studied, and may predict sensitivity to anthracyclines at high or low dose, although confirmatory prospective data are needed.[1-3] Mutation in p53, an important gene involved in cell cycle regulation, may also predict response to cytotoxic drugs, and is the focus of this chapter.

The choice of adjuvant chemotherapy regimen and the optimal target population have been the subject of numerous previous and ongoing randomized trials. The Oxford group meta-analysis established a highly significant benefit of adjuvant chemotherapy in both young and older women with node-negative or node-positive breast cancer.[4] Moreover, compared with CMF (cyclophosphamide, methotrexate, 5-fluorouracil), anthracycline-based regimens were associated with a greater reduction in relative risk of relapse (12%; $2p = 0.006$) and death (11%; $2p = 0.02$, SD 4), which translates into a 2.7% (SD 1.4) absolute survival advantage. It must be noted that the majority of women (70%) in these randomized comparisons were less than 50 years old and that the results of some large comparative trials were not available for inclusion in the analysis. Several such trials that have since been reported support a modest advantage for anthracyclines in both node-negative and node-positive disease, again particularly in premenopausal women.[5,6] Although this additional survival advantage with anthracyclines appears real, it is modest, and comes at the expense of slightly higher toxicity, notably neutropenia, emesis, and small risks of cardiotoxicity and secondary leukaemia. Weighing all of these factors, an increasing tendency to recommend anthracycline-based chemotherapy is evident, particularly in younger women with a high recurrence risk.

New on the adjuvant chemotherapy scene are the taxanes, inhibitors of microtubule disassembly. Early results of an Intergroup study have shown a modest survival advantage in patients treated with four cycles of doxorubicin/cyclophosphamide followed by four cycles of paclitaxel compared with four cycles of doxorubicin/cyclophosphamide alone.[7] At 18 months, the disease-free survival rates were 90% and 86% ($p = 0.0077$), and the overall survival rates were 97% and 95% ($p = 0.0390$), respectively. Longer follow-up and confirmation from similar ongoing trials are clearly necessary before adjuvant combinations of or sequential anthracyclines and taxanes can be recommended routinely. Nevertheless, if other trials corroborate these results, and toxicity is tolerable, a substantial change in adjuvant chemotherapy for breast cancer will ensue, with early estimates of a survival improvement with taxanes and anthracyclines of 3–5% over anthracyclines alone.

Adjuvant chemotherapy is being recommended for a widening spectrum of breast cancer patients, based on the observed survival benefits from large individual trials and the Oxford meta-analysis, even in populations with very low relapse risk.[4,8] Of growing importance is the need to more selectively individualize chemotherapy in order to avoid overtreatment. On the one hand, refinements in prognostic factors in low-risk disease are necessary to better select those for whom risk is greatest and therefore chemotherapy justified. As important, however, is a better understanding of factors predictive of chemoresistance and chemosensitivity, which will enable tailoring of chemotherapy drugs and treatment strategies to the needs of the individual patient/tumor.

p53

Experimental studies have repeatedly demonstrated that anticancer agents achieve their cytotoxic effect in large part through induction of apoptosis.[9,10] DNA damage, such as that induced by cytotoxic drugs, triggers a complex cascade of reactions involving damage sensors, signalling kinases, repair proteins, cell cycle regulators, and apoptosis inducers.[11] p53, which has been labelled the guardian or watchdog of the genome, sits at a crossroads in this pathway. When the p53 protein detects a DNA damage signal, particularly in tumor cells containing activated oncogenes, it strongly activates expression of genes mediating cell cycle arrest and apoptosis. The main effector of p53-dependent cell cycle arrest is the p21 cyclin-dependent kinase inhibitor, which directly blocks the activity of cdk2/cyclin E, producing arrest at the G_1/S boundary.[12] There is no agreed mechanism through which p53 induces apoptosis. Numerous different mediators have been proposed, none of which appears universal. The most commonly cited mechanism is induction of the pro-apoptotic Bax protein.[13]

Mutations in the p53 gene provide a putative mechanism by which neoplastic cells can evade lethal damage from cytotoxic drugs, enabling damaged cells to survive and proliferate. p53 mutations can occur through various mechanisms, resulting in loss of protein expression, alterations in tertiary protein structure, or expression of truncated protein. The biological effect common to all p53 mutations found in tumours is the loss of the transcriptional activator function of p53, which is consistent with the proven role of p53 as a tumor suppressor gene. Mutants expressed at high levels have demonstrable activity in cell culture that could enhance the malignant behavior of some tumors. Collectively, these activities are known as gain-of-function effects, and may be unrelated to the normal function of p53. Since they appear to be specific to particular mutations, their biological significance is hotly debated. p53 mutations have been established as an adverse prognostic factor in numerous cancers. In breast cancer, the prognostic value of p53 mutation is less well documented; however, emerging data support its role as a predictive factor for response to chemotherapy.

p53 STATUS AND CHEMORESISTANCE OR SENSITIVITY: EXPERIMENTAL DATA

Potential interactions between p53 status and response to anthracyclines

In vitro data have shown that doxorubicin activates p53 and, as a result, leads to cell cycle arrest and apoptosis.[14] In vitro experiments also suggest that, compared with their wild-type (wt) counterparts, cell lines and tumors with p53 mutations are relatively resistant to anthracycline-based chemotherapy and radiotherapy.[15,16] In 1994, Lowe et al[17] published seminal data on the relationship between p53 status and the efficacy of cancer therapy in tumour xenografts. Athymic nude mice were injected with transformed embryonic fibroblasts cells that differed primarily in their p53 status (transplantable fibrosarcoma model). Subsequent treatment with doxorubicin resulted in a rapid regression of tumors with wt p53 ($p53^{+/+}$), but not of tumors with mutated p53 ($p53^{-/-}$). Moreover, cells in regressing tumors had morphological and physiological features of apoptosis. These data provide a strong link between p53 mutation, failure of apoptosis induction, and drug resistance.

Potential interactions between p53 status and response to taxanes

The relationship between p53 and sensitivity to paclitaxel (a taxane) is more complex. Paclitaxel blocks cells in mitosis, either by freezing microtubules in a polymerized state or, at lower doses, by preventing microtubules from finding unattached chromosomes.[18] A large NCI study recently examined the dependence of paclitaxel sensitivity on p53 status.[19] Sixty human cancer cell lines with either wt or mutated p53 were exposed to a wide range of DNA-damaging agents, gamma radiation, and paclitaxel. Less growth inhibition was observed in the mutant p53 than in the wt p53 cell lines on exposure to DNA-damaging drugs or radiotherapy. In contrast, no difference in growth inhibition was found when the cell lines were exposed to paclitaxel, suggesting that p53 plays no role in growth inhibition by paclitaxel. The effect of p53 disruption on paclitaxel sensitivity was explored further in MCF-7 breast carcinoma cells, which had been stably transfected with either an HPV16 E6 gene or a dominant-negative mutant p53 gene to inactivate the endogenous wt p53. Again there was no correlation between growth inhibition by taxanes and p53 status. Other experimental studies have also failed to detect a correlation between p53 status and the response to taxanes.[20–25]

In contrast, one influential study found that p53 mutation increased the response to paclitaxel.[26] There is a plausible biological mechanism for this, at least when cells are treated simultaneously with both DNA-damaging agents and taxanes. By activating wt p53, DNA-damaging agents should arrest cells in G_1 and G_2, which in turn prevents cells from entering mitosis, the cell cycle phase in which taxanes are active. When p53 mutations are present, cell cycle arrest does not occur, and mitosis is initiated, thus providing greater opportunity for taxanes to act in cells with p53 mutations. In practice, as noted above, the situation is far less clear than this elegant model suggests, and some results even indicate that in tumors with mutant p53 the response to taxanes is attenuated.[27,28] Thus the predictive role of p53 mutation in response to taxanes is uncertain, and may be influenced by the exact timing and dose of taxane, as well as by concurrent delivery of other drugs or radiotherapy.

p53 AS A PREDICTIVE FACTOR FOR RESPONSE TO CHEMOTHERAPY: CLINICAL DATA

Retrospective clinical studies suggest that p53 mutations detected at the gene level are associated with a worse prognosis and a poor response to adjuvant and neoadjuvant chemotherapy and radiotherapy.[29-31] In patients with locally advanced breast cancer treated with neoadjuvant anthracyclines, the rate of progression during chemotherapy was 22% (4/18) in patients with p53-mutant tumors and only 4.4% (2/45) in patients with wt p53 tumors $(p < 0.05)$.[31] The rates of progression and/or relapse were 69% (11/16) and 8% (3/40) in women with mutant and wt p53 tumors, respectively. Specific p53 mutations in the L2/L3 domain were hypothesized to confer resistance to doxorubicin, but the small numbers, lack of randomization, and retrospective nature of the study mean that, although this conclusion represents a useful starting point for new studies, it cannot be accepted as an established fact. In a small clinical study of neoadjuvant chemotherapy, p53-mutated tumors (assessed by complete direct sequencing) had a low response rate to anthracyclines and a high response rate to taxanes.[32] Unfortunately this study is small and there are no prospective confirmatory studies; thus no definitive conclusions can be drawn based on this single observation.

A major difficulty in clinical studies is in distinguishing prognostic from predictive factors. The problem with p53 is double difficult because p53 is thought to influence both the innate aggressiveness of the tumor and its response to particular treatments. Given the known functions of p53, it is reasonable to expect p53-mutant tumors to be intrinsically more aggressive, for example because of greater aneuploidy or a higher mitotic fraction. To determine whether p53 status predicts response to a particular therapy, one must first weed out these prognostic effects. The only sure way to do this is to prospectively randomize patients with both wt and mutated p53 tumors or two different treatments. Ideally, one group should receive no treatment, but for obvious ethical reasons this is rarely possible. The lack of prospective randomized studies is one of the key reasons why p53 studies have had so little clinical impact to date. We describe below a phase III trial designed specifically to remedy this problem.

p53 ASSESSMENT METHODS: IMMUNOHISTOCHEMISTRY, PCR, FUNCTIONAL TEST IN YEAST

There is a higher risk of false-negative and false-positive results when p53 is assessed by immunohistochemistry (IHC) as compared with sequencing.[33,34] This is partly because IHC fails to detect unstable or truncated proteins, which commonly result from nonsense, frameshift, and splicing mutations. These types of mutation are relatively common in breast cancer, and have been reported in up to 47% of cases.[35] Despite attempts to standardize IHC scoring systems, p53 assessment remains semiquantitative and partly subjective. In a Swedish study, only 75% agreement between two pathologists was obtained using a six-point score.[34] When the medium and high scores were combined and compared with low scores, the level of agreement rose to 92%. However, in the low-scoring group (scores 1 and 2), agreement was only 54%. Clearly, IHC is not the best method to assess p53.

These methodological problems may explain the contradictory results regarding the prognostic value of p53 in breast cancer as assessed by IHC. There seems to be a similar number of studies supporting[1,36–41] as those refuting[34,42–44] the independent prognostic value of p53 mutations or expression. The only confident conclusion that arises is that the correlation of p53 status with prognosis in early breast cancer is best established using RNA- and DNA-based techniques rather than IHC.[33,34]

Simpler DNA structure-based techniques, particularly denaturing gradient gel electrophoresis, are sensitive, but require confirmatory sequencing to exclude polymorphisms and silent mutations. This has led to the belief that p53 sequencing is the gold standard against which new p53 assessment methods should be compared. Sequencing is not without its own limitations, however, not the least of which is that it is expensive. Furthermore, contamination with normal (non-neoplastic) tissue can obscure a mutant peak, so reliable sequencing results can only be obtained with samples containing a high percentage of tumor cells. To achieve this often requires labor-intensive additional tumor enrichment techniques, such as microdissection.

Simple and objective methods for assessing p53 status are clearly needed. Transcriptional activation, a function of normal p53, is abrogated by p53 mutations. A functional test of this transcriptional competence has been developed in yeast.[45,46] This test is simpler to perform than sequencing, in particular because it does not call for microdissection of samples or the use of expensive automated sequencing equipment, and it has the added advantage of providing direct information about p53 function (it detects only biologically important mutations). The test is more sensitive than sequencing of unmicrodissected material because it is not compromised by contamination, even with relatively large amounts of normal tissue. The method can be summarized as follows. RNA is extracted from 100 μm frozen sections. A complementary DNA is made using reverse transcriptase, amplified by polymerase chain reaction (PCR), and transformed into yeast together with a linearized expression vector. The yeast clone the PCR product into the vector by homologous recombination (gap repair), and recombinants are selected on medium lacking leucine. The p53 cDNA is expressed from a constitutive promoter in the plasmid, so all of the yeast colonies contain human p53 protein. The strain also contains an integrated ADE2 reporter gene regulated by a p53-responsive promoter. When the expression plasmid encodes wt p53, the cells express ADE2, grow normally, and form white colonies. When the plasmid encodes mutant p53, the cells fail to express ADE2 and form small red colonies. If desired, sequencing of p53 from plasmids rescued from red yeast colonies can be used to identify the specific mutation. In addition to testing p53 for biologically important mutations, this technique avoids sequencing of p53 genes that do not have mutations, thus saving resources. The assay tests p53 codons 52–364, which includes the entire DNA binding and oligomerization domains.

A PROSPECTIVE STUDY TO ADDRESS THE p53 HYPOTHESIS

Thus experimental data suggest that p53-mutated tumors are less sensitive to anthracyclines, but remain sensitive to taxanes. Is this true in clinical practice? A multicenter randomized neoadjuvant chemotherapy trial is being developed that will prospectively compare a non taxane regimen (with anthracycline) versus a taxane regimen (with anthracycline). This so-called 'BIG-p53' trial will address two questions:

- A classic question: is a treatment including taxanes superior to an anthracycline-based regimen (without taxanes)?
- An innovative question (translational research question): do taxanes offer a greater advantage in tumors with mutant than with wt p53?

Patients with large operable, locally advanced, or inflammatory breast cancer are eligible for this study. In this subgroup of patients with a high risk of distant micrometastases, primary (neoadjuvant) chemotherapy seems preferable in order to treat these micrometastases early. Randomized studies have shown that neoadjuvant chemotherapy in large primary breast cancer enhances the breast conservation rate[47–50] without compromising survival.[47,48,50,51] In locally advanced breast cancer, the addition of adjuvant chemotherapy and hormonal therapy has been shown to improve local control and survival (hormonal therapy) when compared with radiotherapy alone.[52]

Potentially eligible patients will have an incisional or a trucut biopsy to establish the histological diagnosis and provide traditional prognostic information. A portion of the biopsy will be analyzed for p53, using the previously described yeast functional assay. Following biopsy, patients are randomized to six cycles of an epirubicin-containing regimen or an epirubicin/docetaxel combination and definitive locoregional therapy, and are then followed for relapse and survival.

Several different epirubicin-containing combinations will be allowed in the non-taxane arm: although not designed to test the optimal dose intensity of epirubicin, it is recognized that a suboptimal anthracycline dose might compromise outcome. The regimens allowed are FEC100 (recommended for EORTC centers),[53] Canadian CEF,[6] and the tailored FEC as developed by the Swedish group.[54] Despite their heterogeneity, these three regimens share a high dose intensity of epirubicin, and enable various collaborating groups with different policies to participate in the trial while ensuring that an adequate dose of epirubicin is delivered.

It is not clear whether the best strategy is to give anthracyclines and taxanes concomitantly or sequentially; various randomized trials are currently exploring this question. In this study, patients randomized to the taxane-containing arm will receive three cycles of docetaxel 100 mg/m^2 every 21 days (an extensively studied schedule in the metastatic setting[55]), followed by three cycles of epirubicin/docetaxel at doses of 90 mg/m^2 and 75 mg/m^2, respectively, without granulocyte colony-stimulating factor (G-CSF). The schedule for the combination is derived from phase I trials (the French Anti-Cancer Centers Group recommended docetaxel/epirubicin doses of 100/75 mg/m^2 and the International Breast Cancer Study Group (IBCSG), 90/75 mg/m^2, both schedules being given day 1 q21 days).[56,57] The IBCSG study was subsequently extended into phase II: a total of 70 metastatic breast cancer patients were treated (20 in phase I and 50 in the phase II extension).[58] Febrile neutropenia (ANC $< 0.5 \times 10^9$/l with at least one oral temperature of $>38.5°C$ or three oral temperatures of $38°C$ in a 24-h period) occurred in 11% of cycles; 52% of these episodes were managed on an outpatient basis with oral antibiotics. G-CSF support (150 µg/m^2/day subcutaneously from day 2 to day 11) was given in subsequent cycles after febrile neutropenia, or after failure of adequate ANC recovery by the planned day of retreatment. G-CSF was given with 44% of the cycles, predominantly because of febrile neutropenia. Prophylactic oral antibiotics were strongly recommended in patients whose ANC nadir was below 0.5×10^9/l. This is the regimen to be used in the BIG-p53 study.

With multicenter international participation in this study, accrual of the planned 1400 patients should proceed quickly. It is hoped that this prospective study will provide a definitive answer about the predictive role of mutated p53 in response to taxanes and anthracyclines in early breast cancer. Prospective trials are also stratifying for c-ErbB-2 overexpression, and thus bold steps are being taken to narrow the gap between our current approach to adjuvant chemotherapy and a highly individualized treatment strategy that takes into account not only the prognostic profile of the tumor but also its unique sensitivity to systemic cytotoxic drugs.

REFERENCES

1. Thor AD, Berry DA, Budman DR et al, ErbB-2, p53, and efficacy of adjuvant therapy in lymph node-positive breast cancer. *J Natl Cancer Inst* 1998; **90**:1346–60.

2. Paik S, Bryant J, Park C et al, ErbB-2 and response to doxorubicin in patients with axillary lymph node-positive, hormone receptor-negative breast cancer. *J Natl Cancer Inst* 1998; **90**:1361–70.

3. Clark GM, Should selection of adjuvant chemotherapy for patients with breast cancer be based on erbB-2 status? *J Natl Cancer Inst* 1998; **90**:1320–2.

4. Early Breast Cancer Trialists' Collaborative Group, Polychemotherapy for early breast cancer: an overview of the randomised trials. *Lancet* 1998; **352**:930–42.

5. Hutchins L, Green S, Ravdin P et al, CMF versus CAF with and without tamoxifen in high-risk node-negative breast cancer patients and a natural history follow-up study in low-risk node-negative patients: first results of Intergroup trial INT 0102. *Proc Am Soc Clin Oncol* 1998; **17**:1a (Abst 2).

6. Levine MN, Bramwell VH, Pritchard KI et al, Randomized trial of intensive cyclophosphamide, epirubicin, and fluorouracil chemotherapy compared with cyclophosphamide, methotrexate, and fluorouracil in premenopausal women with node-positive breast cancer. *J Clin Oncol* 1998; **16**:2651–8.

7. Henderson IC, Berry D, Demetri G et al, Improved disease-free (DFS) and overall survival (OS) from the addition of sequential paclitaxel (T) but not from the escalation of doxorubicin (A) dose level in the adjuvant chemotherapy of patients (pts) with node-positive primary breast cancer (BC). *Proc Am Soc Clin Oncol* 1998; **17**:101a (Abst 390A).

8. Goldhirsch A, Glick JH, Gelber RD, Senn HJ, Meeting Highlights: International Consensus Panel on the Treatment of Primary Breast Cancer. *J Natl Cancer Inst* 1998; **90**:1601–8.

9. Ellis PA, Smith IE, McCarthy K et al, Preoperative chemotherapy induces apoptosis in early breast cancer. *Lancet* 1997; **349**:849.

10. Hickman JA, Apoptosis induced by anticancer drugs. *Cancer Metastasis Rev* 1992; **11**:121–39.

11. Carr AM, Cell cycle. Piecing together the p53 puzzle. *Science* 2000; **287**:1824–7.

12. Dulic V, Kaufmann WK, Wilson SJ et al, p53-dependent inhibition of cyclin-dependent kinase activities in human fibroblasts during radiation-induced G1 arrest. *Cell* 1994; **74**:1013–23.

13. Miyashita T, Krajewski S, Krajewska M et al, Tumor suppressor p53 is a regulator for bcl-2 and bax gene expression in vitro and in vivo. *Oncogene* 1994; **9**:1799–805.

14. Fritsche M, Haessler C, Brandner G, Induction of nuclear accumulation of the tumor-suppressor protein p53 by DNA-damaging agent. *Oncogene* 1993; **8**:307–18.

15. Lowe SW, Ruley HE, Jacks T, Housman DE, p53-Dependent apoptosis modulates the cytotoxicity of anticancer agents. *Cell* 1993; **74**:957–67.

16. Gudas JM, Nguyen H, Li T et al, Drug-resistant breast cancer cells frequently retain expression of a functional wild-type p53 protein. *Carcinogenesis* 1996; **17**:1417–27.

17. Lowe SW, Dosi S, McClatchey A et al, p53 status and the efficacy of cancer therapy in vivo. *Science* 1994; **266**:807–10.

18. Torres K, Horwitz SB, Mechanisms of Taxol-induced cell death are concentration dependent. *Cancer Res* 1998; **58**:3620–6.

19. Fan S, Cherney B, Reinhold W et al, Disruption of p53 function in immortalized human cells does not affect survival or apoptosis after taxol or vincristine treatment. *Clin Cancer Res* 1998; **4**:1047–54.

20. Vasey PA, Jones NA, Jenkins S et al, Cisplatin, camptothecin, and Taxol sensitivities of cells with p53-associated multidrug resistance. *Mol Pharmacol* 1996; **50**:1536–40.

21. Jordan MA, Wendell K, Gardiner S et al, Mitotic block induced in HeLa cells by low concentration of paclitaxel (Taxol) results in abnormal mitototic exit and apoptotic cell death. *Cancer Res* 1996; **56**:816–25.

22. Lanni JS, Lowe SW, Licitra EJ et al, p53-Independent apoptosis induced by paclitaxel through an indirect mechanism. *Proc Natl Acad Sci USA* 1997; **94**:9679–83.

23. Lazarides E, Taxol-induced mitotic block triggers rapid onset of a p53-independent apoptotic pathway. *Mol Med* 1995; **1**:506–26.

24. O'Connor PM, Jackman J, Bae I et al, Characterization of the p53 tumor suppressor pathway in cell lines of the National Cancer Institute Anticancer Drug Screen and correlations with the growth-inhibitory potency of 123 anticancer agents. *Anticancer Res* 1997; **57**:4285–300.

25. Perego P, Romalli S, Carenini N et al, Ovarian cancer cisplatin-resistant cell lines: multiple changes including collateral sensitivity to Taxol. *Ann Oncol* 1998; **9**:423–30.

26. Wahl AF, Donaldson KL, Fairchild C et al, Loss of normal p53 function confers sensitization to Taxol by increasing G2/m arrest and apoptosis. *Nature Med* 1996; **2**:72–9.

27. Wu GS, El-Deiry WS, p53 and chemosensitivity. *Nature Med* 1996; **2**:255–6.

28. Delia D, Mizutani S, Lamorte G et al, p53 activity and chemotherapy. *Nature Med* 1996; **2**:724–5.

29. Bergh J, Norberg T, Sjögren S et al, Complete sequencing of the p53 gene provides prognostic information in breast cancer patients, particularly in relation to adjuvant systemic therapy and radiotherapy. *Nature Med* 1995; **1**:1029–34.

30. Jansson T, Inganäs M, Sjögren S et al, p53 Status predicts survival in breast cancer patients treated with/without postoperative radiotherapy: a novel hypothesis based on clinical findings. *J Clin Oncol* 1995; **13**:2745–51.

31. Aas T, Borresen AL, Geisler S et al, Specific p53 mutations are associated with de novo resistance to doxorubicin in breast cancer patients. *Nature Med* 1996; **2**:811–14.

32. Kandioler-Eckersberger D, Taucher S, Steiner B et al, p53 Genotype and major response to anthracycline or paclitaxel based neoadjuvant treatment in breast cancer patients. *Proc Am Soc Clin Oncol* 1998; **17**:102a (Abst 392).

33. Falette N, Paperin MP, Treilleux I et al, Prognostic value of p53 gene mutations in a large series of node-negative breast cancer patients. *Cancer Res* 1998; **58**:1451–5.

34. Sjögren S, Inganäs M, Norberg T et al, The p53 gene in breast cancer: prognostic value of complementary DNA sequencing versus immunohistochemistry. *J Natl Cancer Inst* 1996; **88**:173–82.

35. Chappuis PO, Estreicher A, Dieterich B et al, Prognostic significance of p53 mutation in breast cancer: frequent detection of non-missense mutations by yeast functional assay. *Int J Cancer* 1999; **84**:587–93.

36. Barnes DM, Dublin EA, Fisher CJ et al, Immunohistochemical detection of p53 protein in mammary carcinoma: an important new independent indicator of prognosis? *Hum Pathol* 1993; **24**:469–76.

37. Bonnefoi H, Diebold-Berger S, Hamilton A et al, A study of molecular markers with potential prognostic and predictive value (c-erb b-2, p53, cyclin D1, MIB1, ER and PgR) in locally advanced breast cancer treated with neo-adjuvant dose intensive chemotherapy in an

EORTC–NCIC–SAKK randomized phase III study. *Eur J Cancer* 1998; **34**(Suppl 5):S10 (Abstract 133).

38. Silvestrini R, Benini E, Daidone MG et al, p53 as an independent prognostic marker in lymph node-negative breast cancer patients. *J Natl Cancer Inst* 1993; **85**:965–70.

39. Silvestrini R, Daidone MG, Benini E et al, Validation of p53 accumulation as a predictor of distant metastasis at 10 years of follow-up in 1400 node-negative breast cancers. *Clin Cancer Res* 1996; **2**:2007–13.

40. Silvestrini R, Benini E, Venerani S et al, p53 and *bcl-2* expression correlates with clinical outcome in a series of node-positive breast cancer patients. *J Clin Oncol* 1996; **14**:1604–10.

41. Thor AD, Moore DH II, Edgerton SM et al, Accumulation of p53 tumor suppressor gene protein: an independent marker of prognosis in breast cancers. *J Natl Cancer Inst* 1992; **84**:845–55.

42. Elledge RM, Who R, Mansour E et al, Accumulation of p53 protein as a possible predictor of response to adjuvant combination chemotherapy with cyclophosphamide, methotrexate, fluorouracil, and prednisone for breast cancer. *J Natl Cancer Inst* 1995; **87**:1254–6.

43. Clahsen PC, van de Velde CJH, Duval C et al, p53 protein accumulation and response to adjuvant chemotherapy in premenopausal women with node-negative early breast cancer. *J Clin Oncol* 1998; **16**:470–9.

44. Broet P, Spyratos F, Romain S et al, Prognostic value of uPA and p53 accumulation measured by quantitative biochemical assays in 1245 primary breast cancer patients: a multicentre study. *Br J Cancer* 1999; **80**:536–45.

45. Ishioka C, Frebourg T, Yan YX et al, Screening patients for heterozygous p53 mutations using a functional assay in yeast. *Nature Genet* 1993; **5**:124–9.

46. Flaman JM, Frebourg T, Moreau V et al, A simple p53 functional assay for screening cell lines, blood, and tumors. *Proc Natl Acad Sci USA* 1995; **92**:3963–7.

47. Fisher B, Bryant J, Wolmark N et al, Effect of preoperative chemotherapy on the outcome of women with operable breast cancer. *J Clin Oncol* 1998; **16**:2672–85.

48. Mauriac L, Durand M, Avril A, Dilhuydy JM, Effect of primary chemotherapy in conservative treatment of breast cancer patients with operable tumors larger than 3 cm. Results of a randomized trial in a single centre. *Ann Oncol* 1991; **2**:347–54.

49. Powles TJ, Hickish TF, Makris A et al, Randomized trial of chemoendocrine therapy started before or after surgery for treatment of primary breast cancer. *J Clin Oncol* 1995; **13**:547–52.

50. Scholl SM, Fourquet A, Asselain B et al, Neoadjuvant versus adjuvant chemotherapy in premenopausal patients with tumours considered too large for breast conserving surgery: preliminary results of a randomised trial: S6. *Eur J Cancer* 1994; **30A**:645–52.

51. Semilglavoz VF, Topuzov EE, Bavli JL et al, Primary (neoadjuvant) chemotherapy and radiotherapy compared with primary radiotherapy alone in stage IIb–IIIa breast cancer. *Ann Oncol* 1994; **5**:591–5.

52. Bartelink H, Rubens RD, van der Schueren E, Sylvester R, Hormonal therapy prolongs survival in irradiated locally advanced breast cancer: a European Organization for Research and Treatment of Cancer randomised phase III trial. *J Clin Oncol* 1997; **15**:207–15.

53. Bonneterre J, Roche H, Bremond A et al, Results of a randomized trial of adjuvant chemotherapy with FEC 50 vs FEC 100 in high risk node-positive breast cancer patients. *Proc Am Soc Clin Oncol* 1998; **17**:124a (Abst 473).

54. Bergh J, Wiklund T, Erikstein B et al, Dosage of adjuvant G-CSF (filgrastim)-supported FEC polychemotherapy based on equivalent haematological toxicity in high-risk breast cancer patients. *Ann Oncol* 1998; **9**:403–11.

55. Chan S, Friedrichs K, Noel D et al, Prospective randomized trial of docetaxel versus doxorubicin in patients with metastatic breast cancer. *J Clin Oncol* 1999; **17**:2341–54.

56. Pagani O, Sessa C, Martinelli G et al, Dose-finding study of epidoxorubicin and docetaxel as first-line chemotherapy in patients with advanced breast cancer. *Ann Oncol* 1999; **10**:539–45.

57. Kerbrat P, Viens H, Roche P et al, Docetaxel (D) in combination with epirubicin (E) as 1st line chemotherapy (CT) of metastatic breast cancer (MBC): final results. *Proc Am Soc Clin Oncol* 1998; **17**:151a (Abst 579).

58. Pagani O, Sessa C, Nolé F et al, Epidoxorubicin and docetaxel as first-line chemotherapy in patients with advanced breast cancer: a multicentric phase I–II study. *Ann Oncol* (submitted).

35

Preoperative chemotherapy

Justin Stebbing, Ian E Smith

INTRODUCTION

The conventional approach to the systemic management of early breast cancer is to give adjuvant chemotherapy postoperatively, after surgical excision of the primary tumor. In preoperative chemotherapy (also called neoadjuvant or primary chemotherapy[1]), the roles are reversed, and chemotherapy is given as first-line treatment to try and achieve tumor regression and downstaging before surgery. The origins of preoperative chemotherapy lie in experience gained in the management of locally advanced inoperable breast cancer. Here, medical treatment has been used increasingly in recent years prior to local radiotherapy to try to improve local control and prolong survival.[2,3]

This approach has now extended to include the management of large but operable breast cancers, where mastectomy has been the only standard surgical option. Such patients tend to have a poor prognosis irrespective of local treatment,[4] and adjuvant treatment would usually be offered anyway.[5] Although the benefits of adjuvant treatment have been established in a number of randomized trials, [6,7] it is administered when patients are clinically 'disease-free' and there is no way of determining whether an

individual patient has micrometastases and if so, whether or not they are sensitive to cytotoxic agents given. An advantage of preoperative chemotherapy is that it allows the primary tumor itself to be used as an in vivo measure of response,[8] thereby affording an opportunity to study the biology of breast cancer during therapy.

BACKGROUND

Historical perspectives

Mastectomy has dominated the approach to the management of primary breast cancer for the past 100 years, influenced largely by the work of William Halstead at Johns Hopkins during the last decade of the nineteenth century.[9] It is interesting to note that some of his predecessors, including Leroy and James Paget, expressed a degree of skepticism over whether surgical removal of the breast en bloc (with regional nodes and the underlying pectoralis muscle) actually prolonged survival.[10,11]

In 1943, Haagensen and Stout used their experiences to establish a list of criteria that they believed indicated incurability.[12] The list included the presence of peau d'orange (more than one-third of the breast), arm edema, inflammatory cancer, satellite skin, or parasternal nodules. In their series, not only was local-regional failure common, but survival rates were reported as less than 35% at five years. Indeed, mastectomy failed to cure any of the 120 patients followed for eight years.

Practice has now changed for two reasons. First, there are data that show that the risk of recurrence and overall survival are unrelated to the nature and intensity of local treatment:[13] it is now established that use of conservative surgery followed by local radiotherapy is as effective as mastectomy in terms of survival.[14] Second, there are increased demands from patients for more conservative treatments. Although there are notable high-profile exceptions to this trend for breast conservation,[15] the climate now significantly favors immediate conservation whenever possible.[16,17]

Preoperative chemotherapy could be considered to be the next logical step in the gradual evolution of breast cancer management over the last 20–30 years. The rationale behind this approach is considered below.

Scientific rationale

The presence of systemic micrometastases in women with a primary breast cancer has been confirmed by immunocytochemical techniques: a recent study of 350 women with primary breast cancer identified their presence in the bone marrow in exactly one-quarter of all patients at the time of initial surgery.[18] These micrometastases detected using antibody to epithelial membrane antigen are significantly associated with the traditional poor prognostic factors of larger tumors and involved lymph nodes,[19] and also with early recurrence.[20,21]

There are a number of theoretical and laboratory-based reasons why preoperative rather than adjuvant chemotherapy might improve survival in patients with breast cancer, irrespective of tumor size. One relates to the effect that surgical removal of the primary may have on residual micrometastatic populations.

Following work by Simpson-Herren et al[22] on subcutaneous Lewis lung tumors in mice, Fisher demonstrated an increase in growth of metastases after removal of a C3H mammary adenocarcinoma.[23] This was later confirmed in six different tumor host systems, when there was an increase in the thymidine labelling index, doubling time, and tumor size of micrometastases 24 hours after the primary tumor's removal. This dramatic effect could be explained by the presence of a transmissible growth factor that caused identical kinetic changes when injected into recipient mice with the same tumor.[24] Importantly, preoperative chemo-endocrine therapy, with cyclophosphamide or tamoxifen given before surgery, prevented these kinetic changes, suppressed tumor growth, and prolonged mouse survival.[25] The mouse tumors themselves could be used to measure response rates in vivo.

Another theoretical benefit for preoperative chemotherapy is based on the Goldie and Coldman hypothesis. This mathematical model contends that the expansion of micrometastatic disease after surgery allows for the emergence of drug-resistant clones of cells.[26] Recent evidence suggests production of an angiogenesis inhibitor by the primary tumor, the removal of which before chemotherapy allows for neovascularization and metastatic growth.[27] Together, these observations supported the rationale for preoperative chemotherapy and refuted the Skipper and Schabel hypothesis, published in 1973, that the primary tumor response cannot predict responsiveness of micrometastatic disease.[28]

The real measure of any benefit, no matter how elegant the theory, can only be determined with clinical trials, which will be summarized below, focusing on two randomized trials: one conducted under the auspices of the NSABP Protocol B-18,[29–31] the other carried out at the Royal Marsden Hospital.[32]

THE CLINICAL RESPONSE OF OPERABLE BREAST CANCER TO PREOPERATIVE CHEMOTHERAPY

Non-randomized studies

One of the first preoperative chemotherapy studies in potentially operable breast cancer was carried out by the Edinburgh group. Patients rather unconventionally received CHOP (cyclophosphamide, doxorubicin, vincristine, prednisone) chemotherapy either as first-line treatment or after failure of endocrine therapy. Their updated results have demonstrated a 70% response rate with a 26% complete remission rate.[33] In addition, this study emphasized the potential of the tumor itself as an in vivo measure of response: 34 (72%) patients achieved 'a significant reduction in tumor volume', with 13 (28%) complete remissions and 8 (17%) with no histological evidence of invasive carcinoma in surgical specimens. None of the patients studied demonstrated tumor progression.

Investigators of 537 patients treated at the Milan Cancer Institute with either CMF (cyclophosphamide, methotrexate, 5-fluorouracil (5-FU)), an anthracycline- or mitoxantrone-containing combination, or doxorubicin alone, for three or four cycles, reported response rates of 74–78% and a complete remission rate of 12–21%. There was no significant correlation between response and drug schedule used or duration of treatment. In these trials, 3% of patients had evidence of tumor progression during treatment.[34,35] Other non-randomized studies reported similar high response rates.[36–39]

Experience at the Royal Marsden Hospital in London began in 1986 in patients whose tumors were of sufficient size for mastectomy to be required as standard management (median dia-meter 6 cm). Sixty-four patients were treated with either CMF or MMM (methotrexate, mitomycin C, mitoxantrone) chemotherapy. The response rate was 69%, including 17% complete remissions.[40] The authors subsequently developed a novel ambulatory infusional schedule consisting of six cycles of epirubicin 50 mg/m^2, cisplatin 60 mg/m^2 both every 3 weeks along with continuous infusional 5-FU 200 mg/m^2 per day via an ambulatory pump and Hickman line. Since 5-FU is rapidly catabolized, the rationale here was to maintain plasma levels, thereby insuring prolonged exposure of this cell-cycle-specific drug to tumor cells in the S phase. Interestingly, myelosuppression had been shown to be less with continuous 5-FU, whereas stomatitis, diarrhea, and palmar–plantar erythema were dose-limiting.[41] In an initial pilot study of 50 patients, 49 patients (98%) achieved an objective response, including 33 complete remissions (66%).[42] With 123 patients entered from the Royal Marsden, response rates have remained high (clinical response rate of 96%, complete remissions at 54%). The results of the non-randomized trials are summarized in Table 35.1.

Randomized studies of preoperative versus adjuvant chemotherapy

A low-toxicity schedule of mitoxantrone, methotrexate, and tamoxifen (MMT) was studied at the Royal Marsden[32] in patients with smaller cancers (≥2 cm in size, median 3.5 cm). Patients were randomized to receive this treatment either preoperatively or in the adjuvant setting. An overall response rate of 85% was observed, with a complete response rate of 19%, in the preoperative arm.

By far the largest study, however, has been carried out by the National Surgical Adjuvant Breast Project (NSABP), who initiated a trial (B-18) to further evaluate the worth of preoperative chemotherapy.[29–31] Patients were diagnosed

Table 35.1   Non-randomized trials of preoperative chemotherapy

Refs	Tumor size	Schedule[a]	No. of patients (no. randomized)	Response rate (%)
36	Operable	Vinblastine, thiotepa, 5-FU methotrexate, prednisolone (+ doxorubicin if ⩾7 cm)	250	75
39	⩾3 cm, operable	Doxorubicin, vincristine, cyclophosphamide, 5-FU, methotrexate	148	97
37	⩾3 cm	Cisplatin, doxorubicin, cyclophosphamide	26	100
38	>3 cm	Methotrexate or epirubicin + vincristine, 5-FU, cyclophosphamide	158	61
34, 35	⩾3 cm	CMF + doxorubicin	537	76
42[b]	3–12 cm	ECF	123	96
33[b]	⩾4 cm	CHOP	94	70

[a] CMF, cyclophosphamide, methotrexate, 5-FU; ECF, epirubicin, cyclophosphamide, 5-FU; CHOP, cyclophosphamide, doxorubicin, vincristine, prednisone.
[b] Updated results.

with breast cancer by fine-needle aspiration or a tru-cut biopsy before stratification by age, clinical tumor size, and axillary lymph node status. Patients were eligible for the study if their tumors (T1–3N0–1M0) were confined to the breast and axilla and their predicted life expectancy was at least 10 years. Tumors had to be movable in relation to underlying tissues, and patients who demonstrated Haagensesen's and Stout's poor prognostic features[12] (e.g. inflammatory cancer, skin fixation, etc.) were excluded.

Between October 1988 and April 1993, 1523 patients were randomized to receive either four cycles of doxorubicin/cyclophosphamide (AC)

Table 35.2   Randomized trials of preoperative chemotherapy

Refs	Tumor size	Schedule	No. of patients	Response rate (%)
43	3–7 cm	Doxorubicin, 5-FU, cyclophosphamide	200 (390)[*]	65
32	Operable	Mitoxantrone, methotrexate	105 (309)[*]	85
44	>2 cm	Thiotepa, methotrexate, 5-FU	134 (271)[*]	57
45	>3 cm	Epirubicin, vincristine, and methotrexate, followed by mitomycin C, thiotepa, and vindesine	138 (272)[*]	81
32, 33, 46 (NSABP B-18)	Operable	Doxorubicin, cyclophosphamide	749 (1523)[*]	79

[*] Numbers randomized to receive pre-operative chemotherapy.

chemotherapy every three weeks followed by surgery (lumpectomy plus axillary dissection or modified radical mastectomy) or the same surgery followed by chemotherapy. Patients aged 50 years or more (approximately 50% of patients) also received tamoxifen 20 mg once daily following completion of chemotherapy.

The primary B-18 study aims focused on determining whether the use of preoperative chemotherapy increased disease-free survival (DFS) and overall survival (OS) compared with the same chemotherapy given in the adjuvant setting. Secondary aims included the evaluation of clinical and pathological response of the primary tumor, thereby determining the down-staging effect of preoperative chemotherapy on axillary lymph nodes, and the determination of whether it allows for greater breast conservation.

In the NSABP B-18 trial, 747 patients were randomized to receive preoperative chemother-

apy. Following administration, 269 (36%) of patients obtained a complete clinical response and 321 (43%) of patients obtained a partial response (overall response rate 79%). Seventeen percent of patients were classified as having stable disease and, as in the Milan studies, 3% had progressive disease. This last finding of rare incidences of tumor progression is a key finding in all studies of preoperative chemotherapy. The riposte to this important finding may be that initial surgery produces a complete remission each time. The results of the main randomized studies are summarized in Table 35.2.

THE AVOIDANCE OF MASTECTOMY AND LOCAL-REGIONAL FAILURE

Non-randomized studies

The latter half of this century has observed a trend away from mastectomy towards conservative surgery, which is justified by similar results.[13,14] For patients with larger tumors, mastectomy is the only conventional surgical option, but for many women this remains unappealing and perhaps emotionally disturbing. Preoperative chemotherapy offers the possibility of downstaging tumors and avoiding radical surgery.

Though the main entry point in the Royal Marsden ECF (epirubicin, cisplatin, continuous 5-FU) study was the need for mastectomy, after infusional chemotherapy only 8% of patients required a mastectomy.[40] Only one patient developed progressive disease. Similarly, in the Italian studies, patients were selected on the basis of needing mastectomies (cutoff >3 cm), but only 15% of patients subsequently required this after doxorubicin–CMF chemotherapy.[34,35] In their experience, the likelihood of conservative surgery was inversely related to the size of the primary breast cancer. Patients whose tumors were less than 4 cm in diameter had a more than a 90% chance of undergoing conservative surgery, compared with around 60–70% in patients with tumors larger than 5 cm in size. Jacquillat et al[36] initiated one of the earlier studies in 1980, with a mixed population of 250 potentially operable patients. Following cytotoxic treatment, only 11 patients required mastectomy. These early studies provided evidence for an immediate and practical benefit of preoperative chemotherapy.

Randomized studies

These confirm data from non-randomized studies, although the results are less striking. In the Royal Marsden MMT trial, the incidence of mastectomy was reduced from 22% in the adjuvant group to 10% with the use of preoperative chemotherapy ($p < 0.003$).[32] Similar results were observed in the randomized study by Scholl et al.[43] Patients who received CAF preoperative chemotherapy were less likely to undergo a mas-

tectomy (23% versus 36% in the adjuvant arm; $p < 0.003$). Another study of 272 patients with primary breast tumors larger than 3 cm showed that patients receiving preoperative chemotherapy had a 38% mastectomy rate, compared with 100% in the primary-surgery arm of the trial.[44] These three studies focused on larger primary breast cancers (unlike B-18), and eligibility criteria included the need for immediate mastectomy if patients were treated conventionally.

Though the randomization process in the B-18 study distributed patients evenly such that tumor characteristics were similar between the two groups, many women (28%) had tumors less than 2 cm in diameter. Only 13% had tumors larger than 5.1 cm. In this trial, lumpectomy was achieved in 68% of patients in the preoperative group, compared with 60% in the adjuvant group ($p < 0.010$). This effect was most evident in the 13% of women with the larger tumors, contradicting the non-randomized data from Milan suggesting higher response rates in smaller tumors. In this subgroup, more lumpectomies were performed (22%) than was originally proposed (3%). In this trial, surgeons were asked to indicate before randomization the type of operation that they would perform. The best evidence to indicate that preoperative chemotherapy leads to an increase in breast conservation comes from the trialists' findings of a *sevenfold* increase in the number of lumpectomies over that proposed, in the patients with the largest tumors.

A further conclusion from the B-18 study was that age was not found to be a factor in the decision to propose breast conservation. This finding was in contrast to previous studies indicating that lumpectomy is less often used in older women because of physician bias.[47]

Local recurrence

Local recurrence rates have become relevant with the avoidance of mastectomy. There are currently

Table 35.3   Local-regional recurrence

Refs	No. of patients	Postoperative chemotherapy (%)	Preoperative chemotherapy (%)	Median follow-up
46	1495	8.2	10.6	5 years
43	390	20	26	5 years
48	272	4.5	11.4	124 months
49	200	2	1	29 months

four randomized trials that compare local recurrence rates in patients treated with preoperative chemotherapy as compared with the adjuvant setting.[43,46,48,49] The trial by Mauriac et al performed at the Institut Bergonie in Bordeaux demonstrated a significant difference between the two treatments as seen in Table 35.3 (31 local recurrences in the preoperative arm, 12 in adjuvant arm); the other three trials do not show significant differences.

Collection of data is complicated by differences in treatment regimens, which do not allow for a direct head-to-head randomized comparison of preoperative and adjuvant treatment. In the study by Mauriac et al, patients were randomized to either mastectomy followed by adjuvant treatment or preoperative chemotherapy followed by adjusted locoregional treatment (33% had breast irradiation alone, 30% lumpectomy, and 37% mastectomy). In their first group, though 100% of patients had a mastectomy, 24% of patients were deemed to have such good prognostic factors (e.g. no nodal involvement) that adjuvant treatment was not given. This is in spite of the fact that eligibility necessitated T2 tumors larger than 3 cm or T3N0–1M0, which, by the St Galen consensus,[5] would require chemotherapy. Chemotherapy consisted of three cycles of epirubicin, vincristine, and methotrexate, followed by

mitomycin C, thiotepa, and vindesine for three cycles. In their follow-up of the preoperatively treated group, patients with breast recurrences did not have the same worse prognosis as patients with a breast relapse who were in the immediate-mastectomy arm, most of whom (11 out of 12 patients) later had metastatic disease. In the preoperative arm, 13 of 31 patients remain free of distant metastases after salvage mastectomy with a 124-month follow-up.

The risk in the B-18 trial of ipsilateral tumor recurrence was almost identical among 'conventional' candidates for breast-conserving treatment (surgeons had considered these patients suitable for lumpectomy pre-randomization) who underwent preoperative chemotherapy (30 of 435, 6.9%) as in patients who underwent lumpectomy before chemotherapy (26 of 435, 6%). The risk of local failure was, however, greater in those patients who originally were thought to require a mastectomy and whose disease was downstaged sufficiently by preoperative chemotherapy to go on to lumpectomy (10 of 69, 14.5%). There is the suggestion here that avoidance of mastectomy may be associated with an increased local recurrence rate.

A further note of caution on the role of surgery after chemotherapy arises from our Royal Marsden randomized series of 185 patients with large operable breast cancer treated with primary chemotherapy (either conventional 5-FU, epirubicin, cyclophosphamide or infusional epirubicin, cisplatin, 5-FU). A complete response was seen in 21% of patients who then had no surgery but radiotherapy commencing after preoperative chemotherapy. This cohort of patients is showing a significant increase in the incidence of local failure compared with those treated with surgery, despite achievement of a complete clinical response (21% versus 7%; $p < 0.02$). In contrast, however, with the B-18 data, there is no difference in the number of local failures post mastectomy or post lumpectomy.[50]

THE EFFECT OF PREOPERATIVE CHEMOTHERAPY ON SURVIVAL

Non-randomized studies

The impact of preoperative chemotherapy on survival cannot be assessed from non-randomized studies. Small studies, however, give useful information on the predictive implications of response (see below). In the Royal Marsden experience, based on 185 patients treated with different forms of preoperative chemotherapy, responders top chemotherapy had a significantly improved DFS rate (63% versus 41% at five years) and OS rate.[50] The 36% of patients who achieved a complete clinical response, however, did not have an increased survival rate over the 46% achieving only a partial response. Other studies have found conflicting results. In a series of 329 patients, only 188 of whom were operable, those who had a complete clinical response to doxorubicin, vincristine, cyclophosphamide and 5-FU had an increased OS rate over those who did not (83% versus 71% at five years).[51]

Hortobagyi et al[52] also found that response correlated with prognosis. Five-year survival rates for 48 potentially operable stage IIIA patients who responded to treatment were 93%

in patients with a complete remission (CR in 14 patients) and 55% for a partial remission (PR in 29 patients), compared with 0% for non-responders. In stage IIIB disease, five-year survival was achieved in 75% of patients with a CR, in 30% with a PR, and in only 14% of non-responders. These results identify non-responders (5–20%, depending on the study), and, in these patients, other treatments, including second-line or high-dose chemotherapy, may improve survival.

Randomized studies

The earliest randomized trials suggested a small survival benefit. In the study by Mauriac et al,[45] a non-significant trend for improved DFS and OS was noted with 34-month median follow-up. Results of median follow-up of over 10 years duration have been recently published:[48] the trend for improved survival has disappeared, and overall (56%), metastasis-free, and recurrence-free survivals are identical when comparing pre-operative chemotherapy with adjuvant treatment. Overall survival was the same when comparing the patients within the preoperative arm treated with lumpectomy, mastectomy, or irradiation, although the local recurrence rate was higher in this last group.[52]

Similarly, the Royal Marsden MMT trial data have failed to show any differences. Here, 309 patients were randomly assigned to receive combined chemo-endocrine therapy (methotrexate, mitoxantrone, and tamoxifen) given preoperatively for three months before and again three months after surgery (preoperative arm) or post-operatively (conventional adjuvant arm). At a median follow-up of 48 months, the relative risk of adjuvant to preoperative chemotherapy was 0.99 and the disease-free relative risk was 1.09.

Updated results of a French trial involving 390 premenopausal women with stage II–III operable tumors demonstrated that the five-year survival rate was 84% for the preoperative group and 78% for the adjuvant group.[53] In keeping with these results, the NSABP B-18 trial has so far not demonstrated any differences in survival outcomes. At five years, overall survival rates were 80% for both arms, distant metastasis-free survival was 73%, and recurrence-free survival was 67% in both arms.

In B-18, there was, however, evidence of a correlation between the clinical response to preoperative chemotherapy and disease-free survival. Patients whose tumors achieved a clinical CR (cCR) fared significantly better (76% DFS at five years) than those achieving a clinical PR (63.5%) or those demonstrating stable or progressive disease (60.3%) ($p = 0.014$). A similar trend was also noted with overall survival. Because of lack of overall survival differences, the authors of the B-18 trial do not recommend the use of preoperative chemotherapy in smaller tumors amenable to lumpectomy as first-line treatment.

Although further studies are needed, our current level of knowledge suggests that it is reasonable to carry out conservative surgery after preoperative chemotherapy if appropriate downstaging has been achieved. Some suggest informing patients that there may be an increased risk of recurrence after breast-conserving surgery.

PATHOLOGIC PREDICTIVE FACTORS; THE INTERPLAY WITH PREOPERATIVE CHEMOTHERAPY

Non-randomized studies

The occurrence of a cCR subsequent to the use of preoperative chemotherapy may be associated with only partial eradication of occult metastatic disease. It has been suggested that distant eradication occurs only with chemotherapy that completely eliminates a primary breast tumor pathologically. If this were the case, a pathologic complete response (pCR) would prove to be of

greater importance than a cCR and would identify a group of patients who have an excellent prognosis thereafter. The same would hold true for nodal status, which remains the most powerful long-term predictor of outcome.

In one of the earliest trials, the Edinburgh group reported an 88% eight-year survival rate for patients achieving a pCR to chemotherapy, compared with 60% for a cCR and 35% for those not responding clinically. In terms of axillary lymph node status, 10-year survival rates were 85% for node-negative patients, 50% with one to three nodes involved, and 0% for involvement of more than three nodes. Similarly, in a Cox multivariate analysis, the number of lymph nodes involved after preoperative chemotherapy was the most significant variable in a retrospective analysis of 507 patients treated for two to four months with anthracycline-containing regimens. Patients with more than seven nodes involved after chemotherapy had a 10-year OS of only 23%, compared with 61% in women with no nodes involved at all.[54] Results from the Milan Cancer Institute were an 86% eight year DFS for those achieving pCR, compared with 58% for clinical remissions and 37% for non-responders.[34,35] The eight-year DFS rate here was 75% for node-negative patients, 51% for one to three nodes involved, and 35% for more than three nodes.

These trials demonstrated that, in contrast to cCR, a pCR after surgery is an excellent predictor of long-term outcome. In addition, there is now evidence that patients who are node-negative postoperatively have a much improved long-term prognosis. Indeed, pCR has the same advantages and disadvantages of pathologic nodal status. Although they both appear to represent a useful prognostic tool, they are late surrogate markers of outcome, available only after the completion of chemotherapy. Table 35.4 summarizes three trials clearly demonstrating the infrequency of a

Table 35.4   Preoperative chemotherapy and pCR

Refs	Chemotherapy[a] (no. of patients	pCR (%)[b]	Survival rate with pCR[c] (%)	Survival rate with cCR or PR (%)	Survival rate in responders (%)	p-value	Median follow-up
33	CHOP (50)	16	88	60	35	0.05	8-yr OS
34, 35	CMF ± A (537)	4 (1% DCIS)	86	58	37	0.03	8-yr DFS
46	AC (749)	13 (4% DCIS)	85	70	58	0.0001	5-yr DFS

[a] CHOP, cyclophosphamide, doxorubicin, vincristine, prednisone; CMF ± A, cyclophosphamide, methotrexate, 5-FU ± doxorubicin; AC, doxorubicin, cyclophosphamide.
[b] DCIS, ductal carcinoma in situ.
[c] Over follow-up time.

pCR but also the improved survival associated with it.

Randomized studies

Pathologic complete responses in breast tissue and lymph nodes appear to identify a subgroup of patients with a much improved prognosis. At the Royal Marsden, all patients with a pCR regardless of type of treatment (infusional or conventional) are showing a non-significant trend towards an improved DFS (80% versus 58%; $p = 0.02$). A pCR was seen to be more likely in patients with T1 or T2 tumors ($p = 0.004$), younger patients ($p = 0.008$) and for patients whose pCR was reached within two cycles of chemotherapy.[55]

One problem with the utility of pCR, however, is that it is rare: in the B-18 trial, for example, patients achieving a pCR made up 9% of the total. They had a statistically significant improvement in DFS and OS compared with those who

had residual invasive carcinoma of the breast on pathologic exam. The five-year DFS rate for patients achieving a pCR was 85%, compared with 70% for those achieving a cCR without a pCR, and 58% for non-responders.

In the B-18 trial, more patients achieved a cCR (36%) than noted in other studies (median 19%). Women with smaller tumors were more likely to have a cCR to preoperative chemotherapy. In the 245 women whose tumors demonstrated a cCR to preoperative treatment, a pCR was observed in 26%. In a further 11%, ductal carcinoma in situ was seen. When the incidence of pCR was related to tumor size, unlike with cCR, there was no correlation with size of tumor, and a pCR was seen as commonly with large as with small cancers, in contrast to experience at the Royal Marsden.

In terms of nodal disease with preoperative chemotherapy, in the B-18 trial there was a 37% increase in the incidence of pathologically negative nodes, i.e. a 29% increase in patients whose nodes were considered to be clinically negative and a 157% increase in patients considered to be clinically node-positive. Forty-eight percent of women with clinically negative nodes were pathologically node-positive and 14% with clinically positive nodes were pathologically node-negative.

The reason for this is not clear, although these results continue to indicate significant inaccuracy in axillary node staging and also that clinical nodal status is a poor measure of pathologic nodal status. This is further evidence for those who support the continued use of axillary dissection. In addition, the analysis of the utility of clinical nodal status in the previous section must be interpreted prudently. When the prognostic effects of cCR and pCR are taken together along with other factors such as nodal status, the clinical and pathologic tumor response is a good predictor of DFS and a borderline significant predictor for OS.

Results from the B-18 trial demonstrate that in patients with operable breast cancer, preoperative chemotherapy using four cycles of AC is safe and results in high rates of cCR, low rates of pCR, axillary nodal downstaging, and increased rates of breast preservation. When compared with conventional adjuvant chemotherapy, preoperative treatment results in an equivalent DFS, distant metastatic DFS, and OS. Complete pathologic breast tumor response to preoperative chemotherapy correlates best with outcome.

The next generation of trials

Because a pCR to preoperative chemotherapy appears to be of greater importance than a cCR, the finding of infrequent pCRs emphasizes the need for better therapies to increase the incidence of a pCR. To address this issue, in December 1995, the NSABP implemented Protocol B-27, a randomized trial that evaluates the efficacy of docetaxel when administered in the pre-operative or postoperative setting following four cycles of preoperative AC chemotherapy. Docetaxel was selected because of its significant activity in the adjuvant or advanced settings. The study aims to accrue 1606 patients over five years, with OS and DFS being the primary endpoints. Secondary endpoints include whether the addition of a taxane top AC will increase the pCR rate and the incidence of breast conservation. With this number of patients, after three years of further follow-up, a 40% reduction in mortality would be detected with a power of 0.80.

Two further ancillary studies to the B-27 protocol attempt to evaluate serum and tumor biomarkers. The first trial evaluates the utility of the serum HER2/neu (ErbB-2) extracellular domain and serum HER2/neu antibodies in predicting response to preoperative chemotherapy and long-term outcome. By obtaining serum at specified times, the investigators aim to evaluate whether levels of HER2/neu and antibodies to it are associated with recurrence. The second trial observes tumor markers obtained by fine-needle aspiration or core biopsy in predicting response to preoperative chemotherapy and predicting long-term outcome. If there is an increase in DFS or OS with docetaxel, the study will examine whether this is associated with the expression of certain biomarkers, thus giving us an insight into the biologic and clinical effects of preoperative chemotherapy.

New trials are looking at the most effective preoperative chemotherapeutic regimens. The first randomized trial to address this (TOPIC I: trial of preoperative infusional chemotherapy) was performed at the Royal Marsden, and compared AC with infusional ECF in 437 patients. The results of this are awaited. Currently, a randomized phase II trial aims to compare two new regimens (vinorelbine plus epirubicin, and vinorelbine plus mitoxantrone) against standard AC (randomized in a 2:2:1 ratio). Patients receive six cycles of preoperative chemotherapy prior to local treatment, with the three arms being compared in terms of efficacy and tolerance. Provided that these levels are acceptable, recruitment will then proceed into a larger phase III study.

One final point here is that, despite the plethora of improvements in general screening, including breast awareness campaigns and refining of mammographic techniques, up to 15% of women with breast cancer in developed countries seek medical attention late, and present with large primary breast cancers.[56] Late presentations and the attendant worse outcomes are commoner in minorities and poorer socioeconomic groups.[57] Owing to global inequalities in health care,[58] these cases probably accounts for over two-thirds of breast cancer cases worldwide, and since there are 800 000 new breast cancers diagnosed each year, there is great scope for larger randomized studies with longer follow-up times.

BIOLOGIC PREDICTIVE FACTORS

In vitro studies have identified a number of determinants that are involved in the cascade of events leading to apoptosis of tumor cells. The significance of these determinants for the response to chemotherapy has not been established, but preoperative chemotherapy is ideally suited to the discovery of these factors. Response is more easily measured in the primary tumor owing to its anatomic location. At the Royal Marsden, programs of biologic research have been an integral part of clinical trials conducted over the last 15 years.

Sampling of the primary tumor

In the molecular assessment of tumor response to chemotherapy, fine-needle aspirates (FNAs) and core-cut biopsies have been routinely used.

FNAs can be taken up to a frequency of every few days, and although the number of cells can vary substantially, this can be of the order of 10^6 or more. The suspension is ideally suited to analytical techniques such as flow cytometry and cytospins. Cytospins can, in many cases, yield several thousand cells per slide. Furthermore, multiple markers can be measured on a single FNA sample, and these have generally good concordance with the same markers assessed histologically.[59] The main disadvantage of FNAs is that they do not allow invasive disease to be distinguished from in situ lesions on morphological grounds. In the near future, advances may allow the analysis of a panel of markers to discriminate between these.

An important component of studies is measures of apoptosis. The low number of apoptotic cells in treated tumors makes this problematic, and the TUNEL assay (terminal UDP-deoxynucleotide end-labeling) is now used at the Royal Marsden, on cells taken from FNA, using flow cytometry for analysis.[60] Approximately 3000 cells require scoring for sufficient statistical confidence. Core-cuts have the advantage of retaining the tumor's epithelial–stromal architecture, and can reveal more than 25 000 cells. Many sections from the same core can be made available, although local trauma to breast tissue does not allow frequent core-cuts to be made, and they are difficult to perform in smaller tumors.

Studies of biomarkers

Apoptotic index (AI), proliferation (Ki67), and Bcl-2 protein expression have been investigated at the Royal Marsden in the primary breast cancers of 40 patients immediately before infusional ECF and in 20 of these patients who had residual tumor at the completion of six cycles.[61] The implication may be that these residual cells threaten long-term survival since they are chemoresistant. Thirteen patients (65%)

demonstrated a greater than 50% reduction in proliferation as measured by Ki67 after preoperative chemotherapy. Eleven patients showed a greater than 50% reduction in AI, with the median prechemotherapy AI being 0.6% and post chemotherapy AI being 0.2%. Thirteen patients were positive for Bcl-2 prior to chemotherapy. After treatment, five of seven patients whose tumors were negative for Bcl-2 became positive, with the median prechemotherapy Bcl-2 score being 56%, compared with 80% afterwards. These data suggested that apoptosis and proliferation were closely related in vivo and that the phenotype of reduced apoptosis and proliferation along with increased Bcl-2 is associated with resistance to cytotoxic agents.

A further study compared AI before and 24 hours after infusional ECF chemotherapy.[62] Serial core-cut biopsies were taken in 17 patients with tumors greater than 3 cm in size, before and 24 hours after receiving ECF. Their initial report showed an overall increase in the percentage of apoptotic cells from a median of 0.47% to 1.02% ($p = 0.009$). Ten patients showed an increase of greater than 50% within 24 h of chemotherapy, and changes of this degree have been confirmed in a further series of 22 patients.[63] Nine of 13 clinical responders (69%) showed a greater than 50% increase in AI, compared with only one of four clinical non-responders to chemotherapy. This indicated for the first time that chemotherapy induced measurable increases in apoptosis in human breast cancer cells within 24 h of starting treatment. This, in turn, provides evidence that immediate changes may relate to response and subsequent outcome. If larger studies confirm this to be the case then early treatment strategies could be modified, though initial rates of apoptosis and proliferation will need to be included in algorithms that predict regression.[64]

Results from 90 patients in the MMT trial[34] demonstrated that tumors that were negative for HER2/neu had a higher response rate (93% versus 57%; $p = 0.007$).[65] This is consistent with previous reports that it predicts for poor response to both chemotherapy and tamoxifen. An intriguing possibility remains that this could select patients for more aggressive treatment, with higher-dose anthracyclines or taxanes.

Further studies resulted in FNAs being taken on days 1, 3, 7, and 21 after the first cycle of chemotherapy. In pretreatment samples, estrogen-receptor expression and the absence of HER2/neu significantly predicted for complete clinical response. Serial FNAs demonstrated that early increases in progesterone-receptor expression by day 7 and late decreases in proliferation indices by day 21 also predicted for complete clinical response.[66] At the end of three months of chemoendocrine therapy, both Ki67 and AI were lower than seen in a control group of untreated tumors. Patients who had shown objective responses had significantly lower values than those who had no change or progressive disease. These results are consistent with earlier observations that substantial falls in proliferation occur in responders but not in non-responders to chemoendocrine therapy. Certain markers such as p53, cyclins, and caspases may reveal themselves to be even earlier and more sensitive markers than proliferation and apoptosis themselves.

Apoptosis markers (e.g. Bcl-2 and AI) and other prognostic indices are now emerging as a tool to predict response. Whether they will be used clinically on a day-to-day basis remains to be seen, and the results of the B-27 trial are eagerly awaited. The potential appears to exist for chemotherapy tailor-made to suit the tumor signature of each individual patient. In addition, the burden of proof is shifting: as well as deciding when to give chemotherapy, which cytotoxics to administer and how information may be provided on which patients have such favorable prognostic features that they do not need chemotherapy at all.

Biologic therapies

Preoperative treatment allows for the in vivo response to new agents to be assessed, at the macroscopic, microscopic, and molecular levels. It is established that angiogenesis is a requirement for tumor growth above a size of around 2 mm. There is evidence that tamoxifen and paclitaxel inhibit angiogenesis in vivo.[67] Previous studies have shown that neovascularization, as quantified by microvessel density in fixed paraffin-embedded sections, is related to the presence of metastases.[68] Patients in the MMT trial arms had assessments of tumor vascularity made without knowledge of the investigators of patient treatment or outcome. Ninety preoperative-arm samples and 105 adjuvant samples were analysed with immunostaining by the CD34 monoclonal antibody before scoring of microvessesls by the Chalkley method. Vascular scores for preoperative patients were significantly lower than those for adjuvant therapy (5.7 versus 6.3; $p = 0.025$).[69]

This result may be related to tumor regression and reduced production of antiangiogenic factors. Antiangiogenic factors are currently being developed in phase I and II studies. The modest reduction in tumor vasculature with adjuvant chemotherapy may be a source of treatment failure in these patients. Encouragingly, Folkman[70] has suggested that because the endothelial compartment is not considered to be mutating, drug resistance to antiangiogenic agents should not develop.

The evidence from the Royal Marsden studies that absence of HER2/neu predicted for a cCR raises interesting questions regarding HER2/neu. Overexpression of this 185 kDa proto-oncogene product is present in 10–35% of patients with breast cancer, and may result in a worse prognosis, though it may indicate increased sensitivity to doxorubicin and taxanes.[71] In addition, the emergence of Herceptin (trastuzumab) as a new therapy in advanced breast cancer raises questions about its use in the preoperative setting. The application of microarray analyses to clinical samples harvested during periods of maximal response to chemotherapy may reveal yet more data. We are now on the verge of harvesting years of research, from basic science to randomized trials, and translating that work into new treatment protocols for our patients.

SUMMARY OF KEY POINTS

Data from the trials highlighted above have shown that the use of preoperative chemotherapy carries neither a survival advantage nor a disadvantage. In addition, there is a direct correlation between the response of a primary breast tumor to chemotherapy and patient outcome, thus rejecting Skipper's hypothesis. Quantifying breast tumor response is biologically important in that it may serve as an indicator of the effect of treatment on micrometastatic disease.

The high response rates of 70–90% may result in downstaging of the primary tumor, allowing for breast conservation as opposed to mastectomy. Tumor progression is extremely rare and surgical morbidity is not increased. Surgeons' early fears that preoperative chemotherapy may delay the institution of effective local treatment appear to be unfounded. Because clinical complete responses do not usually correlate with pathologic complete responses, surgery is still indicated. A pathologic complete response does, however, appear to identify a subgroup of patients with a particularly favorable prognosis.

CONCLUSIONS

As each change occurs in the treatment of breast cancer, new questions remain unanswered. It remains to be seen whether drugs such as taxanes, vinorelbine, and Herceptin, and crossover to different regimens, can increase response rates to such an extent that mastectomies will be rarely needed. A high complete response rate is, however, a prerequisite of cure, as seen with the successes in treatment of lymphomas, testicular cancer, and pediatric malignancies.

The early changes in proliferation and apoptosis that occur within a day of starting preoperative chemotherapy present this as an invaluable in vivo scenario for the investigation of molecular determinants of this change, and also for the development of new treatments. This work, in association with clinical trials of preoperative chemotherapy, will remain one of the most active and potentially fruitful areas of progress in the treatment of breast cancer.

REFERENCES

1. Stephens FO, The case for a name change from neoadjuvant chemotherapy to induction chemotherapy. *Cancer* 1989; **63**:1245–6.

2. Mamounas EP, Overview of National Surgical Adjuvant Breast Project neoadjuvant chemotherapy studies. *Semin Oncol* 1988; **25**(2):31–5.

3. Schwartz GF, Birchansky CA, Komarnicky LT et al, Induction chemotherapy followed by breast conservation for locally advanced carcinoma of the breast. *Cancer* 1994; **73**:362–9.

4. Haagensen DC, Bodian C, A personal experience with Halsted's radical mastectomy. *Ann Surg* 1984; **199**:143–50.

5. Goldhirsch A, Glick JH, Gelber RD, Senn H-J, International consensus panel on the treatment of primary breast cancer. *J Natl Cancer Inst* 1998; **90**:1601–8.

6. Early Breast Cancer Trialists' Collaborative Group, Systemic treatment of early breast cancer by hormonal, cytotoxic, or immune therapy: 33 randomised trials involving 33,000 recurrences and 24,000 deaths among 75,000 women. *Lancet* 1992; **339**:1–15, 71–85.

7. Budman DR, Berry DA, Cirrincione CT, Dose and dose intensity as determinants of outcome in the adjuvant treatment of breast cancer. *J Natl Cancer Inst* 1998; **90**:1205–11.

8. Forrest AP, Levack PA, Chetty U et al, A human tumour model. *Lancet* 1986; **2**:840–2.

9. Halstead WS, The results of operations for the cure of cancer of the breast performed at The Johns Hopkins Hospital from June, 1889 to January, 1894. *Johns Hopkins Hosp Rep* 1894–1895; **4**:297–350.

10. Leroy d'Etoilles JJJ, Une lettre de M. Leroy d'Etoilles sur l'extirpation des tumeurs cancereuses. *Bull Acad Med* 1867; **9**:454–8.

11. Paget J, Statistiek van den kanker (Cancer statistics). *Ned Weekl Geneesk* 1852; **2**:275, 410.

12. Haagensen CD, Stout AP. Carcinoma of the breast. II. Criteria of inoperability. *Ann Surg* 1943; **118**:859–68.

13. Christian MC, McCabe MS, Korn EL et al, The National Cancer Institute audit of the National Surgical Adjuvant Breast and Bowel Project Protocol B-06. *N Engl J Med* 1995; **333**:1469–74.

14. NIH Consensus Conference, Treatment of early-stage breast cancer. *JAMA* 1991; **265**:391–5.

15. Nattinger AG, Hoffman RG, Howell-Pelz A, Goodwin JS, Effect of Nancy Reagan's mastectomy on choice of surgery for breast cancer by US women. *JAMA* 1998; **279**:762–6.

16. Tasmuth T, von Smitten K, Kaslo E, Pain and other symptoms during the first year after radical and conservative surgery for breast cancer. *Br J Cancer* 1996; **74**:2024–31.

17. Hack TF, Cohen L, Katz J et al, Physical and psychological morbidity after axillary lymph node dissection for breast cancer. *J Clin Oncol* 1999; **17**:143–9.

18. Mansi JL, Gogas H, Bliss JM et al, Outcome of primary breast patients with micrometastases: a long-term follow-up study. *Lancet* 1999; **354**:197–202.

19. Redding WH, Coombes RC, Monoghan P, et al. Detection of isolated mammary carcinoma cells in patients with primary breast cancer. *Lancet* 1983; **ii**:1271–3.

20. Cote RJ, Rosen PP, Lesser ML et al, Prediction of early relapse in patients with operable breast cancer by detection of occult bone micrometastases. *J Clin Oncol* 1991; 9:1749–56.

21. Mansi JL, Berger U, Easton D et al, Micrometases in bone marrow in patients with primary breast cancer: evaluation as an early predictor of bone metastases. *BMJ* 1987; 295:1093–6.

22. Simpson-Herren L, Sanford AH, Holmquist JP, Effects of surgery on the cell kinetics of residual tumour. *Cancer Treat Rep* 1976; 60:1749–60.

23. Gunduz N, Fisher B, Saffer EA, Effect of surgical removal on the growth and kinetics of residual tumor. *Cancer Res* 1979; 39:3861–5.

24. Fisher B, Gunduz N, Coyle J et al, Presence of a growth-stimulating factor in serum following primary tumor removal in mice. *Cancer Res* 1989; 49:1996–2001.

25. Fisher B, Saffer EA, Ruddock C et al, Effect of local or systemic treatment prior to primary tumor removal on the production and response to a serum growth-stimulating factor in mice. *Cancer Res* 1989; 49:2002–4.

26. Goldie JH, Coldman AJ, A mathematical model for relating drug sensitivity of tumors to their spontaneous mutation rate. *Cancer Treat Rep* 1979; 63:1727–33.

27. Fidler IJ, Ellis LM, The implications for angiogenesis for the biology and therapy of cancer metastasis. *Cell* 1996; 79:185–8.

28. Skipper HE, Schabel FM Jr, Quantitative and cytokinetic studies in experimental tumor models. In: Holland JF, Frei E III, eds. *Cancer Medicine.* Philadelphia: Lea and Febiger, 1973: 629–50.

29. Fisher B, Rockette H, Robidoux A et al, Effect of pre-operative therapy for breast cancer (BC) on local-regional disease: first report of NSABP B-18. *Proc Am Soc Clin Oncol* 1994; **13**:64 (Abst 57).

30. Mamounas E, Fisher B, Rockette H et al, Clinical and pathologic local-regional response of operable breast cancer (BC) to preoperative chemotherapy. Results from NSABP B-18. Society of Surgical Oncology meeting, March 20–24, 1996, Atlanta, GA.

31. Fisher B, Brown A, Mamounas E et al, Effect of preoperative therapy for primary breast cancer (BC) on local-regional disease, disease-free survival (DFS) and survival (S). Results from NSABP B-18. *Proc Am Soc Clin Oncol* 1997; **16**:127a (Abst 449).

32. Powles TJ, Hickish TF, Makris A et al, Randomised trial of chemoendocrine therapy started before or after surgery for treatment of primary breast cancer. *J Clin Oncol* 1995; 13:547–52.

33. Cameron DA, Anderson EDC, Levack P et al, Primary systemic therapy for operable breast cancer – 10 year survival data after chemotherapy and hormone therapy. *Br J Cancer* 1997; 76:1099–105.

34. Bonadonna G, Valagussa P, Zucali R, Salvadori B, Primary chemotherapy in surgically resectable breast cancer. *CA Cancer J Clin* 1995; 45:227–43.

35. Bonadonna G, Valagussa P, Brambilla C et al, Primary chemotherapy in operable breast cancer: Eight-year experience at the Milan Cancer Institute. *J Clin Oncol* 1998; 16:93–100.

36. Jacquillat C, Weil M, Baillet F et al, Results of neoadjuvant chemotherapy and radiation therapy in the breast conserving treatment of 250 patients with all stages of infiltrative breast cancer. *Cancer* 1990; 66:119–29.

37. Lara FU, Zinser JW, Castaneda N et al. Neoadjuvant (NA) chemotherapy (CT) with cisplatin (P), doxorubicin (A) and cyclophosphamide (C) (PAC) in stage II–III breast cancer (BC). *Proc Am Soc Clin Oncol* 1996; 15:A169.

38. Calais G, Berger C, Descamps P et al, Conservative treatment feasability with induction chemotherapy, surgery, and radiotherapy for patients with breast carcinoma larger than 3 cm. *Cancer* 1994; 74:1283–8.

39. Chollet P, Charrier S, Brain E et al, Clinical

and pathological response to primary chemotherapy in operable breast cancer. *Eur J Cancer* 1997; **33**:862–6.

40. Smith IE, Jones AL, O'Brien MER et al, Primary medical (neo-adjuvant) chemotherapy for operable breast cancer. *Eur J Cancer* 1993; **29A**:1796–9.

41. Lokich J, Kinsella T, Perri J et al, Phase I study of protracted venous infusion of 5-fluorouracil. *Cancer* 1981; **48**:2565–8.

42. Smith IE, Walsh G, Jones A et al, High complete remission rates with primary neo-adjuvant infusional chemotherapy for large early breast cancer. *J Clin Oncol* 1995; **13**:424–9.

43. Scholl SM, Fourquet A, Asselain B et al, Neo-adjuvant versus adjuvant chemotherapy in premenopausal patients with tumors too large for breast conserving surgery: preliminary results of a randomised trial. *Eur J Cancer* 1994; **30A**:645–52.

44. Semiglazov VF, Topuzov EE, Bavli JL et al, Primary (neoadjuvant) chemotherapy and radiotherapy compared with primary radiotherapy alone in stage IIb–IIIa breast cancer. *Ann Oncol* 1994; **5**:591–5.

45. Mauriac L, Durand M, Avril A et al, Effects of primary chemotherapy in conservative treatment of breast cancer patients with operable tumours larger than 3 cm. *Ann Oncol* 1991; **2**:347–54.

46. Fisher B, Brown A, Mamounas E, Effect of preoperative chemotherapy on local-regional disease in women with operable breast cancer: findings from National Surgical Adjuvant Breast and Bowel Project B-18. *J Clin Oncol* 1997; **15**:2483–93.

47. Fisher B, Ore L, On the underutilisation of breast-conserving surgery for the treatment of breast cancer. *Ann Oncol* 1993; **4**:96–8.

48. Mauriac L, MacGrogan G, Avril A et al, Neoadjuvant chemotherapy for operable breast carcinoma larger than 3 cm: a unicentre randomised trial with a 124 month median follow-up. *Ann Oncol* 1999; **10**:47–52.

49. Makris A, Powles TJ, Ashley S et al, A reduction in requirements in a randomised trial of neoadjuvant chemoendocrine therapy in primary breast cancer. *Ann Oncol* 1998; **9**:1179–84.

50. Ellis P, Smith IE, Ashley S et al, Clinical prognostic and predictive factors for predictive chemotherapy in operable breast cancer. *J Clin Oncol* 1998; **16**:107–14.

51. Ferriere JP, Assier I, Cure H et al, Primary chemotherapy in breast cancer: correlation between tumour response and patient outcome. *Proc Am Soc Clin Oncol* 1996; **15**:84.

52. Hortobagyi GN, Ames FC, Buzdar AU et al, Management of stage III primary breast cancer with primary chemotherapy, surgery and radiation therapy. *Cancer* 1988; **62**:2507–16.

53. Scholl SM, Asselain B, Beuzeboc P et al, Neoadjuvant versus adjuvant chemotherapy in premenopausal patients with tumors considered too large for breast conserving surgery. An update. *Proc Am Soc Clin Oncol* 1995; **14**:A200.

54. Piegra J-Y, Mouret E, Asselain B et al, Prognostic value of node involvement after preoperative chemotherapy in 507 patients with operable breast cancer. *Proc Am Soc Clin Oncol* 1998; **17**:385.

55. Verrill MW, Ashley SE, Walsh GA et al, Pathological complete response (pCR) in patients treated with neoadjuvant chemotherapy for operable breast cancer. *Breast Cancer Res Treat* 1998; **50**:328.

56. Ackland SP, Bitran JD, Dowlatshahi K, Management of locally advanced and inflammatory carcinoma of the breast. *Surg Gynecol Obstet* 1985; **161**:399–408.

57. Freeman HP, Wasfie TJ, Cancer of the breast in poor black women. *Cancer* 1989; **63**:2562.

58. Stebbing J, Too much life on Earth? *QJM* 1997; **90**:597–9.

59. Fernando IN, Powell TJ, Dowsett M et al, Determining factors which predict response to primary medical therapy in breast cancer using a single needle aspirate with immunocy-

tochemical staining and flow cytometry. *Virchows Arch* 1995; **426**:155–61.

60. Dowsett M, Detre S, Ormerod M et al, Analysis and sorting of apoptotic cells from final needle aspirates of excised human primary breast carcinomas. *Cytometry* 1998; **32**:291–300.

61. Ellis PA, Smith IE, Burton SA et al, Changes in proliferation, apoptosis, and Bcl-2 in breast cancer specimens following neoadjuvant chemotherapy. *Breast Cancer Res Treat* 1995; 37:36.

62. Ellis PA, Smith IE, McCarthy K et al, Preoperative chemotherapy induces apoptosis in early breast cancer. *Lancet* 1997; **349**:849.

63. Archer CD, Ellis PA, Dowsett M et al, C-erb-B2 positivity correlates with poor apoptotic response to chemotherapy in primary breast cancer. *Breast Cancer Res Treat* 1998; **50**:237.

64. Johnston SRD, Boeddinghaus IM, Riddler S et al, Idoxifene antagonises oestradiol-dependent MCF-7 breast cancer xenograft growth through sustained induction of apoptosis. *Cancer Res* 1999; **59**:3646–51.

65. Makris A, Powles TJ, Dowsett M et al, Prediction of response to neoadjuvant therapy in primary breast carcinomas. *Clin Cancer Res* 1997; **3**:593–600.

66. Chang J, Powles TJ, Allred DC et al, Predictive molecular markers for clinical outcome following primary chemotherapy for operable breast cancer. *Proc Am Soc Clin Oncol* 1998; **17**:384.

67. Belotti D, Nicoletti I, Vergani V et al, Paclitaxel (Taxol), a microtubule affecting drug, inhibits tumour induced angiogenesis. *Proc Am Assoc Cancer Res* 1996; **37**:57 (Abst 397).

68. Weidner N, Semple JP, Welch WR et al, Tumor angiogenesis and metastasis-correlation in invasive breast carcinoma. *N Engl J Med* 1991; **324**:1–8.

69. Makris A, Powles TJ, Kakolyris S et al, Reduction in angiogenesis after neoadjuvant chemoendocrine therapy in patients with operable breast carcinoma. *Cancer* 1999; **85**:1996–2000.

70. Folkman J, Antiangiogenic therapy. In: DeVita VT, Hellman S, Rosenberg SA, eds. *Cancer: Principles and Practice of Oncology*, 5th edn. Philadelphia: Lipincott-Raven, 1997: 3075–85.

71. Muss HB, Thor AD, Berry DA et al, c-erb-B2 expression and response to adjuvant therapy in women with node-positive early breast cancer. *N Engl J Med* 1994; **330**:1260–6.

36

Evolution in the management of ductal carcinoma *in situ* through randomized clinical trials

Eleftherios P Mamounas

In the past few years, an evolution even more significant than that which occurred in invasive breast cancer has taken place in the clinical presentation, biological understanding and management of non-invasive breast cancer. The development and widespread use of high-quality mammography was the single most important factor initiating the cascade of events that led to these changes. With the expansion of mammography use, the incidence of non-palpable, mammographically detected, localized ductal carcinoma in situ (DCIS) has steadily increased. This type of DCIS possesses an altogether different natural history from palpable DCIS, which is often associated with microinvasion and occasionally with axillary nodal involvement. The demonstration of a favorable natural history for patients with mammographically detected DCIS has challenged the need for radical surgical management, just as the efficacy of breast-conserving surgery was being established for patients with invasive breast cancer.[1]

Randomized clinical trials initiated in the 1980s in both the USA and Europe aimed initially to explore the role of breast-conserving surgery with or without postoperative breast radiotherapy and subsequently to define the role of tamoxifen in patients with DCIS.

ROLE OF LUMPECTOMY AND BREAST RADIOTHERAPY: THE NSABP B-17 TRIAL

The National Surgical Adjuvant Breast and Bowel Project (NSABP) B-17 trial, the first randomized trial in patients with DCIS, was designed to evaluate the value of breast radiotherapy after lumpectomy. Between 1985 and 1990, 818 patients with localized DCIS detected by either physical examination or mammography were randomized to receive either lumpectomy alone or lumpectomy followed by breast radiotherapy (Figure 36.1). As in previous NSABP studies, for B-17 lumpectomy was considered to be the removal of the tumor and a sufficient amount of normal breast tissue so that the specimen margins were histologically free of tumor. Axillary dissection was mandatory at the beginning of the study, but subsequently it became optional, based on evidence indicating that it was not necessary in the treatment of DCIS. Results, initially after 5 and subsequently after 8 years of follow-up,[2,3] demonstrated that the addition of postlumpectomy radiotherapy significantly improved event-free survival by decreasing the rate of non-invasive and invasive ipsilateral breast tumor recurrence. After 8 years, the incidence of *non-invasive* breast cancer recurrence was 13.4% with lumpectomy alone and 8.2% with lumpectomy plus breast radiotherapy ($p = 0.007$). More importantly, the addition of breast radiotherapy reduced the incidence of *invasive* ipsilateral breast cancer recurrence from 13.4% to 3.9% ($p < 0.0001$). There were no significant differences in the rate of other first events ($p = 0.96$) and no overall survival differences between the two treatment groups (8-year survival rate: 94% and 95%, respectively; $p = 0.84$). Locoregional or distant recurrences were uncommon, with only 12 occurring as first events in the 814 randomized patients with follow-up (five in the lumpectomy alone group and seven in the lumpectomy plus radiotherapy group). Another seven locoregional events occurred after an ipsilateral breast tumor recurrence (three in the lumpectomy alone group and four in the lumpectomy plus radiotherapy group). The overall cumulative incidence of contralateral breast cancer as a first event was 4.5% (3.0% invasive and 1.5% non-invasive). The fact that similar cumulative rates of invasive breast cancer occurred in the ipsilateral and the contralateral breast in patients treated with lumpectomy plus radiotherapy should be considered when physicians discuss with patients surgical options for the treatment of localized DCIS (i.e. breast conservation versus mastectomy).

Several questions were raised once the results of the B-17 trial were reported: do all patients with localized DCIS need breast radiotherapy after lumpectomy, or are there subgroups with such a good prognosis that they can be treated with lumpectomy alone? At the other end, are there patients with more extensive or aggressive disease for whom breast conservation is *not* the best option and who may benefit from total mastectomy? Further, as localized DCIS appears to represent a risk factor for the subsequent development of invasive breast cancer, both in the ipsi-

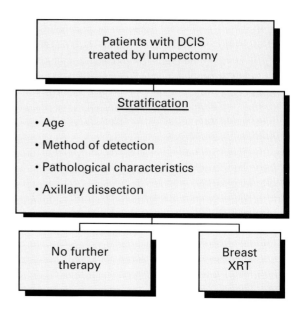

Figure 36.1
Schema of NSABP B-17 comparing lumpectomy alone with lumpectomy plus breast radiotherapy in DCIS patients.

lateral breast (to a greater extent) and in the contralateral breast (to a lesser extent), would these patients benefit from tamoxifen administration?

In an attempt to address the first two questions, the effect of breast radiotherapy after lumpectomy on ipsilateral breast tumor recurrence in subsets of DCIS patients has been evaluated according to prognostic clinicopathologic characteristics. These evaluations have been carried out using data from randomized trials (NSABP B-17)[4,5] and non-randomized cohorts (Van Nuys experience),[6,7] with somewhat discordant results. In the B-17 trial,[4] pathologic characteristics were assessed centrally in a representative subgroup of 573 patients from the total cohort of randomized patients. Tumor characteristics, patient characteristics and outcome were almost identical for the subset that underwent central pathology review and the entire B-17 cohort. After 5 years of follow-up, multivariate analysis identified only the presence of moderate/marked comedo necrosis and uncertain/involved lumpectomy margins as statistically significant independent predictors of risk for ipsilateral breast tumor recurrence, in patients who had been treated with lumpectomy with or without breast irradiation. When hazard rates of ipsilateral breast tumor recurrence were evaluated according to category of margin status and comedo necrosis combined, breast radiotherapy was found to be effective in all patient subgroups, although the absolute benefit was larger in those subgroups that were at higher risk for recurrence. The updated results of central pathology review from the B-17 trial were recently reported after 8 years of follow-up in an expanded cohort of 623 of the 814 evaluable patients.[5] With additional follow-up, the presence of moderate/marked comedo necrosis remained the only statistically significant independent predictor of risk for ipsilateral breast tumor recurrence in both treatment groups. Benefit from radiotherapy continued to be evident both in patients with moderate/marked comedo necrosis and in those with absent/mild comedo necrosis. At 8 years, breast radiation effected a 7% absolute reduction in the rate of breast tumor recurrence in the low-risk group.

The Van Nuys Prognostic Index (VNPI)[6,7] was devised by combining three statistically significant independent predictors of local tumor recurrence in a cohort of DCIS patients who were treated in two institutions. Initially, 254 patients treated with breast-conservation therapy at the Breast Center in Van Nuys between 1979 and 1995 were studied. Subsequently, 79 patients treated at the Children's Hospital in San Francisco between 1972 and 1987 were used to validate the initial results. As comparable patients from both centers revealed almost identical local recurrence-free survival rates in all subsets, the two groups were combined, yielding a final study group of 333 patients with a median follow-up of 79 months. Tissue was processed in a similar manner at both facilities. The margins were inked or dyed, and specimens were serially sectioned at intervals of 2–3 mm. The decision to proceed with mastectomy or breast-conserving surgery and the decision to add further treatment after breast-conserving surgery (i.e. breast radiotherapy) were not randomly assigned or dictated by a set protocol, but were left to the discretion of the treating physician.

By multivariate analysis, three statistically significant predictors of local recurrence were identified – tumor size, margin width and histologic type – and each was given a score of 1 (best) to 3 (worst). A score of 1 was assigned for tumors ⩽15 mm in diameter, 2 for tumors 16–40 mm in diameter and 3 for tumors > 40 mm in diameter. Similarly, a score of 1 was given for margin width ⩾10 mm, 2 for margin width 1–9 mm and 3 for margin width < 1 mm. Finally, a score of 1 was given for non-high-grade tumors without comedo necrosis, 2 for non-high-grade tumors with comedo necrosis and 3 for high-grade tumors, irrespective of the presence or absence of comedo necrosis. The VNPI score was determined by adding the individual scores from each category. Patients with a VNPI score of 3 or 4 had similar outcomes (low risk) as did patients with scores 5, 6 or 7 (intermediate risk), and those with scores 8 or 9 (high risk). However, the three groups (low, intermediate and high risk) had significantly different local recurrence rates. The authors also concluded that patients with VNPI scores of 3 or 4 showed no local disease-free survival benefit from breast radiotherapy after lumpectomy, but patients with VNPI scores of 5, 6 or 7 did. Patients with VNPI scores of 8 or 9 also benefitted from breast radiotherapy, but their local recurrence rate was high with or without radiotherapy, making mastectomy possibly a better choice than breast conservation in this group of patients.

A number of methodologic issues regarding the study of Silverstein have been raised,[8] including the retrospective nature of the study, the inclusion of patients treated at two institutions over a relatively long time period (1972–95), and the potential variation over time in patient selection criteria, mammographic evaluation, extent of surgery, use of radiation and specimen processing. Other investigators have shown that rates of re-excision, specimen radiography and postoperative mammography have increased over time, with a resulting decrease in rates of local recurrence after lumpectomy and breast radiotherapy.[9] The validity of the VNPI has also been called into question because of its retrospective development in a cohort of patients without unified or set local treatment criteria and its lack of independent and prospective confirmation by other groups. Lastly, but perhaps most importantly, the appropriateness of examining and reporting treatment effects in relatively small subgroups of patients in whom therapy is not dictated by a set of protocol has been challenged. A number of biases, some obvious and some more obscure, are introduced by such an approach, making the significance of the results questionable.

Despite these issues, there are more similarities than differences between the NSABP and the Van Nuys studies when it comes to the identification of prognostic factors of recurrence. Both include an assessment of margin status or width (a measure of the distance from the edge of the tumor to the edge of the lumpectomy specimen) and an assessment of grade and/or comedo necrosis (although grade was not an independent predictor in the B-17 study because of its close association with comedo necrosis). Pathologi-cally evaluated tumor size was not an independent predictor in the NSABP study as it was in the VNPI, but *mammographic* tumor size was found to be an independent predictor in the 8-year update of the B-17 results.[3] However, where there are significant differences between the NSABP and the Van Nuys experience is in their respective conclusions relative to treatment effectiveness as outlined above. In such cases of discordance, treatment recommendations resulting from a well-designed and conducted randomized trial bear considerably more weight than those reached by retrospective analysis of an arbitrarily defined cohort of patients, with treatment selection at the discretion of the treating physician.

ROLE OF TAMOXIFEN: THE NSABP B-24 TRIAL

Over the past three decades, a large body of scientific evidence has accumulated that demonstrates the benefit of tamoxifen administration in patients with resected, operable, invasive breast cancer.[10] In these patients, tamoxifen not only reduces the risk of systemic recurrence, but also has a significant impact on reducing the rate of ipsilateral breast tumor recurrence after lumpectomy and breast radiotherapy.[11,12] More importantly, tamoxifen has been found to reduce the incidence of second primary breast cancers in the contralateral breast by about 40%.[10–16] The latter observation – along with preclinical evidence that tamoxifen inhibits both the initiation and the promotion of tumors in experimental animals[17,18] – makes tamoxifen an attractive agent for patients with DCIS treated with lumpectomy and breast radiotherapy, for possibly reducing the rate of development of ipsilateral and contralateral invasive breast cancers.

Several trials have been designed to test this hypothesis. The first to produce results was the NSABP B-24 trial,[19] which evaluated the role of tamoxifen after lumpectomy and postoperative radiotherapy in patients with localized as well as more extensive DCIS (Figure 36.2). Between 1991 and 1994, 1804 women with DCIS treated with lumpectomy and postoperative radiotherapy were randomized to receive either tamoxifen 20 mg or placebo daily for 5 years. Unlike the B-17 trial, in which eligibility requirements included lumpectomy margins free of DCIS, in the B-24 trial patients were eligible whether the lumpectomy margins were free, involved or of unknown status. As a result, in the B-24 trial, about 75% of the patients had lumpectomy margins that were free of DCIS, about 16% had margins that were involved and in about 9% margins were unknown. Otherwise, the distribution of patient and tumor characteristics was similar between the two trials. More than 80% of the tumors in both studies were detected by mammography alone. At 5 years of follow-up, the addition of tamoxifen was shown to have reduced significantly the incidence of all invasive and non-invasive breast cancers at any site by 37% (13.4% in the placebo group vs 8.2% in the tamoxifen group, $p < 0.001$). When the rate of all invasive breast cancer events was evaluated, the administration of tamoxifen was shown to result in a 43% reduction (7.2% in the placebo group vs 4.1% in the tamoxifen group, $p = 0.004$). The addition of tamoxifen also resulted in a non-significant reduction in the rate of non-invasive breast cancers (6.2% vs 4.2% respectively, $p = 0.08$). The effect of the drug in reducing breast cancer events was evident in both the ipsilateral and contralateral breasts. The cumulative incidence of contralateral breast cancers, as first events, was reduced by 52% in the patients who received tamoxifen compared with those who received placebo (3.4% vs 2.0% respectively, $p = 0.01$). Several patient and tumor characteristics were found to increase the rate of ipsilateral breast tumor recurrence: young age (< 50),

involved/unknown lumpectomy margins, presence of comedo necrosis and DCIS presentation with clinical findings. Although, in a small subset of women with clinically apparent DCIS at study entry, ipsilateral breast tumor recurrence rates were similar between the tamoxifen and placebo groups, in general the effect of tamoxifen in reducing ipsilateral breast cancer was evident irrespective of age, margin status or presence/absence of comedo necrosis. Adverse effects from tamoxifen were similar to those observed in other clinical trials of the drug. The rate of endometrial cancer was 1.53/1000 patients per year in the tamoxifen group, compared with 0.45/1000 patients per year in the placebo group.

The results from the B-24 trial indicate a significant benefit from tamoxifen for patients with DCIS. When these results are viewed alongside those demonstrating benefit from tamoxifen for women with prior invasive breast cancer[10–12] and for those with atypical hyperplasia and lobular carcinoma in situ,[20] they support the use

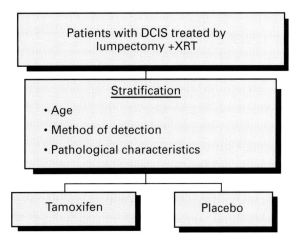

Figure 36.2
Schema of NSABP B-24 comparing tamoxifen with placebo in DCIS patients treated with lumpectomy and breast radiotherapy.

of tamoxifen across the entire spectrum of breast neoplasia.

After the disclosure of the B-24 results, the next logical question is whether the benefit from tamoxifen is limited to subsets of DCIS patients. Given the strong association between estrogen receptor expression and tamoxifen benefit in patients with invasive breast cancer, the possibility of a similar association should be investigated in patients with DCIS. As the effect of tamoxifen in patients with DCIS is evident in both ipsilateral and contralateral breasts, tamoxifen may prove to be of benefit even in patients with estrogen-receptor-negative DCIS.

OTHER CLINICAL TRIALS

A number of other randomized trials that address questions similar to those examined in B-17 and B-24 were initiated in Europe at around the time that the NSABP trials began. Most have recently completed or are in the late stages of completing their accrual, and have no definitive results available yet. The European Organization for Research and Treatment of Cancer (EORTC) trial, which compares lumpectomy with lumpectomy plus breast radiotherapy, closed in 1996 after accruing 1010 patients from 46 centers.[21,22] The Swedish National Trial, comparing sector resection alone to sector resection followed by breast radiotherapy, is also close to completing its accrual.[22] The UK randomized trial, examining the roles of breast radiotherapy and tamoxifen after lumpectomy in a 2 × 2 factorial design, will have preliminary results available in the year 2000.[22]

In the USA, the Eastern Cooperative Oncology Group (ECOG) has initiated a register of observation alone after lumpectomy in patients with low-risk DCIS. Eligible patients must have: (1) low/intermediate nuclear grade, non-comedo DCIS, ≤2.5 cm in greatest diameter or (2) high

nuclear grade, non-comedo DCIS, ≤1.0 cm in greatest diameter. The tumor-free margin width after lumpectomy must be at least 3 mm. In addition, a recently initiated Intergroup study, led by the Radiation Therapy Oncology Group (RTOG), is evaluating the worth of adding breast radiotherapy to tamoxifen in patients with unicentric, mammographically detected, low/intermediate-grade DCIS, ≤2.5 cm in greatest diameter, with a tumor-free margin of width ≥ 3 mm after lumpectomy. Both these trials should be useful in answering whether there are subsets of DCIS patients for whom breast radiotherapy can be omitted without increasing the rate of local recurrence in the ipsilateral breast.

CONCLUSION

Randomized clinical trials have contributed significantly toward the establishment of the value of lumpectomy, breast radiotherapy and tamoxifen for patients with DCIS. This has resulted in new questions being raised, most importantly about which patients do and which patients do not benefit from a certain intervention. Research efforts so far have focused on identifying patients who do not benefit from breast radiotherapy or who may need a mastectomy. The relationship between estrogen receptor expression and tamoxifen benefit is currently being investigated in the NSABP B-24 trial. Future research efforts will concentrate on the molecular characterization of these tumors so that therapy can be tailored appropriately. New biomarkers such as oncogene expression and tumor-suppressor gene inactivation, as well as the presence of other genomic alterations, will play a significant role in future research, not only as prognostic factors of recurrence and predictive factors of treatment effect, but also as potential targets for novel therapeutic interventions.

ACKNOWLEDGMENT

Many thanks to Barbara Good for her editorial assistance with the manuscript.

REFERENCES

1. Fisher B, Redmond C, Poisson R et al, Eight-year results of a randomized clinical trial comparing total mastectomy and lumpectomy with or without irradiation in the treatment of breast cancer. *N Engl J Med* 1989; **320**:822–8.

2. Fisher B, Constantino J, Redmond C et al, Lumpectomy compared with lumpectomy and radiation therapy for the treatment of intraductal breast cancer. *N Engl J Med* 1993; **328**:1581–6.

3. Fisher B, Dignam J, Wolmark N, Mamounas E et al, Lumpectomy and radiation therapy for the treatment of intraductal breast cancer: Findings from National Surgical Adjuvant Breast and Bowel Project B-17. *J Clin Oncol* 1998; **16**:441–52.

4. Fisher ER, Constantino J, Fisher B et al, Pathologic findings from the National Surgical Adjuvant Breast and Bowel Project Protocol B-17: Intraductal carcinoma (ductal carcinoma in situ). *Cancer* 1995; **75**:1310–19.

5. Fisher ER, Dignam J, Tan-Chiu E et al, Pathologic findings from the National Surgical Adjuvant Breast Project (NSABP) Eight-year update of Protocol B-17: Intraductal carcinoma. *Cancer* 1999; **86**:429–38.

6. Silverstein MJ, Lagios MD, Craig PH et al, A prognostic index for ductal carcinoma in situ of the breast. *Cancer* 1996; **77**:2267–74.

7. Silverstein MJ, Lagios MD, Use of predictors of recurrence to plan therapy for DCIS of the breast. *Oncology* 1997; **11**:393–410.

8. Schnitt SJ, Harris JR, Smith BL, Developing a prognostic index for ductal carcinoma in situ of the breast. Are we there yet? *Cancer* 1996; **77**:2189–92.

9. Hiramatsu H, Bornstein BA, Recht A et al, Local recurrence after conservative surgery and radiation therapy for ductal carcinoma in situ. *Cancer J Sci Am* 1995; **1**:55–61.

10. Early Breast Cancer Trialists' Collaborative Group, Tamoxifen for early breast cancer: An overview of the randomised trials. *Lancet* 1998; **351**:1451–67.

11. Fisher B, Constantino J, Redmond C et al, A randomized clinical trial evaluating tamoxifen in the treatment of patients with node-negative breast cancer who have estrogen-receptor-positive tumors. *N Engl J Med* 1989; **320**:479–84.

12. Fisher B, Dignam J, Bryant J et al, Five versus more than five years of tamoxifen therapy for breast cancer patients with negative lymph nodes and estrogen receptor-positive tumors. *J Natl Cancer Inst* 1996; **88**:1529–42.

13. Nolvadex Adjuvant Trial Organisation, Controlled trial of tamoxifen as a single adjuvant agent in the management of early breast cancer. *Br J Cancer* 1988; **57**:608–11.

14. Breast Cancer Trials Committee, Scottish Cancer Trials Office, Adjuvant tamoxifen in the management of operable breast cancer: The Scottish trial. *Lancet* 1987; **ii**:171–5.

15. Rutqvist LE, Cedermark B, Glas U et al, Contralateral primary tumors in breast cancer patients in a randomized trial of adjuvant tamoxifen therapy. *J Natl Cancer Inst* 1991; **83**:1299–306.

16. CRC Adjuvant Breast Trial Working Party, Cyclophosphamide and tamoxifen as adjuvant therapies in the management of breast cancer. *Br J Cancer* 1988; **57**:604–7.

17. Jordan VC, Effect of tamoxifen (ICI 46,474) on initiation and growth of DMBA-induced rat mammary carcinomata. *Eur J Cancer* 1976; **12**:419–24.

18. Jordan VC, Allen KE, Evaluation of the antitumour activity of the non-steroidal; antioestrogen monohydroxytamoxifen in the DMBA-induced rat mammary carcinoma model. *Eur J Cancer* 1980; **16**:239–51.

19. Fisher B, Dignam J, Wolmark N et al, Tamoxifen in treatment of intraductal breast cancer:

National Surgical Adjuvant Breast and Bowel Project B-24 randomised controlled trial. *Lancet* 1999; **353**:1993–2000.

20. Fisher B, Constantino JP, Wickerham DL et al, Tamoxifen for prevention of breast cancer: Report of the National Surgical Adjuvant Breast and Bowel Project P-1 Study. *J Natl Cancer Inst* 1998; **90**:1371–88.

21. Recht A, Van Dongen JA, Fentiman IS et al, Third Meeting of the DCIS Working Party of the EORTC (Fondazione Cini, Isola S. Giorgio, Venezia, 2–8 February 1994) – Conference Report. *Eur J Cancer* 1994; **30A**:1895–900.

22. Recht A, Rutgers EJ, Fentiman IS et al, The Fourth EORTC DCIS Consensus Meeting (Chateau Marquette, Heemskerk, The Netherlands, 23–24 January 1998) – Conference Report. *Eur J Cancer* 1998; **34**:1664–9.

37

Ductal carcinoma in situ: Grading, biologic implications and clinical outcome

Michael D Lagios

Over the last quarter of a century, ductal carcinoma in situ (DCIS) has evolved from a rare clinical entity to the focus of a paradigm shift in the therapeutics of preinvasive disease.

Currently, surgery remains the most effective treatment for DCIS, either as an adequate segmental resection or as a total mastectomy, with resulting cause-specific survival rates of 98% and 99%, respectively, at 10 years for these two types of treatment. Breast conservation, however, requires an adequate excision, yet the serpiginous anatomy of the ductal system, an anatomy that is unknown for an individual patient preoperatively, frequently limits its usefulness and results in high local (in breast) recurrence rates. With a larger number of patients opting for breast conservation – currently about 50% of those with DCIS in the USA – there will be a stronger focus on chemoprevention.

Treatment for DCIS has many advantages over treatment of patients with even T1N0 invasive disease. Axillary dissection is unnecessary for the usual patient with a mammographically detected DCIS of small extent. Likewise, chemotherapy, irradiation and hormonal therapy provide no benefit for appropriately treated patients with limited disease, and this markedly reduces both the medical costs of treatment and their morbidi-

ties. Most importantly, however, treatment for DCIS as opposed to invasive disease is uniquely effective, with cause-specific survivals hardly different from those for a patient without breast cancer.

As most patients with DCIS eventually develop invasive disease if untreated, the cost-effectiveness of intervention, including the requisite mammographic screening, cannot be overestimated. Treatment for breast cancer over the last two millennia, including most of this century, has been equivalent to bailing a sinking caique with a thimble. In contrast, effective treatment for DCIS results in a boat virtually without leaks.

HISTORY

In situ carcinomas of the breast began to be defined only a century ago, and were initially identified morphologically on the basis of cells cytologically similar to those of invasive carcinomas, but confined to duct structures in areas of invasion. The definitions were arbitrary, and opportunities to study the biology of an in situ carcinoma independent of an invasive component, or after a lesser surgical procedure than a mastectomy, were rare. A number of studies relying on review of archival slide material[1,2] demonstrated basic differences between arbitrarily defined in situ carcinomas that led to the concept of risk markers (e.g. lobular carcinoma in situ or LCIS) that identify subsequent risk essentially equally distributed to either breast, and committed lesions (e.g. DCIS) that identify risks largely confined to the ipsilateral breast and often to the same quadrant. The studies of Wellings et al[3] focused attention on the terminal ductolobular units (TDLUs) as a common anatomical site for the development of hyperplastic changes of both 'ductal' and 'lobular' types, as well as corresponding neoplasia. The terms ductal and lobular carcinoma in situ were once meant to signify separate anatomical origins, one in ducts and the other in lobules, but this terminology is now an anachronism.

An explosive increase in publication on in situ carcinomas of the breast has occurred over the last 20 years, in large part reflecting the impact of mammography and multidisciplinary programs of early detection. This new information relates to the definition, diagnostic criteria, and both short- and long-term risks associated with specific types of in situ carcinoma.

DUCTAL CARCINOMA IN SITU: DEFINITION

Ductal carcinoma in situ comprises a heterogeneous group of non-invasive neoplastic proliferations with diverse morphologies and risks of subsequent recurrence and invasive transformation. DCIS predominantly arises in TDLUs but also involves extralobular ducts. As compared with LCIS, DCIS is generally more variable, with larger and more pleomorphic nuclear morphology and often some evidence of architectural differentiation, at least with intercellular spaces. In some situations, non-invasive neoplastic proliferations may include DCIS and LCIS together. Occasionally, it may be difficult to determine whether the proliferation is DCIS or LCIS; some DCIS is characterized by small uniform cells with a solid growth pattern and simulates LCIS. A few in situ neoplastic proliferations are indeterminate, and in that setting they are presumed to have the prognostic implications of both diagnoses, for example local evolution to invasion for DCIS and increased general risk in each breast for LCIS.

Conventionally, DCIS has been classified predominantly on the basis of architectural features such as comedo, cribriform, papillary, solid and micropapillary types.[4,5] Although comedo-type DCIS generally includes significant nuclear abnormalities within the neoplastic proliferation as part of the definition, in most cases the diagnosis of the specific subtypes of DCIS were based on architecture alone. Most architectural differentiation within DCIS has no clinical or biological implications,[4] with the apparent exception of the micropapillary subtypes.[6]

The increasing use of breast-conservation therapy in the treatment of mammographically detected DCIS, in particular, has permitted studies on prognostic factors that predict local recurrences and invasive events in the remaining breast after attempts at excision biopsy. Before the large number of cases of small mammographically detected DCIS, mastectomy was the only acceptable treatment for DCIS, and it remains a standard treatment today.[7,8]

PROGNOSTIC FACTORS

Three prognostic factors have been shown to be important in local control of DCIS after attempts at breast-conservation therapy (BCT): the extent of disease in the breast (and its corollary the residuum after an attempt at excision); the status of margins (also reflecting residual disease in the breast), and the grade of the DCIS. The most significant of these, uncorrected for margins, is grade.[9,10] High nuclear grade and necrosis together define a group of DCIS at much higher risk of local recurrence and invasive transformation. The grade of a DCIS is largely independent of the conventional classification. For example, high nuclear grade lesions can exhibit any architectural pattern, and likewise low nuclear grade lesions.[11,12] There is a growing consensus that classifications based on nuclear grade and necrosis can identify most DCIS patients at risk for short-term local recurrence and invasive transformation[9,11,13,14] after breast-conserving treatment (BCT) with or without irradiation. Most of these short-term recurrences are associated with DCIS exhibiting nuclear grade III morphology and significant coagulative necrosis. Such lesions would be conventionally classified as comedo DCIS. Studies utilizing conventional classification schemes have shown that the majority of short-term failures relate to comedo-type DCIS.[15] It should be recalled that comedo DCIS is not synonymous with high nuclear grade. Some lesions exhibiting comedo-type necrosis and a solid growth pattern are comprised of intermediate- and, in a few cases, low-grade nuclei.

Very little information is available regarding the potential of low-grade (i.e. non-comedo-type) DCIS after biopsy or BCT. It is clear that, in the short term (5–10 years), few local recurrences or invasive transformations occur, but Page et al[16] in a recent upgrade of the only study of low-grade DCIS with adequate follow-up,[2] note a substantial delayed recurrence rate i.e. approximately 37% at 30 years of follow-up. Although the sample is small, it is significant that recurrences were in the same quadrant and in some cases in the site of the prior biopsy – a biology identical to that of higher-grade DCIS and a risk that does not diminish after the menopause. This biology should be contrasted with that of marker lesions, for example atypical duct hyperplasia (ADH), atypical lobular hyperplasia (ALH) and LCIS, which do not predict the side of involvement, and where risk diminishes postmenopausally.[17–19]

GRADE AND CLASSIFICATION

There are several published classifications of DCIS which utilize nuclear grade and necrosis as the major distinguishing features of specific subtypes. The separations achieved by these classifications are different, and in part may impact on interpretation of outcome results. DCIS characterized by grade III nuclear morphology and necrosis is uniformly classified as high grade.[9,11,13,14] The EORTC (European Organization for the Research and Treatment of Cancer) classification,[12] although not utilizing conventional nuclear grade or necrosis as major discriminates, would also regard this as a high grade or, in their terminology, a 'poorly differentiated' DCIS. Fisher et al,[20] summarizing the NSABP (National Surgical Adjuvant Breast and Bowel Project) B-17 pathology analysis, noted that DCIS with grade III nuclei (poor nuclei) and DCIS that exhibited larger areas of necrosis (more than one-third of ducts involved) had a higher local recurrence rate, but reported these results separately, not analyzing the risk associated with two features in concert. Despite the differences in classification, it would appear that high-grade DCIS can be recognized uniformly; all investigators have shown that the high-grade subtype so defined has the highest risk of local recurrence and invasive transformation. The separate classifications are less consistent with regard to the remainder of the heterogenous 'non-comedo' group. DCIS with grade III nuclei but without necrosis, an infrequent association, is classified as high-grade by Silverstein et al,[9] but 'non-comedo' (a lower grade) by Solin et al.[13] Lagios et al[11] and Silverstein et al[9] utilize nuclear grade to separate the remaining DCIS groups;

however, Lagios et al classify low-grade DCIS as grade I nuclei without necrosis and intermediate-grade DCIS as grade II with or without necrosis. Silverstein et al separate DCIS with nuclear grades I and II on the basis of necrosis. Group I (low grade) may exhibit grade I or II nuclei but no necrosis, whereas DCIS with grade I or II nuclei but with any necrosis is classified as intermediate (group II). (Solin et al regard all DCIS without grade III nuclei and necrosis as 'non-comedo'.) Despite these differences in classification, all investigators have shown a substantially diminished local recurrence rate for DCIS not characterized by grade III nuclei and necrosis. Moreover, in those studies in which DCIS are divided into three groups as opposed to the dichotomous comedo/non-comedo, there is a recognizable intermediate group (intermediate grade, group II, intermediately differentiated) that exhibits a morphology and a risk intermediate between low- and high-grade DCIS.

In an analysis of the influence of histologic grading on local recurrence, Solin et al[13] noted recurrence rates of 20% for high-grade DCIS compared with 5% for low-grade lesions at 87 months of follow-up. These results are not dissimilar from the author's study in which recurrence rates were projected as 28% for similarly defined high-grade DCIS and 6% for lower-grade DCIS at 120 months of follow-up. At 124 months of actual follow-up, local recurrences are 33% and 2.3%, respectively, for these two groups.

Silverstein et al[9] have recently confirmed the significance of nuclear grade and necrosis on local recurrence-free survival after BCT for DCIS. With an 8-year actuarial follow-up, DCIS of group I (low or intermediate nuclear grade without necrosis) had a 2% recurrence rate, group II DCIS (low or intermediate nuclear grade with necrosis) a 6% recurrence rate, and group III (any grade III nuclear grade regardless of necrosis) a 16% recurrence rate. Collins et al[21]

corroborated the Van Nuys grading scheme with a 62-month follow-up with figures for low, intermediate and high grade for local recurrence rates of 0%, 8% and 25% respectively. Pertinent to the discussion of the role of radiation therapy was the inability of the study to demonstrate any significant difference in local control with or without irradiation for the two lower-grade groups (group I and II). Only for the high-grade DCIS (group III) did radiation therapy provide a benefit for local control.

A number of papers compare the utility of various existing DCIS classifications, in terms of identifying both subgroups with different outcomes and their reproducibility. Badve et al[22] compared recurrence-free survivals among DCIS subgroups defined by five different classification schemes. Only those schemes based on nuclear grade were able to distinguish subgroups with different risks of recurrence; the conventional architectural classification was unable to do so. The Van Nuys classification, based on nuclear grade and necrosis, achieved the highest p-value (0.001) among those tested. Douglas-Jones et al[23] and Bethwaite et al[24] have found the Van Nuys classification to have the highest level of inter-observer agreement among those tested. Sneige et al[25] compared interobserver reproducibility[25] of the Lagios nuclear grading system for DCIS in a setting of six pathologists with prior training. Complete agreement among the six observers was achieved in 35%, and five of six observers agreed in 36% of 125 cases.

EXTENT OF DISEASE

Clinical concern with the evaluation of size or extent of the area of the breast occupied by DCIS was an early focus during the development of BCT for this disease. Using a serial subgross sectioning technique correlated with specimen radiography, developed by Robert Egan,[26] a clear association was shown between the likelihood of invasive growth and the extent of disease.[27] Egan's technique permitted a correlative radiographic and pathologic mapping of areas of involvement by DCIS. These were extensively sampled from mastectomy material. The initial concern was whether occult invasion might exist in the breast separate from an adequately excised focus of DCIS. This was shown not to be the case. Treatment planning for areas of DCIS of 25 mm or less, which were completely excised by the standards of the day, were not associated with occult areas of invasion in those cases that subsequently went to mastectomy. Silverstein et al[28] demonstrated a similar correlation between the extent of disease and the likelihood of invasion, as did Patchefsky.[6] What was not clearly described at the time was that the invasive focus always occurred within the area occupied by DCIS, and that the area occupied by DCIS had a segmental distribution, as clearly noted subsequently.[29,30]

Using the same serial subgross technique, but applying it to radial segments of the breast, which more closely approximate the true anatomy of the ductal system, Holland and colleagues were able to define more clearly the relationships of DCIS to mammographic microcalcification and to the remaining breast. They identified different distribution patterns among DCIS of different subtypes. DCIS of high grade (poorly differentiated) was more closely defined by the extent of mammographic microcalcifications, and therefore its extent could be estimated with more certainty preoperatively. It was also associated with fewer discontinuities or 'skip areas' in its distribution, and therefore attempts at surgical excision were more likely to be successful. In contrast, DCIS of lower grades (intermediate and well-differentiated) were poorly associated with microcalcification and often exhibited a discontinuous distribution. However, Faverly et al[30] note that 85% of low-grade (well-

differentiated) DCIS would be excised with a 10 mm margin. Despite the greater likelihood of residual disease, lower grades of DCIS have a much lower frequency of local recurrence after attempts at BCT, at least in the first 10 years of follow-up.

MARGIN STATUS

Assessment of resection margins has been a major focus in BCT in the USA since the increasing utilization of that surgical procedure in the mid-1970s. The most common method of margin assessment is based on the use of India ink or some other permanent dye, and selective sampling. This method works well for invasive carcinomas, for most of which a likely area of involved margins can be estimated by palpation. An area of involved margins can be confirmed with few appropriate sections. The method is still practicable but more difficult in DCIS, in which the lesion is generally non-palpable and grossly invisible, and may not be uniformly associated with microcalcification. In these circumstances, margins must be completely examined rather than sampled. This frequently increases substantially the number of tissue samples of cassettes (blocks) prepared; however, neither the margin involvement nor occult microinvasion can be excluded without complete tissue processing. Differences in the kind of tissue processing utilized can contribute significantly to outcome results of BCT in DCIS.[31]

The definitions of an adequate margin initially utilized by several investigators[11,27,32] were too narrow to accommodate the majority of cases of DCIS which exhibited a discontinuous distribution. A standard acceptable margin at the time was 1 mm,[11,32] although the NSABP used anything short of transection of an involved duct as adequate.[33,34] The work of Holland et al[29] and Silverstein et al[35] subsequently documented that a

1 mm margin was inadequate. Silverstein et al, in analyzing the results of initial attempts at excision biopsy, noted that 45% of DCIS that were thought to be adequately excised had residual disease, either at re-excision or mastectomy, and that the size of the free margin was directly related to local recurrence-free survival, all other factors being equal. Even using a definition of an adequate margin of 1 mm, however, achieves a better local recurrence-free survival than did the NSABP B-17 criterion of non-transsection (e.g. 16% of local recurrence at 124 months of mean follow-up[10] versus 22% local recurrence rate at 43 months of mean follow-up.[36]

Margins are one of the three features that are significant predictors in multivariate analyses for local recurrence in DCIS. In the Van Nuys Prognostic Index (VNPI),[35] margins were weighted: $\leqslant 1$ mm (score 3); >1–9 mm (score 2); and $\geqslant 10$ mm or negative re-excision (score 1). The VNPI was an initial attempt at developing a clinicopathologic scoring system to assess the risk of local recurrence among DCIS patients treated with BCT. Analysis of the database clearly showed that there were large differences between DCIS of different nuclear grade as well as subtypes. However, subsequent to its publication, the data were reanalyzed to evaluate the individual contribution of each predictor separately. When DCIS is analyzed by margin status equivalent to $\geqslant 10$ mm or a negative re-excision, the differences between various subtypes defined by nuclear grade or by nuclear grade and necrosis become inconsequential. Local recurrence-free survival rates for high-grade DCIS (nuclear grade III with or without necrosis) with $\geqslant 10$ mm margins, projected to 10 years of actuarial follow-up, are 92%, and for intermediate- and low-grade DCIS virtually 100%.[37,38]

It is clear from this reanalysis that nuclear grade, subtype and size are only pertinent for local recurrence when there is a high risk for residual disease. Given that an estimated 92% of all local recurrences reflect residual (unresected) disease, it is the biology of the residual disease that defines most short-term local recurrences in DCIS.

As the result of the importance of an adequate resection in achieving an outstanding local recurrence-free survival and in obviating the need for radiation therapy, defining the margin status for a patient with DCIS should be of paramount importance in pathology practice. Until practice standards change substantially – and they are beginning to – margins will continue to be poorly defined in cases of DCIS. As a result, DCIS subtyping by nuclear grade and necrosis will continue to be important in estimating the risk of local recurrence for many patients.

VAN NUYS PROGNOSTIC INDEX

Weighting the prognostic factors of grade, extent and margin width has been accomplished in the VNPI,[35] which provides summary scores varying from 3 to 9 for DCIS. In this system, tumor grading is weighted as 1 for low-grade (group I) lesions defined as nuclear grade I and II without necrosis; 2 for intermediate-grade (group II) lesions defined as nuclear grade I or II with necrosis; and 3 for high-grade (group III) lesions, defined as nuclear grade III. Size is weighted as 1, 2, and 3 for $\leqslant 15$ mm, 16–40 mm and $\geqslant 41$ mm, respectively. Margin width is weighted as 1 for margins $\geqslant 10$ mm, or with a negative re-excision, 2 for margins >1–9 mm and 3 for margins $\leqslant 1$ mm. Adding these individual scores produces prognostic groups with summary scores of 3 and 4, 5–7 and 8–9. Local recurrence rates are lowest for VNPI scores of 3 and 4 (5%), and highest for scores of 8 and 9 (60%). Radiation therapy provides no benefit for VNPI scores of 3 or 4, a 13% benefit for scores of 5, 6 or 7 and a large benefit for VNPI scores of 8 or 9. However, despite the large difference in local recurrence rate in the VNPI 8 and 9 groups, dependent on irradiation, both irradiated and non-irradiated patients have such large recurrence rates that radiation therapy is not a practical therapeutic option. Analysis of the data based on margins, however, shows that the differences between different grades of DCIS, all resected with a margin of 10 mm or more, are not statistically significant. An adequate margin eliminates the clinical differences in outcome and the benefit of irradiation for all subgroups.[37] Collins et al[21] have recently corroborated the utility of the VNPI among 96 patients treated only by excision with a median 62-month follow-up. Margins defined as negative, close or positive had the largest impact on 5-year local recurrence rates: 8, 25 and 100%, respectively.

MULTICENTRICITY AND MULTIFOCALITY

The literature on the multicentricity and multifocality of DCIS remains confusing because of the different definitions, methods of tissue processing and sampling techniques employed, and differences in the perspective of the investigators. Two groups of investigators, both of which used Egan's serial subgross technique of examination, exemplify this problem. The focus of Lagios et al[39] was on the question of residual disease after segmental mastectomy (equals lumpectomy), a new and radical direction for American surgeons at the time. They defined as multicentric any focus lying beyond 5 cm of the border of the resection. In most cases, this defined involvement in another quadrant. Holland et al[29] and Faverly et al,[30] although clearly concerned about the success of a surgical resection, were focused more on the distribution of the disease. Multicentricity, by its very definition, required a 4 cm zone of uninvolved breast tissue between the primary and any potential multicentric site. Discontinuous foci of DCIS within 4 cm were defined as multifocal. Holland et al noted that only 5% of DCIS were multicentric using this definition. To what extent these data reflect the large size of DCIS in their patient population remains unknown. However, Faverly et al[30] reported that 63% of the DCIS studied at mastectomy had an extent greater than 5 cm (50 mm), whereas Lagios et al,[11] in a similar mastectomy series, noted that 52% were ≤ 25 mm and 25% ≥ 50 mm. Lagios had previously shown that neither multicentricity nor occult invasion was a feature of the smaller mammographically detected lesions ≤ 25 mm in size.[27]

MICROINVASION

Microinvasion as used in the author's laboratory refers to foci of invasive cancer with maximum diameters of 1 mm or less. This is now officially recognized in the TMN system as T1mic. Larger areas of invasive growth are termed 'minimal invasive carcinoma'. These comprise the original minimal invasive group as defined by Steven Gallagher, those 1–5 mm in maximum diameter (T1a) and the more loosely defined minimal invasive carcinomas, which may measure up to 10 mm in maximum diameter (T1b).

A diagnosis of microinvasion requires all the features of invasive growth, i.e. extension of the lesion beyond the confines of a ductolobular unit, the development of a desmoplastic stroma and an appropriate histology.

Unfortunately, microinvasion can be mimicked by artifact, duct sclerosis, entrapment, etc., and represents one of the most commonly revised diagnoses on review. In speaking with a number of pathologists, the author has noted that there is a philosophy that indicates that it is better to call an equivocal focus of microinvasion than to define the process as DCIS and comment on the equivocal areas. The author's own standard in his laboratory requires that evidence of invasion be present and that equivocal foci of microinvasion not be defined as invasive disease.

Common processes that have led to a misdiagnosis of microinvasion include crush and electrocautery artifact at the edge of a biopsy specimen, colonization of areas of sclerosing adenosis by DCIS, duct sclerosis with entrapment of neoplastic epithelium within the area of the pre-existing duct or ductolobular unit, 'cancerization of lobules' with an associated, very striking, lymphocytic host reaction, and larger ducts showing desquamation of ductal epithelium misinterpreted as 'vascular' invasion. Included with such processes are the implantation of neoplastic epithelium along needle tracts after both fine-needle aspiration and stereotactic core biopsy procedures.

Technical problems related to tissue handling, processing and sectioning contribute significantly to misinterpretation of microinvasion. A number of simple and inexpensive procedures can reduce this error rate. First, surgeons should be cautioned to avoid higher electrocautery voltages when excising diagnostic biopsy material. 'Frying' tissue can not only preclude a diagnosis, but will make a margin evaluation and receptor and other immunohistochemistry impossible.

Second, adequate fixation time will avoid many sins. For diagnostic problems in well-fixed tissue, several superficial levels of the block can often clarify the process. The addition of markers for the epithelial–stromal junction (e.g. actin immunoperoxidase procedures for myo-epithelial elements) will resolve most equivocal lesions.

A diagnosis of microinvasion has serious implications for the probable treatment that the patient may receive. Patients with DCIS are not candidates for adjuvant chemotherapy or radiation therapy after mastectomy and certainly, for most currently detected cases, they are not candidates for axillary dissection.

Being aware of the possible pitfalls in interpreting artifact and other benign distorting processes as microinvasion may permit the pathologist to avoid misdiagnosis. In addition, appropriate use of levels and occasionally simple special stains may permit clarification of an equivocal focus (see the Addendum at the end of the chapter).

TREATMENT: EXCISION VERSUS IRRADIATION

Clinical experience with treatment options other than mastectomy for this group of patients is very recent. Before 1982, there was virtually no published literature on small, mammographically detected foci of DCIS, yet clinical concerns have continued to dwell on questions of multicentricity and occult invasion, features generally associated with the type of DCIS encountered before the introduction of high-quality mammography.

We first reported on a small series of patients with DCIS treated by planned lumpectomy without irradiation in 1982, and the first reports of lumpectomy and irradiation for this disease appeared the following year. Since that time, a small number of studies[11,15,40] have appeared, which have shown a variable success rate in terms of local control, but have not demonstrated an adverse effect on survival by the choice of breast conservation without irradiation.

The author's experience with DCIS of limited extent[10,11,27] has shown that mammographically detected lesions that are adequately excised and documented to be less than 25 mm in extent are not associated with occult invasion or axillary metastasis at mastectomy. The short-term benefits of radiation therapy in reducing the number of local recurrences after excision biopsy for DCIS have been well documented in numerous studies. However, this benefit appears to decrease with longer follow-up. In those studies with follow-up in excess of 5 years[13,41] (Silverstein MJ, personal communication, 1993), recurrences double between 5 and 8 years and are greater still at 10 years of follow-up. Solin et al[13] reported an overall actuarial local recurrence rate of 16% at 10 years of follow-up.

A more recent update by the Van Nuys database of 443 patients with DCIS not randomized, but with significant numbers treated by excision alone and irradiation, has shown that the local recurrence rates are essentially identical at 10 years of follow-up, and that the irradiation benefit at 5 years has largely disappeared by this time.

NSABP B-17

The initial published results of NSABP B-17, a 'multi-institutional' trial of 'lumpectomy' for DCIS, randomized to irradiation or no irradiation, had shown substantial irradiation benefit with a mean follow-up of 43 months (projected to 60 months).[36] However, the actuarial rate of local recurrences in both the irradiated (7%) and the non-irradiated arms (21%) is substantially higher than that reported in non-randomized prospective studies of comparable follow-up. In a recent update of NSABP B-17[42] with 90 months of mean follow-up, total ipsilateral breast recurrences were 12.1% in the irradiated and 26.8% in the non-irradiated arms. These results should be compared with non-randomized studies that exercised more careful attention to margin status. Lagios,[10] who permitted minimum margin widths of 1 mm at the time, reported a 16% local recurrence rate among 79 non-irradiated patients in an updated, mean, 120-month follow-up of the original series reported in 1989.[11] Among DCIS patients with a margin of ≥10 mm or a negative re-excision in the combined Van Nuys–Children's database, the actuarial 10-year

local recurrence rate was 4% (82 months of mean follow-up).[35,37,38] Solin et al[13] reported a 16% local recurrence rate among a multi-institutional group of irradiated DCIS patients at a mean follow-up of 84 months – but for many of the patients, the margin status was unknown. In a recent update with a mean 15-year actuarial follow-up Solin et al[43] reported an 18% local recurrence rate for high-grade DCIS defined as nuclear grade III and comedo necrosis. A direct comparison between the Van Nuys database and that of NSABP B-17 is not possible, but an approximation can be made. Taking the mean size of DCIS as determined by the NSABP in its B-17 study as 90% ≤ 10 mm and segregating out a population of ≤10 mm DCIS from the Van Nuys database reveals a local recurrence rate in breast of 12.2% compared with 26.8% in B-17 patients treated by lumpectomy alone.

The much lower invasive recurrence rate in NSABP B-17 in the irradiated arm and the much higher rate of local recurrence in the non-irradiated arms are in sharp contrast to all other studies of breast conservation in DCIS, with or without irradiation. A possible clue to the differences can be obtained by examining the number of locoregional and/or distant metastases that appear as 'first' events after treatment in NSABP B-17. Of 814 patients, 12 developed a first post-treatment event of either locoregional or distant metastasis. Moreover, there were six subsequent distant metastases after an initial locoregional first event. Therefore, 18 locoregional or distant metastases developed among the 814 patients (2.2%) within the 90-month follow-up, and most of these died of disease.

Lagios[10] reported no locoregional or distant metastases as first events among the small group of 79 patients at 120 months of mean follow-up, and none was observed among 361 conservatively treated patients in the Van Nuys database.[44] Lagios et al[11,27] accepted DCIS for BCT up to 25 mm in extent (size), and Silverstein et al[38] accepted some patients with DCIS over 40 mm in size. In contrast, Fisher et al[42] noted that 90% of all 814 patients in NSABP B-17 had DCIS measurable at $\leqslant 10$ mm in size, and yet all recurrences in B-17 are greater than in the cited non-randomized studies. These differences – the lower invasive recurrence rate in the irradiated arm, the higher recurrence rate in the non-irradiated arm and the significant number of distant first recurrent events – all suggest that a large number of patients in the B-17 database included unrecognized invasive foci, either unsampled in the lumpectomy or left as a residuum in the breast. The NSABP B-17 protocol, as previously noted by Page and Lagios,[31] cannot exclude invasion or margin involvement in the lumpectomy, and, without prospective correlation between preoperative mammography and specimen radiography, cannot evaluate residual disease in the breast. This conclusion is corroborated by the observation of Fisher et al[42] that 'several' locoregional events, and two patients with distant metastases, occurred '7–15 months' after initial treatment, and two of these died of disease within 12 months. This is manifestly not the biology of DCIS alone. Lagios et al[11,27] reported similar locoregional events, distant metastases and deaths – *but* only among patients with extensive ($\geqslant 50$ mm) DCIS treated by mastectomy in whom invasion was detected by the serial subgross examination of Robert Egan. A significant number of similar patients would have to be included in NSABP B-17 to account for the frequency of locoregional and distant first events reported.

Patients who undergo radiation therapy for DCIS after a complete excision are being treated prophylactically. Given the recurrence rates available from the published literature at 8–10 years, it may be more appropriate to reserve radiation therapy for invasive recurrences should they occur.

TAMOXIFEN AS A CHEMOPREVENTIVE AGENT

Although surgical intervention is currently the most effective tool to apply to DCIS, it clearly has major limitations. For a disease that is largely invisible to the naked eye, and distributed within the markedly variable duct system, it is a crude implement indeed. Chemopreventive strategems have been considered in the treatment of DCIS for some time. An effective chemopreventive agent – being able to target DCIS regardless of its anatomic distribution and 'skip' areas of microscopic size – would be a major advance. Recent press releases concerning the benefits of tamoxifen in preventing breast cancer both in general in women at risk[45] and specifically against DCIS in NSABP B-24[46] provoked an enthusiastic and interested response from both physicians and patients. Has tamoxifen allowed us to enter the new millennium with an effective chemopreventive agent? Are we there yet?

In the NSABP P-1 prevention trial, tamoxifen reduced the incidence of invasive breast cancer by 52% and of in situ cancer by 50%. However, these differences reflect the relative percentage difference between the 3.8 invasive cancers per 100 women in the placebo group and the 2.0 invasive cancers per 100 women in the tamoxifen group, over the 5.75 years of the study. The actual benefit, i.e. the percentage of women over this time period in whom tamoxifen prevented breast cancer, was 1.8%. This represents an annual benefit of 0.33%. It would be necessary to treat 333 women with tamoxifen to prevent a single invasive breast cancer in the first year. Both the 52% reduction in risk and the 0.33% annual benefit are true, but the former presentation is much more likely to induce a woman at risk to chose tamoxifen. Tamoxifen had no benefit for estrogen-receptor-negative breast cancers – which represent 29% of all the invasive cancers that occurred among the study participants. In fact there were 22% more receptor-negative breast cancers among tamoxifen users than among controls.

Despite the actual minute benefit (0.33% per annum), given that tens of thousands of women are at risk, many breast cancers might be prevented by tamoxifen. This is perhaps the case – but true chemopreventive agents would be expected to block genetic mutations or the expression of such mutations, which would lead to suppression of tumor development. Does tamoxifen do this? Apparently not, because its effect was present at 20 months of follow-up, which is far too short a time frame to realize the benefit of 'molecular intervention'. Tamoxifen almost certainly suppresses the growth of pre-existing but subclinical carcinomas. Only longer follow-up will allow us to know how many of these suppressed carcinomas will, after 3–5 years, adapt to accept tamoxifen as an agonist and suddenly flourish; the NSABP P-1 trial was halted before these questions could be answered.

In NSABP B-24, similar remarkable percentage reductions in invasive and in situ carcinomas were observed among the DCIS patients randomized to tamoxifen. However, the difference between the two arms – 19.62% ipsilateral breast recurrence in the placebo arm and 13.75% in the tamoxifen arm at 76 months – was not significant at $p = 0.04$. The cumulative incidence at 5 years was 9.3% in the placebo arm and 6.0% in the tamoxifen arm – most of this benefit occurred by reducing invasive breast cancer incidence. On an annual basis, it represents a benefit of 0.66%.

A perspective of the advantages of the two approaches to DCIS control – surgery versus irradiation and tamoxifen – can be obtained by comparing the best results of each. In comparison with the 7% recurrence rate at 76 months with radiation therapy and tamoxifen in NSABP B-24, selecting low-grade lesions of ≤ 15 mm in size with adequate margins results in an ipsilateral recurrence rate at 8 years of less than 1%. The 8-year recurrence rate for all DCIS of ≤ 10 mm in size regardless of grade or margin status was 12%. No benefit of tamoxifen in preventing ipsilateral non-invasive recurrences were seen in B-24, whereas the 50% decrease in contralateral carcinoma amounted to an annual benefit of 0.4%.

RECEPTOR PROTEINS, ONCOGENES AND PLOIDY

A rapidly expanding literature since 1987 describes the presence and distribution of specific oncogenes and receptor proteins, and measures of ploidy and proliferative activity in DCIS. Initially, there was a muted expectation that such investigations would be able to identify DCIS subgroups that are more at risk for invasive transformation or local recurrence after BCT, particularly among patients at highest risk. In part, these expectations were met – but largely by demonstrating a correlation between specific oncogenes or gene products and DCIS subtypes recognized by conventional morphological analysis as being at high risk, i.e. high-grade (poorly differentiated) and/or 'comedo-type' DCIS.

The clearest association between an oncogene and a DNA subtype is seen with HER2/*neu*, which is largely restricted to DCIS subtypes characterized by large cell type and higher nuclear grade.[47–51] Bartkova et al[52] had shown that, among those DCIS that are of mixed subtypes, HER2/*neu* expression is seen only in the large cell component, and this is dramatically evident in cases in which the mixed cell population occurs within single ductules.

DePotter et al[51] demonstrated a significant association between HER2/*neu*-positive, large-cell-type DCIS and the extent of disease in the breast, independent of mitotic index, and hypothesized that HER2/*neu* has a role in motility of in situ carcinomas within the ductal epithelium.[53]

The *p53* tumor suppressor gene, largely studied by immunoperoxidase techniques, is also correlated with high-nuclear-grade subtypes.[47,49,54] O'Malley et al,[55] among others, noted that *p53* was largely limited to high-grade, comedo-type DCIS, but that immunoperoxidase technology missed some *p53* mutations that were detectable by polymerase chain reaction (PCR) amplification and sequencing in the most highly conserved portion of the gene. Poller et al[54] concluded that there was no relationship between *p53* and HER2/*neu* distribution, but nevertheless noted that almost all *p53*-positive DCIS were large cell: 35.8% of large-cell DCIS and only 4.1% of small-cell DCIS were *p53*-positive. Silverstein et al[56] noted a similar relationship between high-grade DCIS, HER2/*neu* and *p53*. Van der Vijer et al[57] confirmed the association of c-HER2/*neu*, *p53* overexpression, cyclin D1 gene amplification and loss of heterozygosity (LOH) on chromosome 17 limited to intermediate- and high-grade lesions in the EORTC classification. These features were not identified in low-grade (well-differentiated) DCIS, which exhibited LOH on chromosome 16.

Estrogen receptor (ER) and progesterone receptor (PgR) proteins, demonstrable by immunoperoxidase techniques, occur in DCIS subtypes, both high and low grade, large and small cell. There are, however, trends in their distribution noted by several investigators. Bobrow et al[47] noted an association between cytonuclear differentiation and PgR. DCIS with 'poor' cytonuclear differentiation, as opposed to 'good' differentiation, tended to lack demonstrable PgR. Similarly, Poller et al[54] noted ER expression to be related to non-comedo architecture, negative HER2/*neu* status, small cell size and, surprisingly, higher S-phase fraction by flow cytometry. Wilbur and Barrows[58] noted a similar trend between grade (equals cytonuclear differentiation) and receptor status. They noted that 75% of ER-negative DCIS exhibited nuclear grade III morphology (high grade), whereas only 14% of ER-positive DCIS were nuclear grade III. Leal et al[48] and Zafrani et al[49] noted no relationship between DCIS subtype and receptor status. These studies would suggest a weak association between high nuclear grade and negative receptor status similar to that noted in many high-grade invasive ductal carcinomas.

Despite the fact that some investigators utilized two-tiered and others three-tiered classifications, there has been a substantial degree of agreement between the studies. DCIS subtypes characterized by large cell type and high nuclear grade tend to be HER2/*neu*-positive, are more probably *p53*-positive and ER-negative, aneuploid, and are more likely to exhibit a higher S-phase fraction or other measurement of proliferation. They are also more likely to exhibit significant comedo-type necrosis, periductal stromal 'desmoplasia' and a diffuse increase in microvessel density.[14,59] In contrast, DCIS of small cell size and of intermediate and/or low nuclear grade and/or non-comedo architecture tend to be HER2/*neu*- and *p53*-negative, and diploid, and, in most studies, exhibit a lower S-phase fraction and a tendency toward positive receptor status. They also tend to lack significant necrosis and stromal reaction.

DCIS of different grades is associated with corollary differences in ploidy, S-phase fractionation, equivalent Ki67 or thymidine labeling, and the presence of certain oncogenes or tumor suppressor genes. Thus, DCIS characterized by grade III nuclei and necrosis (high grade) is characteristically aneuploid or tetraploid, and may exhibit a substantial S-phase fraction, high Ki67 index and contain immunoperoxidase-demonstrable oncogenes or tumor suppressor genes, especially HER2/*neu* and *p53*. DCIS, characterized by grade I nuclei, in contrast tends to be diploid, low S-phase and, generally, HER2/*neu*- and *p53*-negative.[60] The correlation of findings of abnormal ploidy and oncogenes or tumor suppressor genes with more aggressive behavior in invasive carcinoma appears consistent with the high level of risk of local recurrence and invasive transformation of high-grade DCIS, and, in corollary fashion, diploid, low S-phase, HER2/*neu*- and *p53*-negative DCIS ductal types are associated with low nuclear grade.

Despite concerted efforts employing immuno-histochemical demonstration of oncogenes or tumor suppressor genes, and determination of ploidy and S-phase fraction by flow and image cytometry, identification of a subset of morphologically defined high-grade DCIS at greater risk of invasive transformation remains elusive. Morphologic grading achieves as much separation as do numerous ancillary tests. Recently, however, Susnik et al,[61] using a classification based on nuclear texture features, quantified by high-resolution image cytometry, were able to identify 100% high-grade (comedo) DCIS associated with invasion and 80% non-comedo lesions associated with invasion. The study design was necessarily retrospective, but the results are exciting. If successful, automated quantitative analysis of nuclear texture features in DCIS may be able to identify patients at different levels of risk.

The distribution of DCIS within the breast, its association with microcalcification, the types of microcalcification and the likelihood that DCIS may exhibit an extensive growth pattern, with a substantial risk of residual disease after attempts at excision, are also correlated with grade and subtype. DCIS of high grade with comedo necrosis exhibits a segmental, i.e. contiguous, distribution, it is more closely associated with microcalcifications, and it is less likely to show an intermittent, discontinuous or multifocal dis-tribution in the breast.[30] DCIS of intermediate and low grades, in contrast, is less likely to exhibit a contiguous growth pattern even if its distribution can be understood to lie within a segmental duct system. DCIS of these grades are more likely to exhibit discontinuous or multi-focal growth and to show less association with microcalcification. From a clinical point of view, high-grade comedo DCIS is more likely to be adequately excised, given its association with microcalcification and contiguous growth pattern, but nevertheless it is associated with the greatest risk of local recurrence and invasive transformation. Low-grade DCIS is much more likely to be inadequately excised, with residual multifocal disease in the same quadrant, but nevertheless it is associated with a lower risk of subsequent recurrence and invasive transformation.

Although nuclear grade and necrosis would appear to define most of the risk associated with DCIS, certain architectural patterns appear to carry significance independent of nuclear grade. DCIS with micropapillary architectural features, for example, is strongly associated with multifocal and in some cases multicentric growth, i.e. separate foci in different quadrants.[6,62] This growth pattern makes adequate excision extremely difficult. In some cases, mammographic evidence of disease is present in all four quadrants. As a result, most clinical studies that define DCIS with micropapillary features and local nuclear grade were based on excision without adequate margins.

Conventional classification of DCIS perhaps covers 85% of what is recognized as non-invasive ductal carcinoma. A number of less common subtypes remain to be fully defined, both morphologically and with regard to risk. Proliferations with apocrine features, bridging the spectrum from minimal atypia to frank DCIS, were recently the subject of a proposed classification by O'Malley et al.[63] The author anticipates additional efforts in this and other areas in the future, and present his system here. A recent revision[64] of the original Lagios system of nuclear grading[11] separates out apocrine and pure micropapillary lesions to permit further evaluation of their biology.

ADDENDUM: RECOMMENDATIONS OF THE CONSENSUS CONFERENCE ON THE CLASSIFICATION OF DCIS[65]

Recommended documentation in pathology report:
- Nuclear grade, zonal (comedonecrosis) vs punctuate
- Necrosis
- Polarization
- Architectural pattern(s); cite conventional histology: comedo, cribriform, papillary, micropapillary, solid.

Associated features:
- Margins, closest in millimetres and focal or diffuse if involved
- Size (extent and distribution)
- Microcalcification
- Mammographic–pathologic correlation with mammographic findings and specimen X-ray

Tissue processing – optimal:
- Oriented (to nipple)
- Review specimen X-ray
- Inked margins, selective total sequential processing
- Estimate size

REFERENCES

1. Betsell WL Jr, Rosen PP, Lieberman PH et al, Intraductal carcinoma. Long-term follow-up treatment by biopsy alone. *JAMA* 1978; **239**: 1863–7.
2. Page DL, Duport WD, Rogers LW et al, Intra-
ductal carcinoma of the breast: Follow-up after biopsy only. *Cancer* 1982; **49**:752–8.
3. Bobrow LG, Happerfield LC, Gregory WM et al, The classification of ductal carcinoma in situ and its association with biologic markers. *Semin Diag Pathol* 1994; **12**:199–207.
3. Wellings SR, Jensen HM, Marcum RG, An atlas of subgross pathology of human breast with special reference to possible precancerous lesions. *J Natl Cancer Inst* 1975; **55**:231–73.
4. Azzopardi JG, *Problems in Breast Pathology*. Philadelphia: WB Saunders, 1979: 466.
5. McDivitt RW, Stewart FW, Berg JW. *Tumors of the Breast*. Washington, DC, Armed Forces Institute of Pathology, 1968: 156.
6. Patchefsky AS, Schwartz GF, Finkelstein SD et al, Heterogeneity of intraductal carcinoma of the breast. *Cancer* 1989; **63**:731–41.
7. Winchester DP, Mench HR, Osteen RT et al, Treatment trends for ductal carcinoma in situ of the breast. *Ann Surg Oncol* 1995; **2**:207–13.
8. Ernster VL, Barclay J, Kerlikowske K et al, Incidence of and treatment for ductal carcinoma in situ of the breast. *JAMA* 1996; **275**:913–18.
9. Silverstein MJ, Poller DN, Waisman JR et al, Prognostic classification of breast ductal carcinoma in situ. *Lancet* 1995; **345**:1154–7.
10. Lagios MD, Ductal carcinoma in situ: Controversies in diagnosis, biology and treatment. *Breast J* 1995; **1**:67–78.
11. Lagios MD, Margolin FR, Westdahl PR et al, Mammographically detected duct carcinoma in situ. Frequency of local recurrence following tylectomy and prognostic effect of nuclear grade on local recurrence. *Cancer* 1989; **63**: 619–24.
12. Holland R, Peterse JL, Millis RR et al, Ductal carcinoma in situ: A proposal for new classification. *Semin Diag Pathol* 1994; **11**:167–80.
13. Solin LJ, Yeh It, Kurt J et al, Ductal carcinoma in situ (intraductal carcinoma) of the breast treated with breast-conserving surgery and definitive irradiation: Correlation of pathologic parameters with outcome of treatment. *Cancer* 1993; **71**:2532–42.

14. Sneige N, Mcnesse MD, Atkinson EN et al, Ductal carcinoma in situ treated with lumpectomy and irradiation: Histo-pathological analysis of 49 specimens with emphasis on risk factors and long-term results. *Hum Pathol* 1995; 126:642–9.

15. Schwartz GF, Finkel GC, Garcia JG et al, Subclinical ductal carcinoma in situ of the breast. Treatment by local excision and surveillance alone. *Cancer* 1992; 70:2468–74.

16. Page DL, Dupont WD, Rogers LW et al, Continued local recurrence of carcinomas 15–25 years after diagnosis of low grade ductal carcinomas in situ of the breast treated only by biopsy. *Cancer* 1995; 76:1197–200.

17. Page DL, Dupont WD, Rogers LW et al, Atypical hyperplastic lesions of the female breast: A long follow-up study. *Cancer* 1985; 55:2698–708.

18. Dupont WD, Page DL, Risk factors for breast cancer in women with proliferative breast disease. *N Eng J Med* 1985; 312:146–51.

19. London SJ, Connolly JL, Schnitt SJ et al, A prospective study of benign breast disease and risk of breast cancer. *JAMA* 1992; 267:941–4.

20. Fisher ER, Costantino J, Fisher B et al, Pathologic findings from the National Surgical Adjuvant Breast Protocol B-17; intraductal carcinoma (duct carcinoma in situ). *Cancer* 1995; 75:1310–19.

21. Collins L, Lester S, Cooper A, Hetelekidis S et al, Ductal carcinoma in situ (DCIS) treated with excision alone: Predictors of local recurrence. In: *Proceedings of US–Canadian Academy of Pathology Annual Meeting*, 1997: Abst 80.

22. Badve S, A'hern RP, Ward AM et al, Prediction of local recurrence of ductal carcinoma of the breast using five histological classifications: A comparative study with long follow-up. *Hum Pathol* 1998; 29:915–23.

23. Douglas-Jobes AG, Gupta SK, Attanoos RL et al, A critical appraisal of six modern classifications of ductal carcinoma in situ of the breast: Correlation with grade of associated invasive disease. *Histopathology* 1996; 29:397–409.

24. Bethwaite P, Smithe N, Delahunt B, Kenwright D, Reproducibility of new classification schemes for the pathology of ductal carcinoma in situ of the breast. *J Clin Pathol* 1998; 51:450–4.

25. Sneige N, Lagios M, Schwarting R et al, Interobserver reproducibility of the Lagios nuclear grading system for ductal carcinoma in situ. *Hum Pathol* 1998; 30:257–62.

26. Egan RL, Ellis JR, Powell RW, Team approach to the study of disease of the breast. *Cancer* 1971; 71:847–54.

27. Lagios MD, Westdahl PR, Margolin FR et al, Duct carcinoma in situ: Relationship of extent of noninvasive disease to the frequency of occult invasion, multicentricity, lymph node metastases, and short-term treatment failures. *Cancer* 1982; 50:1309–14.

28. Silverstein MJ, Waisman JR, Gierson ED et al, Radiation therapy for intraductal carcinoma. Is it an equal alternative? *Arch Surg* 1991; 126:424–8.

29. Holland R, Veling SHJ, Marvinac M et al, Histologic multiplicity of T1s, T1–2 breast carcinomas. Implications for clinical trials of breast conserving surgery. *Cancer* 1985; 56:979–90.

30. Faverly D, Burgers L, Bult P, Holland R, Three dimensional imaging of mammary ductal carcinoma in situ: Clinical implications. *Semin Diag Pathol* 1994; 11:193–8.

31. Page DL, Lagios MD, Pathologic analysis of the National Surgical Adjuvant Breast Project (SNABP) B-17 Trial. *Cancer* 1995; 75:1219–21.

32. Silverstein MJ, Waisman JR, Gamagami P et al, Intraductal carcinoma of the breast (208) cases. Clinical factors influencing treatment choice. *Cancer* 1990; 55:102–8.

33. Fisher ER, Costantino J, Fisher B et al, Pathologic findings from the National Surgical Adjuvant Breast Protocol B-17: Intraductal carcinoma (duct carcinoma in situ). *Cancer* 1995; 75:1310–19.

34. Fisher ER, Dignam J, Tan-Chiu E et al, Pathologic findings from the National Surgical Adjuvant Breast Project (NSABP) eight-year update of protocol B-17. *Cancer* 1999; 86:429–38.

35. Silverstein MJ, Lagios MD, Groshen S et al, The influence of margin width on local control of ductal carcinoma in situ of the breast. *N Engl J Med* 1999; **340**:1455–61.

36. Fisher B, Costantino J, Redmond C et al, Lumpectomy compared with lumpectomy and radiation therapy for the treatment of intraductal breast cancer. *N Engl J Med* 1993; **328**:1581–6.

37. Lagios MD, Silverstein MJ, Ductal carcinoma in situ. The success of breast conservation therapy: A shared experience of two single institutional nonrandomized prospective studies. *Surg Oncol Clin North Am* 1997; **6**: 385–92.

38. Silverstein MJ, Lagios MD, Use of predictors of recurrence to plan therapy for DCIS of the breast. *Oncology* 1997; **11**:393–410.

39. Lagios MD, Multicentricity of breast carcinoma demonstrated by routine correlated serial subgross and radiographic examination. *Cancer* 1977; **40**:1726–34.

40. Arnesson LG, Smeds S, Fagerberg G et al, Follow-up of two treatment modalities for ductal cancer in situ of the breast. *Br J Surg* 1989; **76**:672–5.

41. Bornstein BA, Recht A, Conolly JL et al, Results of treating ductal carcinoma in situ of the breast with conservative surgery and radiation therapy. *Cancer* 1991; **67**:7–13.

42. Fisher B, Dignam J, Wolmark N et al, Lumpectomy and radiation therapy for the treatment of intraductal breast cancer: Findings from National Surgical Adjuvant Breast and Bowel Project B17. *J Clin Oncol* 1998; **16**:441–52.

43. Solin LJ, Kurtz J, Fourquet A et al, Fifteen-year results of breast conserving surgery and definitive breast irradiation for the treatment of ductal carcinoma in situ of the breast. *J Clin Oncol* 1996; **14**:754–63.

44. Silverstein MJ, Lagios MD, Silvana M et al, Outcome after invasive local recurrence in patients with ductal carcinoma in situ of the breast. *J Clin Oncol* 1998; **16**:1367–73.

45. Fisher B, Costantino J, Wickerham L et al, Tamoxifen for prevention of breast cancer: Report of the National Surgical Adjuvant Breast and Bowel Project P-1 study. *J Natl Cancer Inst* 1998; **90**:1371–88.

46. Fisher B, Dignam J, Wolmark N et al, Tamoxifen in treatment of intraductal breast cancer: National Adjuvant Breast and Bowel Project B-24 randomized controlled trial. *Lancet* 1999; **353**:1993–2000.

47. Bobrow LG, Happerfield LC, Gregory WM et al, The classification of ductal carcinoma in situ and its association with biologic markers. *Semin Diagn Pathol* 1994; **12**:199–207.

48. Leal CB, Schmitt FC, Bento MJ et al, Ductal carcinoma in situ of the breast. Histologic categorization and its relationship to ploidy and immunohistochemical expression of hormone receptors, p53, and c-erbB-2 protein. *Cancer* 1995; **75**:2123–31.

49. Zafrani B, Leroyer A, Forquet A et al, Mammographically detected ductal carcinoma in situ of the breast analyzed with a new classification. A study of 127 cases. Correlation with estrogen and progesterone receptors, p53 and c-erbB-2 proteins and proliferative activity. *Semin Diag Pathol* 1994; **11**:208–14.

50. De Potter CR, Foschini MP, Schelfhout AM et al, Immunohistochemical study of neu protein overexpression in clinging in situ duct carcinoma of the breast. *Virch Arch A Pathol Anat Histopathol* 1993; **422**:375–80.

51. De Potter CR, Schelfhout AM, Verbeeck P et al, Neu overexpression correlates with extent of disease in large cell ductal carcinoma in situ of the breast. *Hum Pathol* 1995; **26**:601–6.

52. Bartkova J, Barnes DM, Millis RR et al, Immunohistochemical demonstration of c-erbB-2 protein in mammary ductal carcinoma in situ. Philadelphia: WB Saunders, 1990.

53. De Potter CR, The neu-oncogene: More than a prognostic indicator? *Hum Pathol* 1994; **25**: 1264–8.

54. Poller DN, Snead D, Roberts EC et al, Oestrogen receptor expression in ductal carcinoma in situ of the breast. Relationship to flow cyto-

metric analysis of DNA and expression of the c-erb B-2 oncoprotein. *Br J Cancer* 1993; **68**:156–61.

55. O'Malley FP, Vnencak-Jones CL, Dupont WD et al, p53 mutations are confined to the comedo type ductal carcinoma in situ of the breast. Immunohistochemical and sequencing data. *Lab Invest* 1994; **71**:67–72.

56. Silverstein MJ, Barth A, Poller DN et al, Ten-year results comparing mastectomy to excision and radiation therapy for ductal carcinoma in situ of the breast. *Eur J Cancer* 1995; **31**:1425–7.

57. Van der Vijver MJ, Peterse JL, Vos C, ter Haar N, Genetic alterations in ductal carcinoma in situ of the breast: Association with histologic type. In: *Proceedings of US–Canadian Academy of Pathology, Annual Meeting*, 1998: Abst 150.

58. Wilbur DC, Barrows GH, Estrogen and progesterone receptor and c-erbB-2 oncoprotein analysis in pure in situ breast carcinoma: an immunohistochemical study. *Mod Pathol* 1993; **6**:114–20.

59. Guidi AJ, Fischer L, Harris JR et al, Microvessel density and distribution in ductal carci-noma in situ of the breast. *J Natl Cancer Inst* 1994; **86**:614–19.

60. Killeen JL, Namiki H, DNA analysis of ductal carcinoma of the breast: A comparison with histologic features. *Cancer* 1991; **68**:2602–7.

61. Susnik B, Worth A, Palcic B et al, Differences in quantitative nuclear features between ductal carcinoma in situ (DCIS) with and without accompanying invasive carcinoma in the surrounding breast. *Anal Cell Pathol* 1995; **8**:39–52.

62. Bellamy COC, McDonald D, Salter DM et al, Non-invasive ductal carcinoma of the breast. The relevance of histologic categorization. *Hum Pathol* 1993; **24**:16–23.

63. O'Malley FP, Page DL, Nelson EH et al, Ductal carcinoma in situ of the breast with apocrine cytology: Definition of a borderline category. *Hum Pathol* 1994; **25**:164–8.

64. Scott MA, Lagios MD, Axelsson K et al, Ductal carcinoma in situ of the breast: Reproducibility of histological subtype analysis. *Hum Pathol* 1997; **28**:967–73.

65. Consensus Conference On the Classification of Ductal Carcinoma in Situ. *Cancer* 1997; **80**:1798–802.

SECTION 11: Prevention and Screening for Breast Cancer

38

Chemoprevention studies in Italy and the UK

Andrea Decensi, Umberto Veronesi

TAMOXIFEN STUDIES

The striking benefits of the National Surgical Adjuvant Breast and Bowel Project (NSABP) P-1 trial do not seem to be confirmed by the European trials.[1,2] The Italian study was a multicentre, double-blind, placebo-controlled, chemoprevention trial, initiated in October 1992, to evaluate the effect of a daily dose of oral tamoxifen 20 mg for 5 years, on the prevention of breast cancer in healthy women.[1] Eligible subjects were well women aged 35–70 years who had had a prior hysterectomy for non-malignant conditions; the primary end-point of this study was the incidence of breast cancer. Recruitment was stopped on 31 December 1997 with 5408 women randomized.

The preliminary results of the Italian study, after a median of 46 months, show no difference in the incidence of breast cancer between the two arms.[1] Of the 41 cases of breast cancer that have occurred so far, 22 cases were in the placebo group and 19 in the tamoxifen group. Given the very limited number of events observed to date, the power to detect the anticipated 33% reduction of breast cancer occurrence in the tamoxifen arm is only 34%. Therefore, comparison with the Breast Cancer Prevention Trial (NSABP P-1) is not appropriate.

Subgroup analyses provide interesting hypotheses, however. Among women more than 1 year after intervention there was a trend towards a beneficial effect of tamoxifen (11 in the tamoxifen arm vs 19 in the placebo arm, $p = 0.16$). A borderline significant reduction of breast cancer was observed among women who were receiving continuous hormone replacement therapy (HRT) and tamoxifen. Compared with the eight cases of breast cancer occurring among the 390 HRT users who were on placebo, there was one case of breast cancer among the 362 HRT users who were receiving tamoxifen (relative risk or RR = 0.13, 95% confidence interval or 95%CI = 0.02–1.02). There was an increased risk of venous vascular events (38 women on tamoxifen vs 18 women on placebo, $p = 0.0053$), mainly consisting of superficial phlebitis, and 15 vs 2 cases of severe hypertriglyceridemia in the tamoxifen and placebo arms, respectively ($p = 0.0013$).

As the combination of tamoxifen and trans-dermal HRT might reduce the risks and side effects of either agent, their combined effect on several cardiovascular risk factors, including blood cholesterol levels, was tested within the trial.[3] Compared with small changes in the placebo group, tamoxifen was associated with changes in total, low-density lipoprotein (LDL) and high-density lipoprotein (HDL)-cholesterol of −9%, −14% and −0.8%, respectively, which were similar in continuous HRT users and those who never used HRT. By contrast, the decrease induced by tamoxifen of total and LDL cholesterol was blunted by two-thirds in women who started HRT whole on tamoxifen. Thus, the beneficial effects of tamoxifen on cardiovascular risk factors are unchanged in current HRT users, whereas they might be attenuated in women who start transdermal HRT while on tamoxifen.

Although tamoxifen can reduce the risk of breast cancer associated with HRT use, HRT could, on the other hand, reduce tamoxifen's adverse events (i.e. vasomotor and urogenital symptoms and, possibly, endometrial cancer). These findings provide the background for future investigations of the combination of tamoxifen and HRT in order to reduce the risks while retaining the benefit of both agents.

An interim analysis of the UK pilot prevention trial has also been published.[2] In this study, 2494 healthy women, aged between 30 and 70 years, at increased risk of breast cancer because of family history were accrued between 1986 and 1996. Each participant had at least one first-degree relative aged under 50 with breast cancer, or one first-degree relative with bilateral breast cancer, or one affected first-degree relative of any age plus another first-degree or second-degree relative. Women with a history of benign breast biopsy who had a first-degree relative with breast cancer were also eligible. They were randomized in a double-blind fashion to receive tamoxifen 20 mg/day or placebo for up to 8 years. The primary end-point was the occurrence of breast cancer.

After a median follow-up of 70 months, when the study had adequate power to detect a 50% reduction of breast cancer in the tamoxifen arm, the results demonstrate the same overall frequency of breast cancer in both arms tamoxifen 34 events, placebo 36 events, RR = 1.06 [95%CI = 0.7–1.7], $p = 0.8$). Interestingly, women who were already on HRT (mostly by the oral route) when they entered the trial showed an increased risk of breast cancer compared with non-users, whereas the subjects who started HRT while on trial had a significantly reduced risk. However, no interaction was noted between ever having taken HRT and any tamoxifen effect on breast cancer occurrence. There were 12 cancers in the 523 women who had ever used HRT (they mostly started the HRT during the study) on tamoxifen compared with 13 of 507 women who had ever used HRT or placebo. The occurrence of severe adverse events was low. There were four cases of endometrial cancer in the tamoxifen arm vs one in the placebo arm and seven cases vs four of deep vein thrombosis and pulmonary embolism.

Using the definition of drop-out as the number of discontinuations other than major events (including women lost to follow-up) divided by the total number of women included in the analysis,[4] the drop-out rate for the Royal Marsden study was 35.5%, for the NSABP P-1 study 28.8%, and for the Italian study 20.7%. In the Italian study, most women left for voluntary reasons other than side effects (1.5 per 100 vs 0.5 per 100 who did leave because of side effects). Moreover, several factors external to the study contributed to the high rate of withdrawal, including bad publicity in the media after the inclusion of tamoxifen in the list of class A carcinogens by the International Agency on Cancer Research (IARC) in 1996. As this affected the rate of accrual, the Data Monitoring Committee advised that recruitment be stopped before the planned date. However, these data, rather than detracting from the findings, should underline the fact that maintaining compliance in the long term is a formidable task even in an apparently highly motivated group and should be borne in mind when planning studies. Increasing public knowledge and appreciation of the value of chemoprevention trials can only help.

As already noted, comparison of the preliminary results among the three studies[1,2,5] is not appropriate given the limited statistical power of the European trials. Other explanations may include a different efficacy of tamoxifen depending on the type of population. The NSABP P-1 trial recruited high-risk women with a combination of genetic and reproductive risk factors for developing breast cancer. The UK study concentrated on younger women with a family history of breast cancer and the Italian study enrolled women who had undergone a hysterectomy and were at a lower risk. For instance, with the actual pattern of event distribution, it is calculated that the Italian study has only a one in five probability of detecting the anticipated 33% reduction of breast cancer incidence in the tamoxifen arm. Given the complexity of the issue, however, further results are clearly necessary. A fourth tamoxifen trial, the International Breast Cancer Intervention Study (IBIS), is currently under way in Europe and Australia.[6] As of February 2000, 6176 women have been recruited. This study is expected to provide an important contribution to the issue of tamoxifen efficacy and safety as a preventive agent.

The broad use of tamoxifen as a chemoprevention agent may be problematic because of the risk of endometrial cancer. This risk appears to be dose and time dependent. A trend to a dose–response effect is suggested in the meta-analysis of the three Scandinavian trials of adjuvant tamoxifen. The RR of endometrial cancer was 5.6 in the Stockholm trial of 40 mg/day and 3.3 and 2.0 in the Danish and south Swedish trial of tamoxifen 30 mg/day, respectively.[7] In the NSABP B-14 trial using the daily dose of 20 mg/day, the RR of endometrial cancer is approximately two times higher than the general population.[8,9] A relationship between length of tamoxifen treatment and endometrial cancer incidence is evident in the meta-analysis of all adjuvant trials of tamoxifen.[10] Given the apparent dose–response relationship between tamoxifen and endometrial cancer, the effect of three doses of tamoxifen on the change in biomarkers regulated by the estrogen receptor has recently been studied.[11] Indeed, a comparable potency of a lower dose of tamoxifen would provide strong support for assessing the preventive efficacy and the safety of low-dose tamoxifen in a larger trial.

A total of 127 healthy hysterectomized women aged 35–70 years were assigned to one of the following four treatment arms: placebo, tamoxifen 10 mg on alternate days, tamoxifen 10 mg/day or tamoxifen 20 mg/day. Comparison between baseline and 2-month measurements of the following parameters was performed: total cholesterol (primary end-point), HDL-cholesterol, LDL-cholesterol, triglycerides, lipoprotein(a), blood cell count, fibrinogen, antithrombin III, osteocalcin and insulin-like growth factor I (IGF-I). After adjustment for the baseline values, there were reductions in circulating levels of total cholesterol, IGF-I and most of the other parameters of the same magnitude in all three tamoxifen arms.[12] When blood concentrations of tamoxifen and its main metabolites were measured, no evidence for a concentration–response relationship was observed on most of the biomarkers, suggesting that a 80% reduction in blood levels from the conventional dose (i.e. from a mean ± SD [standard deviation] of 136.0 ± 52.7 ng/ml attained with 20 mg/day to 26.8 ± 15.1 ng/ml attained with 10 mg every other day) does not affect the biological activity of tamoxifen in a substantial way.[12]

Therefore, a mean tamoxifen concentration of approximately 25 ng/ml was associated with comparable changes in most end-point biomarkers. As tamoxifen has a very high tissue distribution, ranging from 5 to 60 times its blood concentration,[13,14] the breast tissue level attainable with 10 mg on alternate days still exceeds by several times the growth inhibitory concentration of tamoxifen in breast cancer cell lines, which is approximately 35 ng/ml.[15,16] In addition, the concomitant activity of metabolite X, which has a significant growth inhibitory activity in breast cancer cell lines,[16] may further contribute to the total drug inhibitory activity. Finally, recent in vivo studies in a spontaneous rat mammary tumour model indicate that a daily dose corresponding approximately to tamoxifen 1 mg/day has high preventive efficacy on mammary tumor formation.[17]

The issue of tamoxifen dose has also been raised in a recent epidemiological study. A cross-sectional study conducted in older, nursing home residents in the New York State long-term facilities has shown a significant reduction of bone fracture rate among women with breast cancer taking tamoxifen 10 mg/day.[18] During the 1.5-year period for which bone fractures were documented, the fracture rates were 7.6% in 5196 untreated control women, 3.2% in the 125 women receiving tamoxifen 10 mg/day and 6.7% in the 1248 women receiving tamoxifen 20 mg/day. The odds ratio (OR) for 20 mg/day compared with controls is 0.92 (0.72–1.16), whereas for 10 mg/day vs controls it is 0.31 (0.11–0.87, $p = 0.025$). The hip fracture rates were 5.0% in 5196 untreated control women, 2.4% in the 125 women receiving tamoxifen 10 mg/day and 4.6% in the 1248 women receiving tamoxifen 20 mg/day. The OR for 20 mg/day compared with controls is 0.96 (0.72–1.29), whereas that for 10 mg/day vs controls is 0.31 (0.10–1.02, $p = 0.054$). All these considerations

provide a strong rationale to assess a lower dose of tamoxifen in a preventive context.

FENRETINIDE STUDIES

Natural retinoids play a crucial role in cellular proliferation and differentiation, but their poor clinical tolerability has prevented the use of these compounds as cancer preventive agents. Toxic symptoms, which may be acceptable in treating established cancer, are not considered acceptable for reducing cancer risk. One of the less toxic vitamin A analogues studied for breast cancer chemoprevention is fenretinide, a synthetic amide derivative of all-*trans*-retinoic acid.[19] The inhibition of chemically induced mammary carcinoma in rats by fenretinide was first described in 1979.[20] On this basis, fenretinide was proposed for chemoprevention trials in human breast cancer. This compound has been studied extensively and proved to be less toxic than many other retinoids.[19] In contrast to retinoic acid, fenretinide selectively induces apoptosis rather than differentiation in several tumor cell systems[21,22] and maintains a stable plasma concentration during prolonged administration.[23] Although its mechanism of action still remains unclear, recent studies indicate that fenretinide may function both through receptor-dependent and -independent mechanisms.[23–25]

Moreover, fenretinide appears to be a potent inhibitor of the IGF system in breast cancer cell lines and this is an important mechanism of tumor cell growth inhibition by the retinoid.[26]

On the basis of the selective accumulation of fenretinide in the human breast,[23,27] and good tolerability in humans,[19] a phase III trial was started in 1987 aimed at reducing contralateral breast cancer. Briefly, 2972 women with a history of stage I breast cancer were randomized to fenretinide 200 mg/day or no intervention for 5 years. The primary end-point of the study was the occurrence of contralateral breast cancer as the first malignant event. The eligible women were diagnosed with stage I invasive breast cancer or ductal carcinoma in situ (DCIS) within the previous 10 years and had undergone definitive surgery without adjuvant hormone or chemotherapy.

The analysis after a median of 8 years has shown that the number of cases of contralateral breast cancer was comparable in the two arms.[28] At a median observation time of 97 months, there was no significant difference in contralateral breast cancer occurrence between the two arms (65 events in the fenretinide arm vs 71 in the control arm, $p = 0.642$). However, a significant interaction was detected between treatment and menopausal status ($p = 0.045$), with a beneficial effect in premenopausal women (fenretinide, 27 events; control, 42 events; adjusted hazard ratio [HR] = 0.66, 95%CI = 0.41–1.07). There was an opposite trend in postmenopausal women (fenretinide, 38 events; control, 29 events; adjusted HR = 1.32, 95%CI = 0.82–2.15). A similar pattern was observed in ipsilateral breast cancer reappearance (premenopausal women: fenretinide, 58 events, control, 87 events; adjusted HR = 0.65, 95%CI = 0.46–0.92; postmenopausal women: fenretinide, 42 events; control, 34 events; adjusted HR = 1.19, 95%CI = 0.75–1.89; p for the treatment × menopause interaction = 0.045). There was no difference for tumors in other organs, distant metastasis rate and all-cause mortality. Fenretinide was well tolerated and treatment discontinuation caused by severe adverse events was uncommon (4.4%). Interestingly, modulation of plasma IGF-I levels by fenretinide followed a similar pattern, i.e. IGF-I levels were lowered in premenopausal women only.[29] As circulating IGF-I levels are an important risk factor for subsequent breast cancer in premenopausal women,[30] the distinct effect of fenretinide on IGF-I in pre- and postmenopausal women provided the background for testing the clinical effect of fenretinide in the two subgroups. Fenretinide and tamoxifen have an enhancing effect in preventing mammary tumor development in animal models.[31] Further studies of fenretinide and tamoxifen are under way in premenopausal women at increased risk for breast cancer.

REFERENCES

1. Veronesi U, Maisonneuve P, Costa A et al, Prevention of breast cancer with tamoxifen: preliminary findings from the Italian randomised trial among hysterectomised women. Italian Tamoxifen Prevention Study. *Lancet* 1998; 352:93–7.

2. Powles T, Eeles R, Ashley S et al, Interim analysis of the incidence of breast cancer in the Royal Marsden Hospital tamoxifen randomised chemoprevention trial. *Lancet* 1998; 352:98–101.

3. Decensi A, Robertson C, Rotmensz N et al, Effect of tamoxifen and transfermal hormone replacement therapy on cardiovascular risk factors in a prevention trial. Italian Chemoprevention Group. *Br J Cancer* 1998; 78:572–8.

4. Veronesi U, Maisonneuve P, Costa A, Rotmensz N, Boyle P, Drop-outs in tamoxifen prevention trials. *Lancet* 1999; 353:244.

5. Fisher B, Costantino JP, Wickerman DL et al, Tamoxifen for prevention of breast cancer: report of the National Surgical Adjuvant Breast and Bowel Project P-1 Study. *J Natl Cancer Inst* 1998; 90:1371–88.

6. Cuzik J, Continuation of the International Breast Cancer Intervention Study (IBIS). *Eur J Cancer* 1998; 34:1647–8.

7. Rutqvist LE, Johansson H, Signomklao T, Johansson U, Fornander T, Wilking N, Adjuvant tamoxifen therapy for early stage breast cancer and second primary malignancies. Stockholm Breast Cancer Study Group. *J Natl Cancer Inst* 1995; 87:645–51.

8. Fisher B, Costantino JP, Redmond CK, Fisher ER, Wickerman DL, Cronin WM, Endometrial cancer in tamoxifen-treated breast cancer patients: findings from the National Surgical Adjuvant Breast and Bowel Project (NSABP) B-14. *J Natl Cancer Inst* 1994; **86**:527–37.

9. Fisher B, Commentary on endometrial cancer deaths in tamoxifen-treated breast cancer patients. *J Clin Oncol* 1996; **14**:1027–39.

10. Early Breast Cancer Trialists' Collaborative Group, Tamoxifen for early breast cancer: an overview of the randomised trials. *Lancet* 1998; **351**:1451–67.

11. Decensi A, Bonanni B, Guerrieri-Gonzaga A et al, Biologic activity of tamoxifen at low doses in health women. *J Natl Cancer Inst* 1998; **90**:1461–7.

12. Decensi A, Gandini S, Guerrieri-Gonzaga A et al, Effect of blood tamoxifen concentrations on surrogate biomarkers in a trial of dose reduction. *J Clin Oncol* 1999; **17**:2633–8.

13. Johnston SR, Haynes BP, Sacks NP et al, Effect of oestrogen receptor status and time on the intra-tumoural accumulation of tamoxifen and N-desmethyltamoxifen following short-term therapy in human primary breast cancer. *Breast Cancer Res Treat* 1993; **28**:241–50.

14. Lien EA, Solheim E, Ueland PM, Distribution of tamoxifen and its metabolites in rat and human tissues during steady-state treatment. *Cancer Res* 1991; **51**:4837–44.

15. Sutherland RL, Watts CK, Hall RE, Ruenitz PC, Mechanisms of growth inhibition by nonsteroidal antioestrogens in human breast cancer cells. *J Steroid Biochem* 1987; **27**:891–7.

16. Reddel RR, Sutherland RL, N-Desmethyltamoxifen inhibits growth of MCF 7 human mammary carcinoma cells in vitro. *Eur J Cancer Clin Oncol* 1983; **19**:1179–81.

17. Maltoni C, Minardi F, Belpoggi F, Pinto C, Lenzi A, Filippini F, Experimental results on the chemopreventive and side effects of tamoxifen using a human-equivalent animal model. In: Maltoni C, Soffritti M, Davis W, eds. *The Scientific Bases of Cancer Chemopre-vention.* Amsterdam: Elsevier Science, 1996: 197–217.

18. Breuer B, Wallenstein S, Anderson R, Effect of tamoxifen on bone fractures in older nursing home residents. *J Am Geriatr Soc* 1998; **46**: 968–72.

19. Costa A, Formelli F, Chiesa F, Decensi A, De Palo G, Veronesi U, Prospects of chemoprevention of human cancers with the synthetic retinoid fenretinide. *Cancer Res* 1994; **54**: 2032s–7s.

20. Moon RC, Thompson HJ, Becci PJ et al, N-(4-Hydroxyphenyl)retinamide, a new retinoid for prevention of breast cancer in the rat. *Cancer Res* 1979; **39**:1339–46.

21. Lotan R, Retinoids and apoptosis: implications for cancer chemoprevention and therapy. *J Natl Cancer Inst* 1995; **87**:1655–7.

22. Sun SY, Li W, Yue P, Lippman SM, Hong WK, Lotan R, Mediation of N-(4-hydroxyphenyl)retinamide-induced apoptosis in human cancer cells by different mechanisms. *Cancer Res* 1999; **59**:2493–8.

23. Formelli F, Clerici M, Campa T et al, Five-year administration of fenretinide: pharmacokinetics and effects on plasma retinol concentrations. *J Clin Oncol* 1993; **11**:2036–42.

24. Clifford JL, Menter DG, Wang M, Lotan R, Lippman SM, Retinoid receptor-dependent and -independent effects of N-(4-hydroxyphenyl)retinamide in F9 embryonal carcinoma cells. *Cancer Res* 1999; **59**:14–18.

25. Fanjul AN, Delia D, Pierotti MA, Rideout D, Yu JQ, Pfahl M, 4-Hydroxyphenyl retinamide is a highly selective activator of retinoid receptors [published erratum appears in *J Biol Chem* 1996 Dec 27; **271**:33705]. *J Biol Chem* 1996; **271**:22441–6.

26. Favoni RE, de Cupis A, Bruno S et al, Modulation of the insulin-like growth factor-I system by N-(4-hydroxyphenyl)-retinamide in human breast cancer cell lines. *Br J Cancer* 1998; 77:2138–47.

27. Metha RG, Moon RC, Hawthorne M, Formelli F, Costa A, Distribution of fenretinide in the

mammary gland of breast cancer patients. *Eur J Cancer* 1991; **27**:138–41.

28. Veronesi U, De Palo G, Marubini E et al, Randomized trial of fenretinide, a vitamin a analog, to prevent second breast malignancy in women with early breast cancer. *J Natl Cancer Inst* 1999; **91**:1847–56.

29. Torrisi R, Pensa F, Orengo MA et al, The synthetic retinoid fenretinide lowers plasma insulin-like growth factor I levels in breast cancer patients. *Cancer Res* 1993; **53**:4769–71.

30. Hankinson SE, Willett WC, Colditz GA et al, Circulating concentrations of insulin-like growth factor-I and risk of breast cancer. *Lancet* 1998; **351**:1393–6.

31. Ratko TA, Detrisac CJ, Dinger NM, Thomas CF, Kelloff GJ, Moon RC, Chemopreventive efficacy of combined retinoid and tamoxifen treatment following surgical excision of a primary mammary cancer in female rats. *Cancer Res* 1989; **49**:4472–6.

39

Prevention of invasive breast cancer in women at increased risk

Bernard Fisher

Little consideration was given to the prevention of invasive breast cancer[1-3] before the mid-1980s. At that time, the theory was promulgated that dietary fat might be associated with the occurrence of the disease and that restricting fat intake could, perhaps, reduce its incidence.[4] A trial to test that hypothesis has, however, only recently been implemented. The use of retinoids for the prevention of breast cancer was proposed in 1987, when a study was initiated to evaluate the effectiveness of fenretinide (4-HPR),[5] but, to date, no information about the outcome of that study has been reported. During that time, two independent pathways of investigation carried out by the National Surgical Adjuvant Breast and Bowel Project (NSABP) had their origins.

Beginning in November 1984, the group expressed interest in conducting a study to evaluate the worth of tamoxifen as a preventive agent for breast cancer. It was hypothesized that there might be a link between the finding of a decrease in cancer of the contralateral breast after administration of the antiestrogen tamoxifen to women with invasive cancer and the potential of that drug to prevent breast cancer in healthy women. The use of tamoxifen to treat patients with clinically detectable breast cancer had been among the most successful therapeutic efforts of the 1980s. Studies had demonstrated that, when used alone or in combination with chemotherapy for the treatment of advanced breast cancer[6-10] or as postoperative adjuvant therapy in stages I and II disease,[11-15] tamoxifen reduced tumor recurrence and prolonged survival. Of particular importance was the observation that women who received the drug had a significantly lower incidence of contralateral breast cancer than women who received placebo[14-18] and experienced only minimal side effects. Tamoxifen had also been shown to interfere with the initiation and promotion of tumors in experimental systems and to inhibit the growth of malignant cells by a variety of putative mechanisms. Moreover, the extensive literature available with regard to the pharmacokinetics, metabolism and anti-tumor effects of tamoxifen in experimental animals, as well as in humans, further supported the propriety of evaluating the worth of the drug as a preventive agent for breast cancer.[19-22] As a result of these considerations, on 1 June 1992 the NSABP implemented the Breast Cancer Prevention Trial (BCPT), subsequently known as the NSABP P-1 trial, the first study of its kind to be conducted in the USA.

In 1985, a situation had arisen that led the NSABP to undertake a second line of clinical investigation. As a result of the first report of findings from NSABP B-06 – a randomized clinical trial indicating that lumpectomy followed by breast irradiation was as effective as modified radical mastectomy for the treatment of women with invasive breast cancer[23] – breast preservation was being advocated for the management of invasive disease, whereas mastectomy was being used for the management of non-invasive breast cancer. This paradox resulted in uncertainty about the clinical management of women with small, localized ductal carcinoma in situ (DCIS) that was being detected by mammography. That circumstance prompted the NSABP to conduct a randomized controlled trial (B-17) to investigate whether excision of localized DCIS with tumor-free margins of excised tissue (referred to as a *lumpectomy*, although most women had no palpable mass) followed by radiation therapy was more effective than lumpectomy alone in the prevention of a second ipsilateral breast tumor (IBT), in particular one that was invasive. After completion of patient accrual in 1991, another trial (B-24) was begun by the NSABP to test the hypothesis that, in patients with DCIS, especially in women who had either tumor-positive specimen margins or mammographic evidence of scattered calcifications that were unlikely to be associated with invasive cancer, lumpectomy, postoperative radiation therapy and tamoxifen would be more effective than lumpectomy and radiation alone in preventing both invasive and non-invasive cancer.

Those two investigative efforts – one that evaluated the effect of tamoxifen for preventing invasive breast cancer in women at increased risk for the disease and the other that determined the most appropriate treatment for DCIS – remained independent until the findings from each strategy were reported.[24-25] It then became apparent that, because both of the DCIS trials, just as P-1, were related to the prevention of invasive breast cancer in women at increased risk for the disease, the two pathways of investigation had converged.

This report provides an overview of findings obtained from the clinical trials conducted to carry out the two investigative strategies and considers the significance of their convergence into a single guiding principle for addressing the breast cancer problem. The reader is referred to previous reports of P-1,[24,26,27] B-17[28,29] and B-24[25] for additional information about the design and implementation of the trials, conditions for participant eligibility, breast cancer risk assessment, risk–benefit estimates, statistical methods, secondary aims and the study findings.

THE PREVENTION TRIAL

About the study

The aim of the P-1 trial was to determine whether tamoxifen reduced the incidence of breast cancer in women at increased risk for the disease. In addition, the study was designed to evaluate whether tamoxifen influenced a woman's risk of coronary artery disease and whether it had a beneficial effect on women with osteoporosis. It also provided an opportunity to obtain genetic information about breast cancer from a population at increased risk. This report is concerned with the relationship of tamoxifen to breast cancer prevention. Details about the effect of tamoxifen on altering the risk of coronary artery disease and osteoporosis have been presented elsewhere.[24]

In the P-1 trial, women at increased risk for breast cancer were randomly assigned to receive either placebo or tamoxifen 20 mg/day for 5 years. Participants were considered to be at increased risk if they were aged 60 years or more, were between 35 and 59 years of age and had a 5-year predicted risk for breast cancer of at least 1.66%, or had a history of lobular carcinoma in situ (LCIS). An algorithm based on a multivariate logistic regression model employing combinations of risk factors was used to estimate the probability (risk) of the occurrence of breast cancer over time.[30] The variables included in the model were a woman's age, race, number of first-degree relatives with breast cancer, nulliparity or age at first live birth, number of breast biopsies, pathologic diagnosis of atypical hyperplasia and age at menarche. The 1984–88 Surveillance, Epidemiology, and End Results (SEER) rates of invasive breast cancer were used as the rates that were expected to occur. The total US mortality rates for the year 1988 were used to adjust for the age-specific competing risk of death from causes other than breast cancer. The mean time on the study for the 13 175 participants who were included in the analysis was 47.7 months; 73.9% had a follow-up exceeding 36 months, 67.0% were followed for more than 48 months and 36.8% had a follow-up exceeding 60 months. The median follow-up time was 54.6 months.

Of the women 39% were aged 35–49 years at randomization, 31% 50–59 years and 30% 60 years or more. Only 3% of the participants were aged 35–39 years and 6% were aged 70 years or more. Almost all participants were white (96%), more than one-third (37%) had had a hysterectomy, 6% had a history of LCIS and 9% had a history of atypical hyperplasia. The distribution of participants among the placebo and tamoxifen groups relative to these characteristics was similar. Almost a quarter (24%) of the participants had no first-degree relatives with breast cancer, more than a half (57%) had one first-degree relative with the disease, 16% had two and 3% had three or more. About a quarter of the women had a 5-year predicted breast cancer risk of 2.00% or less. Almost three-fifths (58%) had a 5-year risk of between 2.01% and 5.00%, and 17% had a risk of more than 5.00%.

Benefits of tamoxifen

There was a highly significant reduction in the incidence of invasive and non-invasive breast cancer as a result of tamoxifen administration. There was a 49% reduction in the overall risk for invasive breast cancer: 175 cases of invasive cancer in the placebo group, compared with 89 in the tamoxifen group ($p < 0.00001$) (Figure 39.1). The cumulative incidence of invasive breast cancer through 69 months of follow-up was 43 per 1000 and 22 per 1000 women in the placebo and tamoxifen groups, respectively. When the rate of invasive breast cancer was examined according to age, a decrease was observed in all age groups after tamoxifen administration (Table 39.1). The rate decreased by 44% in women aged ≤49 years, 53% in women aged ≥50 years, 51% in women aged between 50 and 59 years and 55% in women ≥60 years. In women with a history of either atypical hyperplasia or LCIS, the risk of invasive cancer was reduced by 86% and 56%, respectively. A reduction in risk was also observed in women with any category of predicted 5-year risk. The reduction ranged from 32% to 66%; a 63% reduction was observed in women with a 5-year predicted risk of ≤2.00 and a 66% reduction in women with a risk of ≥5.01. Of particular interest was the observation of a similar reduction in the rate of invasive breast cancer among women who received tamoxifen, regardless of whether they had no, one, two or three or more first-degree relatives with breast cancer. There was a 54% reduction in women with no first-degree relatives with the disease; in women with three or more, the reduction was 49%. Additional evidence of the effectiveness of the drug was provided by the observation that, during each of the first 6 years of follow-up, tamoxifen administration resulted in a significant reduction in the risk of invasive cancer. The rates of decrease in years 1 through 6 were 35%, 55%, 39%, 49%, 69% and 55%, respectively

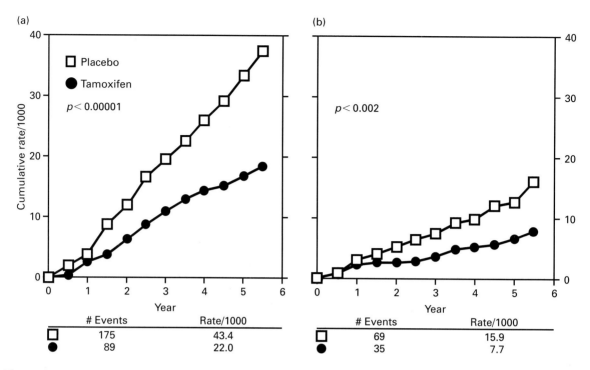

Figure 39.1
Cumulative rates of invasive (a) and non-invasive (b) breast cancers in all participants who received placebo or tamoxifen. The *p*-values are two-sided.

(Figure 39.2). No survival differences were observed between the group receiving placebo and that receiving tamoxifen; six deaths occurred in the former and three in the latter.

When the invasive breast cancers that occurred were related to selected tumor characteristics, particularly important was the finding of a 69% reduction in the rate of estrogen-receptor (ER)-positive tumors in the group that received tamoxifen. No such reduction was observed, however, in the rate of breast cancers that were ER-negative. Similarly, the rate of invasive breast cancer among women in the tamoxifen group was less than that among women in the placebo group in all categories of tumor size. The greatest difference was noted in the occurrence of tumors that were 2.0 cm or less

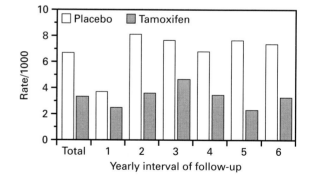

Figure 39.2
Risk of invasive breast cancer in participants who received placebo or tamoxifen, by yearly interval of follow-up.

Table 39.1   Rates of invasive breast cancer by age, 5-year predicted breast cancer risk, number of first-degree relatives with breast cancer, history of lobular carcinoma in situ (LCIS), or history of atypical hyperplasia

Patient characteristic	Rate per 1000 women per 5 years		Risk ratio	95% confidence interval
	Placebo	Tamoxifen		
Age (years)				
≤49	33.5	18.9	0.56	0.4–0.9
50–59	31.4	15.5	0.49	0.3–0.8
≥60	36.7	16.6	0.49	0.3–0.7
5-year predicted risk (%)				
≤2.00	27.7	10.3	0.37	0.2–0.7
≥5.01	66.4	22.6	0.34	0.2–0.6
No. of first-degree relatives with breast cancer				
0	32.3	14.9	0.46	0.2–0.8
1	30.0	15.2	0.51	0.4–0.7
2	43.4	23.8	0.55	0.3–1.0
3	68.6	35.1	0.51	0.2–1.6
History of LCIS				
Yes	65.0	28.5	0.44	0.2–1.1
No	32.1	16.5	0.51	0.4–0.7
History of atypical hyperplasia				
Yes	50.6	7.2	0.14	0.0–0.5
No	32.2	18.1	0.56	0.4–0.7

in size at the time of diagnosis. The rate of occurrence of tumors 1.0 cm or smaller was reduced by 42% as a result of tamoxifen administration; the rate of tumors sized 1.1–2.0 cm was reduced by 62%. A similar reduction, i.e. 50% and 57%, respectively, was observed in the rates of breast cancer in women who had either no nodal involvement or one to three nodes involved with tumor.

There was a 50% reduction in the risk of non-invasive breast cancer ($p < 0.002$). Through 69 months, the cumulative incidence of non-invasive breast cancer among the placebo group was 15.9 per 1000 women versus 7.7 per 1000 women in the tamoxifen group. The reduction was related to a decrease in the incidence of both DCIS and LCIS.

Benefit from a public health perspective
According to National Cancer Institute estimates, approximately 29 million women in the USA would have been potentially eligible for the P-1

trial and would, thus, have been expected to respond to tamoxifen in a manner similar to that of P-1 participants. The number of women in that population who have the potential to benefit from receiving tamoxifen might be estimated by using the data reported in the recent publication of the P-1 findings. As the average annual rate of the occurrence of invasive breast cancer in each 1000 participants in the placebo group of P-1 was 6.76, it might be estimated that, in the population of 29 million women, almost 1 million would, during a 5-year period, have the potential for being diagnosed with such a tumor. In the tamoxifen group of P-1, where the rate of such tumors was 3.43/1000 women per year, approximately 500 000 invasive breast cancers might be detected during that time. Thus, almost half a million invasive breast cancers would be prevented in the expanded population. A similar estimate indicates that almost 200 000 non-invasive tumors (either DCIS or LCIS) would be prevented. In view of these estimates, the benefits that might be achievable by more widespread use of tamoxifen cannot be viewed as trivial.

It needs to be emphasized that, the higher the risk of breast cancer in women who make up a population, the greater the number of breast cancers that will occur and, thus, the greater the number who will benefit from tamoxifen administration. A broad spectrum of risks existed among women who participated in the P-1 study. In some, the risk of developing invasive breast cancer was just high enough to make them eligible for the trial whereas, in others, the risk was much higher. If, for example, the 5-year predicted risk in all of the women comprising the population of 29 million were ≥5.01%, it would be estimated that almost 2 million invasive cancers would have occurred in the placebo group and 650 000 in the tamoxifen group during a 5-year period. Thus, approximately 1.2 million invasive breast cancers might have been prevented.

On the other hand, if the 5-year predicted risk in all 29 million women were ≤2.0%, then approximately 500 000 tumors could possibly have been prevented. Consequently, expanding the findings from the P-1 trial to a larger population of putatively similar women vividly demonstrates the potential impact that the wider use of tamoxifen, or of a similar drug of proven efficacy, could have in diminishing the extent of the breast cancer problem. The P-1 findings support the axiom that small benefits attained in a disease that occurs frequently can result in an advance of major proportions. (These statements do not imply, however, that tamoxifen should be administered to all 29 million women.)

Adverse effects of tamoxifen

The magnitude of the beneficial effects from tamoxifen prompted an appraisal of the magnitude of the adverse effects of tamoxifen with regard to decision-making about whether its benefit exceeded its undesirable side effects to an extent that would warrant its use within, as well as outside, the clinical trial setting. There was considerable concern, both before and during the conduct of the P-1 study, that liver damage, hepatoma, colon cancer and retinal toxicity might be associated with tamoxifen. However, no liver cancers have been observed in either the placebo or the tamoxifen groups of P-1 and, although posterior subcapular opacities were more frequently observed in women who received tamoxifen,[31] there has been no evidence of either macular degeneration or vision-threatening toxicity in that group. There have been too few ophthalmic toxicities from tamoxifen administration in the P-1 trial to warrant making a recommendation that the drug be withheld from women such as those who participated in that study.

Even greater concern was expressed about the risks of endometrial cancer and vascular-related

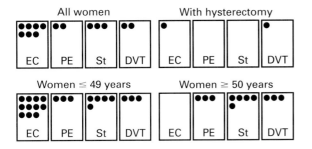

Figure 39.3
Rates of increase in endometrial cancer (EC), pulmonary embolism (PE), stroke (St), and deep-vein thrombosis (DVT) in women at increased risk for breast cancer. Each dot represents one woman per 1000 in 5 years in the P-1 study who experienced the event over 5 years.

toxic events, predominantly in postmenopausal women who participated in the P-1 trial. The issue has been raised, primarily in the lay press, about whether the benefit that was achieved by a reduction in the incidence of breast cancer was sufficiently great to justify the use of tamoxifen as a chemopreventive agent despite the risk of those events. Figure 39.3 presents a concise summary of the risks of endometrial cancer and vascular-related events that appeared in the published report of the P-1 study.[24] Each dot represents a single individual among 1000 P-1 participants who developed either an endometrial cancer, a pulmonary embolus, a stroke or a deep vein thrombosis over a 5-year period, i.e. the rate per 1000 women per 5 years. About 7 of 1000 women, or less than one woman per 100 (0.7%), in the tamoxifen group developed endometrial cancer over a 5-year period. The findings that all invasive endometrial cancers were stage 1 and that no deaths from endometrial cancer were reported were of clinical significance. Although no data are currently available to indicate that women who take tamoxifen should have regular endometrial biopsies or undergo vaginal ultrasonography, all those who take the drug should be advised to undergo an annual gynecologic evaluation and to report any abnormalities that might be evident. Regardless of all other considerations, these findings indicate that concern about the incidence and nature of endometrial cancer as a result of tamoxifen administration has been exaggerated. The results from a meta-analysis conducted by the Early Breast Cancer Trialists' Collaborative Group (EBCTCG), which are practically identical to the NSABP findings, support that view.[32]

When the undesirable vascular events attributable to tamoxifen were evaluated, the findings revealed that, over a 5-year period, 0.2–0.3% of women experienced a stroke, about 0.2% had a pulmonary embolism and between 0.2% and 0.3% exhibited a deep vein thrombosis. Those events occurred less frequently in women aged ≤49 years but were somewhat more frequent in women aged ≥50 years. In the latter group, the rate of endometrial cancer was about 1% over 5 years; for each of the vascular-related events, it was less than 1%. As women who had had a hysterectomy were not at risk for endometrial cancer, the major undesirable side effects in that population consisted only of vascular-related events. The rate of these was similar to the rate of such events in women who had not had a hysterectomy.

When P-1 participants were evaluated with regard to undesirable events from tamoxifen that could have an effect on their quality of life (Table 39.2), it was found that 12% more women in the tamoxifen, than in the placebo, group experienced some degree of hot flashes and 20% more reported vaginal discharge. Of those women who had hot flashes, only about 8% more women in the tamoxifen group than in the placebo group reported that their hot flashes were extremely bothersome; about 2% more described their vaginal discharge in the same manner. A recently

Table 39.2   Distribution of P-1 participants in the placebo and tamoxifen groups by highest percentage of hot flashes, vaginal discharge and depression reported

Symptom	Participants (%)	
	Placebo (*n* = 6498)	Tamoxifen (*n* = 6466)
Hot flashes, bothersome		
No	31	19
Slightly	18	14
Moderately	22	22
Quite a bit	19	28
Extremely	10	18
Vaginal discharge, bothersome		
No	65	45
Slightly	22	26
Moderately	8	17
Quite a bit	3	9
Extremely	1	3
Depression (CES-D)[a]		
0–15	65	65
16–22	16	16
23–29	10	10
30–36	5	5
≥37	4	4

[a] CES-D refers to a self-administered scale of depression developed by the Center for Epidemiological Studies.[12]

published report on the health-related quality-of-life component of the P-1 trial provided information to indicate that weight gain and depression, two clinical problems that have been anecdotally associated with tamoxifen treatment, did not increase in frequency in the women who participated in the study.[33] Moreover, overall rates of sexual activity remained similar for women in both the placebo and tamoxifen groups.

In view of the impressive benefits and low rates of adverse events experienced by women in the tamoxifen group, it is reasonable to consider the way in which the benefits and risks associated with the drug are related to each other. From a clinical perspective, it is not appropriate to make a decision about the net worth of tamoxifen by simply 'trading' one event for another, i.e. by subtracting one undesirable event from one cancer prevented. Although the net benefit from tamoxifen may be quantified statistically, clinical consideration must also be included in any risk–benefit determination. The morbidity and mortality from a hysterectomy for endometrial cancer are likely to be less than those resulting from the use of surgery, radiation and chemotherapy for a breast cancer that would have occurred in the absence of tamoxifen administration.

NSABP B-17 AND B-24 TRIALS IN WOMEN WITH A HISTORY OF DCIS

About the studies

A detailed description of patient eligibility requirements, study design, surgery, and radiation therapy, as well as study end-points and statistical analyses, are included in the reports of NSABP B-17[28,29] and B-24.[25] Women with small, localized DCIS, which had been detected by either physical examination or mammography, were eligible for the B-17 study. Women underwent a lumpectomy with removal of the tumor and a sufficient amount of normal breast tissue so that specimen margins were histologically tumor free. Women with a histologic diagnosis of DCIS whose mammograms showed scattered calcifications were eligible if no tumor was demonstrated upon histologic examination of tissue that contained the calcifications. After they had undergone lumpectomy, women were randomly assigned to receive either ipsilateral breast irradiation or no radiation therapy. The eligibility criteria of patients admitted to the B-24 study were similar in all aspects to those in B-17, except that, in B-24, patients with positive specimen margins or with mammographic findings unlikely to be related to invasive cancer were eligible. The similarity between the two studies is also indicated by the concordant distribution of patient age, method of detection and tumor type

among the two studies (Table 39.3). The size of tumors in B-17 patients was, however, slightly greater than that of women enrolled in B-24, and the incidence of specimen margins that contained tumor in B-24 patients was, as anticipated, greater than that observed in B-17, where eligibility criteria required that the margins be tumor free. After women had undergone lumpectomy, they were randomly assigned to receive either radiation therapy to the ipsilateral breast and placebo ($n = 902$), or radiation therapy and tamoxifen ($n = 902$).

The protocols of both studies stipulated that radiation therapy (50 Gy) be started no later than 8 weeks after surgery. The technique used was similar to that which has been described for previous NSABP studies.[23] Patients in B-24 received either placebo or tamoxifen 10 mg twice daily for 5 years. No dose modifications were made for either agent. In both studies, a tumor detected at a local or regional site after the initial operation was considered an event only when a tissue biopsy of the lesion was positive. A tumor detected at a distant site was considered an event when clinical, radiographic or pathologic findings indicated that tumor was present.

A total of 818 women were entered into the B-17 trial (Table 39.4): 405 women were randomly assigned to the group treated with lumpectomy alone and 413 to the group treated with lumpectomy followed by radiation therapy. In the B-24 study, 902 women were randomly assigned to receive lumpectomy followed by radiation therapy and placebo; 902 were randomly assigned to the group treated with lumpectomy, radiation therapy and tamoxifen (Table 39.4). All women for whom follow-up information was available, including those who failed to meet the entry criteria, were included in the analyses. The mean follow-up time in B-17 was 90 months; in B-24, it was 74 months. No differences between treatment groups in the distribution of selected

Table 39.3   Patient and tumor characteristics in the B-17 and B-24 trials

	B-17		B-24	
	L (403 patients) (%)	L + XRT (411 patients) (%)	Placebo (899 patients) (%)	Tamoxifen (899 patients) (%)
Age (years)				
≤49	35	33	33	34
50–59	29	33	31	30
≥60	37	35	36	37
Detection				
Mammogram	81	80	84	81
Clinical	8	8	8	9
Both	11	12	8	9
Clinical size (cm)				
≤1.0	74	74	83	85
1.1–2.0	15	13	12	9
≥2.1	8	9	4	5
Type				
DCIS	94	97	94	96
DCIS + LCIS	6	3	6	4
Margins				
Initially free			53	54
Free after second operation			17	15
Not free	<1	<1	15	14
Unknown			16	18

L, lymphectomy; XRT, radiation therapy.

patient and tumor characteristics were observed in either study (Table 39.3).

Physical examinations were performed every 6 months and mammography once a year. The primary end-points of both studies were the occurrence of invasive or non-invasive tumors in either the ipsilateral or contralateral breast; tumors detected at local or regional sites were accepted as events only if tissue biopsy of the lesion was positive. Tumors detected at distant sites, i.e. before a local or regional invasive cancer was noted, were considered to be events if clinical, radiographic or pathologic findings showed that a tumor was present. Ipsilateral or

Table 39.4   Study information

Patients	B-17		B-24	
	L	L + XRT	L + XRT + placebo	L + XRT + tamoxifen
Randomized	405	413	902	902
Analyzed	403	411	899	899

L, lumpectomy; XRT, radiation therapy.

contralateral breast tumors, regional or distant metastases, second primary tumors other than a breast tumor that occurred as a first event, or deaths in the absence of evidence of recurrent breast cancer were included in the analyses.

The nature of the DCIS that was diagnosed in the B-17 patients was best characterized by the pathologic and mammographic assessment of the lesion. Pathologic examination revealed that 692 of the 797 resected specimens evaluated (87%) had either no gross tumor or gross tumors that were reported as being ≤1.0 cm in size. Only 2% of all specimens examined had gross tumors of ≥2 cm.

Of the 730 mammograms (90% of all patients in B-17 included in the analyses) that were centrally reviewed, a tumor was identified in 117 (16%). The mass was greater than 2.0 cm in only 15 (2%) of all mammograms examined. Almost 80% of mammograms demonstrated either scattered (7%) or clustered (70%) microcalcifications but no mass. An additional 3% of mammograms demonstrated architectural distortion with no mass or calcifications. There were no mammographic abnormalities in 4% of cases. The mammographic characteristics were distributed uniformly among the two groups. Reports from mammograms unavailable for central review showed similar characteristics: approximately

20% demonstrated the presence of a tumor mass and 80% showed microcalcifications. Most of the masses and microcalcifications were, however, small.

The findings that are available from patients in the B-24 study have indicated that the clinical size of the tumors is slightly smaller than that noted for those in B-17. As anticipated, the incidence of specimen margins that contained tumor in B-24 patients was greater than that observed in B-17, where eligibility criteria required that margins be tumor free.

Benefit from radiation therapy after lumpectomy and added benefit from tamoxifen

As the NSABP B-17 and B-24 studies were similar except for inclusion in B-24 of women with more extensive DCIS, the findings from the B-24 trial may be considered within the context of the B-17 findings. The fact that, for the 5 years, the cumulative incidence of all breast cancer events, invasive or non-invasive, in the group of patients that received lumpectomy, radiation therapy and placebo in B-24 was almost identical to that in women who were treated with lumpectomy and radiation therapy in B-17 (Figure 39.4) further establishes the validity of interrelating the two studies. The spectrum of results from the two

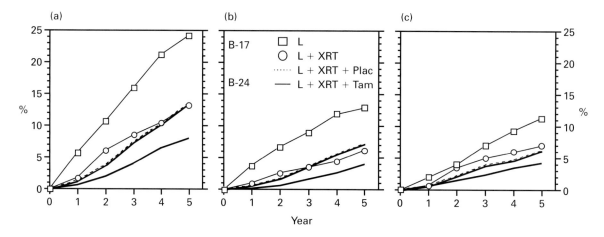

Figure 39.4
Cumulative incidence of all (a), invasive (b), and non-invasive (c) events in the ipsilateral and contralateral breast in the B-17 and B-24 studies. All and invasive cancers include cancers at regional and distant sites. L, lumpectomy; XRT, radiation therapy; Plac, placebo; Tam, tamoxifen.

studies clearly depicts the advantage from radiation therapy, as well as the added benefit from tamoxifen. In the B-17 study, the cumulative incidence of all breast cancer-related events in women treated with lumpectomy alone was about 25% for the 5 years of follow-up whereas, when radiation therapy was given after lumpectomy, it was 13%. It was also 13% in those women in B-24 who received radiation therapy but, when tamoxifen was also given, it was 8%. The benefit from tamoxifen was partly the result of the lower rates of contralateral breast cancer and invasive cancer at regional and distant sites. Thus, when compared with the cumulative incidence of all breast cancer events after treatment with lumpectomy alone in B-17, the administration of tamoxifen and radiation therapy to women in B-24 led to a 68% lower incidence of all breast cancer events for the 5 years of follow-up. Compared with women who underwent lumpectomy alone, the tamoxifen group showed a 77% reduction in the cumulative incidence of all invasive breast cancer events and about a 64% reduction of all non-invasive events.

Linkage of the NSABP DCIS studies and the NSABP P-1 trial

The findings from the B-17 and B-24 studies may be related to those of the NSABP P-1 trial, which showed that the administration of tamoxifen to women at increased risk for breast cancer resulted in 50% fewer non-invasive tumors (both DCIS and LCIS) and 49% fewer invasive breast tumors than observed in the group that received placebo. In B-17, women with a history of DCIS who were treated with lumpectomy were at a greater risk for invasive breast cancer than women in P-1 who had a history of either atypical hyperplasia or LCIS (Figure 39.5). In women with a history of DCIS who were treated with lumpectomy alone in B-17, the rate of the occurrence of an invasive breast cancer was 158/1000 women per 5 years, whereas it was found that the rates of atypical hyperplasia or of LCIS in P-1 were 65 and 51/1000 women per 5 years, respectively. Findings from both the B-17 and B-24 studies showed that invasive cancer rates in DCIS patients who received radiation therapy alone were higher, i.e. about 80/1000 women per 5

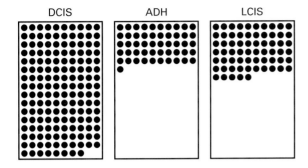

Figure 39.5
Rates of invasive breast cancer in women with a history of either ductal carcinoma in situ (DCIS, B-17), atypical ductal hyperplasia (ADH, B-24) or lobular carcinoma in situ (LCIS, B-24). Each dot represents one woman per 1000 in 5 years.

years, than those in women in P-1 who had a history of LCIS (65/1000 women per 5 years) or atypical hyperplasia (51/1000 women per 5 years) who had received tamoxifen alone.

POTENTIAL TAMOXIFEN RECIPIENTS

Who should take tamoxifen to decrease the risk of developing breast cancer? Women who are younger than 50 and who meet the eligibility requirements of the P-1 trial are likely to be considered highly eligible for tamoxifen because their risk of an adverse event is practically nil, and because the reduction in the incidence of breast cancer for the group overall is reduced by almost a half. Moreover, the greater their risk, the greater the benefit from tamoxifen. Postmenopausal women who have had a hysterectomy are also favorable candidates for tamoxifen because they cannot develop endometrial cancer. As women with a history of LCIS, atypical hyperplasia or DCIS are at particularly increased risk for breast cancer, and because tamoxifen reduces that risk, the level of benefit achieved markedly outweighs the adverse effects that might result from tamox-

ifen administration. As the risk of invasive breast cancer in women with localized DCIS treated by radiation therapy is at least as high, if not higher, than that for women with a history of LCIS or atypical hyperplasia, if consideration is given to administering tamoxifen to women with LCIS or atypical hyperplasia, there can be no justification for withholding its use in women with DCIS.

Although, to date, no information is available to indicate whether women who are at increased risk for breast cancer because they carry *BRCA1* or *BRCA2* mutations should be considered candidates for tamoxifen, these women should be afforded that option, particularly if they are contemplating having a bilateral mastectomy to prevent the disease.

The decision to prescribe tamoxifen for women aged 50 years or more who have stopped menstruating, have not had a hysterectomy and have no history of LCIS, DCIS or atypical hyperplasia is less clear. As the incidence of adverse events remains constant regardless of the cancer risk in these women, it is evident that, the greater the risk, the less controversial the issue. The greater the mortality and morbidity associated with breast cancers that have been prevented by tamoxifen, the greater the benefit from the drug when the benefit is balanced against potential adverse events. A precise level of risk above and below which a woman should or should not be considered a candidate for tamoxifen has not yet been determined and is likely to be difficult to agree on. The probability that an adverse event from tamoxifen will occur in women aged 50 years or more should not prevent the use of tamoxifen in this age group. This recommendation is supported by the following two major considerations:

1. The P-1 study was unblinded by an independent group of investigators from a variety of disciplines so that P-1 participants who took

placebo (including women aged 50 years or more) could choose either to receive tamoxifen or to participate in the NSABP P-2 trial, a new study in which women aged 50 years or more who take tamoxifen will serve as the standard group against which the benefits and adverse effects from the selective estrogen receptor modulator (SERM) raloxifene will be measured.

2. British investigators did not alter their prevention trial because of the adverse endometrial cancer and vascular events reported in P-1.

These circumstances clearly indicate that, in the general population, there must be a substantial number of women aged 50 years and over for whom tamoxifen administration would be appropriate.

It must be emphasized, however, that, before a woman is advised to begin taking tamoxifen, her overall clinical status must be evaluated. Her physical well-being must be assessed to ensure that she does not have co-morbid conditions that make the administration of tamoxifen not only undesirable but inappropriate. Moreover, the task of recommending tamoxifen for women at increased risk for breast cancer should be undertaken only by those individuals who are free of personal bias, possess complete and accurate information about breast disease, know how to determine a woman's risk for breast cancer, and are adept at counseling her about her individual course of action.

COMMENTS RELEVANT TO BREAST CANCER PREVENTION

The findings from P-1 and the two DCIS clinical trials conducted by the NSABP clearly demonstrate that tamoxifen reduces the risk of breast cancer in a substantial number of women at increased risk. As is evident, however, after each demonstration of a therapeutic advance, uncer-

tainty arises with regard to the clinical application of the findings. Failure to resolve all of the issues and to answer all of the questions that have arisen as a result of the NSABP studies does not necessarily detract from either the credibility or the importance of the results, which have opened doors to new pathways for scientific investigation. The following comments address some of the concerns that have arisen subsequent to the publication of the P-1 findings.

Timing and duration of tamoxifen administration

Some researchers have expressed concern about the duration of tamoxifen administration. It has been speculated that, if the drug is given for only 5 years, tumor growth might merely be delayed for a short time and that tumors will subsequently appear when the drug is discontinued. Findings from NSABP B-14, a trial that was conducted to evaluate the worth of tamoxifen for the treatment of patients with node-negative, ER-positive tumors, have not supported this concern.[34] In that study, the benefit from 5 years of tamoxifen administration persisted through 10 years of follow-up. Giving the drug for more than 5 years, however, failed to enhance its effect. Most important, the reduction in the incidence of contralateral breast cancer observed with 5 years of tamoxifen therapy continued up to 10 years of follow-up; a 37% decrease was observed at that time. As the findings from both the B-14 and P-1 trials demonstrated that the breast tumors prevented were ER-positive, it is likely that the benefit noted in the P-1 trial will persist after study participants discontinue taking tamoxifen. Although additional studies are necessary before this issue can be resolved, the value of 5 years of tamoxifen therapy cannot currently be disputed. Another important question concerns the optimal time at which to begin tamoxifen administration. It is likely that alterations were already present in the breast cells of women who developed tumors when they were enrolled in the P-1 study. As these tumors were diagnosed early in the follow-up period, there would seem to be no merit in delaying administration of the drug to women for whom it has been deemed appropriate.

Findings from two European prevention trials

Another issue that has resulted in criticism of the P-1 study arose as a consequence of findings reported from two European prevention trials[35,36] that failed to verify the results obtained from P-1. The simultaneous reports from a British study and an Italian study resulted in a misunderstanding among the public, the media and physicians, who failed to realize that the three studies were too dissimilar in design, population enrolled and other aspects to permit making valid comparisons among them. The disparate findings from each of the three trials relate to differences in boundaries that were initially defined in each study. To view the results of the two European studies as being contradictory to those of P-1 and to contend that the findings from one study either confirmed or rejected the findings of the others is inappropriate, because:

• Fewer breast cancer events occurred in the British and Italian studies than in P-1.
• The criteria for selecting participants were different in the three trials.
• Study participants had different risks for breast cancer.
• There were some differences in protocol compliance among the trials.
• Hormone replacement therapy was used in the two European studies but not in P-1.

Consequently, the value judgment that the two European studies failed to confirm the P-1 study is unwarranted because there was, in actuality, 'no contest' between them.

CONCLUSION

Almost half of the invasive and non-invasive breast cancers in the P-1 trial were prevented, in all age groups, by the administration of tamoxifen. Thus, the findings from that study support the hypothesis that breast cancer can be prevented in women at increased risk for the disease. As thousands of women with invasive breast cancer die each year despite what is viewed as effective treatment, we cannot afford to deny those who do qualify for the drug the opportunity to receive it.

Although more studies are needed to address the issues that have arisen as a result of the P-1 findings, on the basis of the data from that trial, we consider it highly appropriate to offer tamoxifen to women similar to those who participated in the study. To that end, the new NSABP P-2 chemoprevention trial will evaluate postmenopausal women at increased risk for breast cancer who are similar to P-1 participants. In P-2, the toxicity, risks and benefits of the SERM raloxifene will be compared with those of tamoxifen. Although raloxifene has been shown to prevent osteoporosis, its value in reducing the rate of breast cancer without increasing the risk of endometrial cancer has yet to be established. Although science is too complex to permit predictions with regard to future directions for breast cancer research, the findings from P-1 clearly indicate that such research must be related to prevention. Agents that have the ability to prevent the occurrence of ER-negative tumors must be discovered and evaluated, and new, more effective SERMs with different mechanisms of action must be developed. Despite the fact that scientists have failed to eradicate breast cancer in the last millennium, it must be acknowledged that, when viewed in retrospect, the twentieth century was a period during which notable progress was made in the understanding, treatment and prevention of the disease.

REFERENCES

1. Terenius L, Effect of anti-oestrogens on initiation of mammary cancer in the female rat. *Eur J Cancer* 1971; 7:65–70.

2. Jordan VC, Effect of tamoxifen (ICI 46,474) on initiation and growth of DMBA-induced rat mammary carcinomata. *Eur J Cancer* 1976; 12:419–24.

3. Sporn MB, Roberts AB, Role of retinoids in differentiation and carcinogenesis. *J Natl Cancer Inst* 1984; 73:1381–7.

4. Prentice RL, Kakar F, Hursting S et al, Aspects of the rationale for the women's health trial. *J Natl Cancer Inst* 1988; 80:802–14.

5. Veronesi U, DePalo G, Costa A et al, Chemoprevention of breast cancer with retinoids. *J Natl Cancer Inst Monogr* 1992; 12:93–7.

6. Heuson J-C, Current overview of EORTC clinical trials with tamoxifen. *Cancer Treat Rep* 1976; 60:1463–6.

7. Mouridsen H, Palishof T, Patterson J et al, Tamoxifen in advanced breast cancer. *Cancer Treat Rev* 1978; 5:131–41.

8. Legha SS, Buzdar AU, Hortobagyi GN et al, Tamoxifen: use in treatment of metastatic breast cancer refractory to combination chemotherapy. *JAMA* 1979; 242:49–52.

9. Margreiter R, Wiegele J, Tamoxifen (Nolvadex) for premenopausal patients with advanced breast cancer. *Breast Cancer Res Treat* 1984; 4:45–8.

10. Jackson IM, Litherland S, Wakeling AE, Tamoxifen and other antiestrogens. In: Powles TJ, Smith IE, eds. *Medical Management of Breast Cancer*. London: Martin Dunitz, 1991: 51–61.

11. Baum M, Brinkley DM, Dossett JA, et al, Controlled trial of tamoxifen as adjuvant agent in management of early breast cancer. *Lancet* 1983; i:257–61.

12. Nolvadex Adjuvant Trial Organization, Controlled trial of tamoxifen as single adjuvant agent in management of early breast cancer. *Lancet* 1985; i:836–9.

13. Fisher B, Redmond C, Brown A et al, Adjuvant chemotherapy with and without tamoxifen in the treatment of primary breast cancer: 5-year results from the National Surgical Adjuvant Breast and Bowel Project trial. *J Clin Oncol* 1986; 4:459–71.

14. Breast Cancer Trials Committee, Scottish Cancer Trials Office, Adjuvant tamoxifen in the management of operable breast cancer. The Scottish Trial. *Lancet* 1987; ii:171–5.

15. Fisher B, Costantino J, Redmond C et al, A randomized clinical trial evaluating tamoxifen in the treatment of patients with node-negative breast cancer who have estrogen-receptor-positive tumors. *N Engl J Med* 1989; 320:479–84.

16. CRC Adjuvant Breast Trial Working Party, Cyclophosphamide and tamoxifen as adjuvant therapies in the management of breast cancer. *Br J Cancer* 1988; 57:604–7.

17. Rutqvist LE, Cedermark B, Glas U et al, Contralateral primary tumors in breast cancer patients in a randomized trial of adjuvant tamoxifen therapy. *J Natl Cancer Inst* 1991; 83:1299–306.

18. Fisher B, Redmond C, New perspective on cancer of the contralateral breast: A marker for assessing tamoxifen as a preventive agent. *J Natl Cancer Inst* 1991; 83:1278–80.

19. Furr BJ, Patterson JS, Richardson DN et al, Tamoxifen (review). In: Goldberg ME, ed. *Pharmacological and Biochemical Properties of Drug Substances*, Vol. 2. Washington, DC: American Pharmaceutical Association, 1979: 355–99.

20. Adam HK, Pharmacokinetic studies with Nolvadex. *Rev Endocrine-Related Cancer* 1981; (Suppl 9):131–43.

21. Wakeling AE, Valcaccia B, Newboult E et al, Non-steroidal antioestrogens – Receptor binding and biological response in rat uterus, rat mammary carcinoma and human breast cancer cells. *J Steroid Biochem* 1984; 20:111–20.

22. Jordan VC, Fritz NF, Tormey DC, Long-term adjuvant therapy with tamoxifen: Effects on

sex hormone binding globulin and antithrombin III. *Cancer Res* 1987 15; **47**:4517–19.

23. Fisher B, Bauer M, Margolese R et al, Five-year results of a randomized clinical trial comparing total mastectomy and segmental mastectomy with or without radiation in the treatment of breast cancer. *N Engl J Med* 1985; **312**:665–73.

24. Fisher B, Constantino JP, Wickerham DL et al, Tamoxifen for prevention of breast cancer: report of the National Surgical Adjuvant Breast and Bowel Project P-1 study. *J Natl Cancer Inst* 1998; **90**:1371–88.

25. Fisher B, Dignam J, Wolmark N et al, Tamoxifen in treatment of intraductal breast cancer: National Surgical Adjuvant Breast and Bowel Project B-24 randomized controlled trial. *Lancet* 1999; **353**:1993–2000.

26. Fisher B, National Surgical Adjuvant Breast and Bowel Project Breast Cancer Prevention Trial: a reflective commentary. *J Clin Oncol* 1999; **17**:1632–9.

27. Fisher B, Constantino JP, Highlights of the NSABP breast cancer prevention trial. *Cancer Control* 1997; **4**:78–86.

28. Fisher B, Constantino JP, Redmond C et al, Lumpectomy compared with lumpectomy and radiation therapy for the treatment of intraductal breast cancer. *N Engl J Med* 1993; **328**:1581–6.

29. Fisher B, Dignam J, Wolmark N et al, Lumpectomy and radiation therapy for the treatment of intraductal breast cancer: Findings from National Surgical Adjuvant Breast and Bowel Project B-17. *J Clin Oncol* 1998; **16**:441–52.

30. Gail MH, Brinton LA, Byar DP et al, Projecting individualized probabilities of developing breast cancer for white females who are being examined annually. *J Natl Cancer Inst* 1989; **81**:1879–86.

31. Gorin MB, Day R, Constantino JP et al, Long-term tamoxifen citrate use and potential ocular toxicity. *Am J Ophthalmol* 1998; **125**:493–501.

32. Early Breast Cancer Trialists' Collaborative Group, Tamoxifen for early breast cancer: an overview of the randomised trials. *Lancet* 1998; **351**:1451–67.

33. Day R, Ganz PA, Constantino JP et al, Health-related quality of life and tamoxifen in breast cancer prevention: a report from the National Surgical Adjuvant Breast and Bowel Project P-1 study. *J Clin Oncol* 1999; **17**:2659–69.

34. Fisher B, Dignam J, Bryant J et al, Five versus more than five years of tamoxifen therapy for breast cancer patients with negative lymph nodes and estrogen receptor-positive tumors. *J Natl Cancer Inst* 1996; **88**:1529–42.

35. Powles T, Eeles R, Ashley S et al, Interim analysis of the incidence of breast cancer in the Royal Marsden Hospital tamoxifen randomised chemoprevention trial. *Lancet* 1998; **352**:98–101.

36. Veronesi U, Maisonneuve P, Costa A et al, Prevention of breast cancer with tamoxifen: preliminary findings from the Italian randomised trial among hysterectomised women. Italian Tamoxifen Prevention Study. *Lancet* 1998; **352**:93–7.

40
Breast cancer screening: The population and the patient

Heather Bryant

There are few screening interventions that have the same level of evidence as there are for mammographic screening. Randomized trials have been carried out in Canada,[1,2] New York[3] and the UK,[4] along with five locations in Sweden.[5-8] There is general consensus that mammographic screening can reduce the breast cancer mortality rate by about 30% in women aged 50–69.[9,10]

Given this level of evidence, it may be surprising that mammography screening remains exceptionally controversial. In fact, the level of controversy has reached such a high pitch that some observers have suggested that there is little possibility of having a rational public discussion on the issue.[11,12] Some of this debate concerns the evidence itself, and the application of the evidence to particular subgroups of the population. However, an additional layer of confusion is added when public health recommendations are confused with clinical decisions that may be relevant in individual circumstances. Both of these issues are critical to clinicians providing advice to women considering mammographic screening.

CONSIDERATIONS OF THE EVIDENCE

The high degree of consensus noted above has resulted in widespread adoption of mammography screening for women in the 50–69 age group at least, with many countries developing organized public health programs designed to enrol women and to provide them with high-quality mammographic screening.[13] However, this high level of support does not imply that the endorsement is unanimous. Recent reports that there has been no notable breast cancer mortality reduction in Sweden despite the existence of mammography screening for well over a decade led to another meta-analysis, published in 2000.[14] Although this unblinded meta-analysis has been criticized on several grounds,[15-19] the article's conclusion that 'screening for breast cancer with mammography is unjustified' captured the attention of media in many countries.

Even among the majority who agree that the randomized controlled trials have shown the efficacy of screening in the 50–69 age group, there are those who challenge its wisdom on the grounds of opportunity costs.[20] Although Baum, in his opinion piece, supports the extension of the target age group for screening in the UK to include women aged 65–69 (who were not initially targeted by their program), he simultaneously questions whether there would be equal or greater mortality reductions if the money used to finance screening programs was applied to new research or improvements in treatment.

Although this is an important public health question, it is almost impossible to answer. There is generally little detailed information available from which we can estimate compliance of treatments with existing guidelines, and the cost–benefit ratio of incompleted research cannot be assessed. It should be noted, however, that once we start to consider diverting funds from proven, efficacious interventions (such as mammography screening in the 50–69 year old age group), we should be certain that equivalent or greater benefits would accrue to the public. Further, once this discussion is opened, it should not be limited to discussion of breast cancer alone, but to the consideration of what other interventions (from smoking cessation programs to transplant surgery) could benefit the public. Clearly, although this is an interesting academic debate, the current consensus that mammographic screening does reduce mortality in this age group cannot be ignored, and requires its provision in the appropriate age groups.

Perhaps the most contentious debate concerns the value of mammographic screening for women aged 40–49. Current consensus would state that, if there is any benefit for women in this age group, it is a smaller benefit than for women aged over 50, with an estimated reduction of 16% (and confidence intervals of 2–28%).[21] Further, it is delayed for several years; most studies do not show benefit until at least 10 years of follow-up.[21] Mammographic screening appears to be less sensitive in this age group, finding only about 75% of cancers, compared with about a 90% detection rate in older women.[22] Finally, women of any age who go for mammographic screening take some risk that they will have to undergo unnecessary tests, including biopsies; the risk that any biopsies will be benign is higher among younger women.[23]

Several explanations have been put forward for the apparent reduction of efficacy in this age group. Although some of this is probably related to the lower sensitivity noted above, it has also been argued that the studies to date have used similar intervals between screens for women of all age groups, whereas it would appear that pre-clinical tumor progression is faster for younger women.[24] Thus, some have suggested that, if mammography is to be an efficacious screening tool for women in their 40s, it should be performed annually,[25] which was not the case in many of the randomized controlled trials.

However, others have argued that any benefit seen for screening mammography in the 40-year-old age group may in fact have been overestimated in the current randomized controlled trials. This is because the data for individual women are analyzed by their age at randomization, not their age at screening. Thus, many of the screens provided in the trials to women in their 40s at the start of the study were actually carried out after the women were 50 or older. If a portion of the already smaller reductions in mortality seen resulted in fact from screening after the age of 50, it is questionable whether a statistically significant benefit would be seen for screens provided only while a woman was in her 40s.

This has resulted in conflicting recommendations for women in their 40s. The National Cancer Advisory Board in the USA has recommended regular screening for women in this age group.[26] This recommendation was made despite the fact that a consensus panel sponsored by the National Institutes of Health found that the data 'do not warrant a universal recommendation for mammography for all women in their forties'.[21] Instead, they recommended that women aged 40–49 discuss the risks and benefits of screening with their physicians, and make their decisions based on this discussion.

Do these public health recommendations

make sense? What does this remaining controversy mean for the individual physician?

THE PATIENT AND THE POPULATION

In its discussion of its recommendations, the Consensus Panel carefully distinguished between different levels of decision-making, which they classified as personal, interpersonal and large scale.[21] The panel was designed to address this latter, large-scale, public health type of recommendations and, as the panel notes, this requires the most stringent level of evidence.

Why is the level of evidence required higher for this recommendation? Simply put, public health recommendations are aimed at the general public. Once it is decided that such a recommendation will be made, it will generally be promulgated to the general public through mass media, personal invitations and recommendations to physicians that they actively promote these interventions. To have this level of message penetration, one must be confident that the vast majority of reasonable people, if they had all of the information, would agree that the benefits of the procedure outweigh its risks. As the target audience of screening interventions consists of healthy adults, any risk may be seen to violate the premise of 'above all, do no harm', because the individual in question was well before being given the message that she should be screened. Further, the possibilities of benefit, although measurable, are remote: of 1000 women in their 40s screened annually for 10 years, one or two women may have their lives extended, whereas 30% could have had a biopsy to follow up the screening.[12] These one or two women will clearly perceive a benefit (as probably will other women whose breast cancers are detected through screening, even if their clinical course is not altered through the earlier discovery). However, how many of the women with benign biopsies, or

the women who underwent the procedure 10 times, with the attendant personal costs and discomforts and no apparent detection of abnormality, would feel that the risks outweighed the benefits? Although most would probably still not regret the decision to be screened, there may be several women who feel that the risk:benefit ratio did not work in their favor.

This is clearly a question of degree: the same questions can be asked about screening at any age. It would simply appear that the risk:benefit ratio is clearer for women aged over 50 than for those younger. This makes a clear, simple message ('you should be screened') more problematic to deliver to younger women; instead it is more appropriate to provide information and discussion and allow women to make their own decisions based on this. As Ranoshoff[12] notes, this recommendation could be interpreted by some as 'simply passing a very difficult decision on to . . . patients'. He recommends use of the shared decision-making model, in which the physician provides information and the patient shares her own values in order to weigh and decide on the information. A woman who feels at high personal risk for breast cancer, for example, could weigh the same factual information differently from a woman with no particular feeling of increased risk and a strong desire to avoid unnecessary medical interventions. Such a process is clearly desirable; however, there is a real need to develop clear, salient, information tools to support this process, and to provide health-care providers with enough training – and time – to carry this out.

Underlying this recommendation is the assumption that women in their 40s who choose to be screened would have screening made available to them. This may be a difficult decision for health-care planners, because it is clear that screening is less cost-effective in this age group. One estimate, for example, finds that, although there is a 75% chance that screening in the 50–69 age group would cost less than $US50 000 per year of life saved, for women in their 40s, there is only a 7% chance that screening would be this cost-effective.[27] Nevertheless, with some jurisdictions adopting public health recommendations for screening of all women in this age group, it is difficult actively to exclude this group from eligibility.

Screening programs often distinguish between the target population – those who are actively sought out and encouraged to undergo screening – and the eligible population. The eligible population includes both the target group and other women in defined groups who could avail themselves of programmed screening if they chose. The target population should consist of those for whom the risk:benefit ratio is very clear; the rest of the eligible population is the group that could benefit from shared decision-making with their health-care providers.

As the debate currently stands, there still are some clearly defined camps. Some would recommend active public health recruiting and targeting of women in their 40s; a few may actively recommend against screening in this age group. However, there is clear room in the middle for a group that is comfortable with the concept of some women choosing to undergo regular mammographic screening, and others deciding to wait until their 50s or the onset of menopause. Leaving room for this approach allows for the provision of screening for some, without fear of violating the 'no harm' principle for those who would interpret the evidence as providing insufficient benefit for the risks taken in screening.

REFERENCES

1. Miller AB, Baines CJ, To T et al, Canadian National Breast Screening Study, 2: Breast cancer detection and death rates among women aged 50 to 59 years. *Can Med Assoc J* 1992; **147**:

2. Miller AB, Baines CJ, To T et al, Canadian National Breast Screening Study 1: Breast cancer detection and death rates among women aged 40–49 years. *Can Med Assoc J* 1992; **147**:1459–76.

3. Chu KC, Smart CR, Tarone RE, Analysis of breast cancer mortality and stage distribution by age for the Health Insurance Plan clinical trial. *J Natl Cancer Inst* 1988; **80**:1125–32.

4. Alexander FE, Anderson TJ, Brown HK et al, 14 years of follow-up from the Edinburgh randomised trial of breast-cancer screening. *Lancet* 1999; **353**:1903–8.

5. Andersson I, Aspegren K, Janzon L et al, Mammographic screening and mortality from breast cancer: the Malmö mammographic screening trial. *BMJ* 1988; **297**:943–8.

6. Tabar L, Fagerberg G, Chen HH et al, Efficacy of breast cancer screening by age: new results from the Swedish two-county trial. *Cancer* 1995; **75**:2507–17.

7. Frisell J, Lidbrink E, Hellstrom L, Rutqvist LE, Follow-up after 11 years: update of mortality results in the Stockholm mammographic screening trial. *Breast Cancer Res Treat* 1997; **45**:263–70.

8. Bjurstam N, Bjorneld L, Duffy SW et al, The Gothenburg breast screening trial: first results on mortality, incidence, and mode of detection for women aged 39–49 years at randomization. *Cancer* 1997; **80**:2091–9.

9. Fletcher SW, Black W, Harris R et al, Report of the international workshop on screening for breast cancer. *J Natl Cancer Inst* 1993; **85**:1644–56.

10. National Cancer Institute PDQ website, Screening for breast cancer. Accessed at cancernet.nci.nih.gov; access date September 2, 1999.

11. Fletcher SW, Whither scientific deliberation in health policy recommendations? Alice in the Wonderland of breast-cancer screening. *N Engl J Med* 1997; **336**:1180–3.

12. Ranoshoff DF, Harris RP, Lessons from the mammography screening controversy: can we improve the debate? *Ann Intern Med* 1997; **127**:1029–34.

13. Shapiro S, Coleman EA, Broeders M, Codd M, de Koning H, Fracheboud J, Breast cancer screening programs in 22 countries: current policies, administration and guidelines. *Int J Epidemiol* 1998; **27**:735–42.

14. Gotzsche PC, Olsen O, Is screening for breast cancer with mammography justifiable? *Lancet* 2000; **355**:129–34.

15. Duffy SW, Tabar L, Screening mammography re-evaluated (letter). *Lancet* 2000; **355**:748.

16. Moss S, Blanks R, Quinn MJ, Screening mammography re-visited (letter). *Lancet* 2000; **355**:748.

17. Nystrom L, Screening mammography re-visited (letter). *Lancet* 2000; **355**:748–9.

18. Hayes C, Fitzpatrick P, Daly L, Buttimer J, Screening mammography re-visited (letter). *Lancet* 2000; **355**:749.

19. Law M, Hackshaw A, Wald N, Screening mammography re-visited (letter). *Lancet* 2000; **355**:749–50.

20. Baum M, The breast screening controversy. *Eur J Cancer* 1996; **32A**:9–11.

21. National Institutes of Health Consensus Development Panel, National Institutes of Health Consensus Development Conference Statement: breast cancer screening for women ages 40–49. *J Natl Cancer Inst* 1997; **89**:1015–26.

22. Kerlijowske K, Grady D, Barclay J et al, Effect of age, breast density, and family history on the sensitivity of screening mammography. *JAMA* 1996; **276**:33–8.

23. Kerlikowske K, Barclay J, Outcomes of modern screening mammography. *J Natl Cancer Inst Monographs* 1997; **22**:105–11..

24. Tabar L, Duffy SW, Vitak B, Chen HH, Prevost TC, The natural history of breast carcinoma: what have we learned from screening? *Cancer* 1999; **86**:449–62.

25. Feig SA, Increased benefit from shorter screening mammography intervals for women aged 40 to 49 years. *Cancer* 1997; **80**:2035–9.

26. National Cancer Advisory Board, *National Cancer Advisory Board Mammography Recommendations for Women Aged 40–49*. Bethesda, Maryland: National Cancer Advisory Board, 1997. (Available on NCI website at: http://cancernet.nci.nih.gov/news/ncabrec.htm).

27. Salzmann P, Kerlikowske K, Phillips K, Cost-effectiveness of extending mammography guidelines to include women 40 to 49 years of age. *Ann Int Med* 1997; **127**:955–65.

41
Breast screening

Anthony B Miller

It has been recognized for some time that mass screening for breast cancer can reduce mortality from the disease.[1,2] Both single-view mammography alone and double-view mammography combined with physical examination are effective as screening modalities. Current data are insufficient to determine whether appreciable extra benefit, in terms of mortality reduction, derives from adding physical examination to mammography. Further, it is not clear whether mammography adds appreciable extra benefit to screening by physical examination, a question raised by the working group to review the uncontrolled US Breast Cancer Detection Demonstration Projects[3] and under investigation in the Canadian National Breast Screening Study (CNBSS) in women aged 50–59 on entry to the study.[4,5]

The evidence that has accrued to justify the above statements, and the recommendations for national screening programmes that have resulted from them, has been derived, almost uniquely to date for screening, from large randomized phase III screening trials (level I evidence). However, in spite of this, there is no uniformity of view in the interpretation of the data from these trials, especially over screening for women aged 40–49. Part of the problem is that different organizations have accepted differ-

ent levels of evidence in making recommendations for screening. Thus, the American Cancer Society guidelines for breast cancer detection are that every woman should be urged to practise breast self-examination every month from the age of 20 years, that women should have a breast physical examination every 3 years from the age of 20 and every year from the age of 40, and that mammography should be given every 1–2 years from 40 to 49 years and every year from the age of 50.[6] There are in fact no randomized trial data relating to screening women aged under 40, and only one trial included women aged over 69. However, the US Preventive Services Task Force[7] did not recommend mammography screening for women aged 40–49, and the National Cancer Institute, after accepting that scientific evidence does not confirm efficacy of screening in women aged 40–49,[8] reversed that position later, in spite of the recommendations by a consensus conference.[9]

In Canada and several countries in Europe (e.g. Finland, the Netherlands, Sweden, the UK) organized breast screening programmes have been set up, all involving mammography screening for women aged 50–64 (or 69), but only some counties in Sweden actively invite women aged 40–49 for screening. The majority invite women to return every 2 years, but, in the UK, every 3. It is still too early to judge the effectiveness of these programmes. but it is likely that mortality reductions attributable to screening will be seen in those programmes that have achieved the planned (70% or more) level of compliance within a few years.

In the following sections, the evidence that has accrued on screening in the various age groups 40–49, 50–69 and ⩾70 is reviewed.

SCREENING AT AGES 40–49

The hypothesis that the efficacy of screening for women aged 40–49 was less than for women aged 50–69 was raised by the initial report of the Health Insurance Plan (HIP) trial because, at 5 years, there was no evidence that breast screening was effective in women aged 40–49, although the evidence was strong for women aged 50–69.[10] Subsequently, long-term follow-up of the HIP study suggested efficacy in younger women, commencing about 9 years after initiation of screening.[11] However, the numbers of breast cancers detected by mammography screening in women aged 40–49 on entry were low, and the main reason for an apparent reduction of mortality in this age group appears to be a poorer survival of stage I cancers in the control group of the trial, than both the screen-detected cancers and the non-screen-detected cancers in the study group.[12]

As a result of the HIP finding, subsequent trials also examined analytically the efficacy of screening in women aged 40–49, although, with the exception of the CNBSS, none of them had been specifically designed to evaluate this issue. Most of these trials recruited women over the whole of the 40–49 age span, although two, in Edinburgh and Malmö, recruited women only from the age of 45. The initial reports of these trials largely repeated the HIP experience, with no early effect of screening noted, although, as

women aged, benefit began to be seen. Table 41.1 lists the trials, the degree of benefit at the time of the most recent report and the year that the benefit began to be seen. The table includes the UK 'Trial', although this is strictly a quasi-experimental study, only the Edinburgh component being randomized. The Edinburgh trial reports therefore replicate the findings of the UK trial in terms of the Edinburgh screened group; the Edinburgh control group is reported only in the Edinburgh trial reports.

With the exception of the Gothenburg trial, all trials showed delayed efficacy, raising the suspicion that the effect is the result of screening women after the age of 50,[20] especially the Edinburgh and Malmö trials. Even for the Gothenburg trial,[16] there is room for concern over the anomaly of more cancers ascertained in the control than in the screened groups.[21]

An overview analysis of the results of the Swedish trials has been reported,[22] and updated,[23] and meta-analyses of all trials have been performed and updated.[24–30] These are summarized in Table 41.2. Only that of Kerlikowske et al[31] and Kerlikowske[29] specifically addressed the issue of the time after initiation of screening that the effect was noted. In Kerlikowske et al's analysis, the odds ratio (OR) for 7–9 years of follow-up was 1.02, and for 10 or more years it was 0.84. The results of these meta-analyses are similar, but not identical, which is of interest given that they all largely used the same data. Some of the differences relate to different time periods, e.g. that of Cox[24] was restricted to the first 10 years of follow-up. However, the methods used to combine the data varied. This is most strikingly seen for the analysis of Hendrick et al,[27] which produced the greatest estimate of reduction from all seven trials, and a larger estimate of effect for the Swedish trials than Larsson et al,[23] even though they presumably had the same or very similar data to Larsson et al.

Table 41.1   Screening trials of women aged 40(45)–49

Trial	Age range (years)	Year benefit first seen	Latest year of follow-up	RR (95%CI)	Reference
HIP	40–49	7	18	0.77 (NA)	Shapiro et al[11]
Two-county	40–49	8	16	0.87 (0.54–1.41)	Tabar et al[13]
Malmö	45–49	7	17	0.64 (0.45–0.89)	Andersson and Janzon[14]
Stockholm	40–49	10	12	1.08 (0.54–2.17)	Frisell and Lidbrink[15]
Gothenburg	39–49	5	11	0.56 (0.31–0.99)	Bjurstam et al[16]
Edinburgh	45–49	7	14	0.75 (0.48–1.18)[a]	Alexander et al[17]
UK 'Trial'	45–49	7	16	0.70 (0.57–0.86)	UK Trial of Early Detection of Breast Cancer[18]
CNBSS-1	40–49	–	13	1.14 (0.83–1.56)	Miller et al[19]

NA, not available.
[a]Adjusted for socioeconomic status.

Table 41.2   Overview and meta-analyses of screening trials for women aged 40–49

Author	Year	Trials	Period	RR (95%CI)
Larsson et al[23]	1997	Swedish	12.8 years	0.77 (0.59–1.01)
Cox[24]	1997	All 7[a]	10 years	0.93 (0.77–1.11)
Glasziou and Irwig[26]	1997	All 7[a]	To 1996	0.85(0.71–1.01)
Kerlikowske[29]	1997	All 7[a]	7–9 years	1.02 (0.82–1.27)
			10–14 years	0.84 (0.71–0.99)
Hendrick et al[27]	1997	Swedish	To 1997	0.71 (0.57–0.89)
		All 7[a]	Average 12.7 years	0.82 (0.71–0.95)

[a]Not including the UK Trial. Hendrick et al[27] counted the Swedish two-county trial as two trials.

It is unlikely that further follow-up of any of the trials listed in Table 41.1 will solve the question of whether the delayed effect in women aged 40–49 is the result of screening after the age of 50. A further trial has, however, been initiated in the UK, recruiting women aged 40–41, and randomizing them to annual mammography screening for 7 years or unscreened control in a ratio of

1:2. When participants in both the screened and control groups reach the age of 50, they will be included in the UK national programme. No results are expected from this trial for at least 5 years. A similar trial planned for various other countries in Europe (Eurotrial 40) now seems unlikely to proceed.

The studies that have evaluated the cost-effectiveness of screening women aged 40–49 have invariably concluded that the cost-effectiveness is less than for screening women aged over 50.[20,32,33] There are three reasons for this: the lower incidence and detection rates in younger women, a lesser degree of effect and the delay in the effect being seen. However, it seems likely that this differential would be less if screening was initiated at the age of 45.

Only observational data provide some evidence for the efficacy of breast self-examination (BSE) in this age group. Two case–control studies have shown no overall benefit in the reduction of advanced disease,[34,35] but one suggested benefit in BSE compliers.[35] A cohort study of BSE compliers in Finland suggested a benefit in reducing breast cancer mortality,[36] while a case–control study nested within the CNBSS also showed benefit from good BSE practice in reducing breast cancer mortality and cumulative prevalence of advanced (metastatic) breast cancer.[37] The UK quasi-experimental study showed no reduction in breast cancer mortality in the BSE centres, compared with the control, although the proportion of women who attended the BSE classes was low in each area.[18] There are two trials of BSE ongoing, one in Russia[38] and one in China.[39] Neither has yet reached the stage of follow-up at which change in breast cancer mortality would be expected.

There are no randomized trial data that relate to the efficacy of physical examinations of the breast, although there is some evidence that it may be helpful.[40]

SCREENING AT AGES 50–69

The HIP trial showed effectiveness of screening with the combination of mammography plus physical examination annually in women aged 50–64 on entry to the trial.[10,11]

This effect of combined screening was later confirmed by the UK studies[17,18] and a case–control study in the Netherlands.[41] The inference that mammography alone could replicate this benefit was confirmed by several Swedish trials, and case–control studies in Florence[42] and in the Netherlands,[43] and further confirmed by the Swedish overview analysis.[22] The trials of breast screening in this age group are summarized in Table 41.3. Updated data are not yet available for the Malmö and Stockholm trials, and have not yet been published for the Gothenburg trial, but they are included in the Nyström et al[22] overview analysis. It is of interest that, when the data are evaluated by 5-year age at entry group, there is some evidence of lesser effectiveness at age 50–54 than at older ages. This was first seen in one of the case–control studies in the Netherlands,[41] and is suggested by comparing the data for women aged 39–49 for Gothenburg[16] with those published in the Swedish overview analysis for ages 40–59,[22] and is again suggested for Malmö by comparing the data published by Andersson et al[44] for women aged 45–54 with those later reported by Andersson and Janzon[14] for women aged 45–49. This was again seen in the Edinburgh trial,[17] and to a lesser extent in the UK Trial as a whole.[18] The published results of the Edinburgh and UK trials do not provide relative risks (RRs) for the age group 50–64 as a whole, but for the age group 45–64 the RRs were 0.79 (95% confidence interval or 95%CI 0.60–1.02) (adjusted for socioeconomic status)[17] and 0.73 (95%CI 0.63–0.84),[18] respectively.

As, until recently,[46] there has not been any

Table 41.3   Screening trials of women aged 50–69

Trial	Age range (years)	Year benefit first seen	Latest year of follow-up	RR (95%CI)	Reference
HIP	50–64	3	18	0.68 (0.49–0.96)	Shapiro et al[11]
Two-county	50–59	5	14	0.66 (0.46–0.93)	Tabar et al[13]
	60–69	6	14	0.60 (0.42–0.82)	
Malmö	55–69	8	10	0.79 (0.51–1.24)	Andersson et al[44]
Stockholm	50–64	2	7	0.57 (0.3–1.1)	Frisell et al[45]
All Swedish	50–59	3	12	0.72 (0.58–0.90)	Nyström et al[22]
trials	60–69	3	12	0.69 (0.54–0.88)	
Edinburgh	50–54	NA	14	0.99 (0.62–1.58)[a]	Alexander et al[17]
	55–59	NA	14	0.65 (0.43–0.99)[a]	
	60–64	NA	14	0.80 (0.51–1.25)[a]	
UK 'Trial'	50–54	10	16	0.79 (0.62–1.00)	UK Trial of Early Detection of Breast Cancer [18]
	55–59	6	16	0.71 (0.56–0.90)	
	60–64	8	16	0.72 (0.56–0.92)	
CNBSS-2	50–59	–	7	0.97 (0.62–1.52)	Miller et al[5]

NA, not available.
[a]Adjusted for socioeconomic status.

controversy about the efficacy of screening women aged 50–69, there have been far fewer meta-analyses than for screening women aged 40–49. However, Kerlikowske et al[31] reported an RR of 0.74 (95%CI 0.66–0.83) for all studies, with almost identical effects for 7–9 years (0.73, 95%CI 0.63–0.84) to 10–12 years of follow-up (0.76, 95%CI 0.67–0.87).

An intriguing aspect of the results of the trials comparing screening with no screening (i.e. all except CNBSS-2 in Table 41.3) is the failure of the more recent studies, using more modern mammography, to demonstrate greater breast cancer mortality reduction than in the HIP trial, in spite of higher compliance levels. There is some evidence, using surrogate indicators of efficacy, that double-view mammography performs better than the single-view mammography used in most of the early Swedish trials.[47] However, this cannot be the whole explanation. The HIP trial used the combination of mammography of the 1960s with good physical examination. Much of the benefit in that trial was attributable to the earlier detection of advanced cases, probably resulting as much from the physical examinations as from mammography.[48] With the improvement in mammography, many, but not all, of the cancers detected by physical examination but missed by mammography in the HIP era are picked up by modern mammography. However, this does not tell us how much mammography adds to good physical examinations, requiring a specially designed trial to answer.

CNBSS-2 was designed to provide an answer to this question. Thus, in women aged 50–59 the primary objective of the CNBSS was to determine the additional contribution of routine annual mammographic screening to screening by physical examination alone. Screening with yearly mammography in addition to physical examination did detect considerably more node-negative and small breast cancer than screening with physical examination alone, but had no impact on mortality from breast cancer in the first 7 years from entry.[5] Nevertheless, the confidence intervals around this estimate of no effect were wide at 7 years, and an effect of the order seen in the other trials could not be excluded. However, after a follow-up period that ranges from 11 to 16 years from entry, the numbers of events have more than doubled, and there is still no evidence of a breast cancer mortality reduction in the mammography-containing arm, compared with those screened by physical examination and the teaching and reinforcement of BSE.

As to the effect of BSE itself, all the evidence to date is observational, and is as reviewed above for those women aged 40–49.

Most of the studies of the cost-effectiveness of screening for breast cancer have been made to compare screening among women aged 40–49 and those aged 50–69, but some have assessed different frequencies of re-screening.[49,50] The studies that have assessed different frequencies of re-screening have tended to assume a similar degree of efficacy. This seems inherently unlikely, although the conclusion that the marginal benefit of annual screening vs 2-yearly, or 2-yearly vs 3-yearly may be small is probably correct. A trial is under way in the UK assessing different frequencies of screening (annual vs 3-yearly), although it is using surrogate indicators of benefit to estimate the effect, not mortality reduction.

SCREENING AT ≥70 YEARS

Only the Swedish two-county trial included women over the age of 70 (70–74), and it invited them to screening only once, because the compliance was much lower than for younger women. After 14 years, the RR in this age group was 0.79 (95%CI 0.51–1.22).[13]

There is no agreement about whether women aged over 70 should be screened. There is no evidence to suggest that there is likely to be a lesser level of effectiveness in this age group than for those aged 60–69, provided that similar compliance with screening is obtained. However, there is clear evidence that compliance drops off with increasing age, and therefore it is quite likely that the population impact of screening at ages over 70 will be small. Thus, no program currently actively recruits women into screening over the age of 70, although, at least in North America, women who attend for screening over the age of 70 are not turned away. The same types of decisions are made in terms of cessation of screening for women aged 69. There is evidence that the lead time gained from screening is longer for older women, so, even if screening stops at the age of 69, there will continue to be benefit well into their 70s. Therefore in most programmes women are not invited from the age of 69 (some from the age of 65 in Europe), but, in North America, if they continue to attend at older ages they are not turned away.

DISCUSSION

Using the standard criteria, it may be concluded that there is level I evidence for the efficacy of mammography screening for the age group 50–69, given that most studies have shown an early benefit of combined screening with mammography and physical examination, or of mammography alone, although the evidence is strongest for those aged 55–64 on initiation of screening.

For women aged 40–49, the evidence is still at level I, but the interpretation is less certain, largely because of the greater delay to evidence of effect and the suspicion that some at least of the apparent benefit is the result of screening at ages over 50. The NIH Consensus Panel[9] discuss in some depth the various issues, other than economic, that led to their recommendation that, in this age group, the data currently available do not warrant a universal recommendation for mammography for all women in their 40s. Berry later provided some of the statistical underpinning for such a conclusion.[51]

It has often been assumed that the improvement in mammography quality in the last decade or so must inevitably result in a greater degree of benefit. However, Kerlikowske et al[28] have demonstrated the variability that exists in mammographic interpretation, suggesting that the improvement in mammography quality is not being reflected in greater diagnostic efficiency. Further, the cancer detection rates reported for breast screening programmes in the 1990s seem to be no better than from the randomized trials of the 1980s. For example, Wald et al[47] reported a cancer detection rate at the first screening for women aged 50–64 with two-view mammography of 6.84 per 1000. This compares with the CNBSS-2 rate at first screening for women aged 50–59 of 7.20 per 1000. Major improvements in results may therefore await improved technology.

The evidence in support of other modalities of screening is far less than for mammography. So far, BSE has only level III evidence in support of its efficacy. Evidence in support of breast physical examination is even more indirect. However, the CNBSS-2 findings suggest another viable option for screening women over the age of 50. This option may prove to be of substantial interest in countries where breast cancer is an increasing problem, but where mammography services are almost non-existent. Nevertheless, it has to be emphasized that the physical examinations performed in the CNBSS involve far more skilled attention to relatively minor signs than those often rather casually performed by health-care workers, who have not been trained to recognize the signs of minimal breast cancer. The protocol for physical examinations and the teaching of BSE has been fully described by Bassett.[52] Currently, the only breast screening programme that uses this method is the Ontario Breast Screening Program, which, significantly has similar cancer detection rates for women aged 50–59 on initial examination as for CNBSS-2.

REFERENCES

1. Day NE, Baines CJ, Chamberlain J et al, UICC project on screening for cancer: Report of the workshop on screening for breast cancer. *Int J Cancer* 1986; **38**:303–8.
2. Miller AB, Chamberlain J, Day NE, Hakama M, Prorok PC, Report on a workshop of the UICC project on evaluation of screening for cancer. *Int J Cancer* 1990; **46**:761–9.
3. Beahrs O, Shapiro S, Smart C, Report of the working group to review the National Cancer Institute American Cancer Society Breast

Cancer Detection Demonstration Projects. *J Natl Cancer Inst* 1979; **62**:640–709.

4. Miller AB, Howe GR, Wall C, The National Study of Breast Cancer Screening: protocol for a Canadian randomized controlled trial of screening for breast cancer in women. *Clin Invest Med* 1981; **4**:227–58.

5. Miller AB, Baines CJ, To T, Wall C et al, Canadian National Breast Screening Study 2. Breast cancer detection and death rates among women aged 50 to 59 years. *Can Med Assoc J* 1992; **147**:1477–88.

6. Mettlin C, Smart CR, Breast cancer detection guidelines for women aged 40–49 years: rationale for the American Cancer Society reaffirmation of recommendations. *Cancer* 1994; **44**:248–55.

7. Preventive Services Task Force, *Guide to Clinical Preventive Services*. Washington, DC, Department of Health and Human Services, 1989; 26–31.

8. Kaluzny AD, Rimer B, Harris R, The National Cancer Institute and guideline development: lessons from the breast cancer screening controversy. *J Natl Cancer Inst* 1994; **86**:901–3.

9. National Institutes of Health Consensus Development Panel, Consensus statement. *Natl Cancer Inst Monogr* 1997; **22**:vii–xviii.

10. Shapiro S, Strax P, Venet L, Periodic breast cancer screening in reducing mortality from breast cancer. *JAMA* 1971; **215**:1777–85.

11. Shapiro S, Venet W, Strax P, Venet L, Periodic screening for breast cancer. The Health Insurance Plan Project and its Sequelae, 1963–1986. Baltimore, MD: The Johns Hopkins University Press, 1988.

12. Miller AB, Is routine mammography screening appropriate for women 40–49 years of age? *Am J Prev Med* 1991; **7**:55–62.

13. Tabar L, Fagerberg G, Chen H-H et al, Efficacy of breast screening by age. New results from the Swedish two-country trial. *Cancer* 1995; **75**:2501–17.

14. Andersson I, Janzon I, Reduced breast cancer mortality in women under age 50: Updated results from the Malmö mammographic screening program. *Natl Cancer Inst Monogr* 1997; **22**:63–7.

15. Frisell J, Lidbrink E, The Stockholm mammographic screening trial: Risks and benefit in age group 40–49 years. *Natl Cancer Inst Monogr* 1997; **22**:49–51.

16. Bjurstam N, Björneld L, Duffy SW et al, The Gothenburg breast screening trial. First results on mortality, incidence and mode of detection for women ages 39–49 years at randomization. *Cancer* 1997; **80**:2091–9.

17. Alexander FE, Anderson TJ, Brown HK et al, 14 years of follow-up from the Edinburgh randomised trial of breast-cancer screening. *Lancet* 1999; **353**:1903–8.

18. UK Trial of Early Detection of Breast Cancer Group, 16-year mortality from breast cancer in the UK trial of early detection of breast cancer. *Lancet* 1999; **353**:1909–14.

19. Miller AB, To T, Baines CJ, Wall C, The Canadian National Breast Screening Study: Update on breast cancer mortality. *Natl Cancer Inst Monogr* 1997; **22**:37–41.

20. de Koning HJ, van Ineveld BM, van Oortmarssen GJ et al, Breast cancer screening and cost-effectiveness; policy alternatives, quality of life considerations and the possible impact of uncertain factors. *Int J Cancer* 1991; **49**:531–7.

21. Miller AB, Baines CJ, To T, and The Gothenburg Breast Screening Trial. First results on mortality, incidence and mode of detection for women ages 39–49 years at randomization. *Cancer* 1998; **83**:186–8.

22. Nyström L, Rutqvist LE, Wall S et al, Breast cancer screening with mammography: overview of Swedish randomized trials. *Lancet* 1993; **341**:973–8.

23. Larsson L-G, Andersson I, Bjurstam N et al, Updated overview of the Swedish randomized trials on breast cancer screening with mammography: Age group 40–49 at randomization. *Natl Cancer Inst Monogr* 1997; **22**:57–61.

24. Cox B, Variation in the effectiveness of breast

screening by year of follow-up. *Natl Cancer Inst Monogr* 1997; **22**;69–72.

25. Glasziou PP, Woodward AJ, Mahon CM, Mammographic screening trials for women aged under age 50. A quality assessment and meta-analysis. *Med J Aust* 1995; **162**:625–9.

26. Glasziou P, Irwig L, The quality and interpretation of mammographic screening trials for women ages 40–49. *Natl Cancer Inst Monogr* 1997; **22**:73–7.

27. Hendrick RE, Smith RA, Rutledge JH, Smart CR, Benefit of screening mammography in women aged 40–49: A new meta-analysis of randomized controlled trials. *Natl Cancer Inst Monogr* 1997; **22**:87–92.

28. Kerlikowske K, Grady D, Barclay J et al, Variability and accuracy in mammographic interpretation using the American College of Radiology breast imaging reporting and data system. *J Natl Cancer Inst* 1998; **90**:1801–9.

29. Kerlikowske K, Efficacy of screening mammography among women aged 40 to 49 years and 50 to 69 years: Comparison of relative and absolute benefit. *Natl Cancer Inst Monogr* 1997; **22**:79–86.

30. Smart CR, Hendrick RE, Rutledge JH III, Smith RA, Benefit of mammography screening in women ages 40 to 49 years. Current evidence from randomized controlled trials. *Cancer* 1995; **75**:1619–26. (Published erratum appears in *Cancer* 1995; **75**:2788.)

31. Kerlikowske K, Grady D, Rubin SM et al, Efficacy of screening mammography. *JAMA* 1995; **273**:149–54.

32. Eddy DM, Hasselblad V, McGivney W et al, The value of mammography screening in women under age 50 years. *JAMA* 1988; **259**:1512–19.

33. Salzmann P, Kerlikowske K, Phillips K, Cost-effectiveness of extending screening mammography guidelines to include women age 40 to 49 years of age. *Ann Intern Med* 1997; **127**: 955–65.

34. Muscat JE, Huncharek MS, Breast self-examination and extent of disease: A population-based study. *Cancer Detect Prev* 1991; **15**:155–9.

35. Newcomb PA, Weiss NS, Storer BE, Scholes D, Young BE, Voigt LF, Breast self-examination in relation to the occurrence of advanced breast cancer. *J Natl Cancer Inst* 1991; **83**:260–5.

36. Gastrin G, Miller AB, To T et al, Incidence and mortality from breast cancer in the Mama Program for breast screening in Finland, 1973–1986. *Cancer* 1994; **73**:2168–74.

37. Harvey BJ, Miller AB, Baines CJ, Corey PN, Effect of breast self-examination techniques on the risk of death from breast cancer. *Can Med Assoc J* 1997; **157**:1205–12.

38. Semiglazov VF, Sagaidak VN, Moiseyenko VM, Mikhailov EA, Study of the role of breast self-examination in the reduction of mortality from breast cancer: The Russian Federation/World Health Organization Study. *Eur J Cancer* 1993; **29A**:2039–46.

39. Thomas DB, Gao DL, Self SG et al, Randomized trial of breast self-examination in Shanghai: Methodology and preliminary results. *J Natl Cancer Inst* 1997; **89**:355–65.

40. Baines CJ, Miller AB, Mammography versus clinical examination of the breasts. *Natl Cancer Inst Monogr* 1997; **22**:125–9.

41. Collette HJA, Day NE, Rombach JJ, de Waard F, Evaluation of screening for breast cancer in non-randomized study (the Dom project) by means of a case-control study. *Lancet* 1984; **i**:1224–6.

42. Palli D, del Turco R, Buiatti E et al, A case–control study of the efficacy of a non-randomized breast cancer screening program in Florence (Italy). *Int J Cancer* 1986; **38**: 501–4.

43. Verbeek ALM, Hendriks JHCL, Holland R et al, Mammographic screening and breast cancer mortality: Age-specific effects in Nijmegen project, 1975–82. *Lancet* 1985; **i**:865–6.

44. Andersson I, Aspergren K, Janzon L et al, Mammographic screening and mortality from

breast cancer: The Malmö mammographic screening trial. *BMJ* 1988; **297**:943–8.

45. Frisell J, Eklund G, Hellstrom L et al, Randomized study of mammography screening – preliminary report on mortality in the Stockholm trial. *Breast Cancer Res Treat* 1991; **18**:49–56.

46. Gøtsche PC, Olsen O, Is screening for breast cancer with mammography justifiable? *Lancet* 2000; **355**:129–34.

47. Wald NJ, Murphy P, Major P et al, UKCCCR multicentre randomized trial of one- and two-view mammography in breast cancer screening. *BMJ* 1995; **311**:1189–93.

48. Miller AB, Mammography: A critical evaluation of its role in breast cancer screening, especially in developing countries. *J Publ Health Policy* 1989; **10**:486–98.

49. Boer R, de Koning H, Threlfall A et al, Cost effectiveness of shortening the screening interval or extending age range of NHS breast screening programme: computer simulation study. *BMJ* 1998; **317**:376–9.

50. Woodman CBJ, Threlfall AG, Boggis CRM, Prior P, Is the three year breast screening interval too long? Occurrence of interval cancers in NHS breast screening programme's north western region. *BMJ* 1995; **310**:224–6.

51. Berry DA, Benefits and risks of screening mammography for women in their forties: a statistical appraisal. *J Natl Cancer Inst* 1998; **90**:1431–9.

52. Bassett AA, Physical examination of the breasts and breast self-examination. In: Miller AB, ed. *Screening for Cancer*. Orlando, FL: Academic Press, 1995: 271–91.

PART IV
Conclusions

42

The Internet, health professionals and the health consumer

Lewis Rowett

THE INTERNET

Let's take a short cut here: if we want to consider the impact of electronic publishing on health practitioners and the general public, we will do well to cut to the Internet, and fast. That copy of *Best Evidence* on CD-ROM running on your personal computer may be a vital tool to you, but to me, miles away and working on a laptop without a CD drive, it is no use at all. Unless, of course, you have e-mail. . . .

So what's so special about the Internet?

The Internet, as a network of computer networks, has three fundamental components:[1] (1) hardware, the cables, switches, satellites and computers that constitute the physical network; (2) software, the protocols and programs that make the network work; and (3) the people who run the computers, write the programs, create the information, surf the web, etc. There are elements of all three components that are important for our consideration. The widespread nature of the physical networks has made access practically universal: anyone (and here we must acknowledge that we mean anyone with access to a computer, a modem and a phone line, not a majority in world terms) can get on the Net. The

Internet is a peer-to-peer network: unlike a television network, all points on the network can transmit and receive.[2] The standard nature of the protocols and the broadly standard nature of much of the software and publishing languages mean that transmitted information can appear to the reader much as it did to the author. All this has not gone unnoticed: people have been making more and more information available on the Internet,[3] databases, textbooks, practice guidelines and systematic reviews,[4] participating via e-mail, contributing to discussion groups and bulletin boards, and web publishing. It is this last activity and the web surfing that has accompanied it that has driven the recent rapid growth in Internet activities (from barely 200 web servers in September 1993 to more than 7 million in August 1999).[5]

To discover the secrets of the web *click here*

What's so special about the web? Hypertext: the ability to easily link, in context, between documents on the web underpins its functioning and its success.[6] Hypertext itself is not new; the term was coined in the 1960s and the concept is widely credited to Vannevar Bush's 1948 article 'As we may think'; hypertext was already a feature of the Macintosh computer in the 1980s.[7]

But it is in combination with the Internet that hypertext truly shines:[8]

> [H]ypertext and the Internet permit unlimited linkages to related and supplementary material.

Moreover, the hypertext links can stretch across the entire Internet, between documents on the same computer or between documents on different continents,[4] and can link to text, graphics, video, sound, even software, or can be used to call other Internet services such as e-mail and Gopher.[6] That the development of the NCSA Mosaic browser allowed graphics to be displayed in line with text[6] and that the basics of hypertext markup language (HTML), the language that tells a web browser how to display a document, can be learned in a few minutes[9] have probably also contributed to the success of the web.

We have the technology, but what are the issues?

Key issues for any form of academic information on the Internet must be privacy, security, quality, access and archiving.

The issues of privacy and security are probably outside the scope of this chapter, although there are obvious implications for the use of medical information and particularly clinical data. (Those interested in privacy and security issues related to the Internet should consult the CPSR's *Electronic Privacy Guidelines* (http://www.cpsr.org/program/privacy/privacy.8.htm), the *Privacy Resource Center* of the Massachusetts Health Data Consortium (http://www.mahealthdata.org) and Lincoln Stein's *WWW Security FAQ* (http://www.w3.org/Security/Faq/www-security-faq.html).)

The quality of Internet-based medical information has probably been more widely considered than any other issue.[10-12] Here we should remember the distinction between evidence,

which cites original studies or reviews in support of statements, and information, which may not.[8] When considering quality of websites, however, we might also draw a distinction between content and design; the latter is arguably a question relating to access and is considered below. As Coiera[13] has noted, the creation of information content for websites may be the largest single associated cost; higher quality may incur higher costs. In the short term, this may place those who provide high-quality information at a disadvantage, and certainly poor quality health information can be found.[14,15] Nevertheless, in the long term those who can establish a level of trust with their audience should be able to establish a brand identity.[10]

In medicine the development of gateway sites, such as Health on the Net (http://www.hon.ch) and Omni (http://www.omni.ac.uk) and their associated website evaluation criteria, e.g. the HON Code of Conduct (http://www.hon.ch/HONcode), have done much to drive awareness of quality issues, particularly with respect to content. Emerging key criteria are as follows:

- Authorship, which should be clearly indicated with credentials and affiliations.
- Attribution, i.e. clear referencing of source materials and indication of copyright.
- Disclosure of ownership, sponsorship, advertising and privacy policies, and potential conflicts of interest.
- Currency, the freshness of the information and frequency of updates, with clear indications of posting and updating dates.[10,16]

In a study of 29 published rating tools and evaluation criteria for health-related websites, design and aesthetics were the second and sixth most frequently cited points.[16] A strength of the web, if used wisely, is the stability of the user interface:[9] operation of the browser is standard, using browser default colors and fonts for text and links can ease navigation through what may be large and unfamiliar structures. Careful organization of materials within a site, with adequate navigation, in-context links and search facilities, can do much to allow users to find the information that they need. Finding the site on the web in the first place is a still larger issue of access. A recent estimate of the size of the publicly indexable web placed it at 800 million pages, or about 6 terabytes of information.[3] Further, although no search engine was considered to index more than about 16% of the web, only 6% of those 800 million pages are scientific or educational materials. As the electronic journal advocate, Stevan Harnad,[17] has put it: 'In the huge growth of the Internet the relative proportion of research use has shrunk to the size of the flea on the tail of the dog'. It is also important to note that, if currency is a quality issue, search engines can take several months to index updated pages.[3] In such an environment, searching skills will be important to the health professional and reliable, trusted sites will be important to the health consumer.

Archiving is a particularly important access issue: Will we be able to retrieve tomorrow what we have found today? And how about 10, 50, 200 years from now? Anyone who has spent time surfing the web will be familiar with broken links and Error 404 – file not found messages. For research purposes, the long-term availability of electronically published materials is vital. With the oldest, exclusively electronic journals in medicine less than 10 years old,[18] real long-term access has still to be proved. Organizations considering electronic publication must be aware of this issue at the outset of a project and, when necessary, make a commitment to archiving, ideally without changing URLs, the major cause of those broken links.

Underpinning all these issues is the question of cost. If increased quality increases cost, the web may still be the best place to publish because once a site has been established the additional costs related to the publishing of new materials are small relative to those of producing a paper supplement or new CD.

THE EVIDENCE

The web, and the Internet generally, therefore, have many features that make it particularly attractive for practitioners and proponents of evidence-based health care. New materials can be published and distributed cheaply, and existing materials can be similarly updated. Related materials from diverse sources can be linked together, and web-mounted databases, search engines and directories can provide access to journals, abstracts, collaborative tools, and still more databases, search engines and directories. And, as Andrew Booth has noted, evidence-based health care has indeed spawned a minor industry in associated products with the web as a major repository.[19] He should know: his own site, *Netting the Evidence* (http://www.shef.ac.uk/~scharr/ir/netting.html), has links to over 200 sites spread over four continents in several languages. Consequently, strategies for interrogating the web to provide appropriate evidence for specific clinical questions have themselves become a major publishing exercise.[20,21]

It is, however, becoming increasingly apparent that the Internet is, and should be, more than just another publishing system. The combination of global access, peer-to-peer communication and low additional costs for additional materials open up possibilities that have previously been unthinkable.

Where do you want to go tomorrow?

The organization and operation of multicentre clinical trials seem to be a good example of what is possible. Organizations such as the National Cancer Institute (NCI) and the European Organization for Research and Treatment of Cancer (EORTC) already maintain online directories of clinical trials, and a commercial register of randomized trials has been established at http://www.controlled-trials.com. Online patient registration and randomization is being done (see, for example, http://random.eortc.be/). Trials groups may already operate their own password-protected websites, so promoting communication, and data submission via the Internet to a single centralized database is possible. The reduced cost and space constraints associated with web publishing also present an opportunity for extended protocol publication and review. *The Lancet* has, since 1997, offered electronic publication of summaries of randomized trials and systematic review protocols associated with published studies.[22] Meinert[23] has taken this idea further by proposing that authors unwilling or unable to publish their protocol on a website should have their published articles annotated to indicate this. The possibility for pre-publishing protocols under development for extended peer review also exists, and Chalmers and Altman[22] describe this as an opportunity for primary prevention of poor research.

The web may also be a resource where previously unpublished data may be found for systematic reviews. Testing this hypothesis, Eysenbach and Diepgen[24] modified the search strategies of eight recent Cochrane Systematic Reviews to incorporate web searching. These modified strategies identified information on unpublished and ongoing trials relevant to four of the reviews.

Completely new materials have also been generated by the accessibility of the Internet, most notably, perhaps, online groups, often with strong patient involvement, and patient narrative sites, normally developed and maintained by individual patients. A recent survey reports that one-third of people searching on the Internet for disease-related materials are searching for cancer-related content and that a quarter will use online support groups.[25] Certain advantages of online groups are immediately clear: they can draw together geographically dispersed individuals; individuals with limited mobility are not excluded; and rare disease groups can be formed. However, misinformation can be propagated, and the widespread notion that such groups are self-correcting has been challenged by the Internet critic and paediatrician Tim David.[26] Physicians visiting or even using such groups may gain new perspectives on an illness from those most directly affected by it.[27] The proliferation of patient experience sites can also offer different perspectives to physicians, while offering advice and support to fellow patients. See, for example, *Dave's Happy Little Hodgkins Web Site* (http://www.davesite.com/hodgkins/), Dave Kristula's account of his teenage encounter with Hodgkin's disease:

> I got Hodgkins from a curse, most people just get it because. But heck, now we are both in the same boat, so who cares how I got it, let's get to getting rid of it! I was diagnosed with Stage 2b (to my best knowledge) on March somethingith 1997 when I was 15.

He has RealMedia video footage of his stem cell transplantation too.

So we had better not forget that the Internet can give us access to more than just images and text. A good example of this is Gordon Woods's *Palm Pilot Tools for EBM Home Page* (http://www3.mtco.com/glwoods/), which, in addition to a number of useful HTML and document files, also includes spreadsheets and calculators that work within the Palm Pilot personal organizer.

But having said all this, we still recognize that the web is a publishing system and the potential for its use as such in academic publishing is unparalleled. Many journals are available online to subscribers. In 1998 the *British Medical*

Journal announced that it wished its electronic version, which currently has open and free access, to be considered the primary version.[28] Published articles on the site contain links within articles from citations to references and links to MEDline abstracts or online articles, where available, from references; in addition, articles citing the article are noted and linked to, as is related correspondence. As online journals move to rolling publication of electronic articles as they become available, with the increasing use of electronic supplementary materials, such as *The Lancet*'s protocol summaries, increasing numbers of us will use electronic versions of articles without reference to a paper edition.

The Internet also provides ways to speed the editorial process, from fully automated online processing of manuscripts from submission to final decision, to simple communication by e-mail. Even the production of paper journals can be accelerated using the Internet to distribute proofs to authors using Adobe's portable document file (PDF) format, which can preserve the appearance of the printed page when displayed by the Adobe Acrobat software.

The Internet versus the file-drawer effect

More radical solutions to the editorial process also present themselves. Freed from constraints of paper budgets and print runs, why not simply publish everything? Electronic archives of articles not formally peer reviewed already exist and function well in fields such as physics and computer science. The development of an electronic archive for medicine, if it could achieve some respect in the broader medical community, might help to redress the oft-noted publication bias of existing journals towards positive studies. In May 1999, the Director of the National Institutes of Health (NIH), Harold Varmus, proposed E-biomed, a biomedical publishing site on the web that would allow 'instantaneous, cost-free access ... to E-biomed's entire content'.[29] The proposal further called on commercial publishers and learned societies to contribute their journals to that entire content. In addition, the possibility of publication within the system without full, formal, peer review was foreseen. After a 3-month consultation period, during which strong opinions, both for and against, were expressed in many areas, the NIH announced that the site, now renamed PubMed Central, would start operation in January 2000.[30] The peer-review-free element remained intact, but it was made clear that the responsibility for the non-peer-reviewed materials would be devolved to screening organizations. Whether such a system really can promote publication of useful but otherwise neglected materials remains to be seen; the need to finance the system through some form of electronic page charge may reimpose barriers to publication that the system would otherwise remove. Nevertheless, the possibility of linking large numbers of free full-text articles to their MEDline abstracts via the National Library of Medicine's popular PubMed search engine is an exciting one.

THE HEALTH CONSUMER

With all this material available or potentially available on the Internet, what are the consequences for health consumers? What are the consequences for real medical practices? Anecdotal evidence abounds; here a patient self-diagnoses from poor quality information and presents too late to a physician, there a patient finds an important piece of information unknown to his physician. But both scenarios are not specific to the Internet. Despite the wealth and variety of information available on the Internet, no one has yet shown it to have a positive or negative impact on public health outcomes.[13,31]

Implicit in all this is our assumption that

health consumers are everywhere on the Internet. Patients are contributing to support groups and forums, producing their own sites, searching for information in online journals and highly publicized commercial sites such as Drkoop.com and Medscape.com. In the year ending July 1998, over 17 million US adults searched online for health and medical information;[25] the figure is estimated to rise to 30 million by 2000. Indeed, it seems that those medical organizations that open a window on the world through the Internet, but then ignore the possibility of health consumers looking through it, risk their own credibility.

One group of organizations unprepared to take this particular risk is the pharmaceutical industry. Corporates sites with investor information, general company information and information for patients and physicians are commonplace. Direct-to-consumer advertising of prescription medicines is illegal in most countries other than the USA. However, the transnational nature of the Internet makes websites legally mounted in the USA available to the world. Although critics may suggest that notices indicating that pharmaceutical information is 'for US consumers only' are essentially hypocritical, they are not illegal. Companies operating websites outside the USA are still legitimately able to present disease-related material. The International Federation of Pharmaceutical Manufacturers Associations (IFPMA) 'strongly supports the right to use the Internet as a means for providing accurate and scientifically reliable information on medicines in a responsible manner'.[32] Organizations prepared to monitor such reliability and responsibility are also represented on the web. The Food and Drug Administration in the USA maintains an extensive archive of warning letters issued to pharmaceutical companies for breaches of ethical marketing regulations at http://www.fda.gov/cder/warn/; the Estonian State Agency of Medicines maintains a simpler but essentially similar catalogue in Estonian and English at http://www.sam.ee/violations/violations.html.

'I will cause a boy that driveth the plough shall know more of the scriptures than thou dost'

William Tyndale's remark about translating the Bible into English has particular resonance for those who fear that health consumers, with more time and, possibly, greater motivation, will have access to more information than their physicians. Physicians do indeed report feeling poorly prepared to cope with patients armed with information from the Internet.[33] Even so, the fear is surely misplaced and misconstrues the role of the physician in evidence-based practice: health-care practices based on finding, critically appraising and applying evidence appropriately must welcome collaboration from patients in finding information. We must acknowledge that critical appraisal and application will largely remain the preserve of professionals. Professionals must nevertheless take real steps to involve patients by education,[34] engagement and partnership.[35]

Wake up and smell the bouillabaisse!

'The Internet is a veritable bouillabaisse for finding information, with a huge and outrageously expanding pot, and you never know when you stick your fork in what tasty morsel or bit of fish debris you will stab'.[8] And so it will remain. But there is more to do on the Internet than just finding information. The truth may or may not be out there, it's certainly worth a look, but I'm here and so are millions of others. The Internet, seen as a platform for communication and collaboration, will inevitably contribute to the building of communities and partnerships for improved patient care.

REFERENCES

1. Computer Professionals for Social Responsibility, One-planet, one-net fact sheet 1, CPSR (http://www.cpsr.org/onenet/whatis.html, accessed 19 September 1999).

2. Sterling B, *Short History of the Internet*, 1993 (http://www.forthnet.gr/forthnet/isoc/short.history.of.internet accessed 19 October 1999).

3. Lawrence S, Giles L, Accessibility of information on the web. *Nature* 1999; **400**:107–9.

4. Hersh W, Evidence-based medicine and the Internet. *ACP Journal Club*, 1996 (http://www.acponline.org/journals/acpjc/julaug96/jcjedit.htm accessed 22 September 1999).

5. Zakon RB, *Hobbes' Internet Timeline v4.2*, 1999 (http://info.isoc.org/guest/zakon/Internet/History/HIT.html, accessed 22 September 1999).

6. Pallen M, Guide to the internet: the world wide web. *BMJ* 1995; **311**:1552–6.

7. Rockwell G, *Hypertext Places*, 1998 (http://cheiron. humanities. mcmaster.ca/~htp/ accessed 5 November 1999).

8. Sackett DL, Richardson WS, Rosenberg W, Haynes RB, *Evidence-based Medicine – How to practice and teach EBM*. Edinburgh: Churchill Livingstone, 1997.

9. Greenspun P, *Philip and Alex's Guide to Web Publishing*. San Diego, CA: Academic Press/Morgan Kaufmann, 1999 (http://www.photo.net/wtr/thebook/ accessed 19 September 1999).

10. Silberg WM, Lundberg GD, Musacchio RA, Assessing, controlling, and assuring quality of medical information on the internet. *JAMA* 1997; **277**:1244–5.

11. Eysenbach G, Diepgen TL, Towards quality management of medical information on the internet: evaluation, labelling, and filtering of information. *BMJ* 1998; **317**:1496–502 (http://www.bmj.com/cgi/content/short/317/7171/1496 accessed 13 October 1999).

12. Shepperd S, Charnock D, Gann B, Helping patients access high quality health information. *BMJ* 1999; **319**:764–6 (http://www.bmj.com/cgi/content/short/319/7212/764 accessed 21 September 1999).

13. Coiera E, Information epidemics, economics and immunity on the internet. *BMJ* 1998; **317**:1469–70. (http://www.bmj.com/cgi/content/full/317/7171/1469 accessed 13 October 1999).

14. Bower H, Internet sees growth of unverified health claims. *BMJ* 1996; **313**:497.

15. Impicciatore P, Pandolfini C, Casella N, Bonati M, Reliability of health information for the public on the world wide web: systematic survey of advice on managing fever in children at home. *BMJ* 1997; **314**:1875–9.

16. Kim P, Eng TR, Deering MJ, Maxfield A, Published criteria for evaluating health related web sites: review. *BMJ* 1999; **318**:647–9 (http://www.bmj.com/cgi/content/full/318/7184/647 accessed 13 October 1999).

17. Harnad S, How to fast-forward learned serials to the inevitable and the optimal for scholars and scientists, 1997 (http://www.cogsci.ac.uk/~harnad/Papers/Harnad/harnad97.learned.serials.html accessed 18 October 1999).

18. Peek R, The future has arrived. In: *The Impact of Electronic Publishing on the Academic Community*. London: Portland Press, 1997.

19. Booth A, Following the evidence trail (http://www.wellcome.ac.uk/en/1/homlibinfactthiiarc1fol.html accessed 21 September 1999).

20. O'Rourke A, *Finding suitable web sites*, 1999 (http://www.shef.ac.uk/uni/projects/wrp/ebpsem1.html accessed 13 October 1999).

21. Wyatt JC, Vincent S, Selecting computer-based evidence sources. *Ann Oncol* 1999; **10**:267–73.

22. Chalmers I, Altman DG, How can medical journals help prevent poor medical research? Some opportunities presented by electronic publishing. *Lancet* 1999; **353**:490–3.

23. Meinert CL, Beyond CONSORT: need to improve reporting standards for controlled trials. *JAMA* 1998; **279**:1487–9.

24. Eysenbach G, Diepgen TL, Use of the World-Wide-Web to identify unpublished evidence for systematic reviews. *J Med Internet Res* 1999;

1(suppl 1):e25 (http://www.symposium.com/jmir/1999/1/suppl1/e25/index.htm accessed 20 September 1999).

25. Miller TE, Reents S, *The Health Care Industry in Transition: The online mandate to change.* Cyber Dialogue Inc., 1998 (http://www.cyber-dialogue.com/pdfs/white.papers/intel.pdf accessed 21 September 1999).

26. Wellcome Trust, The Internet consultation, 1999 (http://www.wellcome.ac.uk/en/1/homli-binfactthiiarc1con.html accessed 21 September 1999).

27. Lamberg L, Online support groups help patients live with, learn more about the rare skin cancer CTCL-MF. *JAMA* 1997; 277:1422–3.

28. Delamothe T, Smith R, The BMJ's website scales up *BMJ* 1998; 316:1109–10 (http://www.bmj.com/cgi/content/full/316/7138/1109 accessed 22 September 1999).

29. Varmus H, Original proposal for E-biomed (draft and addendum) E-biomed: a proposal for electronic publications in the biomedical sciences, NIH, 1999 (http://www.nih.gov/welcome/director/pubmedcentral/ebio-medarch.htm accessed 1 November 1999).

30. National Institutes of Health, *PubMed Central: An NIH-operated site for electronic distribution of life sciences research reports.* NIH, 1999 (http://www.nih.gov/welcome/director/pub-medcentral/pubmedcentral.htm accessed 1 November 1999).

31. Wyatt JC, Commentary; measuring quality and impact of the world wide web. *BMJ* 1997; 314:1879.

32. International Federation of Pharmaceutical Manufacturers Associations, *The Internet and Pharmaceutical Products: State of the art and the way forward.* IFPMA, 1998 (http://www.ifpma.org/Appendix.htm accessed 13 October 1999).

33. Coiera E, The Internet's challenge to health-care provision. *BMJ* 1996; 312:3–4.

34. Glass RM, Molter J, Hwang MY, Providing a tool for physicians to educate patients, *JAMA* 1998; 279:1309.

35. Jadad A, Promoting partnerships: challenges for the internet age. *BMJ* 1999; 319:761–4 (http://www.bmj.com/cgi/content/full/319/7212/761 accessed 21 September 1999).

43
Summary statement

Jean-Marc Nabholtz, Katia Tonkin, Matti S Aapro, Aman U Buzdar

This book has brought together breast cancer experts from around the globe: in itself an illustration of the current global way in which breast cancer research is heading. Such a global approach can only be of benefit to our patients. As we work together and exchange ideas, we will undoubtedly move more quickly towards our common goal – to make breast cancer an uncommon cause of death rather than the scourge of Western women that it is now.

In Part I we discussed the available tools and their application, and introduced the nature of clinical evidence-based approaches. This is the concept of this publication: clinicians must look critically at the data and decide what is best for their patient population. Often there are insufficient data to answer a question adequately and patients should be encouraged to enter clinical trials. Only by undertaking well-designed and executed clinical trials will we continue to move forward and bring research concepts into the clinical arena. In the future we will have to deal with the explosion of data that will arise from our globalization. If we are not vigilant in our methods of analysis, we might even become victims of our own success.

The available methods of analysis and their limitations have been assessed by experts in these areas. This field is rapidly changing as we recognize the limitations of current systems to encompass new needs. This is especially apparent as we begin to see new gene-based treatments emerging from the laboratory. We will need to look beyond the old phase I, II and III model. Many of the newer therapies that are currently coming out of the laboratory are likely to be chronic treatments. There are, for example, recent data on antiangiogenesis therapy using anti vascular endothelial growth factor (VEGF) antibodies and low-dose weekly chemotherapy. In the laboratory model the tumors can be induced to be resistant to the chemotherapeutic agent prior to antibody and low-dose chemotherapy treatment. Nevertheless, the tumors subsequently decrease in size or disappear. Of course the laboratory success of today will not always result in the clinic success of tomorrow. However, if it does, then we will need a paradigm shift. We will need to assess tumor response, not after the equivalent of two or three cycles of chemotherapy, but maybe after six months or more. Response in the new model is slower than we are used to seeing. This is certainly one of many potential dramatic changes in the way we treat patients with cancer. In the near future we are sure to see treatments that may have to be given chronically for as many as ten years, or possibly for life. Our understanding of toxicity and quality of life, and the instruments we use to measure them, will also have to change.

Part II reviewed a variety of treatment modalities. For each area the authors summarized the data along with the level of evidence, and have therefore given us the level of confidence that we can expect concerning our choices of therapy. We have chosen current areas of therapeutic interest and controversy rather than reviewing all areas of breast cancer treatment historically, as this would not have served our purpose. Our intent was to provide up-to-date information of relevance to the current clinical situation, and in this way stimulate questions for those areas that continue to be controversial. We still have many more areas of uncertainty than we would like. However, that will, by default, help us to design trials that will address these areas. Our really urgent need is to obtain answers as quickly as the patients need them, and at an affordable cost. This is the challenge of the new global model.

Part III discussed the integration of new therapies into the management of breast cancer in the common settings of metastatic and adjuvant breast cancer. It also dealt with the important issues of neoadjuvant treatment for locally advanced or inflammatory disease, and the controversial problem of DCIS and LCIS. Perhaps even more controversial are the more recent conundrums surrounding prevention, and of course, screening issues that continue to be hotly debated, with new follow-up data casting doubt on what had been felt to be resolved issues. Breast cancer remains a complex disease in all its manifestations. If we wish to improve prevention beyond the current prevention trials (e.g. the NSABP STAR trial) we need more agents with dramatically better risk-benefit ratios than are presently to hand. With respect to screening, we may soon see newer and more reliable tech-

niques of imaging, such as magnetic resonance imaging (MRI) or positron emission scanning (PET), which have fewer toxicities than X-ray mammography, become state-of-the-art within the next decade. In the not-too-distant future, when we approach women at high risk for breast cancer, especially those with a family history, we may not only be in a situation where screening is more effective, but we can expect to have the genetic tools to switch off the offending gene(s).

This publication was conceived and brought to fruition as a direct result of the Breast Cancer International Research Group (BCIRG). This new paradigm in breast cancer research stands ready to accept the challenge of globalization and all that this concept entails. One of the obvious ways in which we have almost become globalized is through the 'information highway', the Internet. The Internet has opened up new ways for us to communicate that ignore time zones and almost all the barriers that former communication systems suffered from. The obvious example is of course e-mail. In the making of the book we relied heavily on e-mail communication between authors and editors, and editors and publishers. So far it seems to grab people's attention and usually swift answers follow. Who knows for how long this will continue.

Many of us need the Internet when we research publications because literature searches using sites such as PubMed (US National Institute of Health) have become invaluable. We can use it when we want to find out about clinical trials using sites such as PDQ, also from NIH, and there are lots of sites available when we need help in clinical decision making, such as START from the European School of Oncology (ESO).

However, one of the key issues is site quality and the time it can take to get to the information you want, even if you are specific in your searches. There are a number of sites that have been designed to help the clinician in evidence-based reviews, such as the Cochrane Collaboration. Many journals have on-line versions to speed up communication to readers and complement their paper versions. This is especially useful for those whose mailed copies arrive some time after the published date. New issues concerning communication and medicine will continue to arise, and clinicians and researchers alike will need to address these. Many use on-line journals, and with built-in links we can survey a huge body of literature in a short space of time. This is essential, as there are new journals, some of which are only on-line, appearing each year.

We look forward to the future challenges and hope that this book has served you well in your current practice of oncology for the patient with breast cancer.

Index